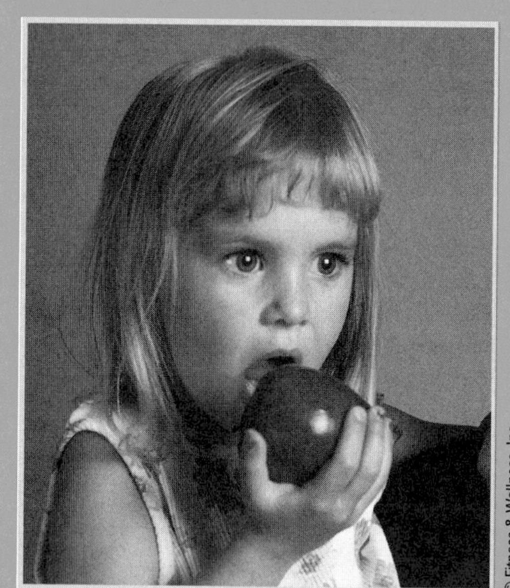

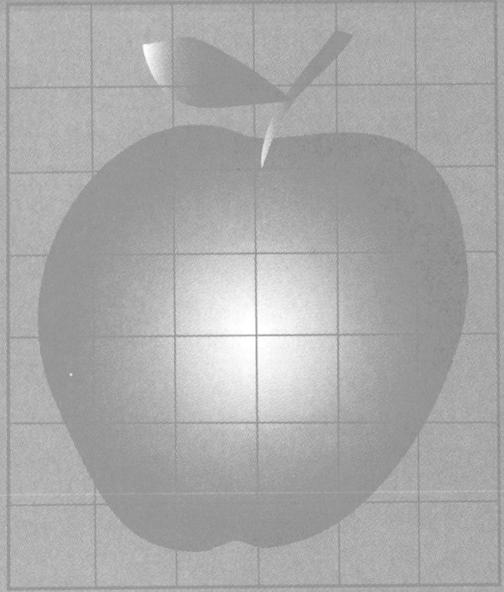

Teaching Children About Health

A Multidisciplinary Approach

2nd Edition

Edited by
Estelle Weinstein, Ph.D.
Hofstra University
Efrem Rosen, Ph.D.
Hofstra University

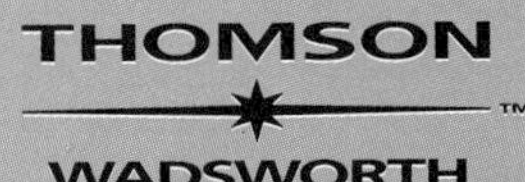

Australia • Canada • Mexico • Singapore • Spain • United Kingdom • United States

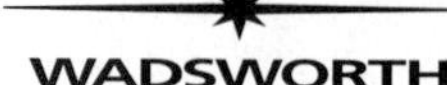

Publisher: Peter Marshall
Associate Editor: April Lemons
Assistant Editor: John Boyd
Editorial Assistant: Andrea Kesterke
Marketing Manager: Jennifer Somerville
Marketing Assistant: Mona Weltmer
Advertising Project Manager: Shemika Britt
Project Manager, Editorial Production: Sandra Craig/Trudy Brown
Print/Media Buyer: Tandra Jorgensen
Permissions Editor: Elizabeth Zuber
Production and Composition: Ash Street Typecrafters, Inc.
Text Designer: Harry Voigt
Photo Researcher: Myrna Engler
Copy Editor: Carol Lombardi
Cover Designer: Larry Didona
Cover Image: © Corbis Stock Market/Jon Feingersh, © Marlen Raabe/CORBIS
Text and Cover Printer: Edwards Brothers

Printed in the United States of America
1 2 3 4 5 6 7 06 05 04 03 02

For more information about our products, contact us at:
Thomson Learning Academic Resource Center
1-800-423-0563
For permission to use material from this text, contact us by:
Phone: 1-800-730-2214 **Fax:** 1-800-730-2215
Web: http://www.thomsonrights.com

Library of Congress Cataloging-in-Publication Data
Teaching children about health: a multidisciplinary approach / edited by Estelle Weinstein, Efrem Rosen.—2nd ed.
p. cm.
Includes bibliographical references and index.
ISBN 0-534-58044-0
1. Health education (Elementary) 2. Interdisciplinary approach in education. I. Weinstein, Estelle, II. Rosen, Efrem

LB1587.A3 T36 2002
372.3'7—dc21 2002022161

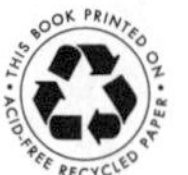

Wadsworth/Thomson Learning
10 Davis Drive
Belmont, CA 94002-3098
USA

Asia
Thomson Learning
5 Shenton Way, #01-01
UIC Building
Singapore 068808

Australia
Nelson Thomson Learning
102 Dodds Street
South Melbourne, Victoria 3205
Australia

Canada
Nelson Thomson Learning
1120 Birchmount Road
Toronto, Ontario M1K 5G4
Canada

Europe/Middle East/Africa
Thomson Learning
High Holborn House
50/51 Bedford Row
London WC1R 4LR
United Kingdom

Latin America
Thomson Learning
Seneca, 53
Colonia Polanco
11560 Mexico D.F.
Mexico

Spain
Paraninfo Thomson Learning
Calle/Magallanes, 25
28015 Madrid, Spain

Dedicated to the memory of Ann Barish and Rose Manson: Your intellect and inspiration has finally found expression in this current generation of women. E.W.

To Sherry: My partner, friend, and confidante, who was there throughout these works. I love you. E.R.

Brief Contents

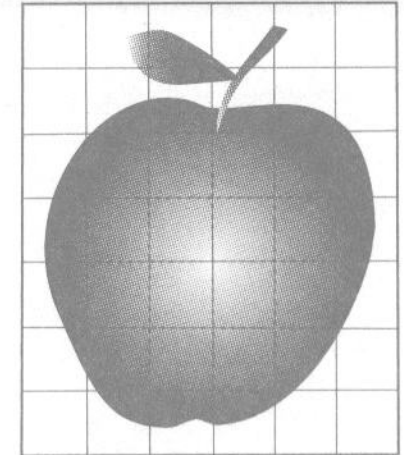

Contents

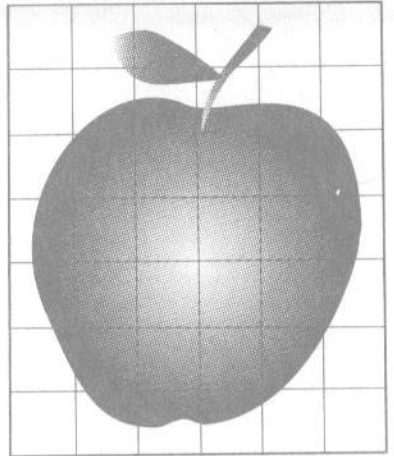

2

The Human Body and Its Development 25

Israel M. Schwartz

3

Nutrition 65

Susan Karp

4

Keeping Kids Active, Keeping Kids Healthy 117

Linda D. Zwiren and Gayle E. Hutchinson

7

Sexual Health, Family Life, and Relationships 225

Estelle Weinstein

8

Childhood Stress 269

Efrem Rosen

9

Preventing School Violence 303

Kathleen Schmalz and Mary Grenz Jalloh

10

Use of Alcohol, Tobacco, and Other Substances 329

Michael J. Ludwig

11

Child Abuse Prevention 375

Alane S. Fagin

Preface

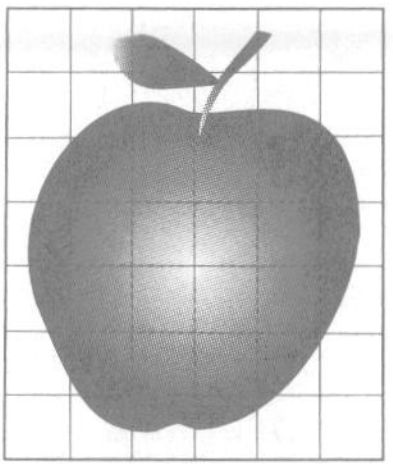

You can't educate a child who isn't healthy and you can't keep a child healthy who isn't educated.

Jocelyn Elders
Former U.S. Surgeon General

This book has been written for elementary school classroom teachers, working alone or in partnership with health educators, in pre-service, professional education, and in-service programs to prepare them to help develop healthy behaviors in their students from the earliest point of education.

Originally, we undertook this book with the greatest of respect for the part health plays in the lives of our children. We have not changed our view. Health, a component of life that sometimes seems so totally manageable and other times so totally elusive, is the foundation upon which the drama of life is enacted. Without health, all else is limited.

Society grapples with the strategies, technologies, and payment systems necessary to support the health of its citizens, but maintaining optimal health must also be a lifetime commitment to healthy behavior choices. That commitment can best be made using knowledge, values, and attitudes about health that begin before children are born, are influenced by their parents or caretakers, and continue throughout their school years until they become mature adults, responsible for their own health and the health status of their community.

In these difficult fiscal times, with accompanying streamlining of curricula, health education must be preserved using a multi-disciplinary approach, so that schools assume their responsibility for supporting healthy children. Granted that the discipline of health education has been responsible for creating national interest in Comprehensive School Health and that more and more state education departments are mandating health education curricula, but health educators' contact time with students continues to be more limited than the time allotted to other disciplines. This limitation sometimes hampers their ability to support students who need to take control of their own health. Moreover, classroom teachers—particularly those in elementary schools, who have the most access to children but limited time in their busy schedules—are often not prepared to include health subjects in their classrooms as a means of complementing and reinforcing the knowledge and messages that health specialists provide.

We created this text to answer this need. It will help teachers become more knowledgeable about, and more comfortable with, health topics, more reflective in their practice of teaching about health, and better equipped with activities for incorporating health subjects into their already overcrowded curriculum.

The Learning Experiences

We strongly believe that unless the classroom teacher partners with the health education specialist in introducing health learning experiences into the curriculum from the many perspectives covered in their other subjects (science, math, language arts, social studies, and so on), health will not become seriously and permanently interesting to students. Further, we think educators will not have a significant influence on the healthy behavior and lifelong choices of their students unless health is integrated into the total learning experience.

Hence, each chapter presents, in addition to the content knowledge base, Learning Experiences that integrate health activities into the standard curriculum. Each chapter provides activities that can be used with the several disciplines found in most elementary school curricula. Each activity identifies the subject area and grade levels for which it was created. These activities are not all-inclusive, but examples with which to begin. They include in-class activities, field trips, projects, and games that will reinforce important concepts in the content area. Each is a complete lesson plan, presented with learning objectives, a step-by-step procedure, homework suggestions, student outcomes, and assessment guidelines.

Although each Learning Experience includes a suggestion for evaluating outcomes, the classroom teacher must assess the level of a particular class to decide upon the developmental appropriateness of each of the outcomes and activities. (We assume that the classroom teacher is trained to determine the developmental level of students and can incorporate appropriate materials and information.)

Classroom teachers also have to consider the values and attitudes of the community in which the school exists. They may have to modify some of the Learning Experiences, and others may be inappropriate because they do not reflect the philosophy of a given school or community. This too is part of the teacher's professional role.

More Resources

Each chapter also provides other resources for additional classroom strategies, media resources, and materials to support this approach. Also new to this edition are Web sites that provide additional information as well as, in some cases, more activities.

Choice of Topics

The topics covered in this book are chosen for their relevance to children's lives. We use a wellness/preventive health model. Each chapter considers health from a physical, social, and emotional perspective—always acknowledging the mind-body connection—and covers basic information in important health areas so that teachers and non-specialists can feel comfortable not only about teaching and answering questions about the material, but also about assessing the developmental appropriateness of the information to their students.

The delivery of the information provided in each chapter would be most effective if it coincides with the health areas the health education specialist is covering. We support this comprehensive team approach and expect that the health education specialist can be a bountiful resource partner with the classroom teacher in the creation of additional activities and materials. This dual and ongoing comprehensive and integrative approach mirrors the process that individuals and their communities need to optimize health.

The Second Edition

It has been only three years since the first edition of this book was published. Based on a strong interest in the book and the comments of reviewers, we agreed to revise its presentation, rewrite extensively, update our sources, and add current Web sites.

Following is an overview of this new edition:

Chapter 1 introduces health education, particularly as it is related to the non–health education specialist in grades K–6. It provides a framework for how health curricula are organized, what their goals and objectives are, and an understanding of the discipline. This chapter also assumes that the reader is familiar with teaching models that are integrative and developmentally appropriate. Hence, we incorporate health into the classroom experience as an integrative model.

The next three chapters—The Human Body and Its Development; Nutrition; and Keeping Kids Active, Keeping Kids Healthy—develop a basic understanding of the bio-physiology of health and of the nutrition and physical activities that sustain the human body. We believe that developing healthy eating and exercise habits early and understanding how they contribute to a healthy state will increase the likelihood of lifelong healthy behaviors.

Chapter 5 presents a brief description of chronic and communicable diseases, especially as they affect children. It is meant to familiarize the classroom teacher with diseases that children and their families commonly encounter. We take a preventive health approach rather than a bio-medical illness and treatment approach. We do not expect the classroom teacher to be an expert on diseases but, rather, to help children understand how they may prevent or delay the onset of illness and live with people who might be ill.

Chapters 6 through 8 present an overview of the psycho-social aspects of health and the mind-body connection. We believe that this bio-psycho-social combination determines people's health status, and that no one of these influences health alone:

> Chapter 6, Mental Health, focuses on developing children's self-esteem, decision-making, and problem-solving strategies. It identifies common emotions (and their relationship to behaviors), mental health services, and some of the more common mental health problems that students have.
>
> Chapter 7, Sexual Health, Family Life, and Relationships, provides a structure for exploring family relationships, other relationships, intimate human expression, and sexuality as integral parts of people's lives. This chapter explores the various ways people relate, the meanings they give to their relationships, and the effects these have on their mental health and physical well-being. This chapter describes the roles of parents and children as important components of family life and as a basis for developing healthy parenting skills. We treat

> sexuality from a health perspective that begins early in child development and also address some of the factors that contribute to social problems associated with it.
>
> Chapter 8 focuses on the interaction between stress and health. We believe stress is no less an issue in childhood than adulthood. We offer an understanding of stress as a change in the state of the body because of a change in the stimuli (stressors) coming from the external and internal environments. How the body copes with stressors and how some stressors are associated with motivation and others with disease are described as they affect children.

Given the recent violent events in schools across the country (the most talked-about being the killings at Columbine High School), where children were hurt, we felt an urgent need to include the experiences of school violence and its prevention. Thus we've added a new chapter—Chapter 9, Preventing School Violence—that includes definitions of the various forms of violence, how they are reported, what the classroom teacher can do, and the several programs that are being implemented to prevent such violence.

Chapters 10 and 11 provide the classroom teacher with information and strategies for helping children deal with the problems associated with the abuse of alcohol and other substances as well as child abuse prevention:

> Chapter 10 presents alcohol and other substances from a preventive perspective, preparing children to deal effectively with their own exposure, abuse in the family, and the peer pressure they may ultimately face. We believe that if children are armed with information, alternatives, strategies for decision making, and resources, they will be able to overcome these problems in their own lives.
>
> Chapter 11 reinforces teachers' training about abused children in their classrooms and prepares them to teach children to recognize abuse, to try to prevent it, and to seek help if it occurs in school or at home.

Children experience grieving and dying in many different ways, which tend to be ignored in the academic setting. Chapter 12 deals with these issues, focusing on helping teachers to teach children about loss as a part of life and to recognize children experiencing loss in their classes.

Chapter 13, Environmental Health, addresses the environment as a significant component of human health. The emphasis is on each person's responsibility in maintaining a healthy environment to sustain the human population and ecosystems of the world. Understanding the nature and sources of pollution and how to prevent the accumulation of pollutants is essential to taking measures that will preserve health. This information is aimed at developing sensitivity in children to these environmental concerns.

Chapter 14, Safety, Injury Prevention, and First Aid, discusses common accidents and injuries that classroom teachers are likely to encounter on the job. This chapter covers suggestions for creating safer environments, on-site interventions that become necessary when an injury occurs, emergency resources in cases of extensive injury and, most important, strategies for preventing violent injury.

Chapter 15, The Consumer of Health Products and Community Health Services, combines Chapters 2 and 15 of the first edition. It prepares teachers to assist students in becoming educated consumers in this highly technical and confusing world of myriad health products and services. It focuses on the complexity of drug information, food labels and how to read them, quackery, and consumer advocacy. It also describes the complexity of health care systems and the extensive list of health professionals so that students will be better able to negotiate the system and improve their health should they need these supports.

We hope that, with this information and integrated classroom activities in hand, classroom teachers will be motivated to structure their curricula to include health topics on an ongoing basis. Involvement by classroom teachers can contribute to the development of children who will have respect for their own health, the health of their family, and the health of their community.

Acknowledgments

To the health educators we have met across the country, and especially in New York State: We thank them for their commitment to children and to education that will support health. Without their expertise, this book could not have been written.

We particularly want to thank all of our contributing authors, old and new. Their scholarship and dedication have allowed the second edition of the book to achieve a diversity of information and pedagogy.

It would not have been possible to complete this project without the day-to-day assistance of Marion Dillon for typing, mailing, telephoning, and just plain listening; without Dean Christman, Dean Johnson, and Hofstra University for all other ancillary supports; or without Alex Andragna and his facility with the computer and formatting. To

Peter Marshall, April Lemons, and the other personnel at Wadsworth Publishing Company—we thank them for their creativity, editorial suggestions, and general guidance and support throughout the publishing process.

We also thank these reviewers for their feedback and guidance regarding the second edition: Mary Hawk, Western Washington University; Debra Hook, California State University, San Bernardino; Claudia Mihovk, State University of West Georgia; Terrence O'Toole, State University of West Georgia; and Adele Ruszak, Millersville University.

Last, but by no means least: to our partners, children, grandchildren, and friends who, for more than two years, put up with our distractions, absences, and long periods of time in front of the computer. We are forever grateful.

List of Contributors

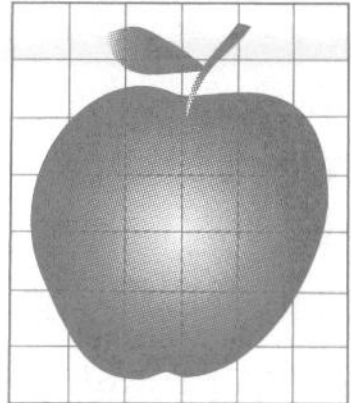

Carol Alberts, EdD

Carol Alberts received her doctorate in Physical Education from St. Johns University and is currently associate professor of Health in the Department of Health Professions and Family Studies in the School of Education at Hofstra University. She has taught First Aid and Safety for 20 years and has worked as a safety consultant for school districts in the greater New York area. She has published several articles related to athletics, legal issues, health, and safety and has presented papers at professional conferences.

Jane Colgan, MA, AC

Jane Colgan is an elementary school health specialist in the Lynbrook School District of New York. She is also an adjunct instructor at both Hofstra University and Nassau Community College, where she teaches courses in Alcoholism and Addictions; Curriculum Design and Development; and Death, Dying and Bereavement.

Alane S. Fagin, MS

Alane S. Fagin is a child development specialist, has been the executive director of Child Abuse Prevention Services on Long Island, NY, and is an adjunct assistant professor at Hofstra University. She has developed child abuse and child sexual abuse prevention curricula and has authored several research articles on child abuse prevention.

Rona Feigenbaum, MA, ACE

Rona Feigenbaum is an assistant professor in the Department of Health, Physical Education and Recreation at Nassau Community College, New York, where she teaches Human Sexuality and Women's Studies courses. She has served as a consultant in sex education curriculum and staff development for local public schools and community agencies and was coordinator of counseling at Planned Parenthood of Nassau County, New York. Ms. Feigenbaum has published several journal articles and presented workshops and seminars at national and regional conferences.

Gayle E. Hutchinson, EdD

Gayle E. Hutchinson received her doctorate from the University of Massachusetts and is an associate professor in Health and Physical Education at California State University. She spent her early career teaching Health and Physical Education in the public schools, then moved into university teaching. She specializes in program and curriculum development, instructional strategies, and diversity issues. She has written several articles, is the co-author of a book, and has presented at state and national conventions.

Mary Grenz Jalloh, MPH, MS, CHES

Mary Grenz Jalloh is the founding director of New York State Center for School Safety. She received her bachelor's degree in Sociology/Anthropology from Oberlin College; a master's in Public Health Education from the University of North Carolina, and master's degree in Rural Sociology from the University of Missouri. She is a certified health education specialist and has served as coordinator of a regional comprehensive health office for the New York State Education Department, public health education administrator in North Carolina, and member of the faculty at the School of Medicine, University of Missouri.

Susan Karp, MEd, RD

Susan Karp is a registered dietitian and has two master's degrees—in exercise physiology and nutrition—from Columbia University. She is an adjunct assistant professor at Hofstra University. She consults and lectures extensively on nutrition and health topics to corporations, health clubs, and teachers throughout the New York City area. She also has a private counseling practice focusing on health and prevention of disease.

Robert B. Lazow, MSW, DrPH

Robert B. Lazow received his master's degree in Social Work from Fordham University and a doctorate in Public Health from Columbia University. He is an associate professor in the Department of Health Professions and Family Studies at Hofstra University, where he teaches courses in preventive health, substance abuse, and administrative and policy issues related to the U.S. health care system. He has a private psychotherapy practice specializing in chemical dependency and is a consultant to health care, educational, and business organizations in the areas of substance abuse and behavioral health.

Michael J. Ludwig, PhD

Dr. Ludwig is an assistant professor in the Department of Health Professions and Family Studies at Hofstra University. He received his PhD from Pennsylvania State University in Health Education. He also holds an MS and BS in Health Education from the State University of New York, College at Cortland. His research focuses on the relationships between and among culture, education, health, and politics. He has published in several peer-reviewed journals, has contributed to edited collections, and has presented his work at local and national conventions. He serves as a reviewer for the *Review of Educational Research* and for the research consortium of the American Association of Health Education (AAHE).

Suanne Maurer, MS, ATC

Suanne Maurer is the coordinator of the National Athletic Trainers Association's approved undergraduate athletic training program and a member of the Department of Physical Education and Sports Sciences at Hofstra University. She is an associate athletic trainer. She has presented papers at the N.A.T.A.'s annual meetings and at the American College of Sports Medicine.

Efrem Rosen, PhD

Efrem Rosen is professor of Biology and coordinator of the Natural Sciences and Master of Arts in Human Sexuality Programs at New College of Hofstra University, New York. He is certified in Sex Education and Counseling by the American Association of Sex Educators, Counselors and Therapists (AASECT). He is a member of the Medical Advisory Committee of Planned Parenthood of Nassau County and a consultant for education and training in human sexuality. He has co-authored a book on sexuality counseling and several articles on adolescent sexuality and AIDS that have been presented at many national and state conferences.

Kathleen Schmalz, EdD, RN, CHES

Kathleen Schmalz is associate chair of the Department of Health and Human Services, College of Mount Saint Vincent, New York. She co-authored *Developing Presentation Skills: A Guide for Effective Instruction* and wrote over 20 publications on current health issues. She is associate editor of a regular column, "Tools of the Trade," which appears in *Health Promotion Practice: A Journal of Health Promotion/Health Education Applications, Policy and Professional Issues*. She is also a non-governmental organization representative, United Nations (associated with the Department of Public Information of the UN-DPI/NGO). She officially represents the American Association for Health Education (AAHE), International Union for Health Promotion and Education (IUHPE), and Society for Public Health Education (SOPHE) at meetings or functions of the UN and serves as a liaison for the UN, NGOs, and the three health promotion and education organizations.

Israel M. Schwartz, PhD

Israel M. Schwartz received his doctorate in Health and Sexuality at New York University and is currently an assistant professor and chair in the Department of Health Sciences and Family Studies at Hofstra University, New York. He has served as a consultant to the New York City Board of Education for Curriculum and Staff Development and has published articles, presented papers, and conducted workshops, nationally and internationally, on adolescent sexual development.

Carole Smitten, MS, NCC

Carole Smitten is an adjunct instructor in Counseling Education at Hofstra University and a guidance counselor at Lynbrook High School, New York. Her specialties are in teaching the theories and principles of counseling and counseling for death, dying, and bereavement.

Andrina Veit, MA

Andrina Veit received her MA at Adelphi University and is currently an assistant professor in the Department of Health, Physical Education and Recreation at Nassau Community College, New York. She is an MSW candidate at Adelphi University specializing in Health, Mental Health and Chemical Dependency.

Kathleen Zammett Walter, MA

Kathleen Z. Walter teaches Health at the Great Neck North Middle School, New York, and Health Pedagogy as an adjunct instructor at Hofstra University, New York. She has been a member of the board of directors and president of the New York State Federation of Professional Health Educators (NYSFPHE) and is co-chair of New York State's new Compact for Learning Curriculum and Assessment Committee for Health, Physical Education and Home Economics. She is also a water safety, first aid and CPR instructor trainer for the American Red Cross.

Estelle Weinstein, PhD

Estelle Weinstein is coordinator of the Community Health Programs in the Department of Health Sciences and Family Studies in the School of Education at Hofstra University, New York. She teaches pre-service and professional preparation undergraduate and graduate courses in School Health Education, Human Sexuality Education, and Counseling and Health Counseling. She is certified in Sex Education and Counseling by the American Association of Sex Educators, Counselors and Therapists (AASECT) and is a clinical member of the American Association of Marriage and Family Therapists (AAMFT) with a private practice in couple, family, and sex therapy. She has consulted with industry, schools, and health service agencies in curriculum and program development, has co-authored a book on sexuality counseling, has contributed several chapters to edited volumes, and has presented workshops at international, national, and regional conferences.

Linda D. Zwiren, EdD

Linda Zwiren received her doctorate from the University of Georgia in Exercise Physiology and is a professor and coordinator of the Exercise Specialist Program in the Department of Physical Education and Sports Sciences at Hofstra University, New York. She is a board member of the American College of Sports Medicine (ACSM) and chair of the Exercise Physiology Academy of the American Association of Health, Physical Education, Recreation and Dance (AAHPERD). Her research focuses on regular activity as preventive medicine for chronic diseases; she has published articles and chapters of books for clinical practitioners, cardiologists, and health and physical educators. She is a professional trainer for fitness leaders in health clubs, corporate fitness programs, and cardiac rehabilitation programs.

1

Health: An Educational Concern

Estelle Weinstein

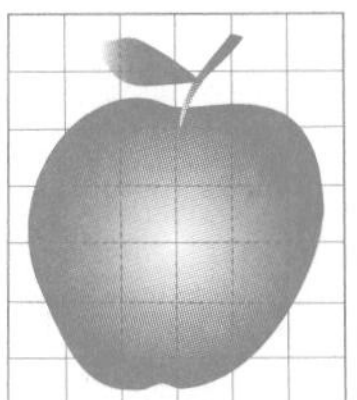

Chapter Outline

The Health of the Nation

The Need for Health Learning: A Historical Perspective

Why Health Education by Classroom Teachers?

The Partnership: Health Educators and Classroom Teachers

Creating Quality Health Education

Health Education Curricula

Theoretical Frameworks Associated with Behavior Change

Some Concepts and Definitions

Prevention Through Promotion

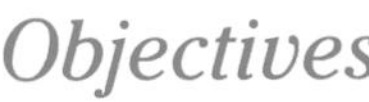

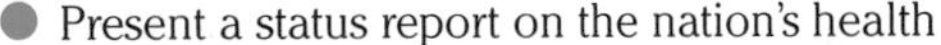

Objectives

- Present a status report on the nation's health
- Make a case for school involvement in health education and promotion
- Identify the roles and shared responsibilities of professionals involved in health education
- Present health competencies identified by AAHE and ASHA
- Describe the role of the federal government in providing standards for health
- Outline general criteria of health education
- Present definitions of the concepts of health, wellness, illness, and disease
- Expand on the concepts of values, beliefs, attitudes, locus of control, and decision-making
- Identify the primary, secondary, and tertiary levels of disease prevention

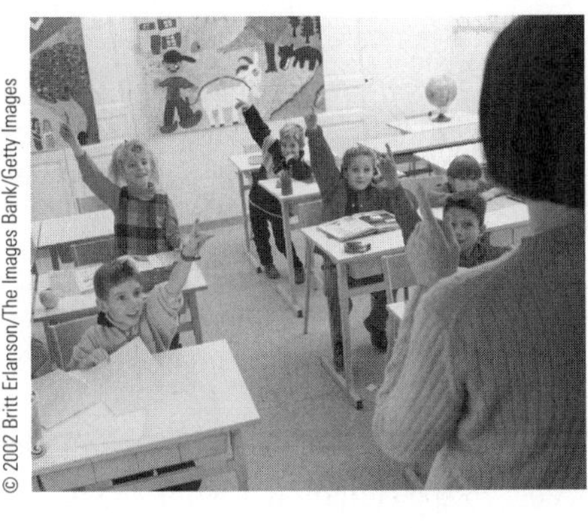

This is the first day of third grade for Cassandra. She is on her way to school with the usual apprehension of an 8-year-old: "Who will be in my class? Will the new teacher like me? Will I be smart enough? What if she calls on me and I don't know the answer?" This year she has lots of questions and lots of things to think about. Her uncle Jack is very sick. Cassandra has heard her mother say that he could die. She isn't sure what is wrong with Uncle Jack or what dying really means or if she could get sick like that and die. And she isn't sure whom she could ask, because her mom gets upset every time someone talks about these kinds of things. She wonders if maybe she could ask her teacher about them.

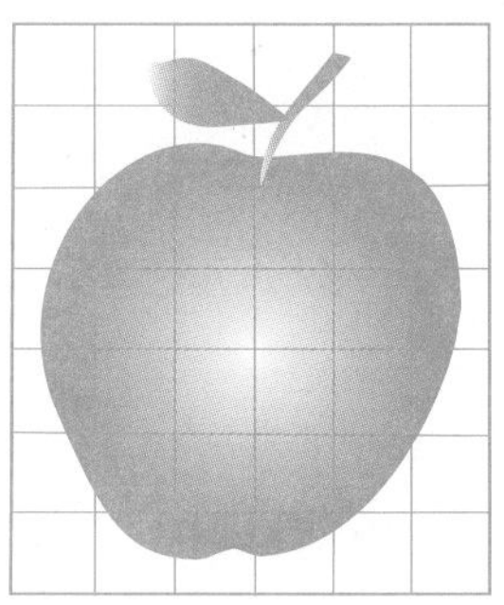

What makes an "askable" teacher? What do teachers need to know about health, wellness and illness, death and dying, to answer children's questions effectively? What should children be learning about health in the school setting, and when should that learning take place?

The Health of the Nation

Each nation, no matter what its customs, wealth, or international status, has as one of its priorities the health of its citizens. The United States devotes money, time, and research to the control of diseases through a system of public health. Yet, despite the vast body of knowledge available, each citizen's health ultimately reflects his or her own behaviors and life choices.

Status of the Nation's Health

As Benjamin Franklin aptly stated, "No nation can ever be stronger or healthier or more understanding than the strength, health, and understanding which it indicates in its youth." In 1900, life expectancy for a baby born in the United States was just under 50 years; babies born today can expect to live approximately 75 years. Moreover, at the turn of the century, surviving the first year of life increased the life expectancy to 56 years, and living to age 20 to 63 years. Today, the risks associated with the first year of life have been reduced such that the life expectancy for a newborn is only 2 years less than that of a 20-year-old.[1] The infant mortality rate in the United States is approximately 12 in every 1,000 live births.[2]

In the United States today, approximately 250,000 children are born each year with birth defects, many of which are the result of the mother's substance abuse, infection during pregnancy, or malnutrition resulting in low birth weight. The leading cause of death in young children is accidents.[3]

Certain sub-populations are associated with greater health problems. Growing numbers of children, particularly those in single-parent families headed by women, remain below the poverty level. Also, ethnic minorities and their children continue to be disproportionately represented in lower socioeconomic groups, which results in their significantly poorer health status. A rather horrific analogy is that a baby born in Cuba has a better chance of surviving his or her first year than does an average African-American baby born in the United States.[4] Moreover, African-American babies who do survive can expect their lifespans to be 6 years shorter than white babies. Disadvantaged minority babies are far more likely to develop a major chronic disease and die than their white counterparts.[5]

The Nation's Health Problems

"Man doesn't die; he kills himself."[6] According to wellness concept pioneer Don Ardell, 8 of the top 10 health killers of people are self-induced diseases related to North American lifestyles. The health problems that face the U.S. population are largely preventable and can be attributed to a few specific behaviors, including those that result in injuries (violence and accidents), poor nutrition, and insufficient physical activity.[7]

Young people are no exception. According to the Youth Risk Behavior Surveillance Survey (YRBSS), three-fourths of deaths among 10–14 year olds are a result of motor vehicle accidents, other unintentional injuries, homicide, and suicide. In addition, high school students participate in behaviors —such as not wearing seat belts, riding with a drunk driver, carrying a weapon, using alcohol and other substances—that increase their risk of death from these same causes. Moreover, the primary causes of death after 25 (cardiovascular diseases and cancer) result from risky behaviors that begin in adolescence or earlier. The YRBSS study suggests that substantial morbidity and other social problems stem from high rates of unintended pregnancies and sexually transmitted diseases (STDs) infections including HIV.[8]

According to the National Commission on the Role of the School and Community in Improving Adolescent Health, for the first time in our history, children are less healthy and less ready to take their place in society than their parents were. With the health status of children as our measure of health, U.S. society, especially people in the educational and allied health communities, have a commitment yet to be fulfilled.[9]

The United States spends more on health care than any other nation in the world. As a nation, we make a powerful commitment to the development of medical technology associated with diagnosis and treatment. At the same time, health is a relatively low priority for our schools, as evidenced by the infrequency of health requirements in the K–12 curriculum. We do not apply the knowledge we have to creating a strong learning component about how students can influence their own health.

Good health is not some mystical phenomenon related to whether people are "good or bad" or even whether they are young or old. It is not something that happens *to* them. Rather, it is something over which they have considerable control. Health results from a combination of knowledge and behavior coupled with a person's heredity. Yet, as a society, we tend to follow the newest fads regarding diet and exercise and worry incessantly about stress levels while doing little to change them. And we succumb to fiscal pressures in determining the effectiveness of our health education initiatives.

The Need for Health Learning: A Historical Perspective

Historically, the maintenance of health, prevention of disease, and health instruction were a function of the family, religious institution, and the community. Family beliefs, habits, and values about health were established early in the home and influenced only indirectly by outside factors. In the 19th century, we came to recognize that children's health was also influenced by the health behaviors, values, and attitudes of peers, teachers, and others in the community. Health was sometimes drastically compromised by epidemics of communicable diseases from unsanitary, and sometimes unsafe, conditions in the school environment. Teachers, nurses, and school physicians were instructed to take some responsibility for the health of children. Subsequent measures included improving sanitary conditions, inspecting students for symptoms of illness, screening for vision and hearing problems, providing nutritional lunches, and, ultimately, delivering some health instruction.

Because of the prevalence and seriousness of childhood communicable diseases, hygiene and basic nutritional subjects were integrated in some schools' curricula. The classroom teacher, often with little (if any) preservice preparation, was expected to take time in a busy school day to include basic health topics in a reactive, or crisis, model of curriculum planning. When a problem arose, the teacher inserted instruction about it. The prevailing notion was that knowing about scientific and health information alone would result in students' changing their health behaviors to prevent serious diseases. Along with increased acceptance of the concept that children with impaired health (physical or mental) could become impaired learners came the emergence of a separate discipline: health education.

Health education professionals were trained and hired to take over these teaching responsibilities from the classroom teacher, eliminating the need to juggle an overfilled curriculum. With acknowledgment that schools must devote attention to the health concerns of their students and in recognition of the part that attitudes and values play in health-behavior choices, health education—once simply a provider of health information—began to change into an instructional model based on disease prevention through health promotion.

Today's educational institutions are increasingly aware of the complex health-related issues facing students and their families. Teachers and administrators are grappling with the degree of responsibility they can and should assume to mediate the problems.[10] According to Marx et al., schools can do much, and they can do it within a "coordinated school health program" model—a model composed of comprehensive health instruction integrated with multiple health services including food services, medical services delivered in school-based health centers, mental health services, and so on.[11]

Why Health Education by Classroom Teachers?

Among the notable changes affecting health education today is the type of illnesses that compromise people's health. With communicable diseases on the wane and, in some cases, completely obliterated, the focus of health education has shifted to **chronic** diseases as the major compromisers of people's health. At first chronic diseases (such as heart disease, diabetes, arthritis, and cancer) were thought to be a result of simply growing old or to be caused primarily by inherited factors. Now, however, they are understood to be influenced by lifestyles and behaviors that begin in early childhood. Furthermore, we now believe that chronic diseases can be controlled or delayed years before symptoms appear by undertaking healthier and more preventive actions. (For more on disease, see Chapter 5.)

Another factor affecting health education is the social change evoked by more single-parent and dual working-parent families. These new realities tend to decrease children's exposure to day-to-day learning about health in the home, leaving the school system with a much more important role in modeling health. As family members hurriedly go their separate ways early in the morning and do not reunite until dinner time, children do not have the opportunity to observe their parents' health habits consistently enough to influence the children's health behaviors. In contrast, health habits of teachers, administrators, and classmates are reinforced repetitively over several hours each and every school day. Also, schoolchildren come from increasingly multi-ethnic communities. Diverse sociocultural and ethnically driven health behaviors influence students' personal lifestyles and behavior choices.

Another change affecting what children learn about health is the sheer number of hours they are exposed to TV and other mass media. They are bombarded by covert and overt misconceptions and misinformation about health and have no way of determining fact from fiction. These experiences have powerful implications for health learning and confirm the need for schools to provide a consistent and comprehensive health education.

For these reasons—current focus on preventive health behaviors, prevalence of single-parent and dual-working parent families, and need to provide reliable information—the classroom teacher is the best candidate for delivering health education.

Working against this need are budgets limited by fiscal constraints. Schools are cutting, if not completely eliminating, specialty positions including school nurse-teachers and health educators. Particularly hard-hit are less affluent, inner-city schools whose communities are marked by a preponderance of drug use and poverty-driven health problems. Such circumstances leave the classroom teacher with, at best, a skeleton health education staff. Additionally, teachers feel responsible, if not state-mandated, to include health subjects in an already overburdened curriculum. This responsibility usually arrives with little professional education or in-service preparation in health issues.

Other changes have transpired in the relationship among schools, students, and health that further compel health educators to reflect on and reformulate the delivery of school health education. Particularly the schools increasingly are playing *en loco parentis* roles.

The Partnership: Health Educators and Classroom Teachers

As an outcome of the dynamic nature of societal problems and living styles, the need for a more comprehensive multi-systemic model has become apparent. The ideal model would be based on a partnership between the health education professional and the classroom teacher, working together with other school personnel, family members, and community leaders. Following is one way this could be implemented.

The Role of the Health Educator

The health educator, much like the medical specialist, has been professionally trained as an educator and, in addition, receives special training in the

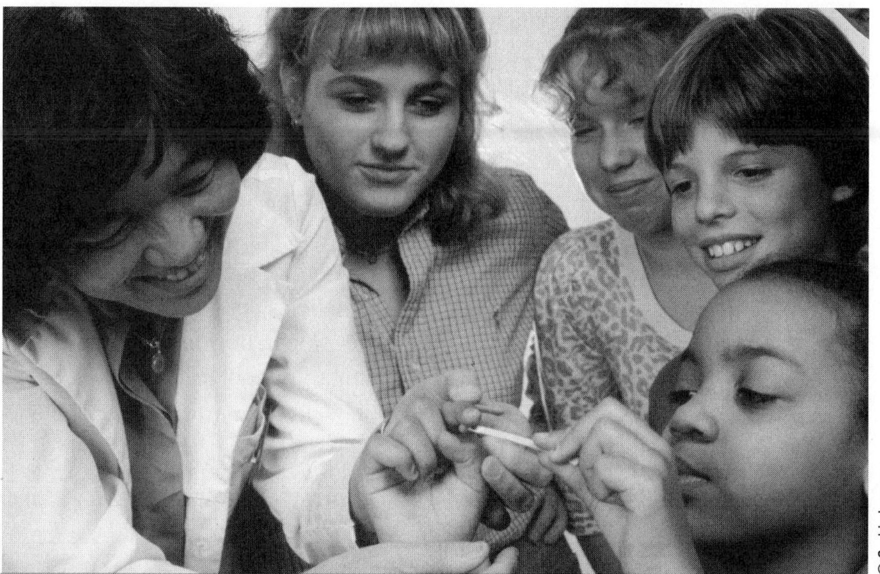

© Corbis Images

Effective health educators have a commitment to students' participatory learning.

discipline of health. The separate disciplines of health promotion, disease prevention, and strategies for health behavior change are the components health educators apply to curriculum development and instruction in comprehensive health education. Training in the delivery of effective health education also requires a commitment to continuous inquiry, self-learning, and reflective and collaborative practice.

This level of commitment by the health educator plus an equal commitment by school administrators and the opportunity to implement effective programs would optimize the health status of schoolchildren and improve their chances of becoming healthy adults.

Unfortunately, sufficient numbers of health educators are not likely to have access to students for more than one or two semesters throughout a student's educational career. Usually, consistent teaching about health does not formally begin until middle school or later. Therefore, elementary schoolchildren who have not yet developed their health habits depend more often upon the classroom teacher for most of their formal learning about health. In this less-than-ideal environment, elementary school classroom teachers, health educators, and allied health personnel (guidance counselors, social workers, and school psychologists) could create team approaches to facilitate the delivery of comprehensive health education.

In addition to formal teaching in separate courses devoted entirely to health education, the professional health educator's role on the team should include

- staying abreast of and sharing information with classroom teachers about new theories, research, technology, and strategies;
- acting as a consultant in planning and implementing supplemental health sessions during regular classes;
- organizing in-service programs; and
- connecting community agencies that have educational materials and programs with classroom teachers.

The Role of the Elementary School Classroom Teacher

Many things influence the commitment of elementary school classroom teachers to health education, including their own personal interest in health, the personal responsibility they feel toward the health needs of their students, the expectations of the school administration, and the effectiveness of teacher-preparation programs to educate classroom teachers about health. The success of programs that classroom teachers deliver is related to the extent of implementation including the depth, range of content covered, and the frequency of health lessons, which, in turn, is related to the amount and length of in-service training.

Teachers are not likely to cover content areas with which they are unfamiliar or uncomfortable. Some teacher-preparation programs offer courses in specific health problems (such as drugs and other substance abuse or AIDS). Others offer health topics in seminar formats scattered throughout the curriculum. Too few programs require formal pre-service training in health education. In sum, then, preparation is usually minimal at best and sometimes leaves classroom teachers feeling inadequate about their ability to effectively teach health subjects.

The commitment of classroom teachers to teaching about health is influenced by many factors:

- Changes in school, community, and social environments, as well as state, county, and district mandates requiring health subjects (such as HIV/AIDS) to be offered on a daily basis (as are English, math, social studies, and so on).
- The federal mandate for "inclusion," which juxtaposes students with disabilities or health-compromising illnesses with students who have little experience with illness or disability. This creates educational opportunities and challenges for learning about living with health problems.
- The rapidly growing aging population and populations in which conditions such as HIV/AIDS, heart disease, cancer, etc., are prevalent have resulted in state mandates for prevention education in K–12.
- Teachers are aware that elementary school children themselves often deal with health-related issues that can covertly affect their behavior and learning.
- Elementary school teachers are seeing considerably more of the social problems expected during adolescence, because the ages of first experience with substance abuse, unintended pregnancy, and sexually transmitted diseases are dropping. Thus, as teachers' tasks have become more complicated in all disciplines, they are being compelled to incorporate health information and developmentally appropriate strategies for prevention—this without compromising the scope of education in any of the disciplines.

We propose that the role (and training) of elementary school teachers be expanded to include a working knowledge of the field of health and the delivery of health education. Further, we propose that they participate, in conjunction with health education teachers, in offering the most current health information and incorporating the most effective methods and materials into a creative and integrated curriculum that encompasses community and parent groups.

The Classroom Teacher as a Role Model

Most teachers have a subtle but powerful impact on students' health behaviors by the examples they set in eating habits, physical activities, responses to stress, substance use (including alcohol, tobacco, and over-the-counter drugs). Teachers are therefore unintentionally health educators of a sort. The health behaviors their students observe in them consistently, over many hours, make teacher modeling especially influential. The classroom environment and health topics that can be infused into the "reading, writing, and arithmetic" curriculum can have subtle but powerful effects on students. These efforts can make a difference in students' ongoing health decision-making and prevention behaviors without compromising traditional curricula. Thus, all the better that teachers be trained in the field of health.

Creating Quality Health Education

Instructor Competencies

The Association for the Advancement of Health Education (AAHE) and the American School Health Association (ASHA) have identified the following competencies, supported by preservice teacher-preparation programs for K–6 elementary school teachers to teach about health. These include the ability to

1. Identify, define, and explain the contemporary concepts of health and health education.
2. Analyze factors influencing the development of health attitudes and behaviors.
3. Identify major causes of illness and death.
4. Cite factors influencing the development and advancement of comprehensive school health education.
5. Define the components of the comprehensive school health program, as currently identified by the Centers for Disease Control and Prevention.
6. Demonstrate the ability to identify creditable sources of information about new developments in areas related to health, education, health education, and health promotion.
7. Identify opportunities for correlation and integration of health information with other subjects and describe ways this can be accomplished.
8. Compare the relationship between growth and development characteristics and appropriate health education lessons.
9. Identify the role of community health agencies in promoting the school health program.

10. Interpret student health information from a given cumulative record.
11. Identify when and how to implement appropriate emergency procedures and first aid, including but not limited to CPR.
12. Identify signs and symptoms of possible student health problems.
13. Describe the process of teacher observation of school-age youth.
14. Select the appropriate actions to be taken when encountering students with health problems.
15. Relate the nutritional needs of school-age children to the school lunch program.
16. Identify motivations for and alternatives to student drug use.
17. Identify the responsibilities of teachers and school personnel for child abuse prevention.
18. Select appropriate educational strategies for health content information based upon the child's age and ability.
19. Demonstrate instructional strategies that foster a wellness lifestyle.
20. Identify appropriate sources of health content information for use in the development of instructional plans.[12]

Defining Coordinated School Health Programs (CSHPs)

Although the teaching of health in the schools can probably be traced back to the early 1800s, not until 1924 was the first comprehensive book published that set standards for the field of health education. Since then, many professional groups have taken leadership roles in framing the discipline of health education and outlining the professional preparation of teachers. These consist of discipline-specific groups (including members of the Coalition of National Health Education Organizations, the National School Health Education Coalition, the American School Health Association, and the Association for Advancement of Health Education) joined by medical associations (American Medical Society, American Pediatric Society), voluntary agencies (American Dietetic Association, American Lung Association, American Heart Association, American Cancer Society), and public health organizations (National Association of State Boards of Education, Department of Health and Human Services, Public Health Service, and local health departments), among others. What has emerged, with agreement from all of these organizations, is a call for a comprehensive approach to the delivery of health education. This comprehensive approach, integrated within a "coordinated school health program" (CSHP) with continuity across grade levels, is what is needed to improve the health of children.[13]

CSHPs are systems or components existing within and around schools that require their related personnel to interact with each other to develop procedures, policies, and activities that ensure the delivery of health education and health services within a healthy school environment. The components of CSHPs are

1. Comprehensive school health education delivered by health coordinators, health educators, classroom teachers, and nurse educators, as appropriate. The role of these health instructors is to deliver health information within a comprehensive school health education (CSHE) program that promotes healthy behaviors, responsible decision making and healthy lifestyles.
2. School health services delivered by doctors, nurses, dentists, and other allied health professionals, as needed. They may provide direct services, assessment, and/or referrals. This health service component includes appraising and protecting students' health, assuring access to allied health services, preventing or controlling communicable diseases, providing emergency care as needed, and maintaining safe conditions in the school facility.[14]
3. A healthy school environment, including physiological and psychosocial factors.[15] This includes proper temperature in the building, well-lit and safe passageways, good air quality, and noise control, as well as a psychosocial climate that supports the development of self-esteem, positive relationships, and a general feeling of safety.
4. School physical education that promotes activities and sports in which students can participate throughout their lives and that, in turn, promote their physical, mental, and social well-being.
5. School nutrition and food services providing students with nutritious and appealing meals that meet the standards of professional nutritional associations such as the Department of Agriculture (USDA), the Department of Health and Human Services (DHHS), and the American Dietetic Association.
6. School counseling, including guidance in the selection of programs, courses, careers, and so on.
7. Psychological and social services drawn from a broad range of mental health professionals attending to students' social, emotional, and general mental health.

8. School-site health promotion encouraging the involvement of advisory boards, coalitions, and parent associations in support of health instruction. These partnerships also involve forging and maintaining relationships with community agencies for the enhancement of children's health. Community involvement encompasses local leaders, direct medical services, and educational services offered by local health agencies to school-aged children and other school personnel.

Defining Comprehensive School Health Education (CSHE) Outcomes

Definitions of health education and descriptions of the role of health educators abound. Nevertheless, it remains, like the discipline itself, a constantly evolving process. The Joint Committee on Health Education Terminology, in 1990, defined "health education" as learning that enables people to voluntarily make decisions and change social conditions in ways that are health-enhancing. (This report is included as Appendix A.)

The Joint Committee on National Health Education Standards, in 1995, produced "Achieving Health Literacy: An Investment in the Future," a document that calls for health literacy as an outcome of effective health education. It defines the health-literate person as one who is a critical thinker and problem solver; a responsible, productive citizen; a self-directed learner; and an effective communicator. Furthermore, it outlines seven standards that describe essential knowledge and skills necessary to be considered health literate. Students will

1. comprehend concepts related to health promotion and disease prevention.
2. demonstrate the ability to access valid health information and health-promoting products and services.
3. demonstrate the ability to practice health-enhancing behaviors and reduce health risks.
4. analyze the influence of culture, media, technology, and other factors on health.
5. demonstrate the ability to use interpersonal communication skills to enhance health.
6. demonstrate the ability to use goal-setting and decision-making skills to enhance health.
7. demonstrate the ability to advocate for personal, family, and community health.

Delivering Comprehensive and Integrated School Health Education

According to the U. S. Department of Education, Comprehensive School Health Education (CSHE) is "a primary prevention strategy for teaching our nation's children and their parents the skills needed for a healthy lifestyle."[16] It involves the development of personal decision-making and problem-solving strategies that children can use to access and incorporate knowledge, clarify personal values, develop and hold attitudes, and choose behaviors that maximize their health and the health of their family and community. For elementary school children, the beginning work is to develop critical thinking skills that result in their ability to comprehend cause and effect, distinguish effective from ineffective strategies, and evaluate risky situations—all resulting in avoidance of dangerous behaviors.

Effective programs no longer emphasize only content knowledge and the physical and psychological consequences of engaging in risky behaviors. Instead, they focus more on intrapersonal factors (such as self-esteem and self-awareness) and inter-personal factors (including peer pressure and significant relationships) to further healthy attitudes and the likelihood of choosing healthier behaviors. More recently, social learning, other behavioral theories, and concepts of multiple intelligences have been incorporated into the curricula. Programs have moved from content-based to skills development, including communication skills and goal-setting activities. Also, a classroom environment that supports various viewpoints and recognizes the multiplicity of values from the home, the teacher, the religious community, and the social group is prerequisite to healthier individual learner outcomes. Figure 1.1 illustrates this changing focus.

Creating Integrated and Developmentally Appropriate Health Education

Integrated health education subsumes health topics within other disciplines. Using integrated formats as an adjunct to courses devoted entirely to health education affords classroom teachers an opportunity to provide health information from historical, cultural, social, scientific, and practical perspectives. Interdisciplinary educational designs reinforce health messages only when they are *not* merely attempts to water down health content, save teaching time, and eliminate discipline-specific health education. Integrated formats can bridge the gap between disciplines, so the content of each becomes more relevant to the lives of students outside of school. Through integrated curricula "students may develop more flexible thinking, adopt multiple points of view, become more adept at generating analogies and improving comprehension."[17]

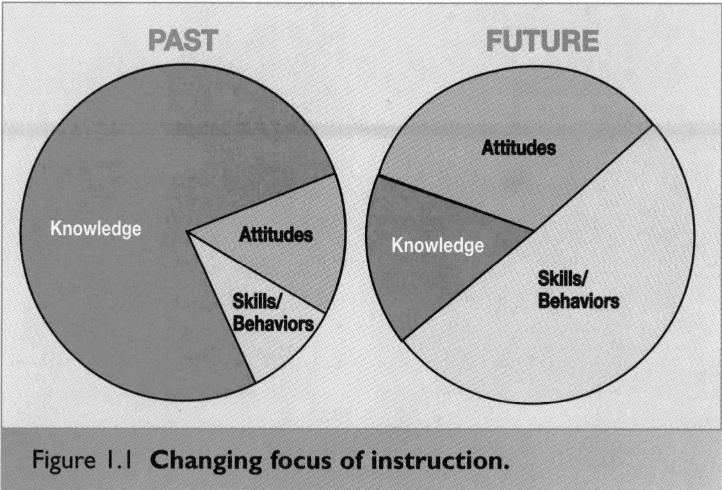

Figure 1.1 **Changing focus of instruction.**

- Learning about health in integrated curricula can broaden personal attitudes and values. Studying the culture and habits of a foreign country could include study of the people's nutritional behaviors, physical activities, patterns of using medical services, and unique cultural factors that influence their health behaviors. This integrated learning opportunity not only increases knowledge about nutrition and social studies but also supports the students' development of cultural sensitivity and cultural awareness.
- When studying the U. S. government and how our laws were established, students could explore agencies that monitor the nation's health, provide health services, govern the use of substances, control communicable disease, and so on, and how these laws ultimately affect their own life choices. Respect for the environment and the complicated issues that surround the protection of health through environmental controls could be included.
- Reading and writing skills can be developed while students research health topics and, in turn, learn about the part research plays in their ability to find appropriate health treatments. Also, as their communication skills increase, they can create more effective patient-provider relationships. Many patients leave doctors' offices with misunderstood information and unanswered questions because of poor listening and weak comprehension skills. Health and other subject matter can be integrated to alleviate these and other concerns.

Health instruction should be developmentally appropriate. Even though enormous variability is present in backgrounds of elementary schoolchildren (in their family, values, attitudes, ethnocultural influences, intelligence, personality, and so forth), general patterns in growth and development can be expected. If the teacher is armed with an understanding of these general patterns and of the uniqueness of the individual children being taught, he or she can plan and implement developmentally appropriate health education. For example, instruction about how health services are paid for is more appropriate in the sixth-grade class than in the K–3 curriculum. Likewise, discussing sexual intercourse as a mode of transmission of the HIV virus is more appropriate for sixth graders, whereas K–3 students might talk about how people "catch" illnesses from one another. (Learning Experiences, placed at the end of each chapter, present developmentally appropriate information by subject area.)

As professional associations and state education departments move toward educational reform within and across disciplines, a new language and new format for organizing curricula and lesson plans is emerging. Each discipline has developed "standards," or learner outcomes, that describe what students should know, what students should be able to do, and what they should be like when they reach commencement, having studied in that discipline. When integrating health education into other disciplines, the classroom teacher will need to be aware of the health education standards as well as standards established by the other disciplines in the integrated model.

Health Education Curricula

The elements of a health education curriculum outlined in the following pages of this chapter include units and lesson plans (presented as Learning Experiences) that encompass elements such as goals and objectives, teaching/learning contexts, procedures (including activities and other strategies that will be used to deliver the lesson), time requirements, and assessment/evaluation methods.

Units

Health education curricula are usually organized by units or sub-discipline content areas to be covered (specific health areas are identified below). The units included in a health curriculum are determined by suggestions from the professional associations, state mandates, local school districts' identified community and family needs assessments, and sometimes input from health service providers. Each unit includes a series of learning experiences that delivers the discipline-specific content and moves the student to achieve the objectives or learner outcomes. Figure 1.2 presents a sample Learner Experience worksheet.

Developing Learning Experiences

Unit information and skills delivered through a sequentially planned set of Learning Experiences (which may be several lessons) relate to one another in an organized manner and build upon each other. Each lesson, like the unit itself, includes the components described above. Although this text assumes that the reader has studied development of lesson plans elsewhere, a format for developing Learning Experiences, including the standards described above, is submitted as a more effective planning tool.

The teacher plans each learning experience by identifying the objective(s) for that day (for example, the students will be able to identify ways by which they can protect themselves from getting the common cold); the content to be learned (for example, the students will know the difference between a virus and a bacterium); specific activities for participation (role plays, story reading, an agency visit, group cooperative activity, homework assignments, and the like); the evaluation assessment strategy(s) that will be used to determine if the objective(s) for the lesson were achieved (a question/answer period, a written test or summary, an activity such as "Something new I learned today about __________ is __________," etc.). The evaluation strategy helps the teacher determine whether the lesson or components of it should be repeated. The evaluation or assessment, if designed as a rubric, also provides students with specific criteria for their grade plus an awareness of how well they have mastered the skills and content.

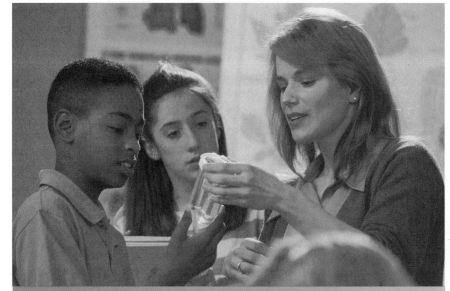

www.comstock.com

Students benefit from hands-on Learning Experiences to reinforce the curriculum content.

Classroom teachers usually attach handouts and other content information to lesson plans, identify audiovisuals that can be used, and prepare a self-reflective instrument that includes the teacher's comments about how effective the teacher thought the lesson was in achieving the objectives; what might be changed, added, or deleted in the future; how effective the audiovisual selection was; and so on. These items will help to strengthen the curriculum for the future.

Sub-Disciplines/ Content Areas/Units

The unit's discipline-specific content areas most frequently subsumed under health education are

- Personal Growth and Development
- Family Life and Human Sexuality
- Environmental Health
- Preventing Violence and Abuse
- Community Health
- Preventing Chronic and Communicable Disease
- Prevention of Alcohol and Other Drug Abuse
- Nutrition
- Mental Health
- Preventing Injury
- First Aid and Safety
- Consumer Health
- Exercise and Physical Fitness

Each of these content areas is usually broken down into subunits that are not mutually exclusive but, rather, build on the overlap between them. Because the technology, information base, and science of health and behavior are constantly changing, the content and subunit areas must constantly be revised to reflect the most current research.

At the elementary-school level, the health content (units) are probably best delivered in a combination of health sessions integrated with other disciplines. The relevance and scope of each topic at the appropriate grade level must be determined.[18] The classroom teacher should feel comfortable

Title of Learning Experience

1. Learning Context

Describe the purpose, objective, or focus of the learning experience, including

- the learning standard(s) and the specific performance indicators being assessed,
- a description of where this experience fits in the school or course curriculum, and
- what students need to know and/or should be able to do to succeed with this learning experience.

2. Procedure

Describe, in narrative form, the actions of students and teachers and the interactions among and between students and teachers, including how the learning experience

- supports student progress toward attainment of the learning standards,
- reflects current scholarship in your field and "best" classroom practice, and
- incorporates technology (when used) into instruction to enhance learning and to assess student performance.

3. Instructional/Environmental Modifications

Describe the procedures used to accommodate the range of abilities in the classroom, including students with disabilities, limited English proficiency, or bilingual students such as

- instructional modifications made and
- physical modifications of the classroom setting.

4. Time Required

For each aspect of the learning experience, state the amount of time for

- planning,
- implementation (note the length of your class period, where appropriate, and the number of days to implement the experience), and
- assessment.

Continued

Figure 1.2 **Sample learning experience worksheets.**

5. Resources

Please note any extraordinary or unique resources (human or material) needed to successfully complete this experience

- for the student and
- for the teacher.

6. Assessment Plan

Describe the

- manner in which students are involved in developing assessment criteria, maintaining an awareness of their progress, and reflecting on their work,
- techniques used to collect evidence of student progress toward meeting the learning standards' performance indicators (e.g., observation, group discussions, journal writing, use of alternative testing techniques), and
- tools used to document student progress (e.g., scoring guides, rating scales, checklists). Please submit these tools.

7. Student Work

Send three or four samples of student work

- that reflect different levels of students performance and
- that include comments reflecting the basis for teacher's assessment.

8. Reflection

Please offer personal comments on the learning experience:

- why this lesson was developed for the specific learning standard(s) and performance indicator(s),
- what you learned from implementing this lesson, and
- how the lesson was reviewed by peers prior to submission and what you learned from the review.

Source: The New York State Academy for Teaching and Learning. Visit: www.nysed.gov. Reprinted with permission.

Figure 1.2 ***(continued)***

with health subjects, especially those with controversial content, and know the most effective strategies for incorporating the information into lessons.

Another organization of content units in health curricula centers on the six adolescent risk behaviors identified by the U.S. Centers for Disease Control (CDC), as follows:

1. Tobacco use
2. Dietary patterns that contribute to disease
3. Sedentary lifestyles
4. Sexual behaviors that result in HIV infection, other sexually transmitted diseases, and unintended pregnancy
5. Alcohol and other drug use
6. Behaviors that result in intentional and unintentional injury.[19]

Some more recent organization of units is in skills-based content areas. The traditional content is delivered through learning experiences that build "skills." The following units in this curriculum are:

Content/Skills and Curriculum Considerations

When developing a curriculum, whether integrating skills across traditional health content units or simply organizing by content alone throughout the K–12 learning experience, students are expected to develop desired competencies as they make choices about their personal lives. Whichever organization of units is selected, it should be delivered sequentially from kindergarten through 12th grade in interdisciplinary formats, it should also incorporate themes that include family and community interests, values, and attitudes. The most effective programs will

- be aimed at increasing cultural sensitivity, respecting diversity while enhancing decision-making and problem-solving abilities;

- include life-cycle perspectives and increase accessibility to health services; and
- maximize the likelihood of students' and teachers' practicing healthy behaviors and choosing healthy lifestyles.

Standards/Goals/ Learner Outcomes

Health education standards or goals that identify what students will know and be able to do must be stated in outcome formats that reflect what is expected of the student—what knowledge they will possess and what skills they will be able to perform. These are usually broad expectations that drive curriculum planning.

Objectives are measures or expectations about what students will be able to do at the completion of an educational experience, unit of study, grade, developmental level, or individual lesson. They identify the means through which goals or learner outcomes are attained.

Educational objectives may be behavioral or instructional. Behavioral objectives are usually those that determine the selection of content, activities, and evaluation procedures for units of study, whereas **instructional objectives** are learner outcomes of a lesson. Classroom teachers should attempt to develop instructional objectives that correspond to planned activities related to health topics and, at the same time, achieve the goals of the more comprehensive school health program. When setting objectives, teachers must ask themselves what is to be accomplished and whether this is realistic within the allotted time and resources.

Evaluation/Assessment

Readers have been or will be trained in testing and measuring their students knowledge and performance. The paper-and-pencil tests (short answer, fill in, multiple-choice, true/false, and essay types) in health education are usually available in hardcopy and CD-ROM as supplements to most school health education textbooks. Tests remain an important part of evaluation of student work, but they do not address the students' ability to use the knowledge constructively to affect their health. Newer assessment concepts are emerging (accompanied by new terminology or jargon) with which teachers have to become familiar. The accompanying box is a sample.

Terms

Current health educators need to measure how students are progressing toward their goals (benchmarks); students' ability to engage in activities that model real-life situations (authentic assessments); students' performance (behaviors) or knowledge in use (performance assessments); and the quality of those behaviors based on established criteria (performance standards). Performance assessments get at the very essence of health education, translating information into action. They describe to the students what they are expected to be able to do *and* how they will do it. The teacher engages the student in his or her own progress and provides constant feedback.

Portfolios

Many health educators are moving toward the portfolio as a project that identifies the student's performance. A portfolio is a collection of the student's work that represents his or her progress through the learning experience, unit, or entire curriculum. It should include an array of work that indicates the student's knowledge, critical-thinking skills, ability to access and evaluate accuracy of research and other health information, ability to engage in reflection, and so on. Criteria for assessing portfolios should be pre-established in consultation with the student.

> **Creating Rubrics for Evaluations**
>
> Where it does not already exist as part of the evaluation of each learning experience that follows, a rubric can be prepared that identifies the mastery of content and skills expected of each student in descending values (from 1–5 or A–F), modified to the appropriate grade or developmental level of the class. A high value is used to indicate a strong grasp of the criteria, a strong ability to perform the task, or a greater number of answers; a lower value represents a weaker grasp, less ability to perform and/or fewer answers. For example, a grade of A means that the student spelled, wrote, or recited all of the new words correctly, and presented 10 of the 10 factors requested; whereas a grade of D means that the student spelled, wrote, or recited only one of the words correctly and presented only one of the factors required.

The contents of the portfolio can be assessed at various times in the curriculum and at the culmination of the entire course of study. The student and his or her parents then have an understanding of how he or she is progressing and what is necessary to achieve more. The emphasis is less on the curriculum and more on the student's progress.

Rubrics

Rubrics—scoring devices that clearly define the criteria and differentiate levels of performance—are an important assessment tool. They also may be instructional. They are most effective when they are generated by the student-teacher partnership. Rubrics clearly define what students will be expected to do maximally and minimally because they are presented in levels of achievement.

Table 1.1
Relationship of the Health Education Content Areas and Adolescent Risk Behaviors to the National Health Education Standards

Health Education Content Areas	National Health Education Standards	Centers for Disease Control and Prevention — Adolescent Risk Behaviors
Community health	1. Student will comprehend concepts related to health promotion and disease prevention.	Tobacco use
Consumer health		
Environmental health	2. Students will demonstrate the ability to access valid health information and health-promoting products and services.	Dietary patterns that contribute to disease
Family life	3. Students will demonstrate the ability to practice health-enhancing behaviors and reduce health risks.	Sedentary lifestyle
Mental and emotional health	4. Students will analyze the influence of culture, media, technology, and other factors on health.	Sexual behaviors that result in HIV infection/other STDs and unintended pregnancy
Injury prevention and safety	5. Students will demonstrate the ability to use interpersonal communication skills to enhance health.	
Nutrition		
Personal health	6. Students will demonstrate the ability to use goal-setting and decision-making skills to enhance health.	Alcohol and other drug use
Prevention and disease	7. Students will demonstrate the ability to advocate for personal, family, and community health.	Behaviors that result in intentional and unintentional injury
Substance use and abuse		

Source: A work of the Joint Committee on National Health Education Standards. Copies may be obtained through the American Health Association, Association for the Advancement of Health Education of the American Cancer Society, Inc., Atlanta, GA: 1995. Reprinted by the permission of the American Cancer Society, Inc.

Using a Likert-type scale, the highest level represents all of the expected work in the highest possible performance for the specific task, and the lowest level represents the least work possible. Rubrics help students clarify what they must do to achieve the highest grade, they can monitor their own progress, and rubrics are understood equally by parents and others who are observing or have a stake in the student's progress, among other benefits.

In addition to setting the stage for more reliable grading, a broad range of assessment techniques provides the teacher with ongoing opportunities to reflect on the curriculum, in both content and teaching strategies, and make the necessary changes to create learning environments and experiences that will successfully move students toward the expected standards/goals.

National Health Goals

A report by the U. S. Department of Health and Human Services, entitled *Healthy People 2000: National Health Promotion and Disease Prevention Objectives,* established broad health goals for the nation, including increasing the healthy lifespan for all Americans, decreasing disparities in sub-populations, and assuring full and equal accessibility to health services. The objectives targeting the health education of the school-age population are presented in Appendix B. These goals can be achieved during elementary school or at the conclusion of high school only if instruction begins early and continues in developmentally appropriate sequences throughout the child's education.

Decreasing and potentially eliminating the health risks defined by the CDC/DASH Youth Risk Behavior Survey (discussed on p. 3) influences the priority goals of health education curricula. The relationship of the health education content areas and adolescent risk behaviors to the National Health Education Standards is shown in Table 1.1.

Each elementary-school classroom lesson that includes health instruction should have as its objectives some specific and measurable contribution to attaining the overall goals of comprehensive health education. For example, an objective of a lesson in community health at the elementary-school level might be "The students will be able to reach emergency health services in their local area" (see Chapter 14). Elementary-school children can be encouraged to develop personal objectives that provide pathways to their goals, increasing the likelihood of commitment to their own lifelong learning and health.

Teaching Styles and Strategies

The experience of health education, whether it is delivered in a discipline-specific course or an interdisciplinary design, is a journey the teacher takes with students. It calls for interacting and learning in a recursive, information-sharing, and experiential manner between students and teacher. Although no single teaching strategy has been identified as most effective with all types of populations, combinations of cognitive and affective models tend to be successful in increasing decision-making and problem-solving capabilities. Much like counselors, teachers are least effective when they are strictly lecturing; giving wrong or right "advice"; or otherwise inhibiting exploration, reflection, critical thinking, and clarification of values.

Strategies that involve the students in active learning through storytelling, role-playing, and other such hands-on activities enhance opportunities for self-discovery. Cooperative learning activities, in which children work in groups to achieve the task, each taking a different component and then merging them to achieve an overall goal, is particularly effective. In health, it increases awareness of the cooperation needed from family, friends, and community in maintaining optimal health.

Guidelines for Health Literacy

Health literacy is the capacity of individuals to obtain, interpret, and understand basic health information and services and the competence to use such information and services in ways which enhance health. Four characteristics were identified as essential to health literacy. The health literate person is a

Critical Thinker and Problem Solver
Health-literate individuals are critical thinkers and problem solvers who identify and creatively address health problems and issues at multiple levels, ranging from personal to international. They utilize a variety of sources to access the current, credible, and applicable information required to make sound health-related decisions. Furthermore, they understand and apply principles of creative thinking along with models of decision-making and goal setting in a health promotion context.

Responsible, Productive Citizen
Health-literate individuals are responsible, productive citizens who realize their obligation to ensure that their community is kept healthy, safe, and secure so that all citizens can experience a high quality of life. They also realize that this obligation begins with self. That is, they are responsible individuals who avoid behaviors that pose a health or safety threat to themselves and/or others or an undue burden on society. Finally, they apply democratic and organizational principles in collaboration with others to maintain and improve individual, family, and community health.

Self-Directed Learner
Health-literate individuals are self-directed learners who have a command of the dynamic health promotion and disease prevention knowledge base. They use literacy, numerical skills, and critical thinking skills to gather, analyze, and apply health information as their needs and priorities change throughout life. They also apply interpersonal and social skills in relationships to learn from others and, as a consequence, grow and mature toward high-level health status.

Effective Communicator
Health-literate individuals are effective communicators who organize and convey beliefs, ideas, and information about health through oral, written, artistic, graphic, and technologic mediums. They create a climate of understanding and concern for others by listening carefully, responding thoughtfully, and presenting a supportive demeanor that encourages others to express themselves. They conscientiously advocate for positions, policies, and programs that are in the best interest of society and intended to enhance personal, family, and community health.

Source: Joint Committee on National Health Education Standards, *National Health Education Standards: Achieving Health Literacy: An Investment in the Future* (American School Health Association, Association for the Advancement of Health Education, and American Cancer Society), Atlanta, GA: 1995.

Theoretical Frameworks Associated with Behavior Change

The notion of behavior and behavior change is an integral part of health education. Hence, knowing the factors that influence how a person might behave and factors that influence changes in those behaviors is important in planning health education activities. Several models and counseling theories have been successful in delivering health education.

Social learning theories are a vital part of teachers' pre-service training. Behavioral theory/cognitive behavioral theory and some of the humanistic psychological theories can be usefully applied to the delivery of health education and incorporated into effective teaching strategies. Also, by acknowledging the importance of values and attitudes to health education, teachers can use values clarification models as an important component of health education. Furthermore, teachers' understanding of multiple intelligences in recognition of individual learning styles enhances the students' success.

The literature is replete with activities for clarifying values—but the emphasis should be on the *learner's* values. The indoctrination of values, especially those of any one teacher, should be avoided. Rather, the strategies that learners can use in clarifying their own values should be stressed.

In addition to the more commonly studied theories mentioned above, important conceptualizations include how health behavior change occurs; what influences a person's ability to adhere to a health or medical regimen; and what factors influence the extent to which people will engage in preventive health activities. Health education specialists study several models, including the PRECEDE model,[20] the Personal Choice Health Behavior model,[21] and the Health Belief Model.[22] The Health Belief Model (HBM) is presented here as an example of how to design a curriculum and classroom activities.

The Health Belief Model

Four major components constitute the HBM as an explanation of the circumstances that will result in actions by individuals to protect their health:

1. Perceived susceptibility to a specific health event: If people believe that the event can actually happen to them (and not just to others), they are more likely to take actions to reduce their susceptibility. Hence, the idea is to teach about the factors that make one more susceptible and then have students participate in activities that apply the general risk factors to their own susceptibility.
2. Perceived severity of the health event: If people believe that contracting a given illness will result in death or permanent disability, they are more likely to engage in behaviors to prevent it. Most professionals, however, have learned that excessive fear tactics do not work over the long run. Fears either immobilize people or cause them to deny the health event and limit action. Hence, the goal in teaching is to achieve a realistic understanding of the severity of a health problem.
3. Perceived effectiveness of adopting certain behaviors to ward off or decrease the health event: If people believe that a behavior or behavior change will affect the severity of the health problem, they are more likely to adopt it. If they believe nothing effective is available, they will not look for it or use it even if suggested. Developing confidence in recognized regimens and witnessing their effectiveness by exposure to people who have been successful often increases their confidence.
4. Perceived barriers to attempts to carry out the desired behaviors: If people believe they can do what is necessary, they will be more likely to do it. If they believe that overcoming the constraints will be too difficult, they will not try. Hence, teachers can have students identify their own personal barriers and develop individual health action plans aimed at overcoming them. This will result in their recognizing their own "internal locus of control."

Assessment

Developing goals and planning objectives, in consultation *with* students rather than *for* students, assures that the learning is relevant to them and maximizes their sense of personal choice and personal responsibility for their own learning. The students' cooperative identification of the assessment rubrics —with the teacher's input—establishes the range of responsibility the students must commit to.[23] Also to be included is the part a community plays in influencing health behavior choices and health services. Then curriculum planning should emerge from an assessment of the students' and the community's needs.

We assume that teachers have had or will have training in assessment strategies. Thus, they will know how to select a representative sample of the population to be assessed; when to select informal groups and appropriate group processes to assess; when to include performance assessment, authentic assessment, or portfolio assessments; and when to use more formal interviews, questionnaires, and other needs-assessment techniques. Moreover, classroom teachers are expected to develop objectives for each lesson and to plan activities that are precise enough to meet those objectives, as well as strategies for measuring them that emerge from their needs assessments, therefore pertinent to their students.

Performance indicators or learning standards expected of students in health education must reflect curriculum activities. These are measured at different grade levels. A learning standard has two components:

1. A content standard (what students know and are able to do)
2. A performance standard (the level or quality of performance the student can exhibit)

The Joint Committee on National Health Education Standards has developed a series of "specific concepts and skills students should know and be able to do by the end of grades 4, 8, & 11".[24] Although these are far more comprehensive than those classroom teachers are likely to use to assess their integrated health lessons, they can be consulted as guidelines for curriculum planning. Some of the long-range outcomes or broad goals of an entire CSHE curriculum are often difficult to measure, and classroom teachers do not usually have the luxury of implementing this level of long-term assessment. However, teachers can review the professional health education literature to determine what those outcomes are and how they are achieved.

Some Concepts and Definitions

Lacey is a 10-year-old girl, physically challenged by congenital blindness. She is a successful runner, a high achiever in school, and generally a happy kid. She is well liked and has lots of friends. She is somewhat restricted in her ability to move around because it takes her a bit longer than sighted children to learn about her environment. She probably would not agree with this description. She often gets impatient with her parents, who are highly protective of her—more protective than other parents, she thinks, and that frustrates her from time to time.

Jeanne is a thin but physically fit early adolescent who loves sports and is, according to her friends, "obsessed with her diet." Her mom and her older sister (17 years old) are overweight, even obese, and their eating habits are awful. They eat a hearty breakfast and a big dinner together every night, and the foods are rich in fat and sugars. Snacks include ice cream, chocolate, potato chips, and other junk food. The family doesn't exercise much. All except Jeanne dislike sports and think Jeanne ought to be softer and more "feminine," less worried about what she eats, and more worried about her school grades. Jeanne diets constantly and exercises vigorously in an attempt to keep her weight down.

Sebastian is a 7-year-old whose dad is a physician. Whenever members of the boy's family have the slightest ailment, they seek the doctor's advice and are usually supplied with the appropriate medicines. They believe the earlier they get treatment, the less likely things will get serious. Sebastian's grandfather died of heart disease at a young age, and so did two uncles on his father's side. Family members are worried about the high level of stress under which they live, and they fear for the life of Sebastian's father. They are all careful about what they eat and how much exercise they get. Sometimes Sebastian's dad is irate if he is not able to get in his hour at the gym on any given day. Sebastian is a worried child.

Sasha's family comes from a foreign country. The members do not speak English very well. In their country, herbs, meditation, and religious and spiritual factors were considered major factors in healing people who were ill. The family does not believe that Western medicine is effective. Recently, when Sasha was entering public school for the first time, the school required her to get vaccinated. The family was reluctant but finally acceded. Basically, Sasha is healthy, and when she doesn't feel well, the family turns to members of the small community from the old country. Rarely does anyone go to the doctor or the clinic, even with a pregnancy. Sasha's family members are strict vegetarians, and the foods they eat are ethnically prepared.

If you were asked to identify which of the situations above were healthy and which family members were healthy, how would you respond? What criteria would you use to come to your conclusions? Would your assessment of these situations be the same as others'? How do you believe your students would respond?

In the first scenario, Lacey's blindness could be considered her major health problem. Or is her major problem associated with her impatience with her parents and frustration with their over-protectiveness, which may compromise her self-esteem and, therefore, her mental health later in life? In the second scenario, are Jeanne's exercise and diet habits indicative of an

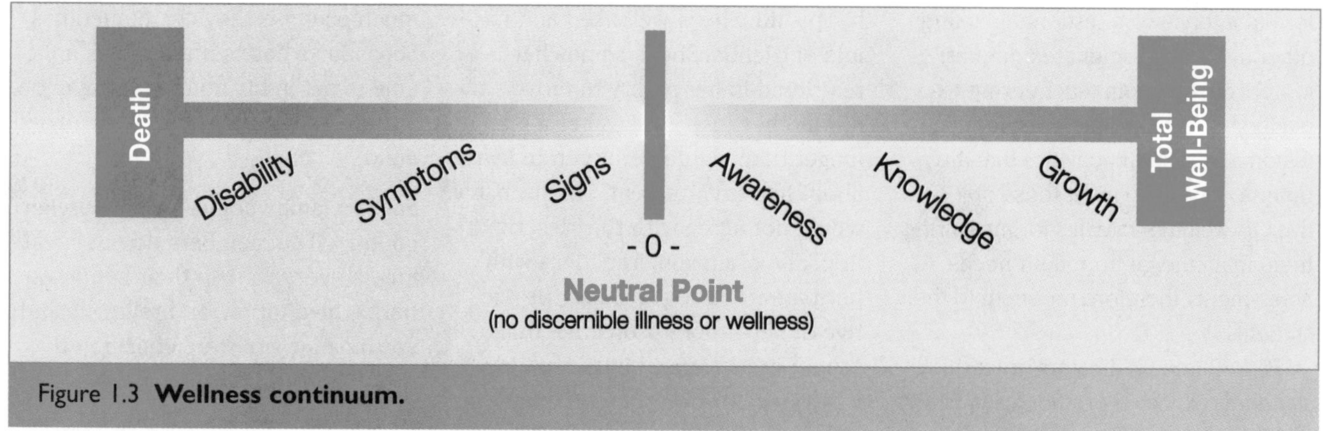

Figure 1.3 **Wellness continuum.**

obsessive-compulsive behavior or eating disorder, or is it her family's influence over her eating behaviors that will create her future health challenge? Is Sebastian's family's use of the health care system effective, or is this evidence of anxiety, fear, and the "worried well" syndrome? How will these behaviors influence Sebastian's notion of control over his own health?

What part will ethnocentric and cultural influences have on Sasha's health, and will they pose health risks? Will real-life situations similar to these examples affect the children in your classrooms?

Your evaluation of such situations will depend in part on your own ideas of health, wellness, and related concepts. These important ideas are discussed below.

What Is Health?

Accepted definitions of **health** range from feelings of wellness and not showing signs of sickness to the absence of symptoms of sickness. The World Health Organization was the first to define health, in 1947, as "a state of complete physical, mental and social well being and not merely the absence of disease and infirmity."[25] The inclusion of "complete" creates difficulty in the definition. Other researchers defined health in terms of an individual's quality of life encompassing social, mental, and biological well-being resulting from his or her ability to adapt to the environment.

"Health" describes a person whose physical body functions efficiently and is generally able to resist the onset of disease or readily heals itself; whose mental well-being copes well with stress and has high self-esteem and a sense of control over life's events; whose social well-being supports positive relationships, maintains a career and sense of community; and whose sense of spirituality supports the person's understanding of life and peacefulness.

Most often, when people feel well, they define themselves as healthy. Using that yardstick, they think they can tell when others are healthy simply by looking at them. Conversely, people know when they are ill because they feel sick, and they also think they know when others are sick. These simplistic notions about health are sometimes faulty, yet they are factors in determining health; how health education is implemented; and what constitutes prevention, research, and interventions.

Clearly, defining health so it is measurable and precise is difficult and is subject to differing views. Although we could probably agree on the components that constitute health, we do not have a universal definition, nor can we precisely state what "healthy" is and exactly how to achieve it. This challenge of definitions is common to the many disciplines (medicine, science, religion, and so on) that determine health and the factors that influence it.

A helpful and useful conceptualization sees health as existing on a continuum from optimal health to premature death, in which are degrees of wellness and illness. We are all "terminal cases," but as long as we are alive, we are in some state of health. Figure 1.3 presents this continuum of health.

A continuum concept of health suggests an individual's continuous balancing of the physical, emotional, social, intellectual, and spiritual components to produce happiness and a higher quality of life. This concept also provides for people taking responsibility for their own health through their actions and the attitudes they hold.

What Is Wellness?

Wellness has been defined as "the constant and deliberate effort to stay healthy and achieve the highest potential for total well-being."[26] High-level wellness is synonymous with optimal health and is often described as an ability to have a purposeful and enjoyable experience of living. (A more extensive discussion about wellness/fitness appears in Chapter 4).

What Is Illness?

Illness can be described as the experience of sickness or lack of well-being. People's perception of themselves as having something wrong with their body (usually accompanied by symptoms, physical or emotional) signals illness. The feeling of illness is frequently what directs people to a medical provider. Illness behaviors consist of activities undertaken by people who consider themselves ill, sometimes before they have been diagnosed, for the purpose of getting well.

Many health professionals agree that health, wellness, and illness are states of being resulting from a mind-body connection—the interrelationship among biophysiological, psychological, and social factors. The effect of the mind on the body must not be underestimated, because our emotions and beliefs have a profound influence not only on our ability to stave off disease but also on our ability to get well.

What Is Disease?

Diseases have specific etiologies, manifestations, and risk factors. **Disease** is usually the culmination of an interaction of factors including genetic predisposition, lifestyle or health behaviors, infectious agents (such as bacteria and viruses), and environmental toxins. A person can have an overall feeling of illness without having a specific disease, and a person can have a disease without having a feeling of illness. For example, the early stages of cancer are usually symptom-free, and the people affected, if asked, would probably describe themselves as healthy.

What Is Spirituality?

Spirituality is thought to have important implications for an individual's health status. Spirituality can be explained in several ways—a personal code of ethics, a moral structure, a person's center, his or her feelings of oneness with his/her surroundings. The spiritual component provides meaning and direction to a person's life through nature, science, religion, morals, values, and ethics.

Some people experience this "wholeness" or connectedness through their relationship with established religion. Others experience it through their personal philosophy of life. A positive spiritual self is a subjective idea, thought to support peacefulness, healthy interpersonal relationships, motivation, and self-nurturing. These qualities are believed to increase the level of wellness.

Health Behavior

Health behavior is a major factor in determining health. Health behavior has been defined as "any activity undertaken by a person believing himself/[herself] to be healthy, for the purpose of preventing disease or detecting it in an asymptomatic stage."[27] Lumped together, our health-related behaviors contribute to our health status.

Health Risk Factors

Health risk factors are characteristics or patterns of behavior that are associated with the potential for developing an illness or a disease. A risk factor does not necessarily cause a disease or illness, but it increases the likelihood of its occurrence. Certain risk factors are within a person's control and can be modified. These include insufficient exercise, poor diet and eating behaviors, smoking, and substance abuse, among others. Risk factors not within a person's control include age, sex, and genetic predisposition. People with noncontrollable risk factors for a certain disease have to be more diligent in modifying their lifestyle by decreasing controllable risk factors so they can decrease their overall risk. For example, a person with a genetic risk for heart disease, as demonstrated by family history, may have to be considerably more diligent about diet and exercise than a person with no such family history.

A Healthy Lifestyle

Lifestyle consists of choices, actions, habits, and patterns that are within our control and that increase or decrease our risk for illness or disease. For example, if we live a "partying" lifestyle, our behaviors are likely to include some extent of alcohol and drug use. If we lead a "workaholic" lifestyle, our behaviors are likely to include long hours of stressful and nonrestful periods with little time for recreation. If we are leading a physically fit lifestyle, we are participating in one of the components of wellness. Our lifestyle and the behaviors that constitute it can make an important contribution to our well-being and longevity.

Locus of Control

The notion of individual control over health has come to the fore. Development of a sense of control over oneself and one's life events begins early in life and continues throughout the lifespan. People who have a strong sense of control exhibit healthier habits, incur less illness, and are more likely to be able to rehabilitate themselves or adjust to serious illness. Childhood experiences, including those learned in the schools, can support a strong sense of control or can foster the opposite, "learned helplessness."

Locus of control in health-related matters occurs on three levels: an "internal locus of control," a "powerful-other locus of control," and a "chance locus of control."[28] People with an **internal locus of control** believe in their own ability to affect their health.

They say things like, "If I take care of myself, I will feel well." People who have a **powerful-other locus of control** believe that their health is under the control of someone other than themselves, such as their physician, parent, dietitian, or religious leader. They take these others' opinions and suggestions as gospel rather than as counsel and do not take responsibility for themselves. They say things like, "If I do exactly as I am told, I will be well." People who have a **chance locus of control** believe that luck or fate determines their health status. If they are lucky, they will not become ill or they will recover quickly. Or they believe that "it is written somewhere" and nothing they can do will change it.

Teachers can foster a strong internal locus of control in students that allows them to feel that what they themselves do is a main force in their ability to be well. With this belief system, children are more likely to choose behaviors that will positively influence their own health. They will seek medical opinion, ask lots of questions, and incorporate the information into their healthy choices. They will not be as likely to follow the pack or the newest fad.

Values, Attitudes, and Belief Systems

Values, attitudes, and beliefs are the underpinnings of thoughts, feelings, and actions. They also affect our ability to make decisions and think critically.

Values are things that individuals hold in high regard. Some values are more universally held. Others are more personal and are held dear by that individual. A person's values may change from time to time. They are influenced by learning, exposure to others, and sociocultural factors, among others. Values influence attitudes, belief systems and, ultimately, behaviors. They are what we weigh when we make decisions or solve problems in our daily lives.

Elementary schoolchildren are just beginning to develop a value system. The values they first evidence reflect their family's values. As children's outside exposure increases, their values reflect those of the community, including cultural and religious groups. As time goes on and children are more heavily exposed to the values of the broader community, especially the media, their values are influenced accordingly.

Pioneers Raths, Harmin, and Simon explained a process whereby people can clarify their values and establish a system of values that supports healthier behaviors.[29] Recognizing what one's true values are and reevaluating them periodically will quiet intrapersonal and interpersonal conflict (times when we act or are pressured to act against our values). According to Raths and his colleagues, several factors have to operate for something to be a value. It has to be freely chosen, chosen from alternatives with awareness of the consequences, and prized and cherished by the individual. Furthermore, a value is one that a person is willing to publicly affirm or acknowledge as valuable to him or her and one that he or she will act upon and repeat consistently.

We can clarify our values by these criteria. Are we willing to state aloud, for all to hear, one of our values? Do our behaviors related to the value support the value? For example, in a school where students' good health is valued, we could expect the principal to affirm the importance of health education, see evidence of it as an integral part of the curriculum, provide healthful meals and snacks, provide medical screening, and hire personnel that respond to health needs.

Attitudes are a group of related beliefs. Our **beliefs** are our acceptance of something as "true or real." Some of our beliefs are stronger than others, and we have held some longer than others. The underlying organization of our beliefs (how long we have held them and how many there are) about a given issue will influence the strength of our attitude about it and, ultimately, our decisions and actions. Our attitudes largely determine our health-related behaviors.

Decision-making is a powerful and important skill. It is the mechanism by which people take responsibility for their own behavior. We choose what we do based on what we determine to be the alternatives. How we act is a result of a combination of many things, including environment, genetic predisposition, intelligence, self-image, opportunity, socioeconomic status, cultural norms, religion, and gender experiences. These are affected by behavioral influences including awareness, value judgments, and risk-taking.

Critical thinking is another important skill that provides students with a framework for making the important decisions that drive their behavior. Critical thinking is self-directed, self-disciplined, self-monitored and self-corrective thinking. A critical thinker is able to

1. raise vital questions in a clear and precise manner;
2. gather and assess relevant information using abstractions to interpret effectively;
3. derive well-reasoned conclusions and solutions by testing them against relevant criteria and standards;
4. think openmindedly, recognizing and assessing (as need be) assumptions, implications, and practical consequences; and
5. communicate effectively with others in figuring out solutions to complex problems.[30]

For Your Health

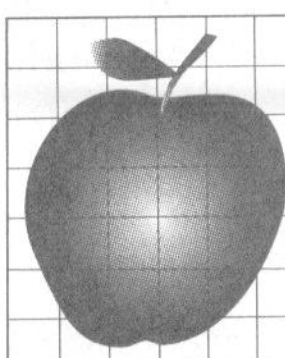

A Decision-Making Process

Good health decisions have lifelong effects. These decisions are not easy to make. Being aware of healthy behaviors and the values that lead to them will make the decision-making process easier. This, in turn, will make for healthier, happier, and less hazardous lives.

The strategies for "good" decision-making can be learned and, therefore, should be incorporated into school curricula. Several decision-making processes are available. The following is one example.

- Ask yourself the question, "Is there a decision to be made?" If the answer is yes, "Is it my decision to make?" The implications here are important. "Does a 10-year-old have to decide whether the drug his mother purchased is the right drug for his symptoms?" There is a decision to be made. He has symptoms. "Is this my decision?" Probably not. Adults make these decisions. The 10-year-old should not spend too much time fretting over it.
- If the answers to the first two questions are yes, gather information including options and alternatives. Use every available source and write down anything and everything pertaining to the decision. If possible, divide the information into facts that are for and facts that are against the decision.
- Weigh the facts by examining the "give ups"—the things you will give up if you make one decision versus the "gets"—what you will get by making that decision. A simple example is smoking a joint. Will it damage my health or well-being? Will it be good for the people who are important to me? Will it affect my judgment? Is it legal? If not, what are the consequences? Can I afford to purchase it? Am I doing it to impress someone else or to belong? If I am, is it worth it? Or will I really be belonging because I am me or because I am smoking?
- Make a decision, determine if you have what you need to carry it out, then act on it. Take a reasonable time (longer for big decisions, shorter for smaller ones) to examine the results of your choice, using your own views and feedback from those you respect.
- Reevaluate the decision and its outcomes and consequences. If you are happy with your decision, go on with your life. If not, do what you can to make positive changes. Few decisions are irrevocable. Revisit the process and decide on one of the other alternatives considered earlier. *A "no" decision is a decision.*

If there is a decision to be made and it is yours to make and you do not make it, someone else might make it for you. Avoiding decisions is usually not productive.

One might apply these concepts to explain and reflect on the cases described on page 17. For example, in describing Lacey, one might say: While she is physically challenged with blindness, she has a high level of wellness and a strong internal locus of control. She believes strongly in herself and her ability to participate in activities that will maintain her as physically fit.

Prevention Through Promotion

The goal of health education is health promotion and disease prevention. Health promotion promotes the elimination of poor health habits and adoption of health behaviors that increase health status. It has been defined as "all of the means by which healthy behavior may be encouraged."[31] Prevention activities can take place on three levels: primary, secondary, and tertiary.

Primary Prevention

Primary prevention means choosing actions that are most likely to prevent a health problem from occurring at all. Early health education consists of increasing knowledge and promoting initial behaviors that are health-supporting and health-enhancing. Children who eat a balanced diet, exercise well, get sufficient rest, and minimize stress as part of their earliest habits will be the most successful "primary preventers." Immunization is another example of a primary prevention activity. Because changing fixed behaviors and ways of living are more difficult than developing initial habits that are healthy, the choice for school health education is primary prevention.

Secondary Prevention

Secondary prevention—early identification and treatment of a health problem either to stop it from getting worse or to reverse it entirely—requires more input from health services. In secondary prevention, health education increases awareness of symptoms and teaches when to seek medical care, how to choose a health care system, and how to effectively access it.

Also, secondary prevention entails developing and implementing a medical plan suggested by the physician or other health provider to prevent a situation from getting worse. For example, secondary prevention can involve changing dietary choices after a diagnosis of high cholesterol as a means of preventing cardiovascular disease or decreasing salt intake to control hypertension.

Tertiary Prevention

Tertiary prevention refers to actions taken to contain or minimize irreversible damage or contain and slow the disease progression while maximizing adjustment and resumption of life's activities. Tertiary prevention is mostly a function of rehabilitation programs and rarely falls within the realm of school health education. An example of tertiary prevention is a rehabilitative exercise program designed to reverse or minimize the effects of a heart attack or injury.

The success of school health education programs rests primarily in their ability to enable students to engage in primary and secondary prevention activities and access tertiary prevention resources, if indicated, in the pursuit of healthy lifestyles.

Summary

Changes in the American family, the ever-increasing responsibility of schools in children's lives, the changing social and work environments, and the influence of the media on children's earliest health behaviors point to the need for effective health promotion and prevention activities in the schools. Moreover, effective health instruction raises student awareness about their own health, and increases their "readiness to learn, improves the health of future generations, and reduces costs to society of caring for those whose illnesses might have been prevented through early education and behavior modification."[32] The complex system and territorial issues that surround delivery of health education as part of a coordinated school health program must be revisited if schools are to help children develop into healthy adults. Classroom teachers can contribute greatly to the likelihood that students will choose a healthy lifestyle.

Schools that embrace coordinated and comprehensive programs focus on key risks to health and learning; welcome and receive help from the adults and students in the school and surrounding community; draw from several disciplines, groups, and agencies; include multiple programs and components; provide staff development; and use inclusive and broad program planning.[33] Developmentally appropriate health education can be delivered without compromising the traditional and required elementary school curriculum, if instructional strategies and content are integrated into the primary disciplines.

A risk assessment and risk reduction conceptualization of curricula can be considered along with the various content areas.[34] Goals and objectives can be carefully planned, and ongoing evaluation of the methods and materials undertaken to assure expected learner outcomes for each lesson and for the entire program. Opportunities for in-service and other professional development in health should be made available to classroom teachers in support of their efforts toward delivery of health education. The result of classroom teachers' commitment to health instruction will be students who have the skills and knowledge to decrease their health risks and optimize their health status throughout the lifespan.

Web Sites

Alan Guttmacher Institute
www.agi.usa.org

American Alliance for Health, Physical Education, Recreation & Dance
www.aahperd.org

American Association for Health Education
www.aahperd.org/aahe

American Health Network
www.ahn.com

American Public Health Association
www.apha.org

American School Health Association www.asha.org

Association for Supervision and Curriculum Development
www.ascd.org

CDC's Morbidity & Mortality Weekly Report
www.cdc.gov/mmwr

CDC's Behavioral Risk Factor Surveillance System
www.cdc.gov/nccdphp/brfss

Census data/kidscount
www.aecf.org/kidscount

Centers For Disease Control (CDC)
www.cdc.gov

Child Health Care
www.wellchild.org

Children Now
www.childrennow.org

Children's Health Care
www.che-peds.com

Classroom Connect
www.classroom.net

Department of Health & Human Services (DHHS) Healthy People 2010
www.health.gov/healthypeople/

Harvard Center for Children's Health
www.hsph.harvard.edu/children

Health Care Financing Administration
www.hcfa.gov

Health Finder
www.healthfinder.org

Healthy Child
www.healthychild.com

Institute for Child Health Policy
www.ichp.edu

Journal of the American Medical Association
www.ama-assn.org.

National Center for Statistics
www.cdc.gov/nchs/

National Clearinghouse for Alcohol and Drug Information
www.health.org/

Centers For Disease Control's (CDC), Division of Adolescent and School Health (DASH)
www.cdc.gov/nccdphp/dash

The Foundation for Critical Thinking
www.criticalthinking.org

U. S. Public Health Service, Healthy People 2000 Progress Review
odphp.osophs.dhhs.gov/pubs/hp2000

U. S. Public Health Service, Healthy People 2010 Objectives: Draft for Public Comment
web.health.gov/healthypeople2010D.

United Nations
www.unsystem.org

World Health Organization
www.who.org

Notes

1. U. S. Department of Health and Human Services, *Healthy People 2000: National Health Promotion and Disease Prevention Objectives* (Washington, DC: Government Printing Office, 1991).
2. U. S. Department of Health and Human Services, *Americans Assess Their Health: United States, 1987* (Washington, DC: Government Printing Office, 1990).
3. See note 1.
4. See note 1.
5. U. S. Bureau of The Census, *Statistical Abstracts of the United States: 1991* (111th ed.) (Washington, DC: Government Printing Office, 1991).
6. D. B. Ardell, *A Contemporary Fable: Upstream/Downstream* (Emmaus, PA: Rodale Press, 1997).
7. U. S. Department of Education, *Comprehensive School Health Education Programs: Innovative Practices and Issues in Setting Standards* (Washington, DC: Office of Educational Research and Improvement, 1993).
8. L. Kann, S. A. Kinchen, B. I. Williams, J. G. Ross, R. Lowry, J. A. Grunbaum, and L. J. Kolbe, State and Local YRBSS Coordinators, "Youth Risk Behavior Surveillance System" *MMWR* 49, ss-5 (1999): 1–34.
9. *Code Blue: Uniting for Healthier Youth* (Alexandria, VA: National Association of State Boards of Education, 1990).
10. E. Marx and D. Northrop, "Partnerships to Keep Students Healthy," *Educational Leadership* 57 (6): 1–4. Available from http://www.ascd.org/reading room/eedlead/0003/marx.html

11. E. Marx, S. F. Wooley, and D. Northrup, *Health Is Academic: A Guide to Coordinated School Health Programs* (New York: Teachers College Press, 1998).
12. J. Varnes, "Preservice Education: Providing Health Knowledge for All Teachers," in *The Comprehensive School Health Challenge: Promoting Health Through Education*, ed. P.C. and K. Middleton (Santa Cruz, CA: ETR Publishing, 1994), 799–800. Reprinted with permission.
13. L. W. Greene, M. W. Kreuter, S. G. Deeds, and K. B. Partridge, "Thoughts from the School Health Education Evaluation Advisory Panel," *Journal of School Health* 55, no. 8 (1985), 335.
14. Centers for Disease Control and Prevention, National Center for Chronic Disease Prevention and Health Promotion, Division of Adolescent and School Health, *Developing Comprehensive School Health Programs to Prevent Important Health Problems and Improve Educational Outcomes* (Atlanta: CDC), 1999.
15. D. Allensworth and L. Kolbe, "The Comprehensive School Health Program: Exploring an Expanded Concept," *Journal of School Health* 57, no. 10 (1987), 409–473.
16. See note 6, p. 1
17. See note 6, p. 57
18. Joint Committee on National Health Education Standards, *National Health Education Standards: Achieving Health Literacy: An Investment in the Future*, American School Health Association, Association for the Advancement of Health Education, Atlanta, GA: American Cancer Society, 1995.
19. Center for Disease Control, Division of Adolescent and School Health (DASH). Available from http://www.cdc.gov/nccdphp/dash/.
20. L. W. Greene, M. W. Kreuter, S. G. Deeds, and K. B. Patridge, *Health Education Planning: A Diagnostic Approach* (Palo Alto, CA: Mayfield Publishing, 1980).
21. D. Horn, "A Model for the Study of Personal Choice Health Behavior," *International Journal of Health Education* 19 (1976): 2.
22. M. H. Becker, ed., *The Health Belief Model and Personal Health Behavior* (Thoroface, NJ: Charles B. Slack, 1974).
23. L. Burak, "Independent Activities Teach Skills for Lifelong Learning," *Journal of Health Education* 24, no. 5 (1993): 376–378.
24. See note 18.
25. World Health Organization, *Chronicles of the World Health Organization*, vol. 1 (Geneva, Switzerland: WHO, 1947), 3.
26. W. W. K. Hoeger, *Lifetime Physical Fitness and Wellness: A Personalized Program* (Belmont, CA: Wadsworth, 2003).
27. S. V. Kasl and S. Cobb, "Health Behavior, Illness Behavior, and Sick Role Behavior in Health and Illness Behavior," *Archives of Environmental Health* 12 (1966): 246–266.
28. K. Wallston, B. S. Wallston, and R. DeVellis, "Development of the Multi-dimensional Health Locus of Control (MHLC) Scales," *Health Education Monographs* 6 (1978): 161–170.
29. L. Raths, M. Harmin, and S. B. Simon, *Values Teaching: Working with Values in the Classroom*. (Columbus, OH: Charles E. Merrill, 1966).
30. R. Paul and L. Elder, *The Miniature Guide to Critical Thinking: Concepts and Tools*. (Dillon City, CA: The Foundation for Critical Thinking, 1999). Available from http://www.criticalthinking.org
31. D. Duncan and R. Gold, "Health Promotion: What Is It?" *Health Values* 10, no. 3 (1986), 47–52.
32. J. Tomlinson, "A Changing Panorama," *Health and Education* 17 (May 1999): 1–11. Available from http://www.ascd.org/readingroom/infobrief/9905.html
33. D. Allensworth, (1995). "The Comprehensive School Health Program: Essential Elements," in J. Tomlinson, (1999) "A Changing Panorama." *Health and Education*, 17, p. 1–11.
34. Joint Committee on National Health Education Standards, *National Health Education Standards: Achieving Health Literacy*. Atlanta, GA: American Cancer Society, 1995).

2

The Human Body and Its Development

Israel M. Schwartz

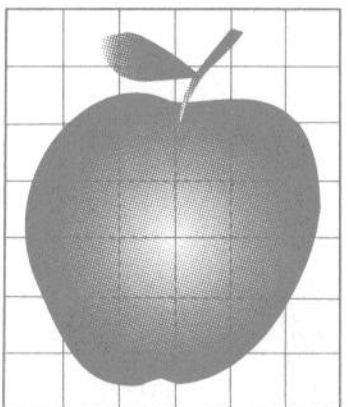

Chapter Outline

The Skeletal System
The Muscular System
The Integumentary System
The Respiratory System
The Circulatory System
The Lymphatic System
The Digestive System
The Urinary System
The Nervous System
The Sensory System
The Endocrine System
The Reproductive System

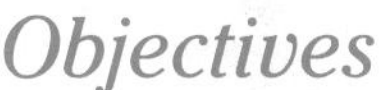

Objectives

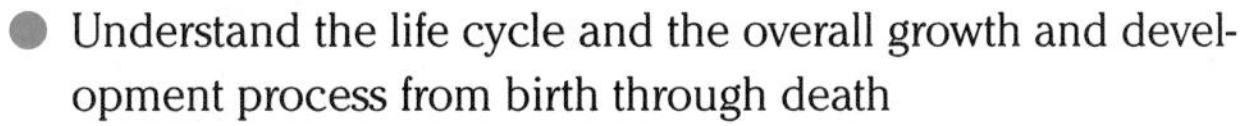

- Understand the life cycle and the overall growth and development process from birth through death
- Describe the interaction of body systems that contribute to a healthy whole
- Explain the skeletal system, development of bones and teeth, and how to keep them healthy
- Explain the types of muscles and muscular development and maintenance
- Identify components of the integumentary system and how they function to promote health
- Explain how the respiratory system works
- Identify the components of the circulatory system and describe the cardiovascular process
- Trace the path of the digestive system and identify its components
- Explain how the urinary system works
- Describe the nervous system, its components, and their roles
- Name the five senses and explain their functions
- Explain the overall role of the endocrine system and the functions of its specific glands and organs
- Describe the male and female reproductive systems

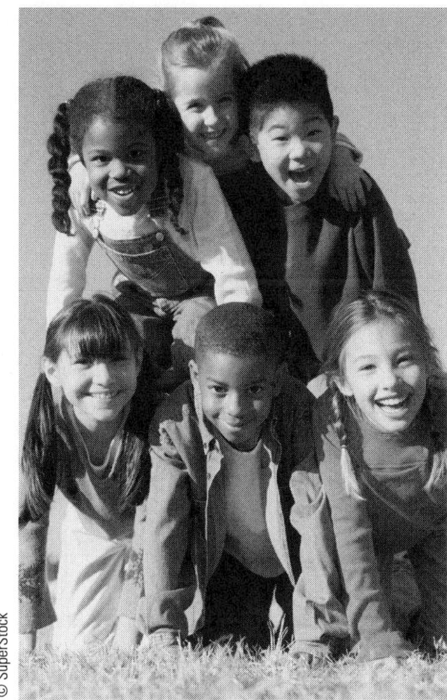

Emilio, Jason, and Santos, three first graders, wanted to play football with their older schoolmates, but they were never included. They practiced hard every day after school, figuring that, if they were good enough, their schoolmates would let them play. One day, as they were roughhousing in the park, Emilio tripped and fell down the hill, holding on to the football tightly as he rolled and rolled. When he landed at the bottom, his lower arm was twisted in a strange way, and he was screaming and crying.

Jason and Santos were scared that something was terribly wrong. They ran for help. One park attendant went to help Emilio, and the other called Emilio's mother, who lived just across the street. As Jason and Santos listened to their friend cry, they heard Emilio's mother say that she thought the arm was badly broken and that he needed to go to the hospital. The park attendant said he was afraid to move Emilio because that could do further damage. They called an ambulance, which took Emilio away.

Jason and Santos waited for their friend to come home. They were hiding behind the bushes when he got out of his mother's car a few hours later. They wondered if his mother would bring the broken arm home with them or just throw it away. How would Emilio look without his arm attached? "Broken arms do fall off, don't they?" thought Jason and Santos. Santos remembered that his sister went to the hospital last year to have her appendix taken out. Even though he wasn't sure what an appendix was or even where it came from, he knew they did not bring it home.

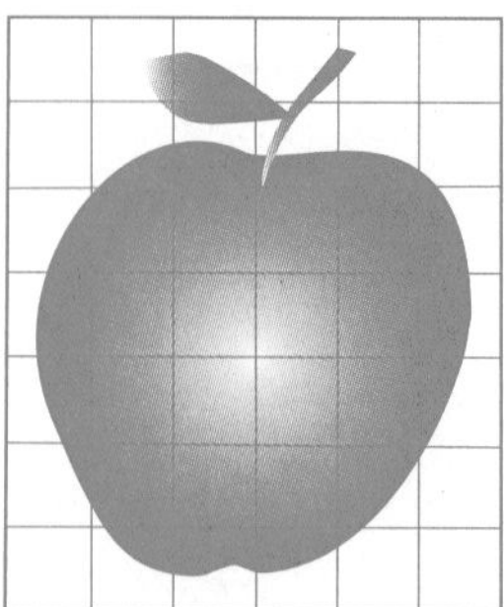

What attacked Grandpa's heart, and where is the heart? How does an arm break? Where is the baby inside the mother's stomach? Where does the food go when it is swallowed? Jason's and Santos's concerns about their friend's arm are a symptom of confusion and of the kind of inquisitiveness that children have about how their body works long before puberty and the lifelong changes their body will undergo.

The myths and misconceptions that begin in early childhood fantasy often continue until people become knowledgeable about their body parts and functions. Teachers in early education can dispel these myths by helping children understand their body parts and how they function.

For teachers to be effective and for children to feel empowered to maximize their health status, both should become aware of the developmental process and how body systems develop and function, particularly from a life cycle perspective. This enables teachers to present the information clearly and children to understand the immediate effects of their actions and behaviors on the major body systems. Such early education will help students maintain a harmonious balance among the various body systems, called **homeostasis**, and promote their bodies' optimal functioning as a central component of personal good health.

All living organisms, including humans, begin life as a single cell and continue through many developmental stages that are known collectively as the life cycle. **Growth** refers to the division and enlargement of cells, which occurs most rapidly during the early stages of life. After only 9 months of cellular growth and differentiation (the formation of cells that become specialized for specific functions), what began as a single human cell becomes a complex set of systems made up of trillions of cells—a newborn baby.

Development is the maturation process whereby the body systems increase in complexity and ability to perform more complicated functions. For example, brain development in the period between infancy and childhood facilitates better coordination and motor movement, as well as the ability to engage in more difficult mental tasks.

As development progresses and cells become more specialized in their function, the growth rate slows. In the later stages of life, growth is barely sufficient (and sometimes insufficient) to replace lost cells and, therefore, the body systems begin to function less efficiently. This is part of the aging process that ends in death as the final stage in the life cycle.

The unique interaction of genetic inheritance, patterns of behavior, and environmental surroundings—all of which have a tremendous impact on growth and development—determines an individual's personal health. Because little can be done to change genetic inheritance, the most effective way to influence personal health is to develop and practice positive health-related behaviors. Personal health is also influenced by environmental surroundings, which include family relationships, cultural norms, and economic resources, as well as the quality of an individual's physical environment.

The human body is made up of trillions of cells. Groups of similar cells form tissues that, in turn, group together to form organs. A group of organs that works together to perform a specific function in the body is referred to as a **body system**. Even though body systems each have distinct and specific functions, each is dependent upon and interrelated with the others. For example, the heart, which is the major organ of the circulatory system, and the lungs, which are the major organs of the respiratory system, work together closely to provide the other body systems with the oxygen and nutrients necessary for life. Similarly, the skeletal and muscular systems work closely for body structural support and movement, in addition to providing protective and supportive functions for other organs and systems in the body. The body systems are described in this chapter.

The Skeletal System

At birth the human skeleton consists of 350 soft bones. As an individual grows and develops, many of these soft bones (made of cartilage) fuse into larger and more rigid single bones. The adult human skeletal system contains 206 bones. Bones range in size from the large thigh bones (femurs), which account for approximately one-quarter of the body's height, to the small bones in the ear, which are only a fraction of an inch long.

Bones have several functions:

1. They support the body.
2. They maintain posture.
3. With the assistance of joints, they allow for movement.
4. They protect the vital organs (for example, the skull protects the brain, the spine protects the spinal cord, and the breastbone and rib cage protect the heart and lungs).
5. Some of the larger bones produce blood cells in their marrow.

The two main skeletal groups are the axial skeleton, which includes the skull (29 bones), spinal column (26 bones), rib cage (24 bones) and breastbone, and the appendicular skeleton, which includes the hands (27 bones in each), feet (26 bones in each), arms (3 bones in each), legs (5 bones in each), shoulder blades (2 bones), and pelvis (2 bones). Figure 2.1 illustrates the human skeleton.

Development of Bones and Teeth

During growth, bones increase in size but maintain the same shape. For example, the jawbone of an adult is nearly twice the size of a child's, but its shape is the same. This change in jawbone size allows room for permanent teeth to replace baby teeth. Baby teeth begin to develop during the first year of life and usually are all in place by age 3. Baby teeth total 20: 10 in the upper jaw and 10 in the lower jaw. Teeth grow in different shapes and sizes because of their different functions. The front teeth (incisors) are for biting; the side teeth (canines) are for tearing; and the back teeth (premolars and molars) are for chewing and grinding. As the individual grows, baby teeth are replaced by the larger, stronger, and more numerous permanent teeth needed for adult eating needs.

Starting at approximately age 6, the baby teeth begin to fall out and permanent teeth begin to grow in. The teeth farthest back in the jaw (the third molars, or the "wisdom teeth") are the last permanent teeth to grow in. At about age 25, most people have a full set of 32 permanent teeth (16 in the lower jaw and 16 in the upper jaw).

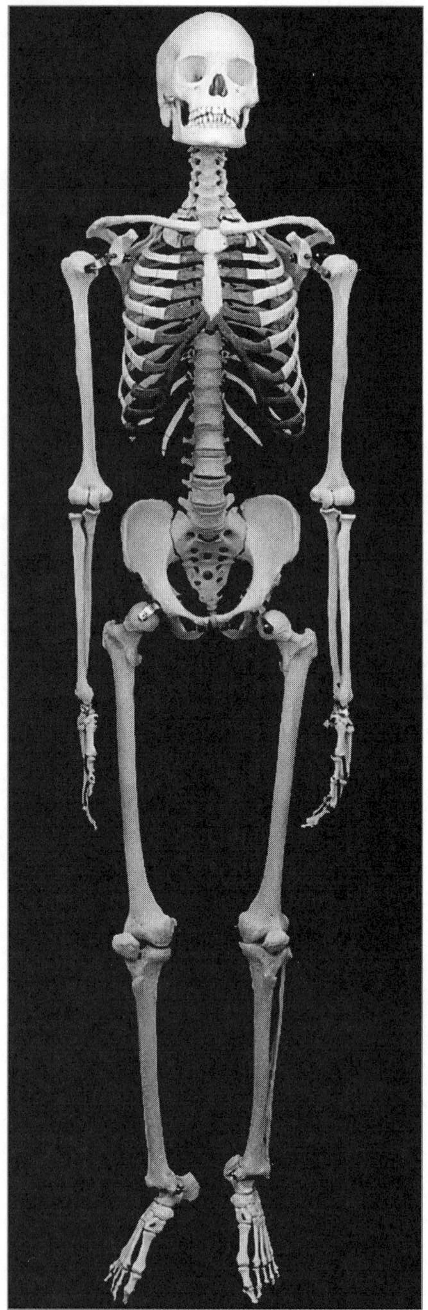

Figure 2.1 **The human skeleton.**

The most rapid periods of skeletal growth and development are during infancy, and secondarily during puberty (the beginning of sexual maturation). Until about age 11, boys and girls grow at generally the same rate. Between ages 11 and 13, girls are often taller than boys. By age 14 or 15, the reverse is generally true. This is because puberty, which is accompanied by a growth spurt, generally occurs about 2 years earlier in girls than in boys.[1] By about age 20, the skeleton reaches its final size. After that, the emphasis switches from growth of bones to their maintenance.

A common skeletal disorder in children is scoliosis, a lateral curvature of the spine. Structural deformities that appear in childhood often can be detected by a physical examination. Some schools provide screening examinations to help detect early cases of scoliosis.

Skeletal Injuries

Dislocating a bone from its joint or breaking a bone (fracture) are common injuries in active children and adults. If properly treated, the injuries generally heal with no permanent damage. As the body ages, however, bone mass begins to decrease, making them weaker and thus more prone to fracture and more difficult to heal. This happens in both sexes but is more common in women after menopause and is associated with the disease called osteoporosis.

Calcium is an essential nutrient needed for strong and healthy bones and teeth. Calcium is found in dairy products, dark green vegetables, and some fish. Bones also can be strengthened through strength-training exercises. Sufficient calcium and regular exercise throughout life, particularly in childhood, adolescence, and young adulthood, are needed to maintain strong bones and help prevent osteoporosis later in life.[2]

Problems with Teeth

Dental caries (cavities) caused by tooth decay, constitute the most frequent dental problem in children. If left untreated they can result in tooth loss. Because teeth play an important role in digestion as well as in speech and overall physical appearance, proper dental care is essential to promote strong and healthy teeth at every life stage.

Dental care may include brushing teeth at least twice a day (preferably after each meal); flossing daily to remove plaque; avoiding sweet and sticky candies; eating a balanced diet with adequate amounts of vitamins C and D; drinking water and using toothpaste with fluoride; and going for regular preventive dental examinations for early detection and treatment of caries and other dental problems.

The Muscular System

Whereas the skeletal system provides the structural framework, the muscular system (shown in Figure 2.2) actually moves the body's parts. Muscle tissue consists of fibers that have the ability to contract. The approximately 650 muscles in the body are divided into three groups:

1. Skeletal, or voluntary, muscles.
2. Smooth, or involuntary, muscles.
3. Cardiac, or heart, muscles.

Skeletal Muscles

The skeletal muscles are attached to the bones. These muscles hold the bones in place, give the body its shape and, most important—together with ligaments and tendons (elastic connective tissue) —move the bones in the face, neck, torso, arms, legs, hands, and feet. Skeletal muscles also are called **voluntary muscles** because they can be controlled consciously. They enable us to run, smile, ride a bicycle, play baseball,

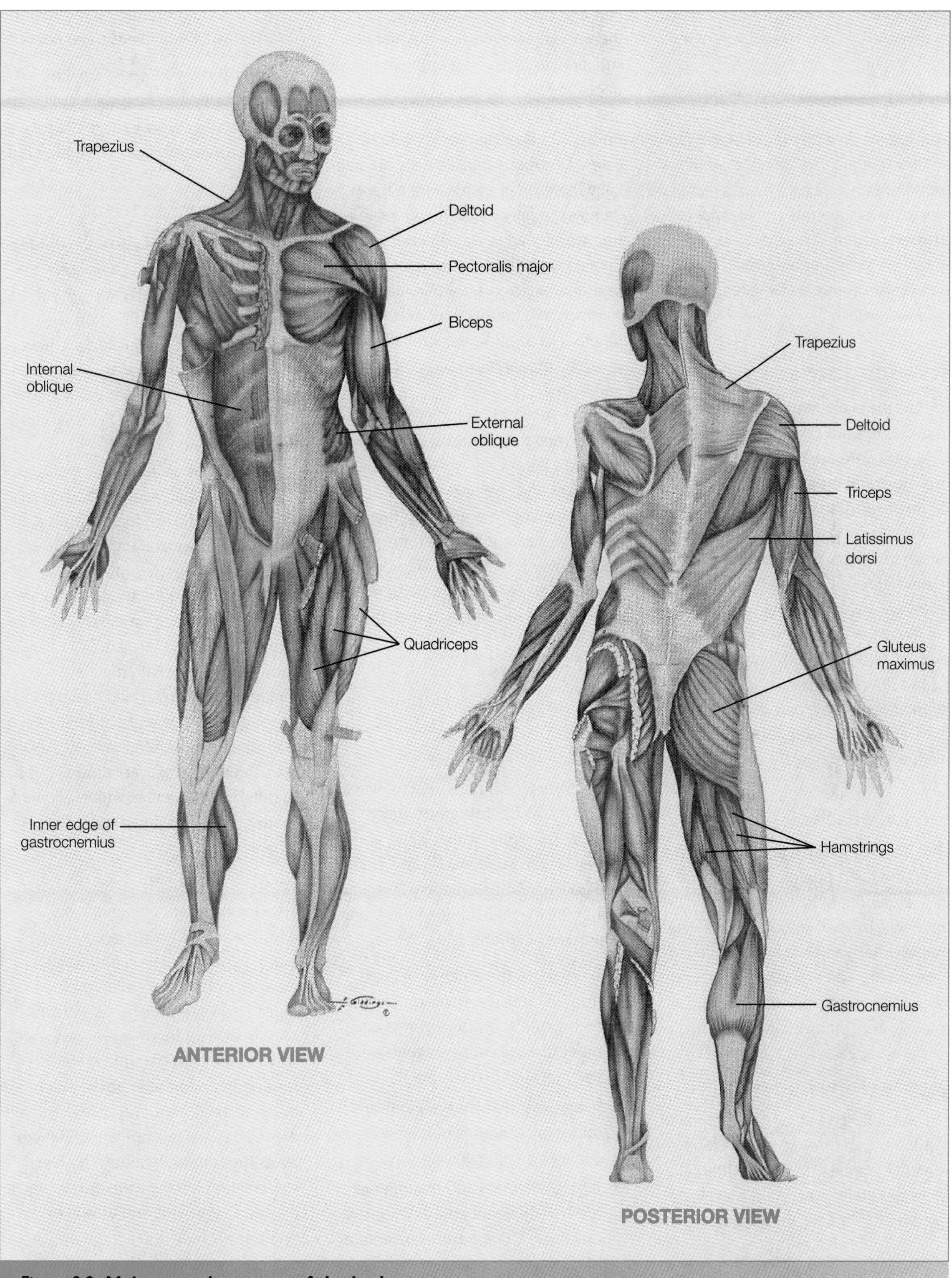

Figure 2.2 **Major muscle groups of the body.**

write letters, and do any other activity that requires some type of voluntary movement.

At least two muscles working in opposition are needed for any skeletal movement. To either bend or straighten a limb, one muscle contracts while another muscle relaxes. Muscles that bend the joints in the arms and legs are called **flexors**, and muscles that straighten the joints are called **extensors**. Thus, when the flexors contract, the extensors relax, and vice versa.

Smooth Muscles

Unlike the skeletal muscles, the smooth muscles are not consciously controlled and, therefore, are referred to as the **involuntary muscles**. They are found in the walls of many of the body's internal organs such as the stomach, lungs, intestines, and blood vessels. By contracting and relaxing, the smooth muscles—which are regulated automatically by the autonomic nervous system—control digestion, breathing, and blood flow. Although smooth muscles work more slowly than skeletal muscles, they are able to work for longer periods without tiring.

Heart Muscles

The heart or cardiac muscles, which keep the heart pumping nonstop during a person's entire lifetime, combine the characteristics of smooth and skeletal muscles. Like smooth muscles, they are involuntary and work constantly. Like skeletal muscles, they can respond quickly and change pace when needed.

Muscle Development

As muscular growth and development (along with neurological development) steadily progress in early childhood, so does the ability to control bowel and bladder movement, tie shoelaces, comb hair, and catch a ball. Maturation of the eye muscles at age 6 is generally sufficient to give children the apparatus necessary for reading.[3] Manipulative and coordination skills develop rapidly during a child's elementary school years. At puberty, muscle cells dramatically increase in males, with a lesser increase in fatty cells. The opposite is true with females. This difference, attributable primarily to a surge in hormone production (testosterone in males and estrogen in females), accounts for the differences in muscular strength and physical appearances between men and women.

Once growth is complete—sometime during the early 20s—the body begins to deteriorate slowly. Muscles lose mass and strength. As the muscles age, the person becomes less flexible and more susceptible to strains, pulls, and cramps. Regular and vigorous physical activity can slow the loss of muscle mass and strength over the lifespan.

The Integumentary System

The skin, hair, and nails are collectively referred to as the **integumentary system**. The skin—which is the body's largest organ, weighing about 7 pounds and covering approximately 20 square feet in the average adult—has several important functions:

1. It separates the inner body parts from the outside environment, protecting the body from germs and other disease-causing agents, while keeping vital fluids inside.
2. It excretes dissolved mineral salts and small amounts of body wastes (urea and lactic acid).
3. It helps regulate and maintain an ideal body temperature of approximately 98.6 degrees by constricting blood vessels and pores to reduce heat loss when the body needs to be warmed and producing perspiration when the body needs to be cooled.
4. It converts ultraviolet rays from the sun to vitamin D.
5. It contains sensory receptors for pressure, touch, pain, heat, and cold.

Outer Layer of Skin

Skin cells at the surface of the **epidermis** are dead (because this layer contains no blood vessels) and get rubbed off by movement and friction, as when washing. Just below the surface, however, new cells are produced continuously to replace the millions of skin cells that are shed daily. Each skin cell is replaced once a month.

The epidermis has small openings called pores that lead to glands (see discussion of the endocrine system on page 41). **Melanin**, a dark brown substance that helps determine a person's skin color, is also found in the epidermis. Melanin is responsible for freckles and helps protect the skin from the sun's rays. People with high levels of melanin have darker skin and the accompanying greater natural protection against harmful ultraviolet (UV) rays. Melanin levels vary among people of different ethnicities, which accounts for the different skin colors.

Inner Layer of Skin

The **dermis**, just beneath the epidermis, contains sweat glands (for temperature regulation and waste removal), oil glands (to help keep skin moist and waterproof), hair follicles, muscle fibers, blood vessels, and sensory nerve endings (which relay information to the brain about touch, pressure, pain, heat, and cold). Beneath the dermis is a layer of tissue that connects the skin to the body. This layer stores fat, which insulates and protects the internal organs and also helps retain body heat.

Other Skin Structures

Both hair and nails are outgrowths of the skin. They are similar, too, in that both are produced by special skin cells that are dead when they reach the surface. This is why cutting hair and trimming nails do not hurt. Nails protect the sensitive surfaces of the fingertips and toes. Hair, which grows out of follicles in the dermis, also functions as a protector. For example, eyelashes protect the eyes, and hair on the head protects against overexposure to ultraviolet rays in the summer and against loss of body heat in the winter.

Most people have approximately 100,000 hairs on their head. These hairs grow about half an inch per month until they reach their natural length, which varies among individuals. Hairs that stop growing fall out and are replaced by new growing hairs. This is why people often find several loose hairs on their brush or clothing every day.

Hair grows in three basic shapes—straight, wavy, and curly—and several colors—black, brown, blonde, or red, and shades thereof. Both shape and color are determined by heredity. Because melanin in hair decreases in many people as they grow older, their hair begins to gray and eventually turns white.[4]

Skin Care

Proper care of the skin, hair, and nails enhances a person's physical appearance and contributes to overall personal health. Skin care requires washing with soap daily and limiting exposure to harmful UV rays. Nail care includes cutting and cleaning fingernails and toenails as needed. Healthy hair is maintained by daily combing or brushing, and shampooing at least once a week. Also important to healthy skin, hair, and nails are sleep, exercise, and a balanced diet.

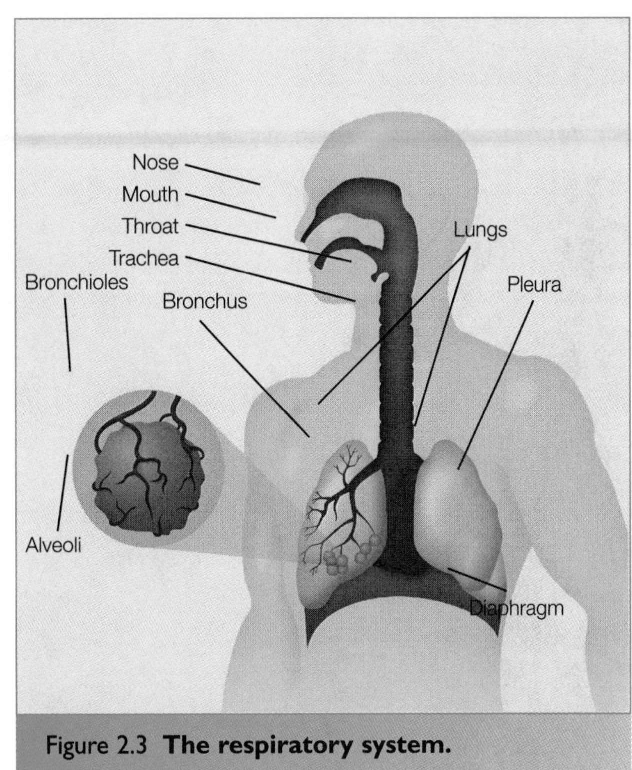

Figure 2.3 **The respiratory system.**

The Respiratory System

The respiratory system, working in conjunction with the heart, supplies body cells with oxygen and disposes of the waste product carbon dioxide. The cells require oxygen to convert food into the energy needed to sustain life. This process, called cell **metabolism**, creates carbon dioxide as a waste product.

The major organs of the respiratory system are the nose and mouth, throat, **trachea** (windpipe), bronchial tubes, lungs, and tiny air sacs called alveoli. The **diaphragm** (a muscle at the bottom of the chest cavity) and the rib cage also play an essential role in **respiration**. When the diaphragm contracts, the rib cage expands, enlarging the chest cavity and thereby pulling air into the lungs (inhalation). When the diaphragm relaxes, the chest cavity shrinks, forcing air out of the lungs (exhalation).

During inhalation through the nose or mouth, oxygen travels into the windpipe and then into the **bronchus** of each lung. In the lungs, the oxygen travels into smaller tubes, the **bronchioles**, which lead to the **alveoli** (tiny air sacs). These air sacs are surrounded by small blood vessels—and here the oxygen crosses the cell membranes from the alveoli into the blood. Thus, inhaling brings oxygen into the bloodstream via the alveoli, after which it is carried to all the cells in the body. Similarly, carbon dioxide, taken from the cells, leaves the bloodstream via the alveoli and is expelled from the lungs by exhaling. The parts of the respiratory system are illustrated in Figure 2.3.

The body adjusts the volume and flow of air into the lungs according to its oxygen needs. For example, exercise increases the need for oxygen, so the amount of air inhaled with each breath during exercise may be as much as four times greater than when the body is at

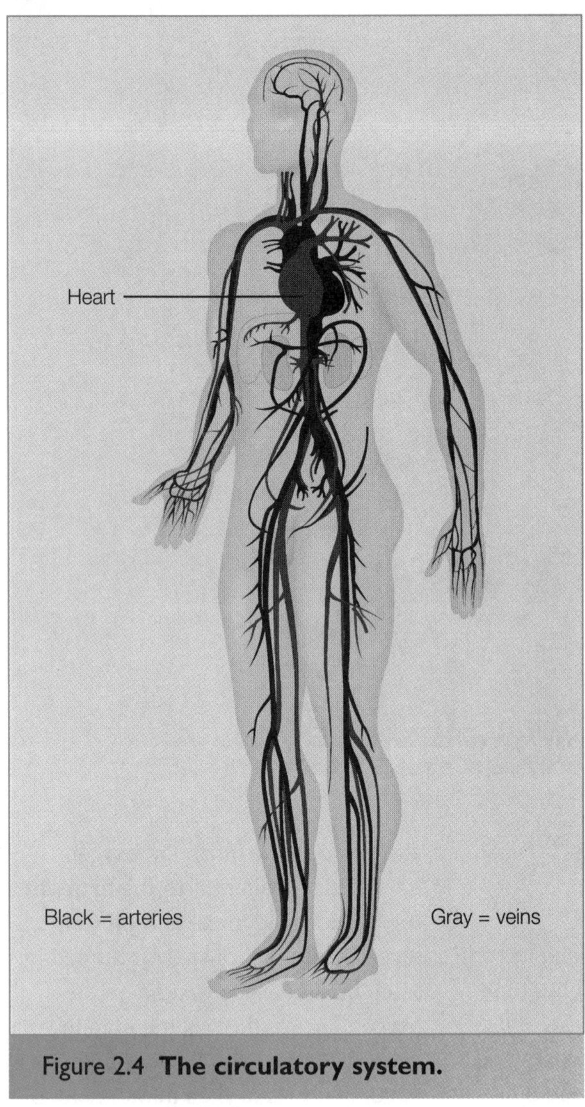

Figure 2.4 **The circulatory system.**

rest. Breathing rates differ between children and adults. Children breathe approximately 15 times a minute, whereas adults breathe approximately 12 times a minute.[5] Respiration is vital for life. The body can survive without food or water for days, but death would occur without oxygen within a few minutes.

The body has a number of mechanisms that help protect the respiratory system and maintain proper functioning. For example, coughing and sneezing are reflexive or involuntary actions that help keep the respiratory passages clear by expelling foreign particles. Voluntary ways to protect the body include practicing hygiene to impede the spread of germs, not smoking, and controlling air pollution (see Chapter 13). In addition, respiratory functioning can be enhanced by cardiorespiratory endurance conditioning, which enables the body to take in, transport, and use oxygen in the most efficient way possible.[6] Examples of activities that develop cardiorespiratory endurance are swimming, jogging, and aerobic dancing.

The Circulatory System

The circulatory system, which consists of the heart, the blood vessels, and the blood, is responsible for continuously moving blood through every part of the body. It delivers fresh oxygen-rich blood to all the cells in the body and takes away carbon dioxide and other waste products to be disposed of by the lungs and kidneys. The blood flowing through the circulatory system also carries regulating hormones and chemicals, as well as a network of cells that defend the body against invading pathogens. Figure 2.4 shows the heart and major arteries and veins in the circulatory system.

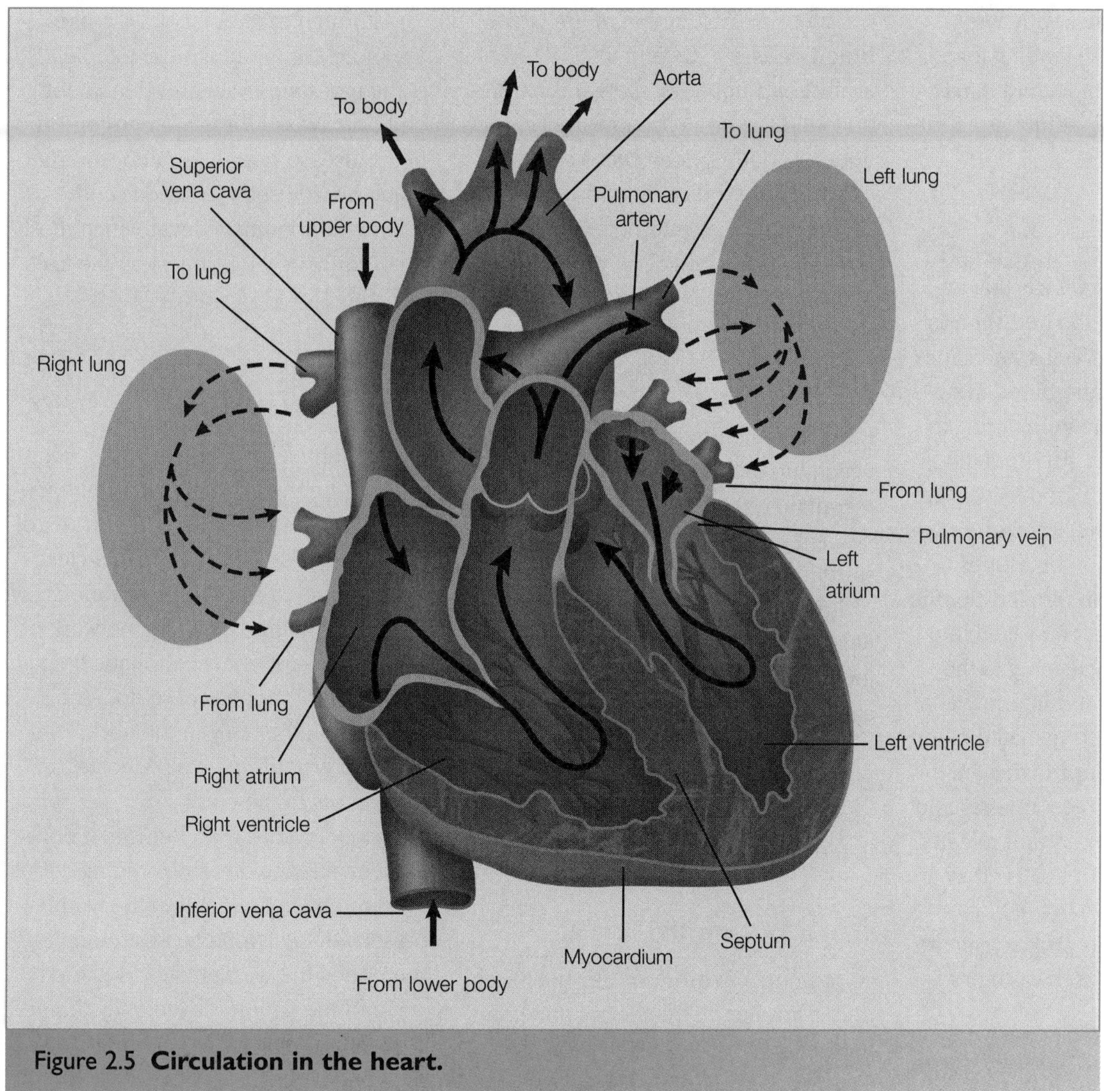

Figure 2.5 **Circulation in the heart.**

The Heart

The heart (illustrated in Figure 2.5) is fist-sized and has two pumps. Each pump is divided into two chambers: an upper atrium (**auricle**) and lower ventricle. The auricles receive blood from the veins and pass it to the ventricles through a valve. From the ventricles, blood is forcefully pumped into the arteries. The two right-side compartments form the right chamber of the heart, and the two left-side compartments form the left chamber of the heart.

The right and left chambers are separated by a wall of muscle called the **septum**. The right side of the heart receives deoxygenated blood from the veins and pumps it to the lungs for carbon dioxide disposal and oxygen replenishment. The oxygenated blood is then passed to the left side of the heart, which pumps it into the main artery, called the **aorta**, leading to the network of arteries throughout the body. When the blood returns through the veins, the cycle begins again. The heart muscle receives oxygen-rich blood to sustain its own functioning from the coronary arteries, which feed into branches leading to the wall of the heart, the **myocardium**.

The heart pumps in a rhythmic cycle, the heartbeat, of muscular contractions. At rest, the heart beats approximately 70 times a minute, pumping about 5 quarts of blood. As activity increases, so does the heart rate and amount of blood pumped. Measurement of the force of circulating blood against the wall of the blood vessels is called **blood pressure**. As the heart contracts and relaxes, the pressure changes. Hence, blood pressure is expressed as a fraction (values are in millimeters of mercury) of **systolic pressure** during contraction over **diastolic pressure** during relaxation.

Blood pressure varies with age. An average blood pressure reading for a baby may be 70/50. For a child it may be 100/60. For a young adult it is about 120/80.

Blood Vessels

The network of blood vessels that extends to every part of the body consists of three types: arteries, veins, and capillaries. The **arteries** carry blood away from the heart, and the **veins** bring it back. Arteries range in size from the aorta (through which blood leaves the heart), the largest, to the **arterioles**, the smallest in a succession of arteries branching off the aorta. Similarly, for the return journey, smaller veins feed into larger ones, ultimately leading to the main veins (superior and inferior vena cava), which carry deoxygenated blood back into the heart. **Capillaries** are tiny blood vessels that connect arteries and veins. These play an important role in the circulatory system, because they are the points of exchange in the bloodstream where nutrients and oxygen are delivered to the cells and waste products are picked up.

Blood

Blood, the fluid component of the circulatory system, constitutes approximately 7 percent of the total body weight. For example, a child weighing 75 pounds has about 2.5 quarts of blood, whereas an adult weighing 150 pounds has about 5 quarts.

Blood consists of red cells (41 percent), white cells (1 percent), platelets (3 percent), and a liquid called plasma (55 percent), made up mostly of water. The **red blood cells** contain the protein, **hemoglobin**, which carries oxygen from the lungs throughout the body and also gives blood its red color. Red blood cells are produced in the bone marrow and have a lifespan of about 120 days.

The primary function of the **white blood cells** is to defend the body against harmful foreign organisms. Produced in the bone marrow, the lymph nodes, and the spleen, these cells seek out, engulf, and destroy **pathogens** (bacteria, viruses, and other agents of disease) in the body. The **platelets** maintain the walls of the blood vessels. When a vessel is injured, they plug up holes by forming insoluble clots, thereby curtailing the loss of blood. **Plasma** is the liquid component in which the blood cells are suspended. It contains 90 percent water and 10 percent proteins, minerals, and other substances.

Information gathered by measuring types and quantities of substances found in the blood can help detect disease and provide clues about the condition of the body's various systems. Hence, blood tests are an important part of preventive health care at every stage in the life cycle.

Cardiovascular Health

To promote **cardiovascular** health, an understanding of the factors that contribute to cardiovascular disease is essential. Some risk factors—heredity, race (African Americans are at greater risk than whites), gender (men are at greater risk than women), and age (risk increases with age for both sexes)—are uncontrollable.[7] Other risk factors—high-fat diet, inactivity, smoking, high blood pressure (consistent readings of over 140/90), and obesity—are controllable. Adopting healthy lifestyle habits when one is young—such as a low-fat diet, regular exercise, weight management, no smoking, and skills to cope with stress—can help reduce the risk for developing cardiovascular disease later in life.

Although cardiovascular diseases are more common in older people, some types are more prevalent among children. Two of these are **congenital** heart disease, present at birth, and rheumatic heart disease, a serious consequence of rheumatic fever, which most commonly develops between the ages of 5 and 15.[8]

The Lymphatic System

The lymphatic system (shown in Figure 2.6) has been called the "other circulatory system."[9] It consists of a network of artery-like vessels that contain a clear, watery fluid called lymph. At various points along this branching network of vessels are clusters of lymphatic tissue called lymph nodes. These nodes are concentrated mainly in the neck, armpits, and groin, but are also located in other parts of the body.

Lymph comes from fluids that ooze from capillaries, thereby draining debris from the bloodstream into the lymph vessels. As the lymph passes through the nodes, the waste matter is filtered out and the lymph is eventually drained back into the bloodstream through a network of vessels that lead to the veins in the neck. The lymphatic system does not have a pump. The pressure from the adjacent circulatory system and muscular movements drive the lymph through the system, and valves ensure a one-way flow.

The lymph nodes play a crucial role in fighting infection. White blood cells gather in the nodes and do battle with invading pathogens. Hence, the lymph nodes swell during illness, and they can be felt in the neck, armpits, and groin. When the illness is gone, the nodes return to their normal size.

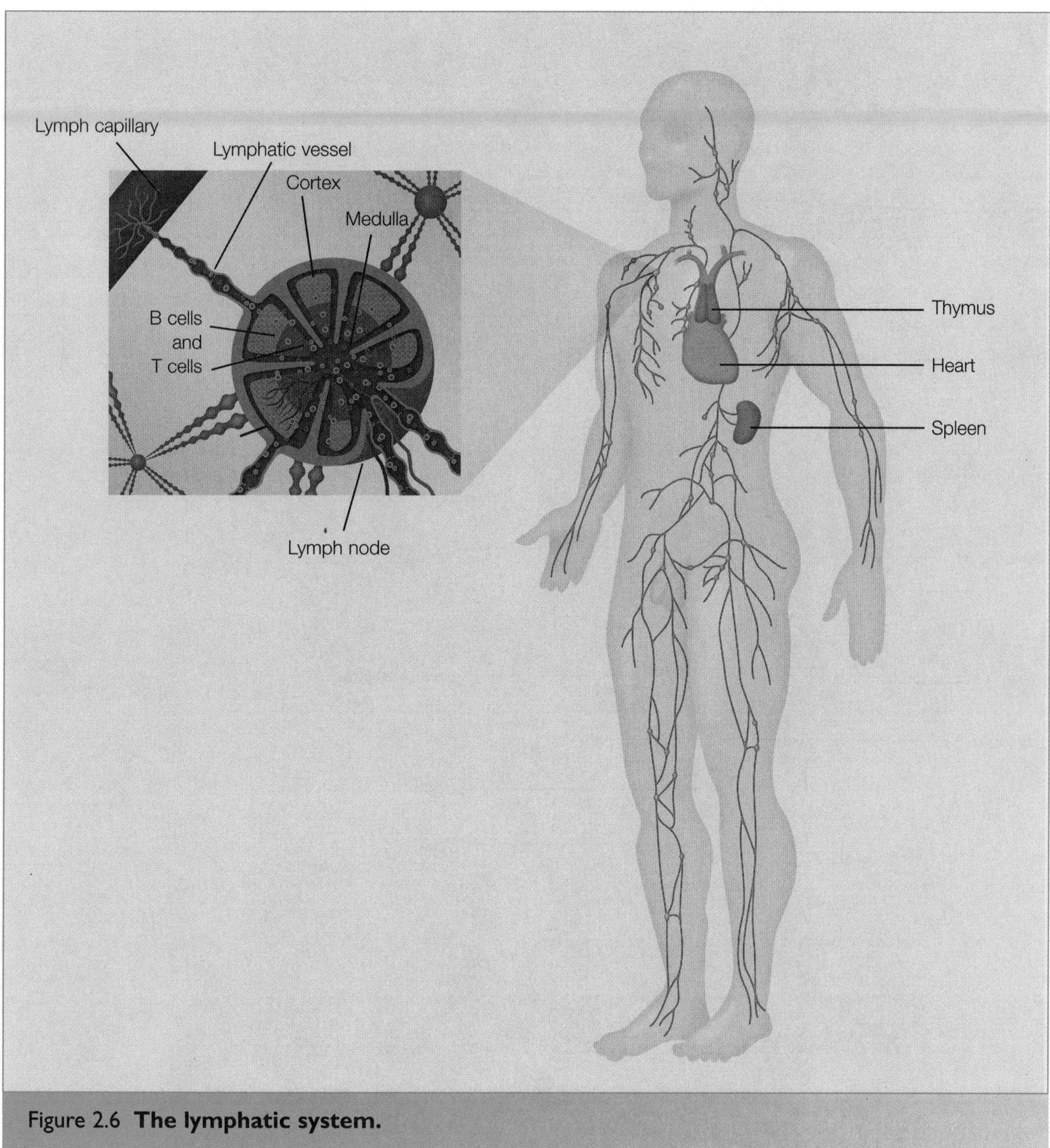

Figure 2.6 **The lymphatic system.**

Immune Reactions

The body's natural defense against invading pathogens is produced by a collaborative effort between the blood and the lymphatic system. Together they create a complex network of cells that form the **immune system.** The white blood cells, produced primarily in the bone marrow and the spleen, are the primary elements in immune reactions. Several types of white blood cells play a role in trying to neutralize foreign invaders. They include the macrophage, T4 cells, T8 cells, and B cells. (See Chapter 5 for more detail.)

During infancy and childhood, the lymphatic system plays an essential part in the development of immunity—the body's natural defense against infection—through its role in the production of antibodies. By adolescence, the build-up of antibodies is substantial enough to make the body much more resistant to infection than it was during early childhood.

The Digestive System

The digestive system is responsible for breaking down food into substances that can be absorbed into the bloodstream and distributed to the body's cells as fuel for life-sustaining functions. The system is mainly a hollow muscular tube, the **alimentary canal**, which begins at the mouth and, following a convoluted path, ends at the anus. The canal, if extended, would measure several times the body's height. It is divided into several specialized

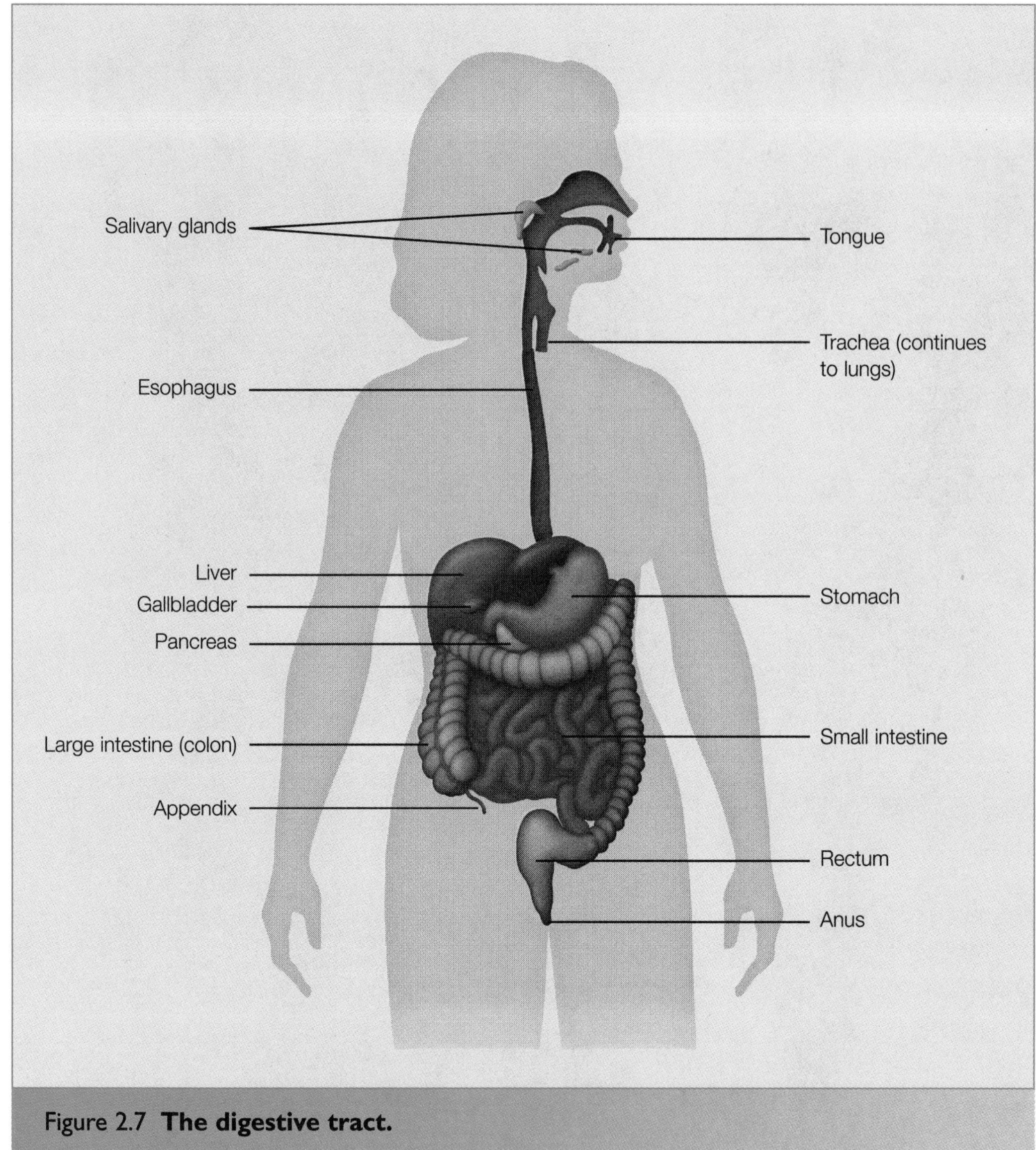

Figure 2.7 **The digestive tract.**

sections differing in shape, size, and task to be performed. The parts of the canal are the mouth, **esophagus**, stomach, small intestine, large intestine, **rectum**, and **anus**. Other components of the system are the teeth, salivary glands, pancreas, **liver**, and **gallbladder**. Hence food enters through the mouth, usable nutrients are processed and absorbed along the canal, and solid wastes are expelled through the anus. The digestive system is illustrated in Figure 2.7.

Digestion of Food

The process of digestion actually begins in the head.[10] The thought, sight, or smell of food may instigate the flow of saliva and other digestive juices in anticipation of food about to enter the system. After food enters through the mouth, the teeth cut, grind, and mash the food into manageable pieces, which then pass down the esophagus into the stomach. While the food is still in the mouth, **saliva**, which contains the enzyme **amylase**, begins breaking down starches into sugars, as well as moistening dry food about to be swallowed. The body produces approximately a quart of saliva daily.

The Stomach

In the stomach, **peristalsis**, involuntary rhythmic muscular contractions, mixes the food with acid and enzymes to begin the process of digesting protein. After approximately 1 to 2 hours of mashing and churning, the food in the stomach turns into a pasty substance called **chyme**. The stomach—which can expand to accommodate about two quarts of food—processes an average of about 1,100 pounds of food a year.[11]

The Small Intestine

From the stomach, chyme is moved at intervals into the **duodenum**, the first section of the small intestine, where **bile** (made in the liver and stored in the gallbladder) aids in the breakdown of fat and pancreatic juices assist in digesting proteins and carbohydrates.

The small intestine is the place where nutrients are absorbed into the body's circulatory system. The sites of absorption are the fingerlike projections from the intestinal wall called **villi**. The villi, in turn, are covered with even smaller fingerlike projections, called microvilli, thereby greatly enlarging the surface area for absorption.

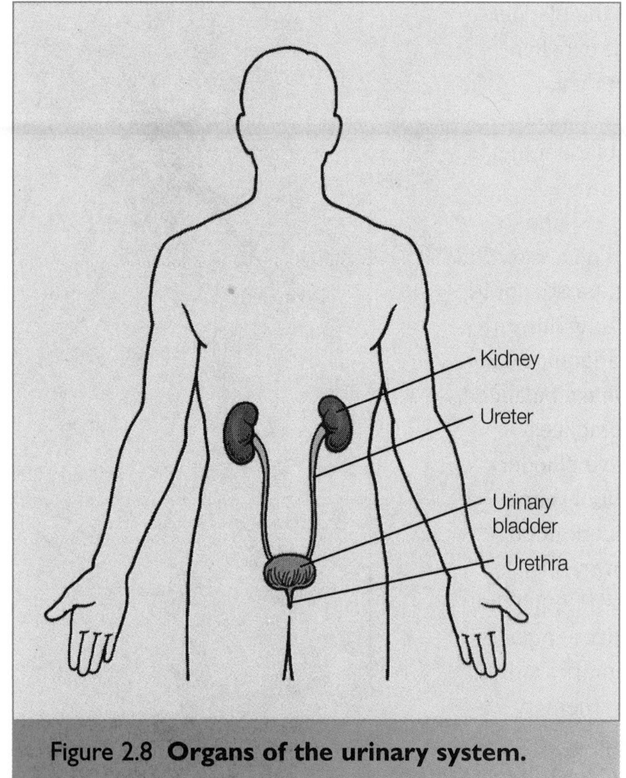

Figure 2.8 **Organs of the urinary system.**

The Large Intestine

Undigested substances collect in the large intestine, where water is squeezed out and peristaltic contractions move the solid waste through the **colon**. In addition to the water, some remaining minerals are absorbed through the colon before the solid waste is excreted through the rectum and anus.

Development of the Digestive System

The most rapid growth and development of the digestive system occur during the preschool years. Maturation of the sphincter muscles in the anus and bladder occurs around age 2, enabling a child to begin bowel and bladder control, which is usually mastered completely during the preschool years. Growth is gradual during middle childhood and as with most other body systems accelerates again during adolescence.

Childhood disturbances of the digestive system usually are accompanied by symptoms and signs. Common symptoms of individuals with digestive disturbances include nausea, pain, fever, headache, and irritability. Typical signs that can be observed in children with digestive disturbances include restlessness, flushed skin, facial grimaces, and red, watery eyes.[12] Symptoms and signs may reflect either a mild temporary condition or a more serious condition and, therefore, should be checked by a health-care professional.

Maintaining a well-balanced diet that includes fiber, along with good eating habits that begin at an early age, promote a healthy digestive system. Sound nutrition (discussed in Chapter 3) reduces the risk of disorders of the digestive tract later in life.

The Urinary System

Whereas the digestive system disposes of solid waste, the urinary system disposes of waste from the body's blood. The urinary system consists of the bladder, the urethra, two kidneys, and two ureters (shown in Figure 2.8). The kidneys filter wastes, unwanted minerals, and excess water from the bloodstream and form a yellowish fluid called urine. Urine contains more than 90 percent water. Urea, salts, phosphoric acid, and other wastes account for the remainder.

Blood enters the **kidneys** through the renal arteries and leaves through the renal veins. The blood that passes through the kidneys (approximately 400 gallons a day), after being filtered, is reabsorbed into the bloodstream. The filtered waste passes out of the body as urine. The urine produced by the kidneys passes down through the **ureters**, one from each kidney, to the bladder. There it is stored until it is expelled from the body via the **urethra**.

When approximately 6 ounces of urine accumulate in the bladder, the person feels the urge to urinate, although the bladder can expand to hold twice that amount, if necessary. On the average, an individual passes about 1½ quarts of urine daily. A healthy urinary system requires an adequate daily intake of fluids, a nutritionally balanced diet, and good hygienic practices.

Children usually achieve bladder control during the preschool years. A common condition in childhood in both boys and girls, however, is **enuresis**, or bed-wetting. Although the majority of children are dry at night by age 4 or 5, a significant number are still bed-wetting during the elementary school years. Children typically gain control as they grow older, and it is rarely a problem past puberty.

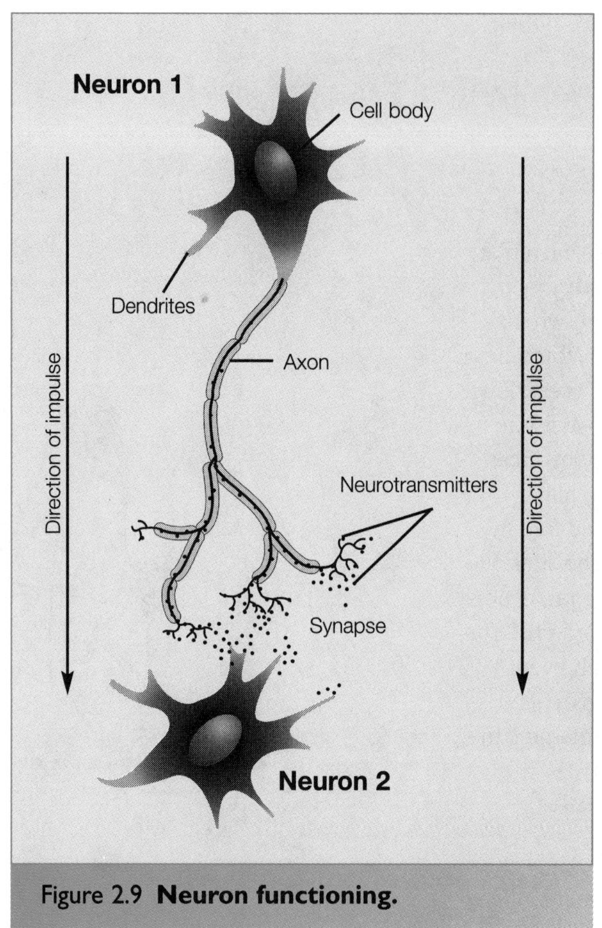

Figure 2.9 **Neuron functioning.**

The Nervous System

The nervous system is the body's communication network. It processes thoughts, stores information and coordinates all of the body's actions, both voluntary and involuntary. The **central nervous system** is made up of the brain and spinal cord. Peripheral nerves branch off from both.

Nerve Functioning

The basic units of the nervous system are nerve cells called **neurons**. Impulses are transmitted, with the assistance of **neurotransmitters**, from one nerve cell to another at a gap between the **axon** of one cell and the dendrite of another. This gap or space is called a **synapse**. Billions of neurons form a communication network that extends to all parts of the body. Sensory neurons pick up information about the internal and external environment and carry it to the interneurons in the spinal cord and brain, which, in turn, send responses to the motor neurons, prompting action. Messages can travel along these neurons at a speed of about 360 feet per second, enabling quick responses.[13] Collections of neurons or nerve fibers form the nerves of the body. Figure 2.9 depicts neuron functioning.

The Brain and Spinal Cord

The brain, weighing around 3 pounds and located inside the upper part of the skull, is a complex organ containing approximately 10 billion nerve cells. These cells require a great supply of oxygenated blood and are responsible for thought, memory, feeling, movement, and the control of vital body functions. Each specialized function is controlled by a distinct area of the brain, depicted in Figure 2.10.

The **cerebrum**, the largest part of the brain, is divided into a right and left hemisphere, each with a surface that resembles a walnut shell. The cerebrum controls intellectual abilities (reasoning, thinking, remembering, writing, and speaking), muscular movement, sensory perception (smell, sight, taste, touch, and sound), and the expression of emotion. Because of nerve fiber crossovers, messages from the right hemisphere control the left side of the body and messages from the left hemisphere control the right side of the body. Most people are right-handed because the left hemisphere usually is more dominant.

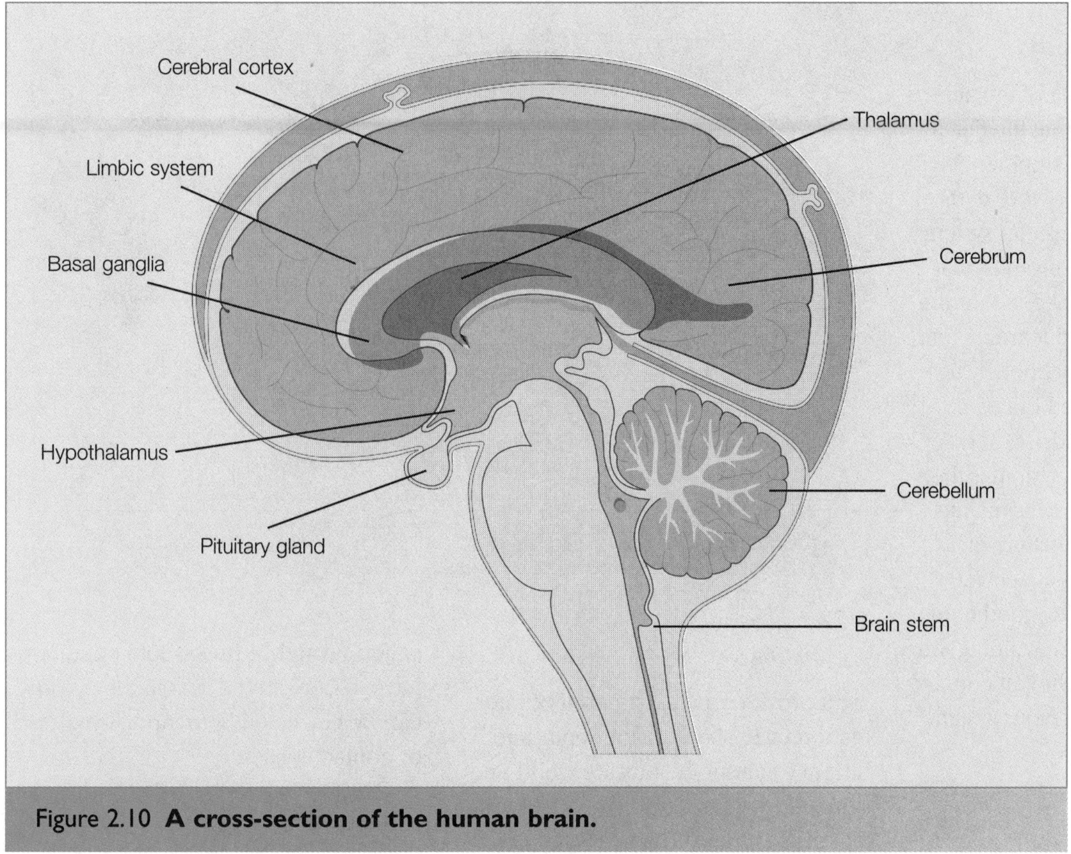

Figure 2.10 **A cross-section of the human brain.**

The **cerebellum**, located behind and beneath the cerebrum, coordinates the fine-motor control over muscular movement and balance. Activities such as playing the piano, walking, running, riding a bicycle, and picking up an object would be impossible without assistance from the cerebellum. Once learned, these activities are done automatically without really thinking.

The brain stem is located at approximately the center of the skull, connecting the cerebrum to the spinal cord. It is divided into three parts: the midbrain, the pons, and the medulla. The **midbrain** is involved in regulating sleep and wakefulness and controls eye movement and pupil size. The **pons**, a bundle of nerve fibers that link the spinal cord to the brain, also plays a role in eye movement, as well as the regulation of breathing. The **medulla**, located just above the spinal cord, controls vital functions such as breathing, heart rate, blood pressure, and swallowing.

The spinal cord, running through the protective vertebral column, is about 18 inches in length and about 2 ounces in weight. The spinal cord connects the brain and carries information to all the parts of the body.

Peripheral Nerves

The **peripheral nerves** consist of 31 pairs of spinal nerves (which branch off from the spinal cord) and 12 pairs of cranial nerves (which emerge directly from the brain). Each pair controls a specific part of the body. Peripheral nerves that control voluntary actions form the **somatic nervous system**. These nerves control all voluntary movement and activity. They are also responsible for sensations such as pain, pressure, and temperature.

Peripheral nerves that control involuntary responses (such as breathing, heartbeat, and digestion) form the **autonomic nervous system**, which consists of two parts: the sympathetic and the parasympathetic. **Sympathetic nerve impulses** adjust body functions—heart rate and breathing rate are increased, pupils dilate, adrenal glands secrete hormones, digestion is inhibited, and more glucose is released into the bloodstream—when the body is under stress, excited, or engaged in strenuous physical activity. The **parasympathetic nerve impulses** reverse the effects of the sympathetic impulses after the stress or excitement is over, bringing body functions back to normal and thus maintaining homeostasis. The interplay between these two components of the autonomic nervous system enables the body to adapt to a variety of situations and circumstances.

Development of the Nervous System

Growth and development of the nervous system is rapid during the first 5 years of life. Its early development facilitates the development of other parts of the body, such as the muscular system. This sets the stage for neuromuscular coordination and skills needed for the activities, challenges, and learning that children experience in school. By age 10, the child has achieved the adult brain's weight of 3 pounds.

Because the nervous system is the control center of the body, its maintenance is essential for a lifetime of optimal health. Intellectual activity, leisure activity, safety rules, good nutrition, regular exercise, and avoiding the abuse of drugs and alcohol all contribute to keeping the nervous system healthy.

The Sensory System

The sensory system consists of the organs that provide the nervous system with information about the outside world. The five senses are seeing, hearing, tasting, smelling, and touching. The organs that collect sensory information are the eyes, ears, tongue, nose, and skin. These organs contain nerve endings called **receptors**, which collect information and send it to the brain. The brain interprets the information and immediately sends messages back to the body for appropriate action. For example, if a person touches something hot, the sensory receptors in the skin send the information to the spinal cord, which in turn sends a message to the arm to pull away (a reflex).

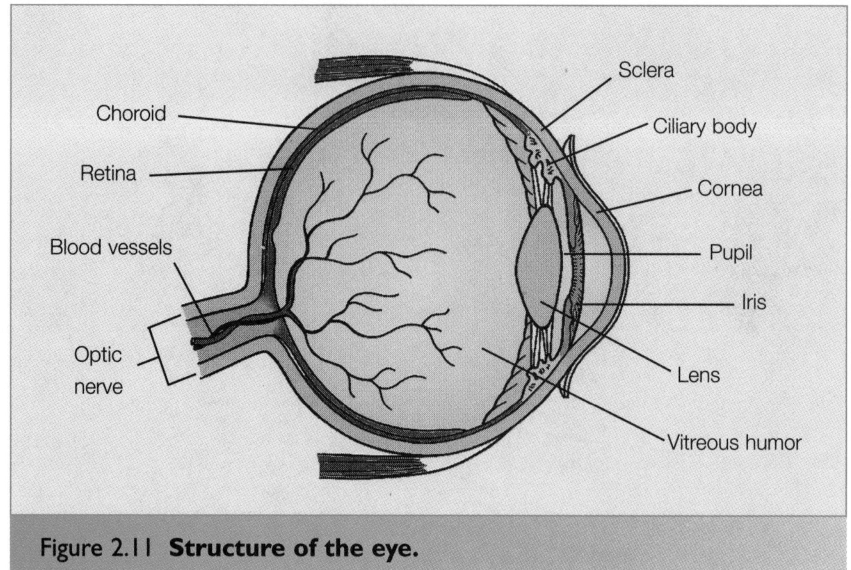

Figure 2.11 **Structure of the eye.**

Eyesight

Sight provides a great amount of information (size, shape, color, depth, and distance) about the outside world and is therefore considered the most important sense of all.[14] The eye is the organ responsible for sight. Major parts of the eye are the cornea, pupil, iris, lens, retina, and optic nerve. Light enters the eye through the **cornea**. Too much light will damage the eye, so the muscles of the **iris** regulate the amount of light that enters. For example, in dim light the iris relaxes and the **pupil** widens, allowing more light to come in. In bright light the iris contracts and the pupil becomes smaller to let in less light.

Inside the eye, light passes through the **lens**, which focuses light on the **retina**, which is lined with millions of light and color receptors. The **optic nerve** carries the information from the retina to the brain, which produces the images one sees. The extrinsic muscles of the eye allow for coordinated movement of both eyes, so that, along with head movements, scanning the environment in all directions is possible. Figure 2.11 shows the parts of the eye.

Some people are born with or develop conditions in which they cannot see distant objects clearly, called **nearsightedness**, or close objects clearly, called **farsightedness**. Both conditions have to do with the lens in the eye and can be corrected by wearing eyeglasses or contact lenses.

Proper eye care includes having regular vision check-ups (at 1- to 4-year intervals), wearing safety goggles when engaged in activities that may send foreign objects into the eye, avoiding staring at the sun, not touching or rubbing the eyes with unwashed hands, and having proper lighting when reading or doing other close work.

Hearing

The ear, depicted in Figure 2.12, is the organ that senses sound. The process of hearing begins at the outer ear, which picks up sound and directs it into the **auditory canal**. From there the sound reaches the **eardrum**, which vibrates when sound waves hit it. The hammer, anvil, and stirrup—three small bones, or **ossicles**, inside the ear—magnify vibrations from the eardrum. The cochlea picks up vibrations from the ossicles and, through auditory nerves, sends the information to the brain, which interprets the sound. The ear also contains

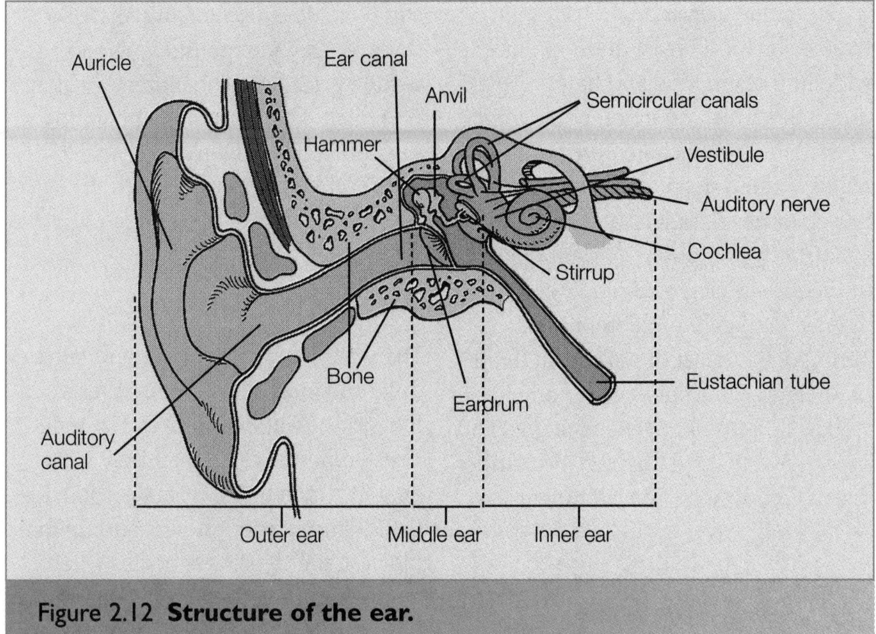

Figure 2.12 **Structure of the ear.**

three **semicircular canals**, which provide the brain with information needed to maintain a sense of **equilibrium** or balance.

Proper care of ears and hearing includes avoiding exposure to loud noises over 80 decibels, not inserting objects into the ear, and promptly seeking treatment for ear infection—a common condition in young children.

Taste

The tongue is the organ that senses taste. Thousands of **taste buds**, grouped in specific areas on the upper part of the tongue, are sensitive to four basic tastes:

1. sweet (front of tongue)
2. bitter (back of tongue)
3. sour (sides of tongue)
4. salt (sides of tongue)

When food is placed into the mouth, the taste buds send signals to the brain, which interprets the taste. The sense of taste is much stronger when it is combined with the sense of smell.

Smell

The organ that senses smell is the nose. When a person sniffs, gases in the air enter the nasal cavity and stimulate special smell receptors. These, in turn, send messages along the **olfactory nerves** to the brain, where the information is interpreted as a specific odor. The sense of smell can be important in detecting dangers such as spoiled food, fire, and poisonous gas.

Touch, Pressure, and Pain

The skin contains nerve endings that pick up sensory information (see "The Integumentary System," page 30). These sensory nerve endings relay information to the brain about touch, pressure, pain, heat, and cold. This information keeps the brain informed about external conditions, enabling it to respond accordingly. Although sensory receptors are all over the surface of the skin, some regions have a higher concentration of receptors and are, therefore, more sensitive. The lips and the fingertips are the most sensitive regions of the skin.

The Endocrine System

The endocrine system, working closely with the nervous system, controls and regulates many body activities. The chemical messengers of this system are called **hormones**, which are secreted directly into the bloodstream by the **endocrine glands**. Traveling through the bloodstream, hormones reach all the cells in the body but stimulate only those cells specifically targeted to respond. The endocrine glands include the hypothalamus—the link between, and a part of, both the nervous and the endocrine systems; pituitary, pineal, thymus, thyroid, parathyroid and adrenal glands; the pancreas; and the gonads (ovaries in females and testes in males).

The **hypothalamus**, a part of the brain located in the center of the head, is the control center of the endocrine system. The hypothalamus sends its messages via hormones directly to the pituitary gland, situated just beneath it, which, in turn, stimulates and regulates other glands to secrete their hormones.

The Pituitary Gland

The **pituitary gland** releases dozens of hormones that regulate the hormonal output of the other endocrine glands. Its anterior (front) lobe releases hormones that regulate the reproductive glands, affect overall growth and development, and regulate adrenal secretions. The hormones released by the posterior (back) lobe control urine output and water balance and affect the smooth muscles in the body.[15]

The Pineal, Thymus, and Thyroid Glands

The **pineal gland** is located in the brain and is involved in the control of the body's internal clock. This gland is influenced by light and is believed to affect sleep. The **thymus** promotes the development of antibodies in children but has no known function in adults.

The **thyroid gland** secretes hormones that regulate the body's metabolic rate, affect growth, and, together with hormones secreted by the parathyroid glands, maintain and control blood calcium levels.

The Adrenal Glands

The two **adrenal glands**, located on top of the kidneys, are each divided into inner and outer layers. The outer layer, called the cortex, secretes hormones involved in the metabolism of carbohydrates, proteins, and fats; hormones that maintain salt and fluid balance; and hormones responsible for the development of secondary sex characteristics. The inner layer, called the medulla, secretes epinephrine and norepinephrine—hormones that prepare the body for "flight or fight" during times of danger or stress (see Chapter 8).

The Pancreas

The **pancreas**, a large gland located near the stomach and opening into the small intestine, produces **insulin**, the hormone responsible for regulating the body's blood sugar level. Diabetes is the condition wherein the pancreas does not produce enough insulin to regulate the level of sugar in the blood (see Chapter 5).

The Ovaries and Testes

The **ovaries** (in females) and **testes** (in males) secrete hormones that promote growth and development of the reproductive organs, as well as secondary sex characteristics and overall physical growth. These hormones, stimulated by the pituitary gland, are responsible for the marked differences in appearance and development between males and females beginning at puberty and for the maturation of the reproductive system to the point at which conception and gestation become possible.

Secondary sex characteristics in females include breast development, widening of the hips, and hair growth under the arms and in the pubic area.

Secondary sex characteristics in males include deepening of the voice, muscular development, and growth of facial, body, and pubic hair. Although the sequence of growth and development is predictable, differences in timing of the onset of puberty and the physical growth spurt vary among individuals as a result of genetic factors and state of health. (See Chapter 7 for further discussion of sexual development.)

Other Glands and Their Functions

The endocrine system has a dynamic influence on the body at every stage in the life cycle. During childhood, and even more dramatically during adolescence, this system regulates body growth and development. Endocrine glands orchestrate the maternity cycle that gives birth to new life and, throughout life, they play essential roles in regulating the functioning of all body systems.

Other glands in the body, unlike endocrine glands, do not release substances directly into the bloodstream. Rather, they release their products into the digestive tract or to the outside of the body. These are called **exocrine glands**. They include gastric, salivary, sweat, tear, and mammary glands. Gastric and salivary glands aid digestion. Sweat glands cool the body, if it becomes overheated from physical exercise, emotional excitement, or stress, by releasing perspiration through openings onto the skin's surface. Tear glands keep the eyes moist and clean. Strong emotions or a foreign particle in the eye can stimulate a greater production of tears, which is what happens when a person cries.

Mammary glands, located in the breasts, do not develop in males. In females these glands become well developed when endocrine hormones stimulate development of female secondary sex characteristics. When a female gives birth, the mammary glands (stimulated by hormones) begin to produce milk to feed the baby.

The Reproductive System

The system in which males and females differ the most, in both structures and functions, is the reproductive system. These differences are precisely what enable a man and a woman to join together and produce a new and unique individual. The process begins when a male reproductive cell, the **sperm**, unites with a female reproductive cell, the **ovum**, or egg. In this union, called **fertilization**, each cell contributes half of the needed genetic material. Hence, a fertilized egg, a **zygote**, contains all the necessary instructions to begin the development of a new human being.

The Male System

The major organs of the male reproductive system, shown in Figure 2.13, are the scrotum, testicles, and penis. The **scrotum** is a muscular pouch that hangs between the legs and contains the two testicles. The **testicles**, or testes, are oval-shaped organs that begin to produce sperm at puberty. In addition to sperm, the testicles produce the male sex hormone **testosterone**. The **penis**, located in front of the testicles, is the organ that transports the sperm out of the male and into the female and also transports urine from the bladder to outside the body.

From the site of production in the testicles, millions of sperm travel through several tubular structures—the epididymis, vas deferens, and urethra—and are joined by a protective and nourishing fluid secreted by the **seminal vesicles**, **prostate gland**, and **Cowper's gland**, before they are finally discharged from the penis in ejaculation.

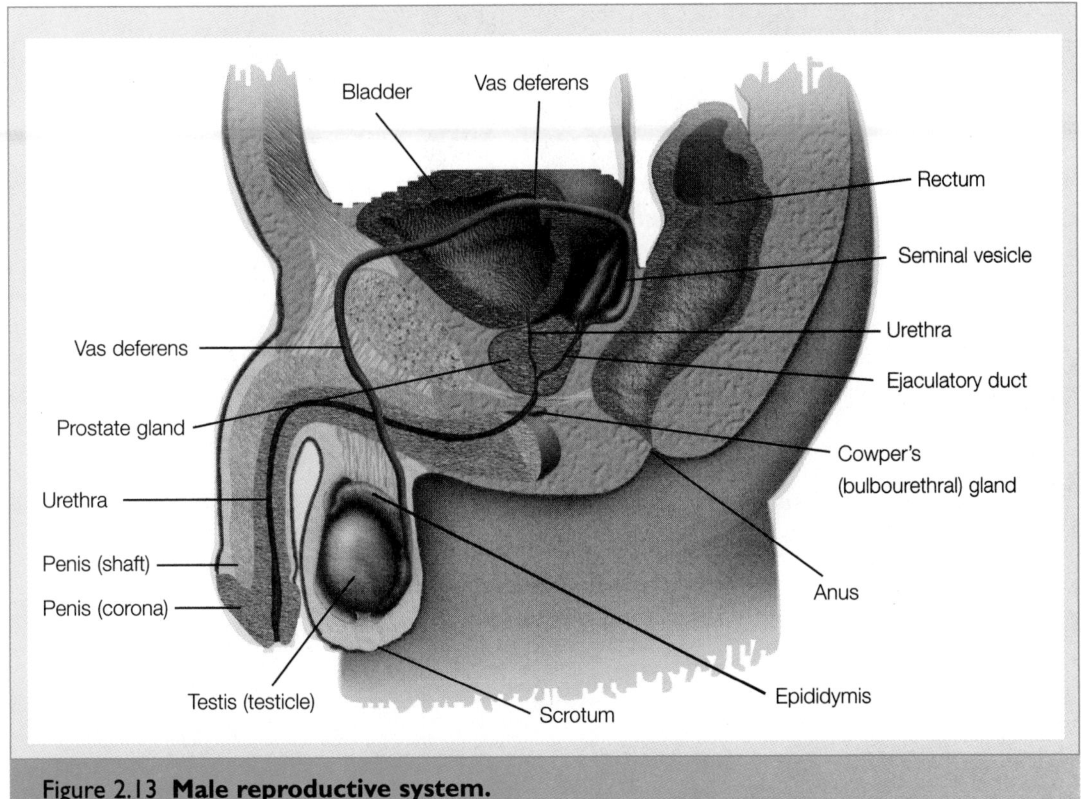

Figure 2.13 **Male reproductive system.**

The Female System

Unlike the male reproductive organs, most of which can be seen outside the body, the organs of the female reproductive system are housed inside and cannot be seen externally. These organs include the vagina, uterus, fallopian tubes, and ovaries, illustrated in Figure 2.14. The **vagina**, located in the groin area, is an elastic muscular canal that leads from the outside of the body to the **cervix**, the opening to the uterus. In addition to being the structure that receives the discharged sperm from the male, the vagina is the passageway called the birth canal, through which a baby leaves the mother's body.

The **uterus** is a pear-shaped muscular organ inside of which the developing baby grows. Branching out from both sides of the uterus are the **fallopian tubes**, which extend to just outside the ovaries. The two ovaries, located in the lower abdomen, each contain up to 20,000 eggs. Beginning at puberty, an egg matures and is released from alternating ovaries once a month. This process, called **ovulation**, is part of the female reproductive, or **menstrual cycle**, the monthly process in which both the egg and the uterus prepare for fertilization and pregnancy.

If fertilization does not occur, the thickened uterine lining, the **endometrium**, where the fertilized egg would have been implanted, begins to break down and passes out of the body in a mixture of blood and other fluids. Called **menstruation**, this discharge usually lasts about 5 days, during which females wear sanitary pads or tampons to absorb the flow of blood.

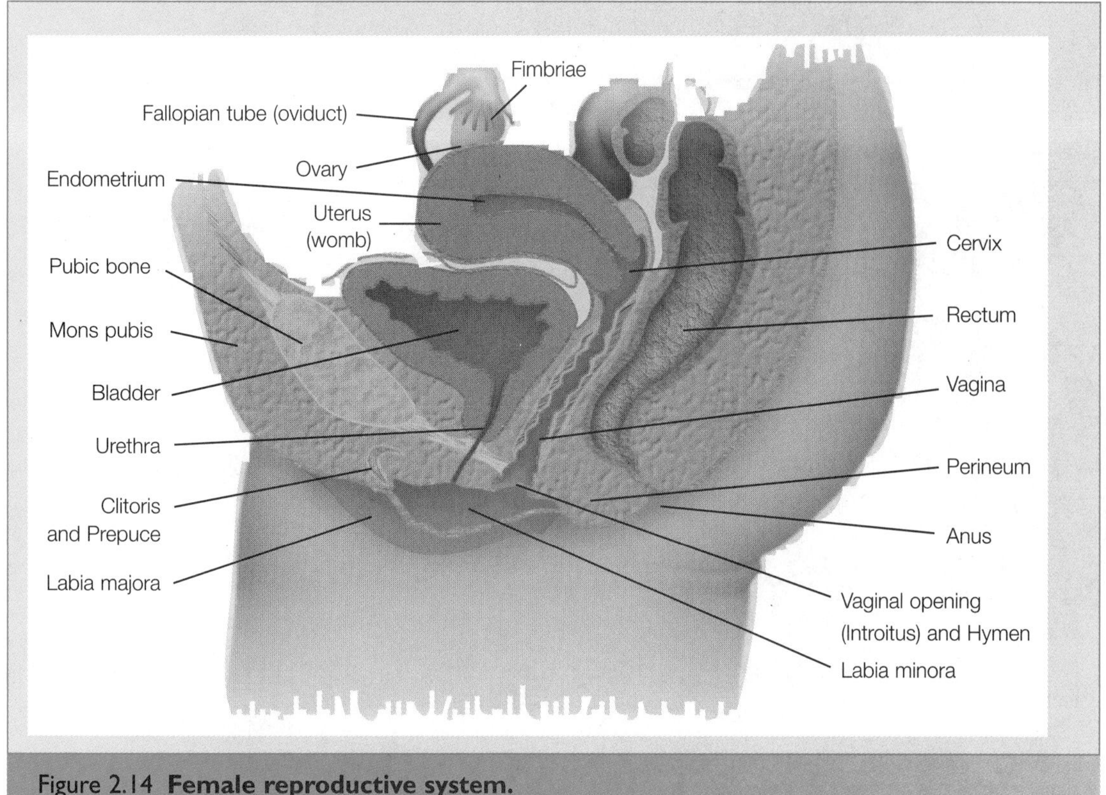

Figure 2.14 **Female reproductive system.**

The Process of Reproduction

In sum, then, reproduction works like this: Sperm, deposited by the penis into the vagina, travel up through the cervix and uterus into the fallopian tubes, where several sperm may meet the egg that has been released from the ovary. If fertilization occurs, the resulting zygote travels to the uterus and attaches itself to the lining where, for about 9 months, it continues to grow and develop into a new human being. At the end of that time, the baby passes through the birth canal and enters the world. A new journey begins and the cycle of life continues. If fertilization does not occur, menstruation follows, and the woman begins another monthly cycle.

Summary

Growth and development occur in a predictable pattern throughout life. This knowledge can be applied to health needs of people at various life stages. Basic to this understanding is the awareness of body systems, their roles and functions, and how they are interrelated.

The skeletal system includes the bones and teeth. The condition of one's teeth, perhaps more than any other body component, reflect the application of health-care principles. The muscular system is composed of voluntary (skeletal) and involuntary (such as heart) muscles. The integumentary system collectively includes the skin, hair, and nails, which serve primarily a protective function and are the first line of defense against disease.

The respiratory system works in conjunction with the circulatory system to deliver oxygen to carry out body functions and dispose of the carbon dioxide waste products of metabolism. The respiratory system is composed of the nose, throat, trachea, bronchial tubes, lungs, and alveoli. Components of the circulatory system are the heart, blood vessels (arteries and veins), and blood. The digestive system is a tract beginning with the mouth, traveling down the esophagus to the stomach, progressing to the small intestine, then the large intestine, and ending with the rectum and anus. Various organs contribute enzymes that digest food along the way.

The urinary system basically consists of the kidneys and bladder. Its purpose is to filter body fluids and eliminate liquid wastes. The body's nervous system is composed of the brain and spinal cord (the central nervous system) and peripheral nerves. The brain is the repository of thought, information, and emotion, and it coordinates all of the body's actions through the nerves. The body has five senses that give us information about the outside world: seeing, hearing, taste, smell, and touch. These make up the sensory system.

The endocrine system works with the nervous system, releasing hormones into the bloodstream to control and regulate body activities. The exocrine glands release their products into the digestive tract or to the outside of the body (as in the case of perspiration). Major organs of the reproductive system include, in males, the penis, scrotum, testicles, and prostate gland; in females, the vagina, cervix, uterus, fallopian tubes, and ovaries.

A basic understanding of these systems will enable the teacher to convey health-related information and plan activities that are appropriate for elementary school students at various levels. This information ultimately can lead to healthier living.

Web Sites

The Amazing Backbone
http://tqjunior.thinkquest.org/4131/

Eye Structure
http://www.exploratorium.edu/xref/phenomena/eye_structure.html

Human Body Adventure
http://www.vilenski.com/science/humanbody/index.html

How Stuff Works
http://www.howstuffworks.com

The Liver
http://tqjunior.thinkquest.org/3782/liver.htm

Lung Association: Especially for Children
http://www.lung.ca/children/

My Body
http://www.kidshealth.org/kid/body/mybody.html

Neuroscience for Kids
http://faculty.washington.edu/chudler/neurok.html

On the Defense: The Immune System
http://biologyabout.com/science/biology/library/weekly/aa040397.htm?terms=immune

The Real Deal on the Digestive System
http://www.kidshealth.org/kid/body/digest_noSW.html

The Skeletal System
http://tqjunior.thinkquest.org/5777/ske1.htm

Notes

1. Creswell, W. H., and I. M. Newman. *School Health Practice.* 10th ed. St. Louis: Mosby-Year Book, 1993.
2. McArdle, W. D., F. I. Katch, and V. L. Katch. *Exercise Physiology: Energy, Nutrition, and Human Performance.* 4th ed. Philadelphia: Lea and Febiger, 1996.
3. See note 1.
4. Greenberg, J., and R. Gold. *Holt Health.* 2nd ed. Austin, TX: Holt, Rinehart and Winston, 1994.
5. Anspaugh, D. J. and Ezell, *Teaching Today's Health.* 4th ed. Boston: Allyn & Bacon, 1995.
6. Payne, W. A., and D. B. Hahn. *Understanding Your Health.* 3d ed. St. Louis: Mosby-Year Book, 1992.
7. Donatelle, R. J. and L. G. Davis. *Health: The Basics.* 4th ed. Boston: Allyn & Bacon, 2001.
8. See note 7.
9. Parker, S. *The Body Atlas.* London: Dorling Kindersley, 1993.
10. Christian, J. L., and J. L. Greger. *Nutrition for Living.* Redwood City, CA: Benjamin/Cummings, 1994.
11. See note 9.
12. See note 1.
13. Getchell, L. H., G. D. Pippin, and J. W. Varnes. *Perspectives on Health.* Lexington, KY: Heath & Co., 1994.
14. See note 5.
15. See note 5.

Learning Experiences

Teaching the processes of growth and development is complex and can be confusing for students. The challenge for the teacher is to keep the technical information accurate, yet simple. In developing a self-image, students need to know about their body systems and how they develop. Learning about the wonder of the human body and how it functions is one step in the direction of long-term health. Students tend to take a keen interest in their bodies and have a natural curiosity about how they grow and change.

Grades K–2

Students in the early grades can learn that they have the power to affect the growth of their body's systems. Their behaviors can make their system strong and healthy or weak and in need of medical attention. They should learn that cleanliness is important to good health. For example, knowing about dental hygiene and caring for their teeth properly can prevent problems later in life.

This is the best time to teach students about exercise, rest, and eating a balanced diet for the development of a healthy body. They will recognize that being healthy makes their body systems work well. By the end of lessons on the development of body systems, the students should be able to

1. list the body systems and describe how they grow and change throughout the life cycle;
2. name and describe the most important parts;
3. describe how they can help their systems grow in a healthy way through exercise, rest, and a balanced diet;
4. demonstrate daily care of the human body, which serves as the basis for personal health and well-being; and
5. identify ways in which people are unique in their growth and development.

Grades 3–4

Students at grade levels 3 and 4 have a great interest in the human body and will build on the information they learned in grades K–2. Good topics for these grade levels include the basic structure and functioning of the body systems—including the respiratory, circulatory, nervous, digestive, skeletal, and reproductive systems—and how these systems can benefit from exercise. By the end of these lessons, students should be able to

1. list names of the body systems and their parts;
2. describe how these parts function and interact so the body functions as an integrated whole;
3. identify how body parts can break down and thereby produce illness;
4. describe the differences in bodies of different people, including men and women and people with various disabilities; and
5. explain why body parts develop at different rates in different children.

Grades 5–6

At grades 5 and 6, students' bodies are beginning to go through puberty—the most rapid period of changes. Girls begin the process first, and boys follow shortly thereafter. The most common question asked is, "Am I normal?" Gender differences come to the fore, and reproductive processes take hold. Respect and care for the body should continue to be emphasized. More information is needed about how the systems work and are integrated into the whole. By the end of these lessons, students will be able to

1. discuss the importance of good health habits and their effects on the body;
2. describe the differences between good and bad health habits and their effects on growth and development;
3. discuss the best ways to care for body systems;
4. describe the changes and gender differences associated with puberty; and
5. describe how protecting the eyes, ears, teeth, and other body parts is essential to personal health.

Learning Experience 2-1

My Body

Grade Level

K–2

Primary Disciplines

Science, Art

Learning Objectives

Following this activity, students will be able to sort and put together the major bone groups in the body.

Time Required

Two sessions (total 90 minutes)

Materials

Crayons, scissors, fasteners, and handout of skeletal parts (Figure 2.1 may be used as a basis)

Description of Activity

Students receive six pictures of bone groupings (skull, rib cage, pelvis, two arms, and two legs), which they cut out and put together in proper human form. Students color parts with crayons and connect using fasteners.

Homework

None

Evaluation

Students will be able to

- Identify the bone groups of the body by name.
- Spell the words correctly.
- Correctly attach the pictures of bone groups to a human form.

Learning Experience 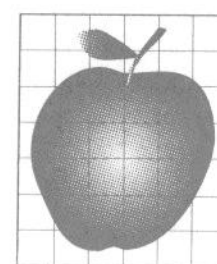 2-2

Crossword Puzzle

Grade Level
K–2

Primary Disciplines
Science, Spelling

Learning Objectives
Following this activity, students will be able to identify eight parts of the head (hair, forehead, nose, mouth, ear, eyebrow, chin, and cheek).

Time Required
15 minutes

Materials
Handout and pencil

Description of Activity
Students receive the crossword puzzle handout and fill in the words using the arrows in the picture as clues.

Homework
Students review the parts of the head and memorize the spelling words.

Evaluation
Students will be able to

- Read and recognize the parts of the human head.
- Correctly spell the parts of the human head.
- Do a simple crossword puzzle.

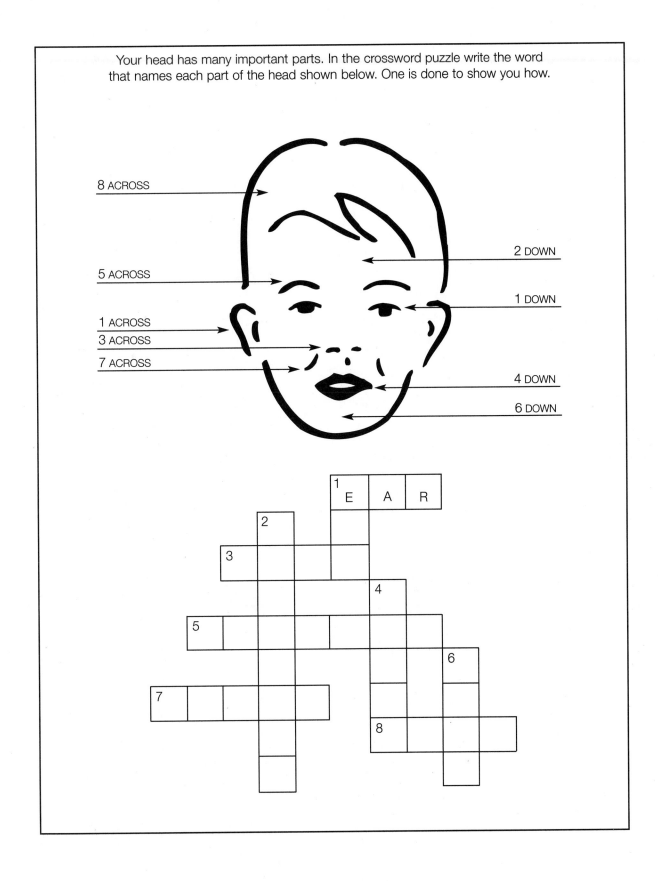
Your head has many important parts. In the crossword puzzle write the word that names each part of the head shown below. One is done to show you how.
8 ACROSS
2 DOWN
5 ACROSS
1 DOWN
1 ACROSS
3 ACROSS
7 ACROSS
4 DOWN
6 DOWN
1
E
A
R
2
3
4
5
6
7
8

Learning Experience 2-3

The Senses

Grade Level

1–2

Primary Disciplines

Science, Spelling

Learning Objectives

Following this activity, students will be able to identify and spell the parts of the body that are related to each of the five senses.

Time Required

10 minutes

Materials

Pencil and paper

Description of Activity

Students receive a handout (example shown above) with a list of the five senses and write the part of the body used for each sense.

A. See ________________

B. Hear ________________

C. Smell ________________

D. Taste ________________

E. Touch ________________

Homework

Students review the five senses and memorize the spelling words.

Evaluation

Students will be able to

- Identify the senses.
- Identify the associated body part with the senses.
- Read, recognize, and spell the body parts and the senses correctly.
- Explain how the body parts and senses are related.

Answers

1. Eyes
2. Ears
3. Nose
4. Tongue
5. Skin

Learning Experience 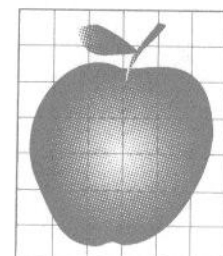 2-4

Unscrambling Body Part Names

Grade Level

3–4

Primary Disciplines

Science, Spelling

Learning Objectives

Following this activity, students will be able to identify and spell nine parts of the body.

Time Required

15 minutes

Materials

Handout and pencil

Description of Activity

Students receive a handout (example shown on next page) with nine scrambled words, each pointing to a part of the body. They unscramble the words and spell each body part correctly.

Homework

Students will review the body parts and memorize the spelling words.

Evaluation

Students will be able to:

- Read, recognize, and spell the names of body parts.
- Unscramble the words for the body parts, spelling them correctly.

Answers

1. Head
2. Neck
3. Shoulder
4. Arm
5. Elbow
6. Hand
7. Leg
8. Knee
9. Foot

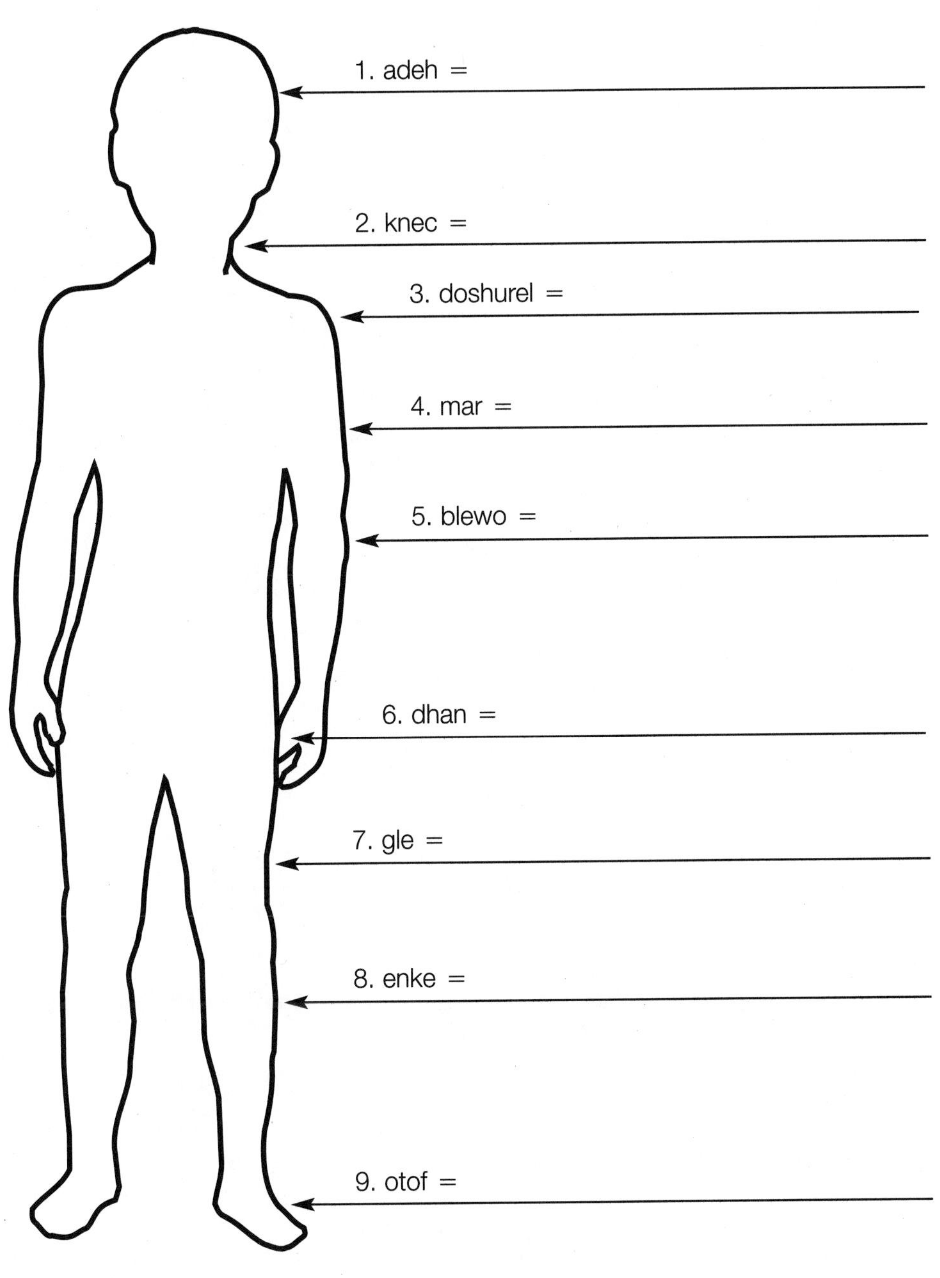
1. adeh =
2. knec =
3. doshurel =
4. mar =
5. blewo =
6. dhan =
7. gle =
8. enke =
9. otof =

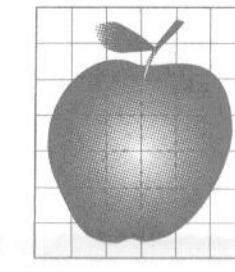

Learning Experience 2-5

Alphabetizing Body Part Names

Grade Level
3–4

Primary Disciplines
Science, Spelling

Learning Objectives
Following this activity, students will be able to alphabetize and list the names of various parts of the human body.

Time Required
30 minutes

Materials
Handout of the list of words to be alphabetized, pencil

Description of Activity
Students list the words in alphabetical order.

nose	tongue	brain	skin	nails	ears	eyes
head	hair	arms	legs	hands	feet	face
heart	liver	blood	lungs	bones	neck	stomach
toes	fingers	skull	spine	mouth	teeth	kidneys

Homework
Using a picture of a person they have cut out of a magazine, students will label each part on the picture.

Evaluation
Students will be able to

- Read, recognize, and spell the names of body parts.
- Alphabetize a list of words consisting of body parts.
- Describe where each body part is on the human body.

Answers

brain	ears	eyes	nails	nose	skin	tongue
arms	face	feet	hair	hands	head	legs
blood	bones	heart	liver	lungs	neck	stomach
fingers	kidneys	mouth	skull	spine	teeth	toes

Learning Experience 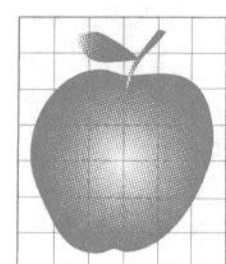 2-6

Personal Health Biography

Grade Level

5–6

Primary Disciplines

Science, English

Learning Objectives

Following this activity, students will be able to use their writing skills to describe important biographical information about their personal health.

Time Required

One session (45 minutes)

Materials

Paper and pencil

Description of Activity

Students write a biographical essay about their personal health. Information to be included should be brainstormed and listed on the chalkboard. Information could include date of birth, place of birth, weight at birth, length at birth, record of immunization, blood type, current height and weight, any childhood surgery, illnesses, allergies, eyesight and hearing, dental care, physical activities, eating and sleeping habits.

Homework

Students will have to gather much of this information from parents, doctors, and others.

Evaluation

Students will be able to

- Identify and recognize what information contributes to a health profile.
- Gather pertinent information about their own health.
- Describe in writing important information about their health using correct spelling and grammar.

Learning Experience 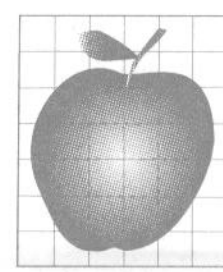 2-7

Strength of a Hair

Grade Level

3–4

Primary Disciplines

Science, Math

Learning Objectives

Following this activity, students will be able to demonstrate the strength of a hair and its ability to stretch.

Time Required

One session (45 minutes)

Materials

Samples of hair (one 7 inches or longer and one about 4 inches long), Scotch tape, ruler, marking pen, rod or wooden clothes hanger, large glass jar with a lid, and key

Description of Activities

1. To demonstrate the strength of a hair, students will tape a long hair to a 12-inch ruler (or any article weighing approximately 2 ounces) and tape the other end of the hair to a rod, from which the object dangles. The hair will not break for several days. Repeat experiment with different colors and/or types of hair to compare results.
2. To demonstrate elasticity of a hair, students will tape one end of a 4-inch hair to a key and tape the other end of the hair to the underside of a glass jar lid, letting the hair and key hang inside the jar (see illustration on next page). On the outside of the jar, mark the spot where the key hangs every day for a week. After several days, the key should descend about 1 inch.
3. Students will brainstorm ways they keep their hair healthy.

Homework

Students write down on a sheet of paper the color, length, and type of hair (curly, straight, or wavy) used in the experiments. Which type of hair stretches most—curly or straight? Does hair color matter? Who in their family has similar hair to theirs, and how is it similar?

Evaluation

Students will be able to

- Describe the various properties of human hair.
- Describe the properties of their own hair.
- Explain how hair types occur in families.
- Describe how to care for hair to keep it healthy.

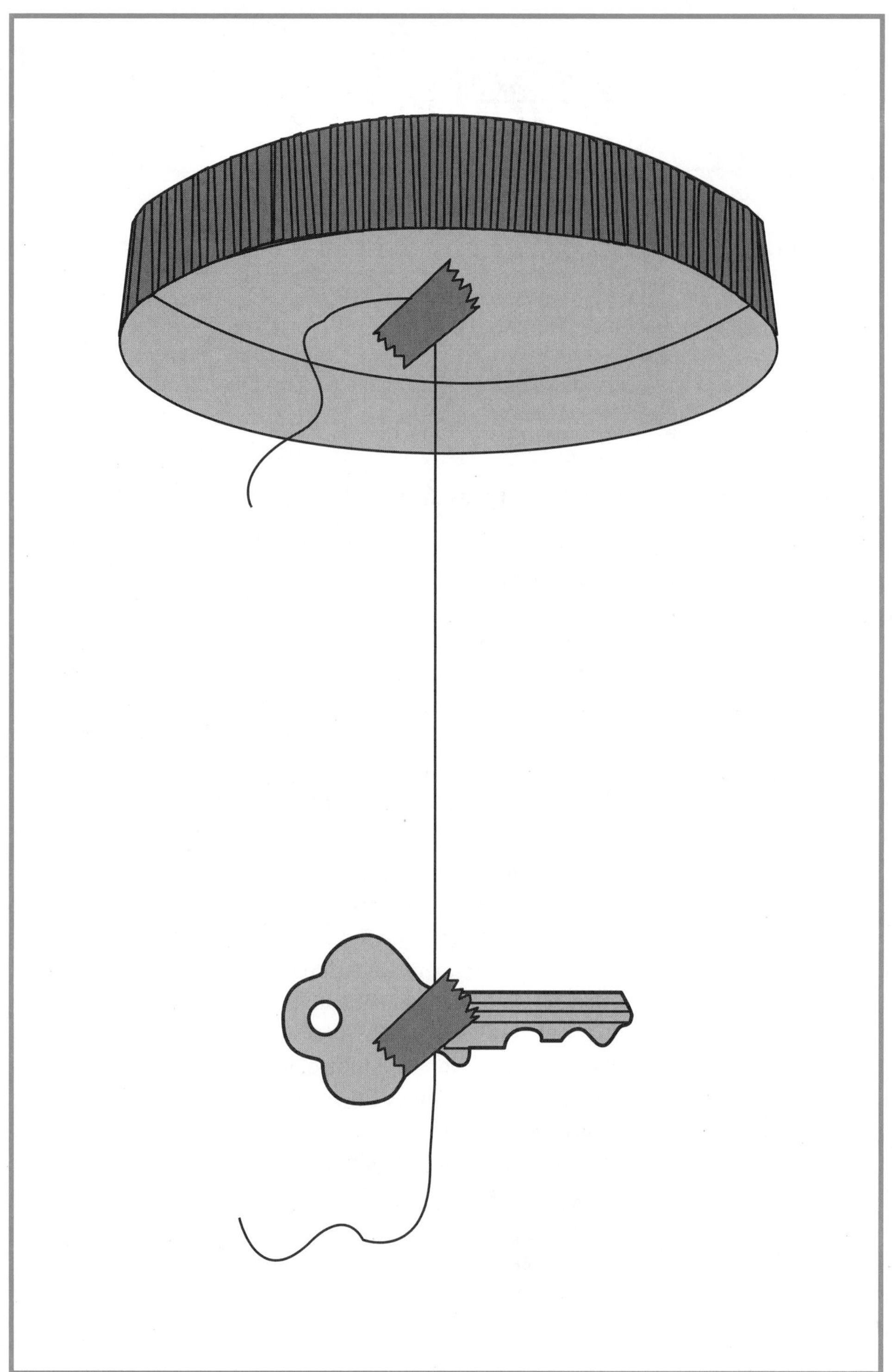

Learning Experience 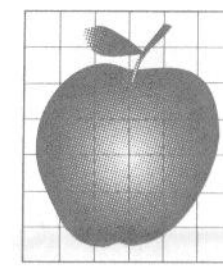 2-8

Taking a Pulse

Grade Level

3–4

Primary Disciplines

Science, Math

Learning Objectives

Following this activity, students will be able to

- measure their heart rate and
- read a simple graph or table.

Time Required

One session (45 minutes)

Materials

Graph paper, pencil, watch with second hand, and enough space for a few students to run or jump in

Description of Activity

Using the graph paper, make a grid for each student like the one shown below. Have the students predict which activities will make their heart beat the fastest and slowest. You may need to separate the activities in Step 5 by at least 30 minutes to allow students' pulses to return to normal.

1. Sit quietly for a few minutes.
2. Count your pulse from the artery on your wrist for 15 seconds.
3. Multiply this number by 4 to get the number of beats in a minute.
4. Place an X under "Resting" on the chart (below) next to the number of your heartbeats.
5. Perform the activities in Columns 3 through 5. Count and record your pulse after each.

Heartbeats per minute	Resting	Walking slowly	Walking fast	Hopping on one foot
140				
120				
100				
80				
60				

Homework

Students repeat this activity with other family members and make a chart for each of them.

Evaluation

Students will be able to

- Take their own pulse rate.
- Take a pulse rate on another person.
- Compare resting pulse rate to activity pulse rates.
- Perform calculations that describe pulse rate changes under different circumstances.
- Explain what a pulse rate measures.
- Create a chart and a graph using pulse rates and make comparison statements from them.

Learning Experience 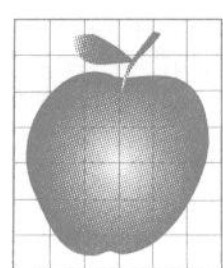 2-9

Small Intestine

Grade Level

3–4

Primary Discipline

Science

Learning Objectives

Following this activity, students will be able to

- describe why the small intestine is so absorbent and
- describe how the small intestine works.

Time Required

One session

Materials

Paper towels, two bread pans, tablespoon, scissors, small pitcher of water

Description of Activity

Cut one paper towel to fit in the bottom of a bread pan and place it there. Fold three other towels into long accordion folds and place into the other. Using the tablespoon, add water slowly to each pan. See how much water each will absorb before water is left standing in the pan. Explain that the absorbent layer inside the small intestine of a grown person would measure more than 300 square yards if stretched out flat.

Homework

None

Evaluation

Students will be able to

- Locate the small intestine.
- Describe the action of the small intestine.
- Relate the purpose of the small intestine to digestion.

Learning Experience 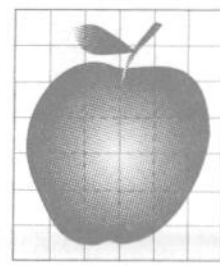 2-10

Genetic History

Grade Level

5–6

Primary Disciplines

Science, Social Studies

Learning Objectives

Following this activity, students will be able to

- trace their family's genetic history and
- describe the relationship between genetic history and health.

Time Required

One session

Materials

Notebook, pen, tape recorder (optional), access to family photo albums and other records of family history (medical records, birth certificates, and the like)

Description of Activity

Have students make a list of all the relatives they know and describe some of their physical characteristics (shape of fingernails, skin color, hair, baldness, height, weight, allergies, eye color, and so on). Then ask "Who else in the family has the same trait?" have students draw a family tree showing how these traits were passed down.

Homework

Preceding the activity, students interview relatives and look at photo albums and medical records to gather information.

Evaluation

Students will be able to construct a family tree and describe how some of their traits were inherited.

3

Nutrition

Susan Karp

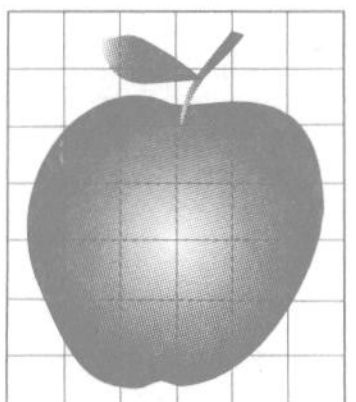

Chapter Outline

Nutrition Education
Nutrients
Phytochemicals
Water
The Food Guide Pyramids
Food Labeling

Objectives

- Offer various definitions of nutrition
- Identify factors that contribute to food habits and preferences
- Summarize the Dietary Guidelines for Americans
- State some of the nutrition objectives from Healthy People 2010
- Classify nutrients
- Identify the types of carbohydrates and their food sources
- Differentiate saturated, unsaturated, and trans fats
- Identify the issues involved in weight management and the associated problems of obesity and eating disorders
- Enumerate the functions of proteins in the body
- List the water-soluble and fat-soluble vitamins and the ramifications for daily intake
- Differentiate the major and trace minerals and identify health problems associated with specific deficiencies
- Explain the Recommended Dietary Allowances (RDAs)
- Describe the USDA Food Guide Pyramid, the vegetarian diet pyramid, and food guide pyramid for young children
- Suggest the value and possible uses of the food label on commercially packaged products

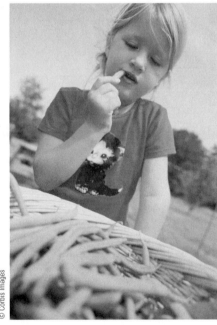

Amy is an 11-year-old fifth-grade student. Amy was about 15 percent above her ideal body weight prior to this year, and during the past year she has gained approximately 7 pounds. She is extremely concerned about her weight and body image and does not want to be overweight in her first year in middle school.

Amy has opted not to eat breakfast because she thinks this will help her lose weight. During the morning hours at school, she finds that she is having trouble concentrating, and she becomes tired and irritable. The elementary school that Amy attends offers after-school intramural sports. She does not participate, because she is uncomfortable about her weight. Amy does not care for many of the foods served for lunch in the school cafeteria.

Outside of school, Amy prefers french fries and snack foods such as potato chips to satisfy her hunger. She normally goes home after school and has a snack before she begins her homework. After she completes her homework, she either talks on the telephone to her friends or watches television.

Amy is interested in nutrition and has begun reading food labels to find out the ingredients, particularly the amount of fat and calories. She has heard that fat is bad for her but doesn't know how much she can eat or that there are different types of fat. Amy is confused by the food labels and the different and conflicting information in the media. She is somewhat aware of the types of foods that are considered healthy but is not certain about what foods are unhealthy. The idea of putting all the information together to have a healthy diet and lifestyle is overwhelming to her.

• • •

Jason is a thin sixth-grader. He wants to be on the high school wrestling team when he gets older. His brother has told him that he will have to be bigger and heavier. He remembers that, when his brother wanted to change his wrestling classification, he was told he had to gain weight quickly. He heard his brother telling his friends how much fun it would be eat lots of cake and candy to gain weight fast. That didn't sound right to Jason, but he plans to do the same thing if he has to, to get onto the high school wrestling team—a major goal for him.

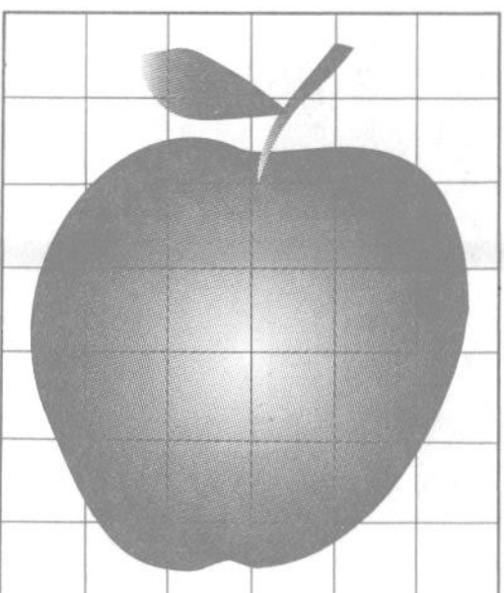

Will Amy's eating pattern result in a constant battle with food and weight throughout her life? What messages about weight control has Jason received?

For some people, eating behaviors emerge from family eating patterns. Others develop eating habits from well-documented information. Others succumb to media hype and advertising. Many people have become obsessed with specific components of food and their relationship to disease. They may want a quick fix. Some people incorporate one piece of information about a food and eliminate or pay no attention to others. For example, some people are proud of eliminating fat from their diet but do not question the chemicals used to replace the fats or the artificial sugar added to food. They have not asked themselves about the health risks associated with crash diets or the stress from worrying about their weight.

People spend a great deal of time eating for reasons other than nutrition. Eating can be a way of making people feel good. Food sometimes has a role in a system of reward or punishment. How often we have heard, "If you eat everything on your plate, you can have dessert." Dessert is the reward for doing something "right." Food has been used as a lesson in social consciousness: "Children in [some location] are starving, so you shouldn't waste food—clean your plate!" Food is also a central component of hospitality. Social planning often centers on the choice of a good restaurant and the quality of its food. That quality rarely has anything to do with nutrition or good health; it simply relates to good taste and presentation.

In some families, eating together is a ritual that defines how well the family is functioning: "A family that eats together, stays together." Food and the roles people play in its preparation are an indication of their culture. Mothers may be considered good mothers because of the way they feed their family. Frequently, dietary habits and foods are chosen or eliminated from diets because of religious tenets. For all these reasons, children and adults should be educated about nutrition.

Nutrition Education

In addition to understanding the biochemistry of food and its relationship to health, the psychological and sociological factors that determine why and what people eat contribute to the monumental task of nutrition education. And not only do teachers have to muddle through the literature to figure out how various foods affect us, but we also have to figure out what information is reliable and what is not. Given all this information, nutrition educators have to assist in the development of habits and lifestyles that support healthy eating by further understanding the effects of mental health, attitudes, and values about how people eat.

The primary goal of the health educator is to incorporate this information into the curriculum in a meaningful way. Helping children make dietary choices that will enhance their health is of critical importance. Frequently, this means making choices that are different from their families and peers. Necessary changes in habits and diets are required as new information about the relationship between health and nutrition continues to emerge.

Dissemination of nutritional information requires that nutritionists, physicians, and educators devise appropriate ways to relay this knowledge to the public in some useful way. Because information about nutrition continues to change, educators who use this information must stay current with the latest findings. The growing cadre of alternative, or complementary, medical and health care providers believe that traditional medicine has not recognized the relationship between nutrition and health beyond a cursory look, and physicians have little formal training in the area.

The general population is increasingly embracing the views of complementary medicine, particularly in the use of vitamin supplements and in nutritional treatments for serious illnesses. Thus, the nutrition educator can no longer ignore these influences on nutritional habits. What follows is a brief summary of what teachers need to know to develop a good nutrition education curriculum for students.

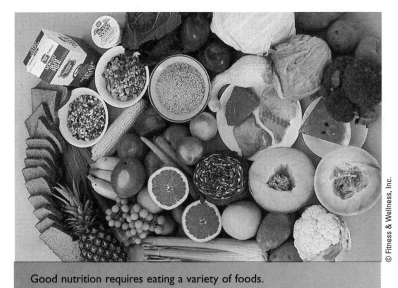

Good nutrition requires eating a variety of foods.

© Fitness & Wellness, Inc.

The Basics of Nutrition

Nutrition has a number of meanings and definitions. According to an early definition, nutrition is the combination of processes by which the living organism receives and utilizes the materials (food) necessary for the maintenance of its bodily processes and for the growth and renewal of its organ systems.[1] For most people, nutrition relates to the foods we eat and, possibly, its nutrient content. Although one major point becomes evident—that proper nutrition is essential for optimal bodily functions—not everyone agrees on what is "proper." In this text, good nutrition is defined as the acquisition and utilization of food, food products, and supplements for the purpose of achieving and maintaining optimal health, growth, and development.

Table 3.1
Dietary Guidelines for Americans

Aim for Fitness	Build a Healthy Base	Choose Sensibly
Aim for a healthy weight. Be physically active each day.	Let the pyramid guide your food choices. Choose a variety of whole grains. Choose a variety of fruits and vegetables daily. Keep foods safe to eat.	Choose a diet that is low in saturated fat and cholesterol and moderate in daily total fat. Choose beverages and foods to moderate your intake of sugars. Choose and prepare foods with less salt. If you drink alcoholic beverages, do so in moderation.

Source: U. S. Department of Health and Human Services (2000).

Incorporating nutrition education into the school curriculum promotes good health for students. Childhood and adolescence are important periods for establishing a healthful diet and good exercise habits that can reduce the onset of obesity and may decrease the development of certain chronic diseases in later life.

The ultimate responsibility of ensuring children's healthy eating falls on their parents or guardians. Therefore, a curriculum designed to develop healthy habits or change the unhealthy eating behaviors of students must be directed simultaneously at children and their primary caregivers, because they are the ones who usually determine what foods are purchased and how they are prepared. Thus, parents or guardians must be included in the nutrition education of their children.

What determines people's food habits? Factors such as taste, economics, ethnicity, peer pressure, and nutrient content contribute to food choices. Fast foods and eating out have become a way of life. Nonetheless, sometimes people do base their food selections on their knowledge of nutrition and its relationship to health and disease. To make this easier, the U. S. Department of Agriculture (USDA) and the Department of Health and Human Services (DHHS) developed the Dietary Guidelines for Americans to provide practical advice for healthy Americans about food choices that will promote health and help to reduce disease.[2] These guidelines are published every 5 years to include the latest scientific findings about links between diet and chronic disease. The most recent edition of the Dietary Guidelines, released in 2000, contains three basic messages: 1. Aim for Fitness, 2. Build a Healthy Base, 3. Choose Sensibly. The 10 new dietary guidelines are clustered into these three groups and are shown in Table 3.1.

For Your Health

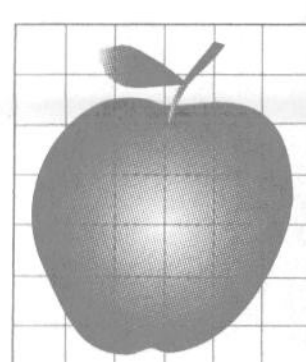

Nutritional Aids to a Healthy Heart

- Eat fiber, found in fruit, vegetables, cereals, and grains.
- Eat beans. Legumes contain a lot of soluble fiber and other cholesterol-lowering components. All kinds of beans work.
- Eat garlic.
- Get enough vitamin C. This means 2,000 mg of vitamin C daily. Orange juice is a good source.
- Get B vitamins. These include folic acid, B_6, and B_{12}. Good sources are green leafy vegetables and orange juice.
- Eat fish. Two or three servings a week supply enough healthy omega-3 oils.
- Eat flavonoids. These denote foods rich in antioxidants and include grapes, onions, apples, and tea.
- Cut back on saturated (animal) fats, contained in meat, cheese, butter, and milk (except nonfat or skim milk). The best fat is the type in olives and olive oil, almonds, walnuts, avocados, and canola oil.

Source: Jean Carper, author of the book *Stop Aging Now.*

In addition, the U.S. Department of Health and Human Services sets 10-year health objectives for the nation. The most recent edition, *Healthy People 2010,* was released in 2000.[3] Educators can incorporate these objectives into educational curricula and furnish students with the means to improve their diets. The nutrition objectives are

- Increase the prevalence of healthy weight and decrease the prevalence of obesity.
- Reduce growth retardation among low-income children.
- Increase the proportion of people aged 2 and older who meet the Dietary Guidelines for fat and saturated fat in the diet.
- Increase intakes of fruit and vegetables to at least five servings a day.
- Increase intakes of grain products to at least six servings a day.
- Increase the proportion of people who meet the recommendation for calcium.
- Increase the proportion of people who limit themselves to the daily value of 2,400–3,000 milligrams or less of sodium a day.
- Reduce iron deficiency in children, adolescents, women of childbearing age, and low-income pregnant women.
- Increase the proportion of mothers who breastfeed immediately after birth, for the first 6 months, and preferably through the infant's first year of life. Increase the proportion of mothers who breastfeed exclusively.
- Increase the proportion of children and adolescents whose intakes of meals and snacks at school contribute to overall dietary quality.
- Increase the proportion of schools teaching essential nutrition topics.

Information about how foods and their ingredients affect the health of people has radically changed over the years. For a long time, we have accepted the relationship of obesity to poor health, but now, more than ever, we associate diseases such as heart disease, high blood pressure, cancer, diabetes, osteoporosis, arthritis, and some birth defects to poor eating habits and/or deficiencies or excesses of specific food components.

Increasing evidence supports the relationship between the immune system and eating behavior. Poor eating habits and insufficient nutrients seem to play a significant role in lowering a person's ability to resist common viral and bacterial infections and in causing illnesses to be lengthier and more severe. Health and well-being also seem to be influenced by specific food components and their combinations.

Nutrients

The human body requires energy to perform its voluntary and involuntary activities. This energy is provided by nutrients in the food we eat. The six classes of nutrients are carbohydrates, fats, proteins, vitamins, minerals, and water. Of these, only fats, carbohydrates, and proteins yield energy for the body. Minerals and vitamins are utilized for regulatory and other bodily functions. Water, although it does not provide energy, is the most important nutrient, and we cannot live long without it. Figure 3.1 outlines the basic functions of nutrients.

The nutrients that the body can synthesize itself are termed **nonessential nutrients**. Others, termed essential nutrients, must be obtained from the

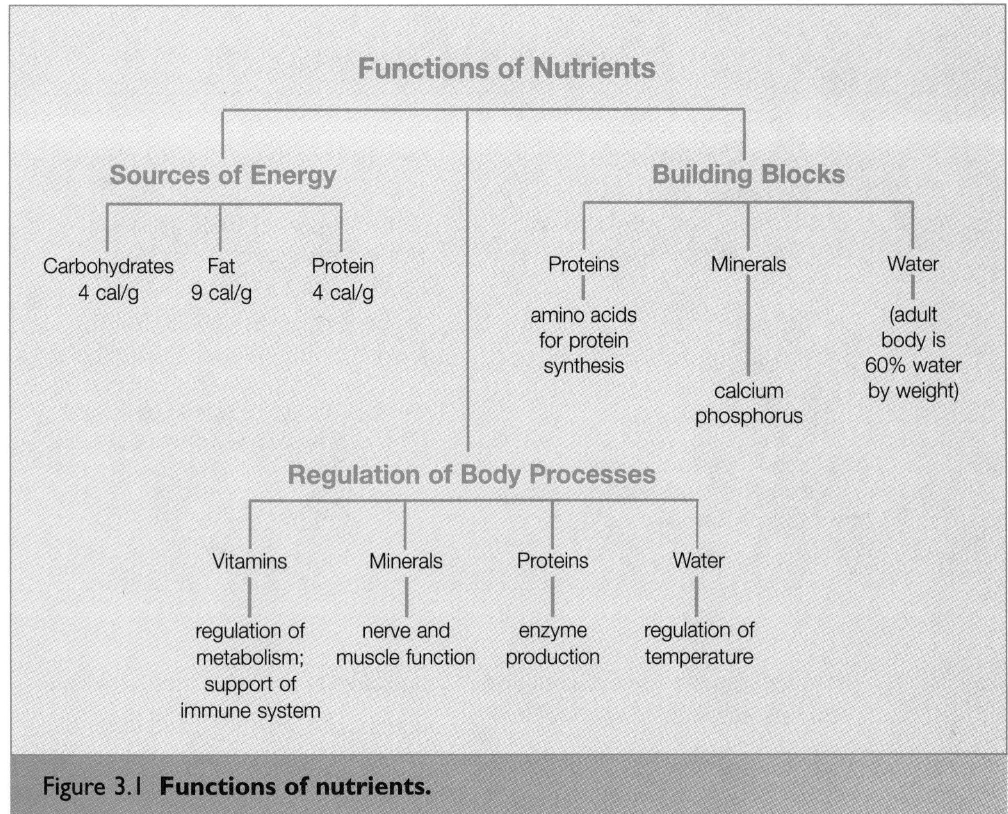

Figure 3.1 **Functions of nutrients.**

food we ingest. If the body does not receive essential nutrients, it can enter a state of deficiency. Therefore, children must eat a variety of foods containing the essential nutrients. Teaching children what food they should eat is an essential component of the curriculum.

Carbohydrates

Carbohydrates are made of carbon, hydrogen, and oxygen and provide a major source of fuel for the body. They contain 4 calories/gram. Our body converts most carbohydrates that we eat to **glucose**, a monosaccharide (one sugar). This glucose is then used as a fuel source for many cells in the body. Our brain, red blood cells, and nervous system use glucose exclusively. This is one reason why carbohydrates are fundamental to a diet.

Other monosaccharides of nutritional importance include **fructose** (found in fruit) and **galactose**. Monosaccharides can be chemically joined together to form **disaccharides** (two sugars). These disaccharides include **lactose** (milk sugar), **maltose**, and **sucrose** (also known as table sugar). The mono- and disaccharides are also known as the simple sugars. Chains of many glucose units put together form another category of carbohydrates classified as **polysaccharides** (many sugars). These complex carbohydrates include **starch**, (the storage form of glucose in plants), glycogen (the storage form of glucose in animals), and most fibers, such as cellulose, hemicellulose, and pectin. Figure 3.2 outlines the classification of carbohydrates.

Carbohydrates can be obtained by eating a diet rich in grains or starches such as bread, pasta, beans, rice, potatoes, cereal (preferably whole grain), vegetables, fruits, and milk products. The dietary recommendation is to obtain 55 percent to 60 percent of one's overall daily caloric intake from carbohydrates.

The use of sugar has increased during the past century. Many people are consuming as much as a fourth of their calories as sugar. The major problem with this intake is that it displaces foods with high **nutrient density** from the diet. Refined white sugar has been termed an empty-calorie food because it contains no nutrients. The controversies surrounding the relationship of sugar to obesity, diabetes, and hyperactivity have been researched extensively with inconclusive results. However, one area in which sugar definitely has a negative effect is in promoting dental caries. Sugar is the best energy source for bacteria that cause tooth decay. The Dietary Guidelines recommends that people choose beverages and foods that moderate their intake of sugar.

Fiber, indigestible carbohydrates derived from plants, has proven to be extremely important to health. Dietary

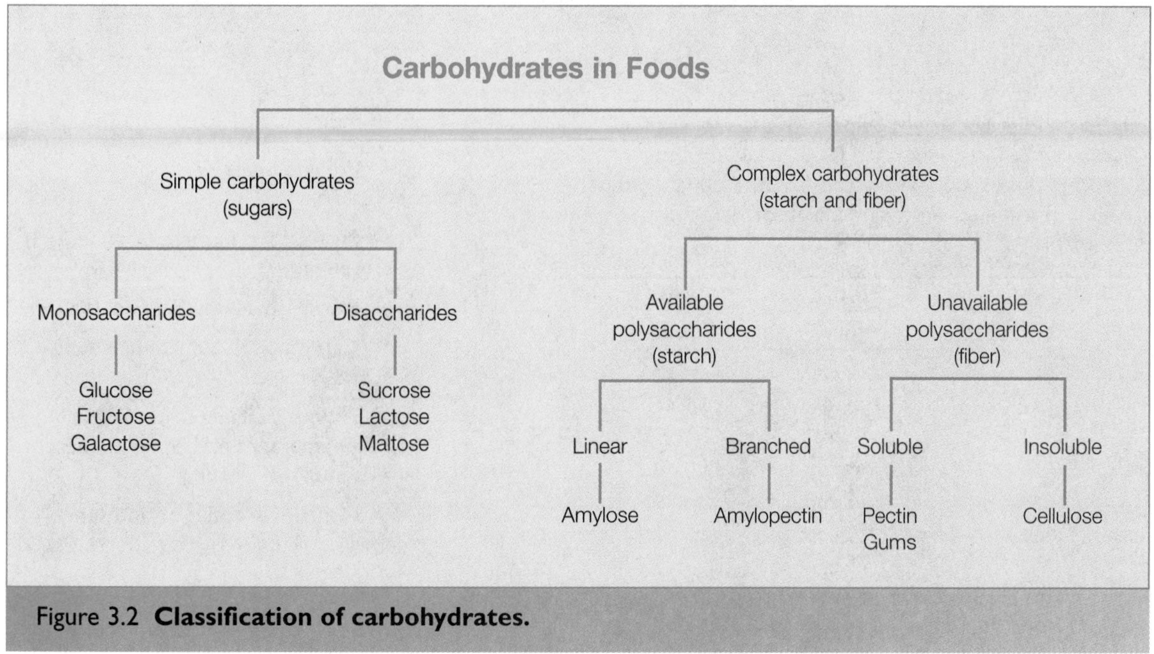

Figure 3.2 **Classification of carbohydrates.**

fiber consists primarily of cellulose, which cannot be broken down by digestive enzymes. Fiber aids in the regular elimination of wastes, contributes to lower blood cholesterol, helps to regulate blood sugar, and has a role in preventing certain types of cancer. The World Health Organization recommends an intake of 27 to 40 grams of dietary fiber daily.[4] To obtain sufficient fiber, a person should consume some fruit, grains, or vegetables at each meal and also as snacks. The box on page 72 lists fiber content of some familiar foods.

Lipids

Lipids, more commonly known as fats, are usually categorized into the following three groups:

- triglycerides (glycerol + 3 fatty acids)
- phospholipids (lecithin)
- sterols (including cholesterol)

The majority of fat that we eat in our diet is in the form of triglycerides. Additionally, excess fat in our bodies, that is stored in our adipocytes (fat cells), is in the form of triglycerides. The three fatty acids that make up a triglyceride can be either saturated fatty acids (containing no double bonds between the carbons), monounsaturated fatty acids (containing one double bond), or polyunsaturated (containing two or more double bonds). The box above lists the main functions of fats.

Triglycerides composed mainly of saturated fatty acids tend to be solid at room temperature. **Saturated fat** is usually found in foods of animal origin such as meat, whole milk, butter, and cheese. Notable exceptions are the tropical oils—coconut and palm kernel oil—that are not derived from foods of animal origin but are highly saturated.

Triglycerides, composed mainly of mono- or polyunsaturated fatty acids, are liquid at room temperature. These include the oils such as olive (monounsaturated), corn, sunflower, safflower and other vegetable oils (polyunsaturated). The fat content of various oils is shown in Figure 3.3.

Oils that have undergone chemical alteration result in the shape of the fatty acid being changed. This process, known as hydrogenation (adding hydrogens to the double bond), produces trans fatty acids, which raise blood **cholesterol**.[5] Trans fatty acids are found in stick margarine, shortening, fried foods, and in many types of processed foods. Foods that contain trans fatty acids are identified by the ingredient list located on the package label. The words "partially hydrogenated" indicate that the product contains these trans fatty acids.

Fats are needed in the diet because they supply the body with the essential fatty acids necessary for vision, immune processes, and production of hormone-like compounds that are necessary for a wide variety of functions.[6] These essential fatty acids cannot be produced by the body and must be supplied by the diet. Certain oils, nuts, seeds and fatty fish are excellent sources of these essential fatty acids. In addition, vitamins A, D, E, and K are fat-soluble and are found in fat-containing foods. Fats lend flavor to foods, as well as contribute to satiety (the feeling of fullness after eating). Storage fat acts as a cushion or padding, protecting vital organs. Fat insulates the body from nerve damage and from extreme hot and cold temperatures.

Dietary Fiber Content of Selected Foods

Fiber is important in the diet because it helps decrease the risk for cardiovascular disease and cancer. Increased fiber intake also may lower the risk of coronary heart disease because saturated fats often take the place of fiber in the diet, increasing the absorption and formation of cholesterol.

Food	Serving Size	Dietary Fiber (gm)
Almonds, shelled	¼ cup	3.9
Apple	1 medium	3.7
Banana	1 small	1.2
Beans, red kidney	½ cup	8.2
Blackberries	½ cup	4.9
Beets, red, canned (cooked)	½ cup	1.4
Brazil nuts	1 oz.	2.5
Broccoli (cooked)	½ cup	3.3
Brown rice (cooked)	½ cup	1.7
Carrots (cooked)	½ cup	3.3
Cauliflower (cooked)	½ cup	5.0
Cereal		
All Bran	1 oz	8.5
Cheerios	1 oz	1.1
Cornflakes	1 oz	0.5
Fruit and Fibre	1 oz	4.0
Fruit Wheats	1 oz	2.0
Just Right	1 oz	2.0
Wheaties	1 oz	2.0
Corn (cooked)	½ cup	2.2
Eggplant (cooked)	½ cup	3.0
Lettuce (chopped)	½ cup	0.5
Orange	1 medium	4.3
Parsnips (cooked)	½ cup	2.1
Pear	1 medium	4.5
Peas (cooked)	½ cup	4.4
Popcorn (plain)	1 cup	1.2
Potato (baked)	1 medium	4.9
Strawberries	½ cup	1.6
Summer squash (cooked)	½ cup	1.6
Watermelon	1 cup	0.1

Functions of Fats (Lipids)

- Provide energy (1 gram = 9 calories)
- Protect and insulate body as stored fat
- Provide essential fatty acids
- Carry fat-soluble vitamins A, D, E, and K
- Provide building materials for cell membranes and other tissues; aids in blood clotting
- Contribute to flavor and satiety

Fats provide a significant fuel source for the body. During rest and light activity, fats provide half of the energy used by the body. The excess energy from food that the body does not utilize is stored as fat. When fat is to be utilized to provide energy, carbohydrates must be also available. This is because a little carbohydrate is needed to properly metabolize the fat. If fat is broken down for use as energy without carbohydrates being available, the body produces ketones. This potentially dangerous condition, called **ketosis**, is likely to result from carbohydrate- and calorie-restricted diets.[7] In ketosis, the acid-base balance of the body becomes disturbed and can lead to further loss of minerals. Ketosis during pregnancy can cause brain damage to the developing fetus.

Because fat contains more than double the number of calories per gram than protein or carbohydrate, many high-fat foods are also high in calories. Protein and carbohydrate provide 4 calories/gram of food, and fat provides 9 calories/gram. Although fats serve important functions in the body, overindulgence has been proven to be detrimental to health. A high-fat diet is more likely to cause weight gain, and obesity is a major contributing factor to many chronic diseases. Additionally,

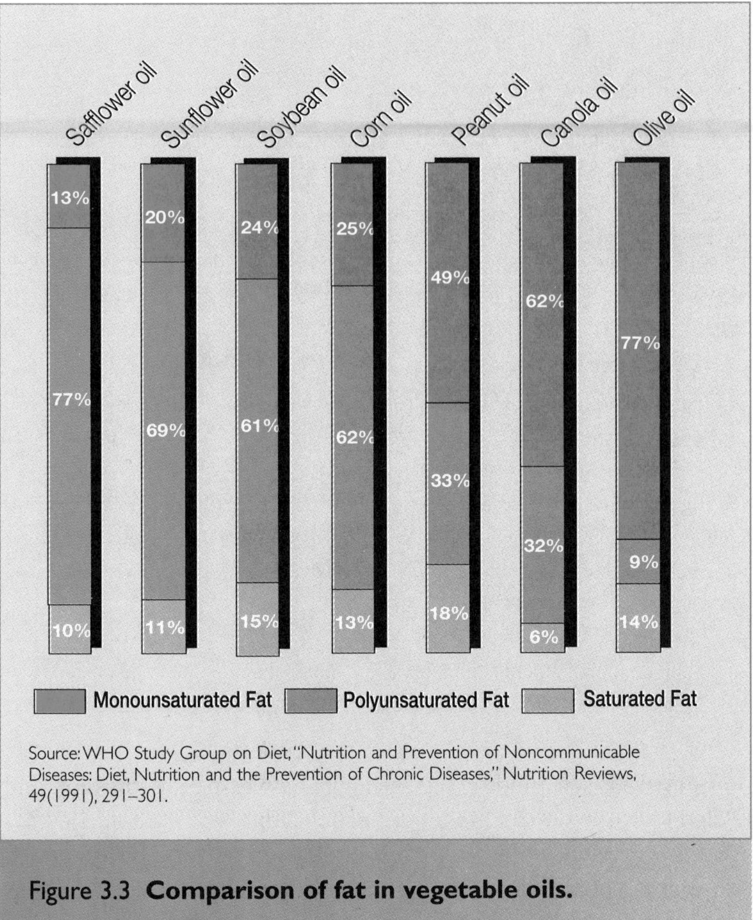

Source: WHO Study Group on Diet, "Nutrition and Prevention of Noncommunicable Diseases: Diet, Nutrition and the Prevention of Chronic Diseases," Nutrition Reviews, 49(1991), 291–301.

Figure 3.3 **Comparison of fat in vegetable oils.**

A Formula For Fat

Here's a handy formula for figuring how many fat calories you should have each day:

Your total calories per day = ____________

multiplied by .30 = ____________

divided by 9 = ____________
(1 gram of fat has 9 calories)

research shows a link between fat intake (particularly saturated fat and trans fat) and blood cholesterol levels.[8] Blood cholesterol is one predictor of a fatal heart attack or stroke. The higher the cholesterol level, the more likely the attack. Finally, a high total fat intake is associated with cancer susceptibility. Table 3.2 shows the relationship between total calories in a healthy diet and the amount obtained from fat.

The World Health Organization recommends an upper limit of 30 percent of total calories from fat in the diet. Only 10 percent of these calories should come from saturated fat. Table 3.2 and the box above present two easy ways to estimate appropriate fat intake.

Table 3.2
Healthy Fat Intake Versus Total Daily Calories

	Total Daily Calories			
Fat intake	1,600	2,000	2,500	2,800
Total Fat (Grams)	53	65	80	93
Saturated Fat (Grams)	18	20	25	31

Weight Management

One of the major health problems in the United States is **obesity**. It results from a **sedentary lifestyle**, excessive calorie intake, and a relatively high proportion of fat in the diet.

Obesity was traditionally defined as being 20 percent or more above the appropriate weight for a related height. However, weight/height tables have limited usefulness. They provide a very narrow range of body weights that are considered acceptable. These tables fail to consider other measures of health and fitness and do not consider body composition.

Presently, nutritionists and physicians are more concerned with body composition, the proportion of fat tissue to lean muscle mass. Two individuals might have the same weight, but one person could have a high percentage of body fat and the other individual could have a high percentage of muscle (lean tissue). Using the weight tables, both might be considered overweight—however, only the individual with the excess body fat is potentially at risk for obesity-related health problems. Measurements of body composition eliminate these types of issues.

Of even greater importance than either weight or body composition is the development and maintenance of healthy eating and exercise habits. If a healthy diet and an active lifestyle are followed regularly and the individual does not have any obesity-related health problems—such as high blood pressure, high blood glucose, elevated cholesterol, or an elevated waist-to-hip ratio (indicating central obesity)—then attaining a particular number on the scale or a specified percentage of body fat becomes less important.

Obesity in Children

Children are not exempt from obesity. The obesity rate in children is rising alarmingly. They are exposed to commercials and advertisements enticing them to eat foods that are high in fat and sugar. In addition, children spend countless hours snacking on high-fat foods in front of the TV set. Extended television watching contributes to physical inactivity—another factor contributing to obesity (see Chapter 4).

Students need to learn that body weight depends on the number of calories the body takes in and burns. To lose weight, a person has to burn more calories than he or she consumes.

Weight loss in obese children has to be monitored carefully by the parents as well as a registered dietitian or pediatrician. Children are still growing, and their growth cannot be compromised by severely restricting calories in their diet. The issue of body image should also be addressed in these children. Children who equate love and self-worth with body size can develop healthier outlooks with proper guidance from teachers.

Eating Disorders

Related to body image is the increasing problem of eating disorders. Anorexia nervosa and bulimia nervosa, the most severe eating disorders, affect approximately 3 percent of young women. Many more young girls have disordered eating, a precursor that includes preoccupation with food and weight.

Some Clues to Eating Disorders

If anyone you know exhibits any of the following symptoms, they may have an eating disorder.

- Excessive weight loss that leaves them 15–25% below recommended weight
- Frequent weight fluctuations (often a result of rollercoaster dieting)
- Unusual eating habits, such as taking tiny bites or moving the food around on the plate
- Excuses for not eating meals with family or friends
- Secretive behavior, especially with regard to eating or to bathroom use
- Excessive use of laxatives or diet pills
- Depression or social withdrawal
- Excessive exercise
- Disruption of menstrual periods
- Increased gum disease or dental cavities (induced by vomiting and malnutrition)
- Extreme sensitivity to cold
- Distorted body image, signaled by continual comments such as, "I'm too fat"
- Increased susceptibility to fractures
- Family or roommates notice food disappearing regularly

Anorexia nervosa is self-imposed starvation related to a severely distorted body image. Even when they are dangerously underweight, people with anorexia nervosa see themselves as fat. **Bulimia nervosa** is characterized by frequent episodes of consuming large amounts of food (**binge eating**) at a single sitting. This is followed by self-induced vomiting, use of laxatives (purging), and/or excessive exercise to avoid weight gain. These disorders, particularly anorexia, affect young girls.[9]

The exact causes of eating disorders remain unclear. Genetic, social, and psychological factors are all thought to play a role. Recent studies have indicated that these disorders may have some basis in brain chemistry. In addition, eating disorders occur more frequently in families with a history of eating disorders as well as other anxiety disorders. Social pressure to attain an unrealistic standard of thinness clearly is an important factor in the development of both disorders. Psychological factors include low self-esteem, striving for control to offset the feeling of helplessness, depression, and perfectionism.

Although no one completely understands why these eating disorders arise in certain people, serious dieting is a powerful predictor that an eating disorder may emerge.[10] Identifying young girls who are dieting inappropriately is necessary to offer early intervention to high-risk students. The box above lists symptoms of eating disorders.

Girls who participate in endurance-based and/or appearance-based athletics are at special risk for developing another type of eating disorder known as the female athlete triad. This condition is characterized by disordered eating, **amenorrhea** (cessation of menstruation), and low bone density. The cycle starts with the athletes adopting harmful eating patterns in an attempt to lose weight. Their low energy intake coupled with the drastic reduction in body fat can trigger the body to stop producing estrogen. This lack of estrogen results in menstrual cycle

Protein Facts

- Amino acids are the building blocks of all living things. About 20 are found in food.
- Essential amino acids must be supplied by diet: They are histidine, isoleucine, leucine, lysine, methionine, phenylalanine, threonine, tryptophan, valine.
- Nonessential amino acids can be manufactured in the body itself, given an adequate diet.

irregularities and can cause loss of calcium from the bones. These athletic young women are then much more susceptible to fractures and may ultimately suffer from osteoporosis.[11] Much of the bone loss may be irreversible.

The elementary years are not too soon to head off tendencies toward eating disorders by promoting a healthy body image, encouraging exercise and activity, and providing factual information about the effects of improper eating patterns. The goal with young people should be fitness, not thinness.

Proteins

As the building blocks of all cells of the body, **proteins** are an indispensable nutrient. First named 150 years ago after the Greek word *proteios* ("of prime importance"), proteins have revealed countless secrets about the way life processes take place. They also account for many nutritional concerns. Proteins are found mostly in muscle tissues, as well as in bones, blood, and body fluids. The box on the next page lists crucial protein functions.

Proteins are made up of strings of amino acids. These **amino acids** contain nitrogen, which is one way that proteins differ from carbohydrates and fats. Nine amino acids cannot be manufactured by the body, so these essential amino acids must be obtained from food. Eleven nonessential amino acids, if not consumed in the diet, are manufactured in the cells in the amounts the body needs.

Proteins have many specific functions:

1. They are used to build tissue.
2. They are used to repair worn-out tissue. (Both of these functions may require extra protein during periods of rapid growth, such as during childhood and after tissue damage.)
3. Some hormones, such as growth hormone, are made from amino acids.
4. Proteins are partially responsible for maintaining proper fluid balance in the body.
5. Proteins can, if necessary, be used for energy if not enough carbohydrates and fats are available. (This will occur when an individual is fasting, eating a very low-calorie diet or a low-carbohydrate diet. It is not, however, considered an ideal source of energy for the body.

Proteins were not designed to be used as a primary energy source. Their main purposes are maintenance, repair, and growth of muscle and other tissues as well as the other functions listed above. Carbohydrates and fats are considered the main sources of energy.

Vegetarians who choose not to consume animal products can meet their protein requirements by eating foods such as grains, legumes, seeds, nuts, and vegetables. The protein needs of children and adults are different, so children should not eat a vegetarian diet without first consulting a medical professional or nutritionist. A vegetarian food guide pyramid (shown in Figure 3.5, page 78) has been developed to help vegetarians with their food choices.

The body's protein needs change depending upon the person's health and growth state. Infants and children, as well as pregnant women, require more protein, as do individuals infected with viruses, bacteria, and other illnesses.

Vitamins

Vitamins are carbon-containing substances that the body must obtain from the diet to maintain health, although only very small amounts are required. Vitamins do not contain any energy, but many help to release the energy stored in the three macronutrients. Vitamins perform a wide variety of functions: Some assist in growth and maintenance by working along with enzymes; others play an active role in supporting the immune system. The regulation of energy metabolism and maintenance in most body systems (see Chapter 2) depends upon various vitamins.

The two major classes of vitamins are water-soluble and fat-soluble. The water-soluble vitamins include the set of B vitamins and vitamin C. The fat-soluble vitamins include vitamins A, D, E, and K. Fat-soluble vitamins are more readily stored in the body, therefore excesses can build up more quickly and reach toxic levels. The body more readily excretes the water-soluble vitamins; therefore toxicity is less likely, but still can result if the vitamin is consumed in large enough quantity.

The issue of vitamin supplementation is extremely controversial. The ideal way for a healthy individual to meet the body's vitamin requirement is to eat a variety of nutritious food daily. The prevailing belief among dietitians and physicians is that the **Recommended Dietary Allowance (RDA)**, set by the Food and Drug Administration, should be the standard for healthy people's energy and nutrient intake. This means that people who eat a balanced diet can get their vitamins from food sources and, preferably, not from a pill.

Minerals

Minerals are essential to health. They are essential to a wide variety of functions, including

1. muscle contraction and relaxation,
2. water and electrolyte balance,
3. metabolism and growth of the body, and
4. the manufacture of genetic chemicals, such as DNA.

Macro-minerals include calcium, phosphorus, potassium, sulfur, sodium, chloride, and magnesium. Microminerals, or **trace minerals**, though no less important, are required in smaller amounts. These include iron, iodine (which may be added to commercial table salt), fluoride (which is added to many community water supplies), zinc, selenium, copper, cobalt, chromium, manganese, and molybdenum. Mineral deficiency has been linked to high blood pressure, cancer, diabetes, tooth decay and osteoporosis (lack of calcium), and anemia (lack of iron).

Of most concern for children at the elementary-age level is iron deficiency anemia, which is relatively common in students. Also, children need sufficient calcium and minerals in general during the growth spurt accompanying puberty. Eating foods from all the food groups daily is the best insurance that an individual is obtaining all of the needed minerals.

Phytochemicals

Food provides us with more than just energy, vitamins, and minerals. A varied diet provides the body with phytochemicals. These chemicals, found in foods of plant origin, are not yet considered essential nutrients, but do have important health functions. A diet high in phytochemicals has been associated with a reduced risk of heart disease, cancer, and many other chronic diseases. There are hundreds of different types of phytochemicals. Eating a diet rich in fruits, vegetables, and whole grains is the best way to ensure a rich intake of these important nutrients.[12]

The following list provides tips to help children increase their intake of fruit, vegetables, and whole grains—and thus of phytochemicals:

- Offer whole grain cereals, breads, and crackers
- Prepare cereal with berries or sliced fruit
- Serve pancakes or waffles with fruit in the batter and on top
- Serve 100 percent fruit juice or vegetable juice instead of soft drinks
- Prepare omelets with vegetables
- Serve yogurt or ice cream with berries on top
- Thicken soups with finely chopped or pureed carrots
- Prepare lasagna with spinach and shredded carrots
- Add different types of vegetables to soups and stews
- Top a baked potato with vegetables and low-fat cheese
- Prepare sandwiches with sprouts, tomatoes, and shredded carrots
- Add dried fruit to rice or stuffing
- Prepare tuna and chicken salad with grated vegetables, raisins, and/or apple chunks
- Offer fresh or dried fruit as snacks instead of chips or candy
- Offer fruit-filled cookies, such as fig, apple, or apricot bars
- Prepare smoothies using frozen bananas and other fruits, fruit juice, non-fat yogurt, and ice cubes

Water

Approximately 60 percent of the body weight consists of water. Bones contain about 20 percent water, and brain tissue is 75 percent water. Water is needed to digest and absorb nutrients, regulate body temperature (especially during exercise), lubricate the joints, remove waste products, transport oxygen and nutrients, and build and repair cells. A loss of even 5 percent of the body's water is called dehydration. A 10 to 15 percent loss can be fatal.

Students should develop the habit of drinking a lot of water—not soda pop or sweetened fruit punches—to maintain optimum health. During exercise sessions, they should take time to replenish the water lost through perspiration.

Most public drinking water supplies in the United States are safe, and the lapses are well publicized. In addition, many families use bottled water.

It should be noted that some bottled water might not contain fluoride, which is necessary to help prevent tooth decay. People who routinely use bottled water should check with their dentist to discuss the best means for their children to obtain the fluoride they need. There are now many other sources of fluoride, including toothpaste, mouthwash, and ready-to-eat infant formulas.

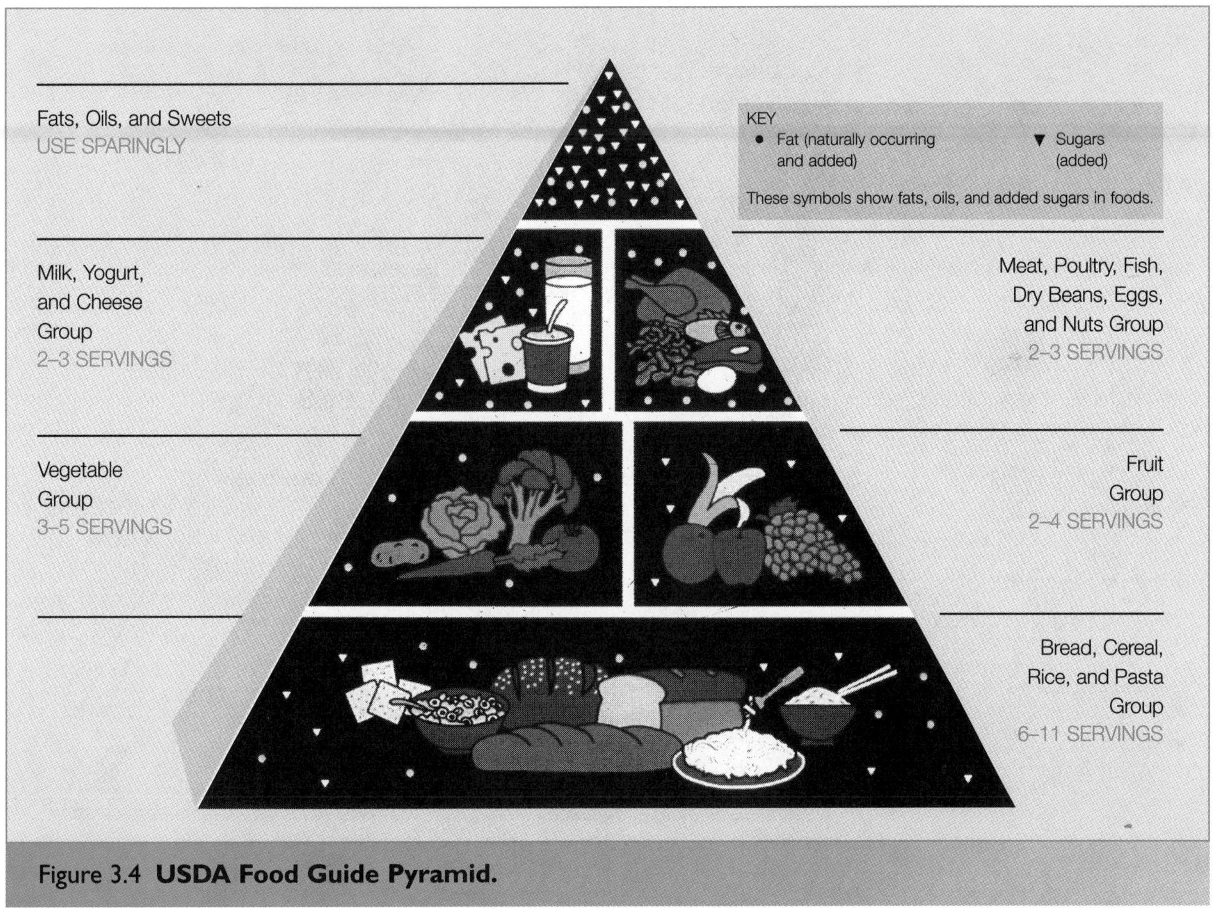

Figure 3.4 **USDA Food Guide Pyramid.**

The Food Guide Pyramids

The Food Guide Pyramid, released by the federal government in 1992, is the official food guide in the United States. This guide follows the principles outlined in the Dietary Guidelines for Americans. The Food Guide Pyramid (see Figure 3.4) gives recommended servings for each of the groups. A person needs to select foods from *all* the food groups daily to obtain the needed nutrients. This conveys one of the strongest messages of the pyramid: variety. The messages of eating food in moderation and avoiding extremes is portrayed in the tip of the pyramid: use fats, oils, and sweets sparingly. The box on the next page shows recommended serving sizes for each food group.

- The bread, cereal, rice, and pasta group forms the base of the pyramid. The recommendation is to eat 6 to 11 servings a day from this group and to select whole grain varieties often.
- The next level contains the fruit and vegetable groups. The foods in these two groups provide the necessary amounts of vitamins A and C, folic acid, and minerals such as iron, potassium, and magnesium. These foods also contain much fiber and little or no fat. The recommendation is to consume 2 to 4 servings of fruit and 3 to 5 servings of vegetables a day.
- Moving up the pyramid, the next category contains meat, fish, dry beans, eggs, and nuts. The foods in this group are essential to getting enough protein, the B vitamins, iron, and zinc. Select 2 to 3 servings from this group for a total of 6 ounces. It is recommended that plant sources of protein, such as beans, be included in the diet on a regular basis.
- In the milk, yogurt, and cheese group, 2 to 3 servings a day are recommended. These products provide calcium, which is particularly important to growing children and teenagers. The recommendation is to choose primarily low-fat and non-fat items.
- The final and smallest group, located at the tip of the pyramid, consists of fats, oils, and sweets. These are to be used sparingly because they provide many calories and few nutrients.

If people follow the recommendations above, their intake of total fat and saturated fat will remain below 30 percent of their caloric intake.

Sample Serving Sizes for Categories in Food Guide Pyramid

Bread, cereal, rice, and pasta

- 1 slice of bread
- 1 oz ready-to-eat cereal
- ½ cup cooked cereal, rice, or pasta
- 1 small tortilla
- ½ bagel

Vegetable

- 1 cup raw leafy vegetable
- ½ cup other vegetables, cooked or chopped raw
- ¾ cup vegetable juice

Fruit

- 1 medium apple, banana, or orange
- ½ cup chopped, cooked, or canned fruit
- ¾ cup fruit juice

Milk, yogurt, and cheese

- 1 cup milk or yogurt
- 1½ oz natural cheese
- 2 oz processed cheese

Meat, poultry, fish, dry beans, eggs, and nuts

- 2–3 oz cooked lean meat, poultry, or fish
- ½ cup cooked dry beans, 1 egg, or 2 tbsp peanut butter counts as 1 oz lean meat
- ⅓ cup of nuts

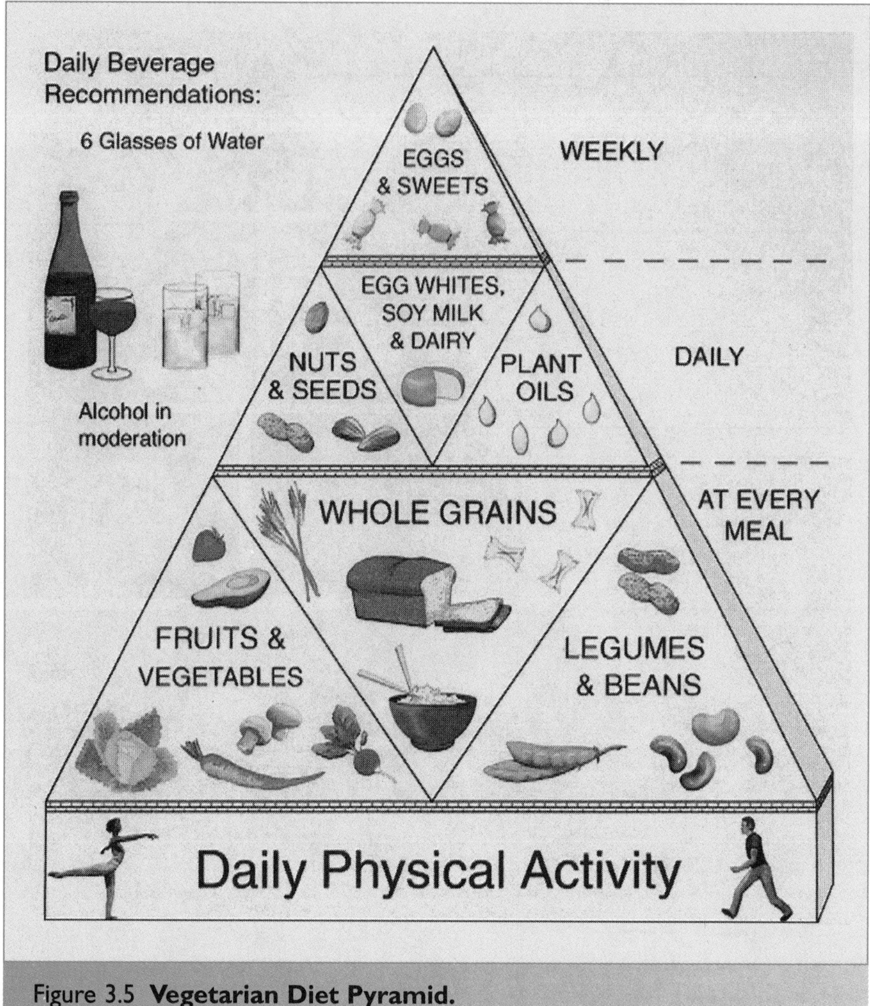

Figure 3.5 **Vegetarian Diet Pyramid.**

The USDA Food Guide Pyramid is based on typical American eating patterns. A variety of other dietary pyramids have been developed for use with various ethnic groups. These include, but are not limited to, the Mediterranean, Asian, Latin American, and vegetarian food pyramids (this is shown in Figure 3.5). Many of these ethnic food guide pyramids were developed by Oldways Preservation and Exchange Trust, a nonprofit company in Cambridge, Massachusetts. These pyramids can help people choose foods that fit a specific ethnic or cultural diet.[13] Educators have a responsibility to develop course materials that address cultural beliefs and preferences regarding food.[14] The pyramid especially for young children is shown in Figure 3.6.

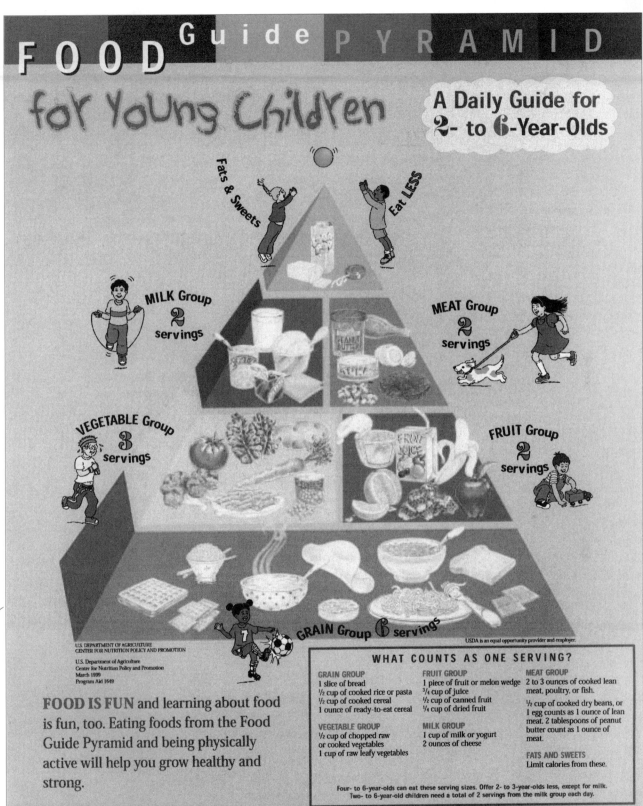

Figure 3.6 **Food Guide Pyramid for young children.**

Cautions in Reading Labels

- Don't be misled by what the manufacturer says on other parts of the product. "Reduced Fat" doesn't mean no fat or low fat.
- Just because a product label says "No Preservatives" doesn't mean other chemicals have not been used in processing.
- When comparing products, make sure to check serving size. A 7-ounce serving will be higher in nutrients simply because it's larger than a 3-ounce serving used by another brand.
- Pull or sell date is the last date on which the product should be sold, assuming that it has been stored and handled properly. The pull date allows for some storage time in the home refrigerator. Coldcuts, milk, ice cream, and refrigerated baked products are examples of foods with pull dates.
- Expiration date is the last date on which the food should be eaten or used. Baby formula and yeast are examples of products that carry an expiration date.
- Freshness date may allow for normal home storage. Some bakery products that have a freshness date are sold at a reduced price for a short time after the date.

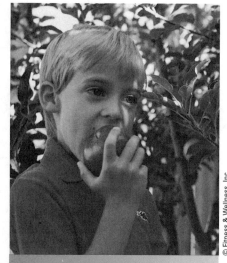

Positive nutrition habits should be taught and reinforced in early youth.

Food Labeling

In response to the Nutrition Labeling and Education Act of 1990, the Food and Drug Administration and the U.S. Department of Agriculture revised the requirements for labels on commercial packaged food products. These rules define a host of permissible nutrient content claims—such as "low fat," "light," "low-sodium," and "high dietary fiber"—and identify permissible health requirements that link diet to health. The intended purpose of the new **food label** is to help consumers choose more healthful diets and to offer incentives to food companies to improve the nutritional qualities of their products. A sample food label is given in Figure 3.7, and the box above contains special cautions about reading food labels.

People can use food labels in planning a healthy diet. In addition, the information on food labels helps people follow a physician's or dietitian's recommendations for a specific diet, such as low-fat or low-sodium, more easily.

Summary

The search for information connecting nutritional intake with health continues. The relationship between specific foods and specific diseases is becoming clearer as the research goes forward. Heart disease, cancer, and diabetes, for example, have been associated with diets high in fat, particularly saturated fat, although exactly how much and in what types of people is not clear. The immune system is affected by nutrition as well. Children with poor nutrition tend to get more respiratory and other infections. They have more serious illnesses and remain sick longer.

A balanced diet seems to be the key to healthy nutrition. It is not difficult to achieve, but it is easily influenced by commercials and advertisements, conflicting food claims, and peer pressure. Thus, maintaining a balanced diet is a product of early experiences and development of sound habits. Teaching children how to achieve a balanced and healthy diet is the challenge of health educators. Classroom teachers and nutritionists can contribute to the quality of their students' eating habits by presenting reliable information in ways that are appropriate and understandable at the various grade levels.

Serving Size
Is your serving the same size as the one on the label? If you eat double the serving size listed, you need to double the nutrient and calorie values. If you eat one-half the serving size shown here, cut the nutrient and calorie values in half.

Calories
Are you overweight? Cut back a little on calories! Look here to see how a serving of the food adds to your daily total. A 5'4", 138-lb. active woman needs about 2,200 calories each day. A 5'10", 174-lb. active man needs about 2,900. How about you?

Total Carbohydrate
When you cut down on fat, you can eat more carbohydrates. Carbohydrates are in foods like bread, potatoes, fruits, and vegetables. Choose these often! They give you more nutrients than **sugars** like soda pop and candy.

Dietary Fiber
Grandmother called it "roughage," but her advice to eat more is still up-to-date! That goes for both soluble and insoluble kinds of dietary fiber. Fruits, vegetables, whole-grain foods, beans and peas are all good sources and can help reduce the risk of heart disease and cancer.

Protein
Most Americans get more protein than they need. Where there is animal protein, there is also fat and cholesterol. Eat small servings of lean meat, fish, and poultry. Use skim or low-fat milk, yogurt, and cheese. Try vegetable proteins like beans, grains, and cereals.

Vitamins & Minerals
Your goal here is 100% of each for the day. Don't count on one food to do it all. Let a combination of foods add up to a winning score.

Nutrition Facts

Serving Size ½ cup (114g)
Servings Per Container 4

Amount Per Serving	
Calories 90	Calories from Fat 30
	% Daily Value*
Total Fat 3g	**5%**
Saturated Fat 0g	**0%**
Cholesterol 0mg	**0%**
Sodium 300mg	**13%**
Total Carbohydrate 13g	**4%**
Dietary Fiber 3g	**12%**
Sugars 3g	
Protein 3g	

Vitamin A	80%	Vitamin C	60%
Calcium	4%	Iron	4%

* Percent Daily Values are based on a 2000 calorie diet. Your daily values may be higher or lower depending on your calorie needs:

	Calories	2000	2500
Total Fat	Less than	65g	80g
Sat Fat	Less than	20g	25g
Cholesterol	Less than	300mg	300mg
Sodium	Less than	2400mg	2400mg
Total Carbohydrate		300g	375g
Fiber		25g	30g

Calories per gram:
Fat 9 • Carbohydrates 4 • Protein 4

More nutrients may be listed on some labels.

Total Fat
Aim low: Most people need to cut back on fat! Too much fat may contribute to heart disease and cancer. Try to limit your **calories from fat.** For a healthy heart, choose foods with a big difference between the total number of calories and the number of calories from fat.

Saturated Fat
A new kind of fat? No — saturated fat is part of the total fat in food. It is listed separately because it's the key player in raising blood cholesterol and your risk of heart disease. Eat less!

Cholesterol
Too much cholesterol — a second cousin to fat — can lead to heart disease. Challenge yourself to eat less than 300 mg each day.

Sodium
You call it "salt," the label calls it "sodium." Either way, it may add up to high blood pressure in some people. So, keep your sodium intake low — 2,400 to 3,000 mg or less each day.*

* The AHA recommends no more than 3,000 mg sodium per day for healthy adults.

Daily Value
Feel like you're drowning in numbers? Let the Daily Value be your guide. Daily Values are listed for people who eat 2,000 or 2,500 calories each day. If you eat more, your personal daily value may be higher than what's listed on the label. If you eat less, your personal daily value may be lower.

For fat, saturated fat, cholesterol and sodium, choose foods with a low **% Daily Value**. For total carbohydrate, dietary fiber, vitamins, and minerals, your daily value goal is to reach 100% of each.

g = grams (About 28 g = 1 ounce)
mg = milligrams (1,000 mg = 1 g)

You Can Rely on the New Label

Rest assured, when you see key words and health claims on product labels, they mean what they say as defined by the government. For example:

Key Words	*What They Mean*
Fat Free	Less than 0.5 gram of fat per serving
Low Fat	3 grams of fat (or less) per serving
Lean	Less than 10 grams of fat, 4 grams of saturated fat and 95 milligrams of cholesterol per serving
Light (Lite)	1/3 less calories or no more than 1/2 the fat of the higher-calorie, higher-fat version; or no more than 1/2 the sodium of the higher-sodium version
Cholesterol Free	Less than 2 milligrams of cholesterol and 2 grams (or less) of saturated fat per serving

To Make Health Claims About . . .	*The Food Must Be . . .*
Heart disease and fats	Low in fat, saturated fat, and cholesterol
Blood pressure and sodium	Low in sodium
Heart disease and fruits, vegetables, and grain products	A fruit, vegetable, or grain product low in fat, saturated fat, and cholesterol, that contains at least 0.6 gram soluble fiber, without fortification, per serving

Other claims may appear on some labels.

Figure 3.7 **Food label: Nutrition facts.**

Resources and Web Sites

Consumer and Professional Organizations

American Anorexia & Bulimia Association
165 West 46th Street #1108
New York, NY 10036
www.members.aol.com/amanbu

American Cancer Society
National Home Office
1599 Clifton Road NE
Atlanta, GA 30329-4251
www.cancer.org

American Dental Association
Division of Communications
211 East Chicago Avenue
Chicago, IL 60611-2678
www.ada.org

American Diabetes Association
1660 Duke Street
Alexandria, VA 22314
www.diabetes.org

American Dietetic Association
216 West Jackson Boulevard
Suite 800
Chicago, IL 60606-6995
www.eatright.org

American School Food Service Association
www.asfsa.org

American Heart Association
Box BHG, National Center
7320 Greenville Avenue
Dallas, TX 75231
www.amhrt.org

American Medical Association
515 North State Street
Chicago, IL 60610
www.ama-assn.org

American Public Health Association
1015 Fifteenth Street NW
Washington, DC 20005
www.apha.org

Center for Science in the Public Interest
1875 Connecticut Avenue, NW
Suite 300
Washington, DC 20009
www.cspinet.org

Consumer Information Center
Department 609K
Pueblo, CO 81009
www.pueblo.gsa.gov

FDA Center for Food Safety and Applied Nutrition
200 C Street SW
Washington, DC 20204
www.vm.cfsan.fda.gov

Food and Nutrition Information Center
National Agricultural Library, Room 304
10301 Baltimore Avenue
Beltsville, MD 20705-2351
www.nal.usda.gov/fnic

Daily Apple—Your Expert Guide to Total Health
www.thedailyapple.com/index.htm

National Council Against Health Fraud
P.O. Box 1276
Loma Linda, CA 92354
www.ncahf.org

Society for Nutrition Education
1001 Connecticut Ave. NW
Suite 528
Washington, DC 20036-5528
www.jne.org

Journals and Newsletters

American Council Digest
Berkeley Wellness Letter
Contemporary Nutrition
CNI Nutrition Week
Environmental Nutrition
Harvard Medical School Health Letter
Journal of the American Dietetic Association
Journal of Canadian Dietetic Association
American Journal of Clinical Nutrition
Lancet
Journal of the American Medical Association (JAMA)
Journal of Nutrition Education
Nutrition Action Health Letter
Nutrition Today
Nutrition and the M.D.
Nutrition Research Newsletter
Nutrition Reviews
Tufts University Health and Nutrition Letter

Trade Organizations

General Mills
Nutrition Department
Number One General Mills Boulevard
Minneapolis, MN 55426
www.generalmills.com

Kellogg Company
P.O. Box 3599
Battle Creek, MI 49016-3599
www.kelloggs.com

Mead Johnson Nutritionals
2400 West Lloyd Expressway
Evansville, IN 47721
www.meadjohnson.com

Nabisco Consumer Affairs
100 DeForest Avenue
East Hanover, NJ 07936
www.nabisco.com

Pillsbury Company
Consumer Relations
P.O. Box 550
Minneapolis, MN 55440-9843
www.pillsbury.com

Procter and Gamble Company
One Procter and Gamble Plaza
Cincinnati, OH 45202
www.pg.com/info

Ross Laboratories
Director of Professional Services
625 Cleveland Avenue
Columbus, OH 43215
www.abbot.com

United Fresh Fruit and Vegetable Association
727 North Washington Street
Alexandria, VA 22314
(703) 836-3410

Additional Health and Nutrition Web Sites

5 A Day for Better Health
www.5aday.com

Anorexia Nervosa and Related Eating Disorders (ANRED)
www.anred.com

Healthy People 2010
www.health.gov/healthypeople/document/default.htm

Kids Food Cyber Club
www.kidsfood.org

Kids Cart Smart Food Choices at Home, Shopping and Eating Out
www.ext.vt.edu/pubs/preschoolnutr/348-652/348-652.html

Medline
www.nlm.nih.gov/databases/freemedl.html

The Tufts University Nutrition Navigator
www.navigator.tufts.edu

US Government Healthfinder
www.healthfinder.gov

USDA Dietary Guidelines
www.nal.usda.gov/fnic/dga

USDA Food Guide Pyramid
www.nal.usda.gov/fnic/Fpyr/pyramid.html

Notes

1. D. Turner, *Handbook of Diet Therapy,* 5th ed. (Chicago: University of Chicago Press, 1970).
2. "Nutrition and Your Health: Dietary Guidelines for Americans," 5th ed. *Home and Garden Bulletin* No. 232 (Washington, DC: U. S. Depts. of Agriculture and Health and Human Services, 2000).
3. *Healthy People 2010: National Health Promotion and Disease Prevention Objectives* (Washington, DC: U. S. Department of Health and Human Services, 2000).
4. WHO Study Group on Diet, "Nutrition and Prevention of Noncommunicable Diseases: Diet, Nutrition and the Prevention of Chronic Diseases," *Nutrition Reviews* 49 (1991): 291–301.
5. A. Ascherio and W. C. Willett, "Health Effects of Trans Fatty Acids," *American Journal of Clinical Nutrition* 66 (1997): 1006S–1010S.
6. WHO and FAL Joint Consultation, "Fats and Oils in Human Nutrition," *Nutrition Reviews* 53 (1995): 202–205.
7. R. J. Levi, "Carbohydrates in Modern Nutrition" in *Health and Disease*, 9th ed., edited by M. E. Shils et al. (Baltimore: Williams & Wilkins, 1999).
8. M. Noakes and P.M. Clifton "Oil Blends Containing Partially Hydrogenated Fats: Differential Effects on Plasma Lipids," *American Journal of Clinical Nutrition* 68 (1998): 242–247.
9. A. E. Becker, "Eating Disorders," *New England Journal of Medicine* 340 (1999): 1092.
10. G. C. Patton, R. Selzer, C. Coffey, J. B. Carlin, and R. Wolfe, "Onset of Adolescent Eating Disorders: Population Based Cohort Study over 3 Years," *British Medical Journal* 318, no. 7186 (1999) 765–778.
11. M. L. Rencken, C. H. Chestnut, and B. L. Drinkwater, "Bone Density at Multiple Skeletal Sites in Amenorrheic Athletes," *Journal of the American Medical Association* 276 (1996): 238–240.
12. W. J. Craig, "Phytochemicals: Guardians of Our Health," *Journal of the American Dietetic Association* 97, suppl. 2 (1997): S199.
13. C. Davis, P. Britten, and E. Meyers, "Past, Present and Future of the Food Guide Pyramid," *Journal of the American Dietetic Association* 101, no. 8 (2001): 881–885.
14. American Dietetic Association, "How to Put the Food Guide Pyramid into Practice," *Journal of the American Dietetic Association* 94 (1994): 1030–1035.

Learning Experiences

Although children are resilient and able to bounce back from most noxious influences, studies strongly suggest that their eating habits can affect their ability to concentrate and learn; energy level, self-control, resistance to ordinary illnesses, and athletic ability; as well as their overall stamina and growth. Understanding the basics of nutrition and its contribution to overall health and well-being enables elementary school students to make sound decisions about food choices and to contribute to wise family meal planning at home.

Grades K–2

Children at this level benefit from a hands-on learning experience. The activities suggested teach the relationship between healthy food choices and overall health. The evaluation strategies allow students to apply their new knowledge of nutrition to their lifestyle. By the end of the activities on nutrition, students should be able to

1. identify the types of food that constitute a healthy snack and those that contribute unwanted calories;
2. describe the sensations of tasting, feeling, and smelling foods as applied to trying new foods;
3. identify the role of television and advertising in promoting healthy versus unhealthy eating;
4. describe the role of foods in fueling the body for growth;
5. identify the reason for differences in growth patterns;
6. recognize the importance of eating breakfast;
7. identify the various nutrients in food that help people to grow and stay healthy.

Grades 3–4

In these grades, students understand the various factors that influence their food choices. They recognize the similarities and differences between themselves and their families and other individuals in the community. Students in these grades comprehend the link between eating high-calorie foods and gaining weight. By the end of activities on nutrition, students in grades 3 and 4 should be able to

1. identify reasons for making various food choices (for example, taste, economics, nutrient content);

2. describe the differences and similarities in the cultural food heritage of classmates;
3. identify the components of a balanced meal along with the daily requirement for each, as shown in the Food Guide Pyramid;
4. identify the energy-yielding nutrients (fat, carbohydrate, protein) and their basic functions within the body;
5. identify the relationship between energy input and expenditure, focusing on excess caloric intake and its possible effects;
6. evaluate their caloric intake for a specific meal, identifying high- and low-calorie foods.

Grades 5–6

In grades 5 and 6, students continue to discover the connection between their bodies and the nutrients supplied by foods. They distinguish between the need to incorporate various foods into their daily eating patterns and the desire to eat certain foods based solely on taste. Students become aware of the agricultural industry and its contribution to the history and economy of the United States. They are able to apply their knowledge of nutrition to enriching their health. By the end of activities on nutrition, fifth and sixth graders should be able to:

1. describe body cells' need for nutrients;
2. identify some of the nutrients in various foods and the need to eat a variety of foods;
3. explain the importance of water to the body and estimate water content in various foods;
4. identify different sources of sugar in foods by reading labels;
5. describe the effects of sugar on the body and teeth.

One strategy for evaluating an entire interdisciplinary unit is to have the students collect all of the learning experiences in one folder, or portfolio. This portfolio of work can be graded as a whole, or the activities can be graded individually. It is a good idea to develop lists of the materials you would expect to find in the portfolio and a rubric of criteria that you would use to grade the quality of the materials.

Rubrics can identify groups, individuals, or one entire project. They should be provided before the unit begins so the students can decide the level of work they must do for the grade they are hoping to achieve. For suggestions on creating a rubric with which to evaluate student performance of Learning Experiences, see page 13.

Learning Experience 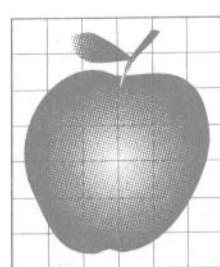 3-1

Different Tastes and Smells

Grade Level

K–2

Primary Disciplines

Science, Language Arts

Learning Objectives

Following this activity, students will be able to identify three of the five senses by tasting a variety of food samples.

Time Required

30 minutes

Materials

Shoebox, bowl, blindfolds, various foods

Description of Activity

1. Select a shoebox or other appropriate container.
2. Select one food to put in the box.
3. Blindfold a student and have him/her reach into the box and feel the food.
4. Give each student a turn to touch the food. [*Caution:* Food that is handled should not be eaten.]
5. Discuss the answers to the following questions: What is the shape of the food? Is it hard or soft? Bumpy or smooth? What do you think it is?
6. Discuss the importance of the sense of smell to the sense of taste.
7. Place in a bowl various foods with distinctive smells, such as apple slice, piece of orange, piece of onion segment, celery leaf, banana slice, and pineapple chunk.
8. Have the students wear blindfolds and see how many of the foods they can identify by smell.
9. Discuss students' favorite foods and how they smell.
10. Introduce new vocabulary words that describe the taste, texture, and temperature of foods. Have students describe various foods using new vocabulary words. For example:

sweet — sugar
sour — lemon
sticky — peanut butter
chewy — raisin
dry — cracker
crispy — apple
crunchy — celery
cold — water
juicy — watermelon
hot — hamburger
solid — cheese
liquid — juice
hard — carrot
soft — mashed potatoes

Homework

Students could bring in pictures of food cut out of magazines to use for items 9 and 10.

Evaluation

Students will be able to identify a variety of foods by smell or taste. They will explain how smell and vision affects their attitudes about food. They will be able to do the following:

- Explain how smell and vision affect their attitudes about food.
- Differentiate colors using food items.
- Recognize how vocabulary words are associated with foods.
- Describe attributes of foods including smell, taste, texture, temperature.
- Recognize different foods from advertisements.

Learning Experience 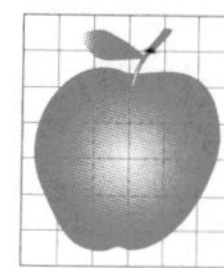 3-2

Healthy Snacks

Grade Level

K–2

Primary Disciplines

Language Arts, Math

Learning Objectives

Following this activity, students will be able to identify nutritious foods by creating a healthy snack.

Time Required

30 minutes

Materials

Celery, peanut butter, raisins, handout

Description of Activity

The teacher and students create the healthy snack called "ants on a log."

1. Stuff celery stalks with peanut butter and place raisins on top.
2. Have each child count the raisins.

Homework

The students will bring in the food items.

Evaluation

Students will be able to

- Demonstrate simple addition skills.
- Differentiate healthy snacks from unhealthy snacks.

Dear Parent,

Your child will be learning about foods and how proper choices can keep us healthy. The following are some suggestions for nutritious snacks. Please review them with your child and eat some of them together:

fruit: bananas, apple slices, orange slices, grapes

low-fat cheeses with crackers

peanut butter with breadsticks

unbuttered popcorn

frozen fruit juice desserts

yogurt with added fresh fruit

milk shakes with added fresh fruit, such as bananas or strawberries

home-made oatmeal or peanut butter cookies

Thank you.

Learning Experience 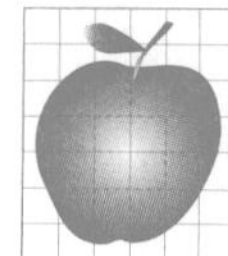 3-3

Food Bingo

Grade Level

K–2

Primary Discipline

Language Arts

Learning Objectives

Following this activity, students will be able to recognize the beginning letter of the names of healthy foods.

Time Required

15 minutes

Materials

Bingo cards and beans or similar food item to be used as markers

Description of Activity

Each student receives a bingo card with various letters on it and beans to cover the letters. The teacher calls out the name of a healthy food (such as "Apple"). The students cover the appropriate beginning letter of the food on his/her bingo card.

Homework

Students will draw pictures of healthy foods beginning with C, D, E.

Evaluation

Students will name three healthy foods beginning with the letters, A, B, C (e.g., apple, banana, carrot). They will also be able to

- Replicate the shapes of various foods.
- Recognize the letters of the alphabet.
- Recognize the correct spellings of foods appropriate to grade level.
- Distinguish healthy foods from other foods.

Learning Experience 3-4

TV Commercials

Grade Level

K–2

Primary Discipline

Language Arts

Learning Objectives

Following this activity, students will be able to classify as healthy or unhealthy foods they see in TV commercials.

Time Required

1½ hours (at home)

Materials

Watching TV at home, handout

Description of Activity

The teacher sends the handout "Children and Television" home with the students. The students are asked to watch one hour of children's afternoon or weekend-morning television with an adult. The parent or child will make a list, to be brought into school, of all the food commercials viewed. The teacher can have the students talk about the foods they saw on television.

Homework

List of foods from TV commercials to be brought into class.

Evaluation

Students will identify subjects of homework commercials as healthy or unhealthy foods. They will be able to

- Identify foods from frequently watched TV.
- Distinguish healthy foods from unhealthy foods in advertisements.

Children and Television

You can help control the effect that television has on your child by doing the following things:

- Watch TV with your child.
- Discuss why you approve or disapprove of items advertised on TV programs.
- Limit the amount of time and the programs your child watches on TV.
- Help and encourage your child to do activities other than watching TV. Play games, cook, draw, and read together.

Learning Experience 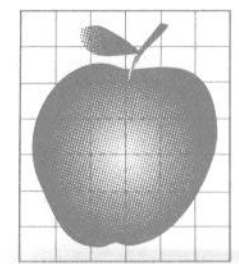 3-5

Food and Energy

Grade Level

K–2

Primary Discipline

Science

Learning Objectives

Following this activity, students will be able to state the importance of eating foods to fuel their body for activity and growth.

Time Required

30–45 minutes

Materials

Magazines, paper, crayons

Description of Activity

1. Collect pictures of cars, trucks, boats, and planes, and of children playing, eating, and sleeping.
2. Discuss with the students what each picture illustrates.

Questions for Discussion

- What do cars, trucks, boats, and planes use for fuel? (A: Gasoline or diesel fuel)
- What happens when a car runs out of fuel? (A: It won't go.)
- What do you use for fuel to make your body go? (A: Food)
- What happens if you do not eat food? (A: You get tired and hungry and don't have any energy.)
- Why? (A: Food gives you energy to work and play just as gasoline gives cars energy to go.)
- Which pictures show children using the most energy? The least?
- What happens if you eat too much? (A: You feel too full or maybe even get sick. You can also get fat.)
- Point out that eating too much can give us more fuel than we can use immediately, so it is stored as body fat. Exercise helps us use extra food energy. If we don't exercise, the fuel is stored as body fat.

Homework

The students might bring in the pictures named previously, cut from magazines.

Evaluation

Students demonstrate three activities that require a lot of energy from food and three activities that do not require as much food energy. They are able to

- Explain the importance of food and exercise.
- Describe what happens to food when it is not used as energy.
- Identify activities that require energy.
- Distinguish between activities that require a lot of energy and those that require little energy.

Source: *Nutrition Comes Alive*, Level 1, Division of Nutritional Sciences, Cornell University, 1986. Reprinted with permission.

Learning Experience 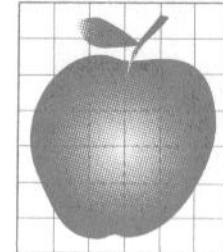 3-6

Pulse Rate Related to Energy

Grade Level

K–2

Primary Discipline

Science

Learning Objectives

Following this activity, students will be able to describe the relationship between activity and energy and what happens when a person exerts energy.

Time Required

45 minutes

Materials

Stop watch

Description of Activity

Students can see how exercise affects the amount of energy their bodies use by feeling their pulse.

1. Ask the students to locate a pulse point by placing three fingers by the side of their windpipe. Explain that what they feel is their heart pumping blood.
2. Time them for 10 seconds and have them count the number of beats they feel. Ask them to write down this number.
3. Have them jump in place 25 times.
4. Have them again take their pulse for 10 seconds and record the number of beats. Did their number increase? By how much?
5. Explain that as they moved faster, their hearts pumped faster and used more energy. The energy came from food they had eaten.
6. Ask the students to name some of their favorite activities. Which ones require a lot of energy? Which require little? Point out that high-energy activities use arms and legs for action.
7. Make a list on the board of high- and low-energy activities.

Homework

Students will record all their exercise for 1 week:

	Amount of Time	**Type of of Exercise**
S	____________	____________
M	____________	____________
T	____________	____________
W	____________	____________
TH	____________	____________
F	____________	____________
S	____________	____________

Evaluation

Students will name three activities that cause their heart to pump faster and thereby utilize more energy. They will be able to

- Describe how to take a pulse.
- Explain what a pulse rate measures.
- Describe how the pulse rate changes with activity.
- Explain how pulse rate and the body's use of energy relate to one another.
- Differentiate activities that require a lot of energy from those that require little energy.

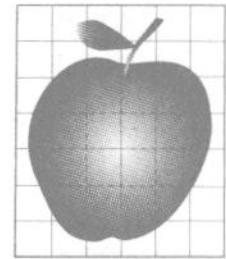

Learning Experience 3-7

Energy from Breakfast

Grade Level

3–4

Primary Disciplines

Health, Math

Learning Objectives

Following this activity, students will be able to state the important contribution that breakfast makes to early morning energy.

Time Required

30 minutes

Materials

Wall clock or hand-held clock, handout

Description of Activity

Use of a clock will help students determine how many hours pass between the last time they eat in the evening and breakfast the next morning, between breakfast and lunch, between lunch and dinner, and between meals and snacks.

1. On the chalkboard write the average number of hours between the meals throughout the day. Emphasize that because of the long stretch between dinner or evening snacks and breakfast, the body gets low in food energy. To have energy for work and play, breakfast is important.
2. Ask the students to name foods they eat for breakfast. Include foods not usually associated with breakfast, such as a piece of cold pizza or, as well as the more usual cereal, eggs, toast, and the like. Assure them that foods eaten for dinner or lunch can also be eaten for breakfast.
3. List the foods on the chalkboard and ask the class to raise hands to show how many have ever eaten each food for breakfast. Record the number of responses for each food.
4. Have the students think of alternative breakfast ideas. Explain that combinations of nutritious foods other than just the so-called breakfast foods can give us good breakfast energy. To avoid a mid-morning slump, students should eat at least one food high in protein, such as peanut butter, milk, cheese, or egg. Also foods that are high in sugar (doughnuts, sweet rolls) and foods high in fat and sodium (bacon and sausage) are not as healthy.

Homework

Handout is sent home to family emphasizing the importance of breakfast. The students should be familiar with what it says and discuss the points in class.

Evaluation

Students will be able to

- Describe the time lapse between meals, including overnight.
- Explain the importance of the breakfast meal to body energy.
- Identify healthy breakfast foods.
- Describe their own eating habits and distinguish healthy ones from unhealthy ones.

Source: *Nutrition Comes Alive*, Level 2, Division of Nutritional Sciences, Cornell University, 1986. Reprinted with permission.

Dear Parent,

We have been talking in class about the importance of breakfast for energy in the morning. Why is breakfast so important? Scientific research shows that eating food in the morning helps a child stay more mentally alert and physically efficient throughout the morning hours. Skipping or skimping on a morning meal can lead to a low blood sugar level, which can bring on feelings of hunger called "mid-morning slump."

The body breaks down foods into glucose, a basic nutrient that blood carries to cells for growth and maintenance. A morning meal that includes both protein and carbohydrate or starch helps maintain blood glucose above the fasting level. Blood glucose falls to a fasting level several hours after we eat. If we do not eat, the level dips farther, forcing the body to draw on its stored sources of energy.

Many foods can supply the carbohydrates and protein the body needs. We need to learn to eat combinations of foods that will supply our needs and help us to avoid a mid-morning slump. Examples of good breakfast choices are:

1. Milk with a peanut-butter sandwich
2. Unsweetened cereal and yogurt topped with fruit
3. Grapefruit juice and leftover pizza slice
4. Orange slices, toast, and cottage cheese
5. Apple slices, peanut butter, bagel, milk
6. Banana milkshake and toast
7. Milk, English muffin with melted cheese and tomato slice, peach

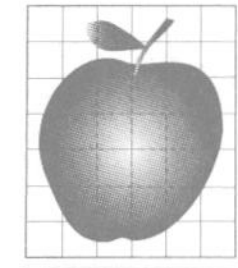

Learning Experience 3-8

Charting Personal Growth

Grade Level

3–4

Primary Discipline

Math

Learning Objectives

Following this activity, students will be able to identify the relationship of food to growth pattern.

Time Required

45 minutes

Materials

Scale (for weighing students), tape measure, large sheet of roll paper

Description of Activity

Introduction

Ask these questions:

- How can you tell you are growing? (A: Clothes are smaller, you weigh more, shoes don't fit, hair and nails get longer.)
- What helps you grow? (A: Food.)
- Does everyone grow at the same rate? (A: People grow differently and at different stages.)

Activity

The students will weigh themselves and measure their height. They make a chart recording the students' measurements. The activity is repeated every 2 or 3 months, followed by a discussion of the changes in growth.

1. Attach a large piece of paper to the wall so that students can line up and mark their height on the paper.
2. Students will create a bar graph on the paper by drawing vertical bars downward and labeling with their names.
3. They each weigh themselves and make a bar next to the height bar, in a different color, representing their weight.

Discussion

- What is the difference in inches between the tallest and shortest students?
- Which students are the same height?
- Are those students the same weight? Why?

Homework

Students will make a bar graph representing the heights of three members of their family.

Evaluation

Students will be able to

- Explain how food relates to growth.
- Describe the signs of body growth.
- Explain why people grow at different rates.
- Recognize that height is not always associated with body weight.
- Use bar graphs to describe growth patterns.

Source: *Nutrition Comes Alive*, Level 1, Division of Nutritional Sciences, Cornell University, 1986. Reprinted with permission.

Learning Experience 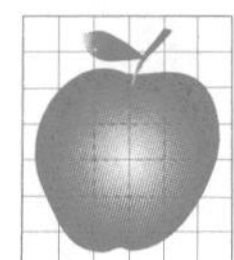 3-9

Invisible Goodness

Grade Level

3–4

Primary Disciplines

Science, Language Arts

Learning Objectives

Following this activity, students will be able to identify the roles of various nutrients in the body.

Time Required

30–45 minutes

Materials

Glass of water, lemon juice, brown paper towels, potato chips, oranges

Description of Activity

Students are introduced to the concept that foods are mixtures of substances called nutrients. The two parts of this activity are:

1. Show the students a glass of water with lemon juice in it. Ask if they can see the lemon juice. Explain that the lemon juice is like nutrients in food. They are there, even though we can't see them. Write the word "nutrient" on the board. Explain that nutrients in food help people to grow and have energy for working and playing.
2. Test for fat: Give each student a brown paper towel, a potato chip, and an orange section. Have them tear the paper towel in half and write "potato chip" on one half and "orange" on the other half. Rub each food on the paper until it leaves a spot. Let the papers dry, then hold them up to the light. If the food contains fat, a translucent spot will appear and light will shine through. Water (and orange juice) produces a translucent spot, but the spot disappears when it dries. A fat spot will not disappear.

Discussion

Which food contains fat? (A: Potato chip). Fat is a source of energy, which you need to work and play. Many foods provide energy. People often get too much energy from foods and not enough important nutrients such as iron. You have to choose foods carefully to get enough nutrients and not too much fat. Too many fatty foods can also contribute to health problems, such as heart disease, later in life.

Homework

Students will bring in three food labels from commercial foods that contain more than 10 grams of fat per serving.

Evaluation

Students will be able to

- Define nutrient.
- Explain how nutrients relate to growth and energy.
- Define fats and identify foods with large amounts of fats.
- Explain how fats relate to energy.
- Explain how to read a label for fat content and identify how much fat is healthy and how much is not healthy.

Source: *Nutrition Comes Alive*, Level 2, Division of Nutritional Sciences, Cornell University, 1986. Reprinted with permission.

Learning Experience 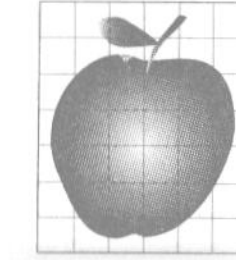 3-10

The Classroom Store

Grade Level

3–4

Primary Disciplines

Math, Health

Learning Objectives

Following this activity, students will be able to exchange play money and identify healthy foods.

Time Required

30–60 minutes

Materials

Pictures of food, poster paper for signs and price tags, construction paper for play money

Description of Activity

Using the materials brought from home, students label each food item with a price. The students can make signs for the "store," stating special prices of food (4 oranges for $1.00). The students make play money for use in the store.

1. Set up a corner of the classroom as the store.
2. Have students take turns being the cashier as well as the customer.
3. Ask the students to read food labels on the empty containers.

Questions for Discussion

- What types of food did you choose to buy? Why?
- How do you know what is in the food?
- If the oranges are 25 cents each, how many can you get for $1.00 (or whatever is applicable)? Review the exchange of money.

Homework

Preceding the activity, students collect pictures of fresh fruit and vegetables and bring these to school along with a clean, empty food carton or container.

Evaluation

Students are given $1.00 of play money each. They must go to the "Classroom Store" and purchase healthy items equaling approximately $1.00.

Additional Criteria

Students are able to

- Identify healthy foods in a grocery store.
- Identify prices of foods.
- Read food labels.
- Select healthier foods instead of unhealthy foods with limited money.
- Explain how many of the same items or how many different items one could purchase with a given amount of money.

Learning Experience 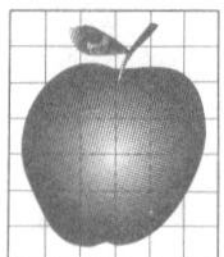 3-11

Dinner at My House

Grade Level

3–4

Primary Discipline

Health

Learning Objectives

Following this activity, students will be able to identify various reasons for making food choices.

Time Required

45 minutes

Materials

Paper and pencils, handout

Description of Activity

Introduction

Why do we make the food choices we do? We have many reasons for selecting different foods. When we're young, we are often affected by taste and what is familiar to us. These choices may be very different from home to home.

Activity

On the back of the handout,

1. Ask students to list all the foods and beverages they consumed during the evening meal the day before.
2. Have several students name some of the foods on their lists. Record these foods on the chalkboard.
3. Have the entire class try to guess why the students chose these foods. Record possible reasons on the board.
4. Have the students match the examples with the general reasons on the handout.

Examples from Students	*General Reasons*
We always have it.	habit
It's Dad's favorite.	family favorite
You need to have vegetables.	nutritional value
It gives you energy.	nutritional value
My mother works.	limited time
It costs less than a roast.	cost
It tastes good.	taste
It's easy to cook.	ease of preparation

5. Help the students see that the reasons they gave match up with the general reasons for food choices on the handout list.

Homework

To personalize food choices at home, the students pick one food from the family meal they listed on the back of their worksheet and write it at the top of the handout. After everyone has completed the handout, the class will report on the following:

- What factors were important to you?
- How might your answers change if you had chosen another food?
- Is your rating similar to those of other students, or are your reasons for food choices very different?

Evaluation

Students will be able to

- Identify factors that determine why people choose the foods they eat.
- Identify the foods they eat and the reasons for eating them.
- Discuss how the reasons people eat certain foods relate to a healthy or an unhealthy diet.

Reasons for Selecting Foods

Pick one of the foods from the list of foods you ate last night. For each of the reasons listed, circle 1, 2, or 3 to indicate how important that reason was to you for eating that food.

Name of Food Selected ______________________________

Reasons for Food Choice	*Very Important*	*Somewhat Important*	*Not Very Important*
1. Taste	1	2	3
2. Smell	1	2	3
3. Color	1	2	3
4. Texture	1	2	3
5. Nutritional value	1	2	3
6. Family favorite	1	2	3
7. Habit	1	2	3
8. Parent's advice	1	2	3
9. Cost	1	2	3
10. Ease of preparation	1	2	3
11. Time of day	1	2	3
12. To try something new	1	2	3

Learning Experience 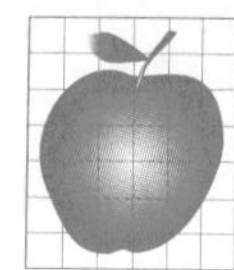 3-12

International Meal

Grade Level

3–4

Primary Discipline

Social Studies

Learning Objectives

Following this activity, students will be able to identify differences and similarities in the cultural food heritage represented in the class.

Time Required

45 minutes

Materials

Paper plates, forks, napkins, handout

Description of Activity

Students bring in one food reflecting their cultural heritage to share with the class. Preferably, the students bring the recipe as well.

Questions for Discussion

- What country is the food originally from?
- Is the recipe from a parent, a grandparent, or someone else?
- Do you eat the food at a certain holiday, or is it part of your typical meal?

Homework

See the handout.

Evaluation

Students will be able to

- Identify food staples that are used in several different countries, such as rice, pasta/noodles, corn meal, and various kinds of beans (soybeans, lentils, pintos, garbanzos).
- Describe the relationship between culture and diet.
- Identify foods that people from their own culture eat often.
- Identify common foods in U.S. culture.
- Identify food staples from various cultures.

Dear Parent,

We are currently studying the cultural heritage of the students in our class. We are tying this unit into the study of nutrition. Each student is requested to bring in a food reflecting his/her ethnic background. Have your child help make the food so he/she may tell the class about how the food is prepared and the ingredients that are used. Please let me know which day you will be able to do this.

____

Thank you for your cooperation.

Learning Experience 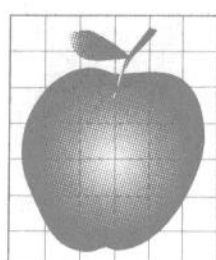 3-13

Food Guide Pyramid

Grade Level

3–4

Primary Discipline

Health and Nutrition

Learning Objectives

Following this activity, students will be able to identify the various foods in the food groups and categorize them according to the Food Guide Pyramid.

Time Required

30–45 minutes

Materials

Food Guide Pyramid poster, pictures of foods

Description of Activity

From a Food Guide Pyramid posted in the room, the class reviews the basic food groups. They affix pictures of the various foods to the appropriate place on the pyramid.

Questions for Discussion

- How many students had food in the bread group? fruit? vegetable? and so on.
- How many students eat foods from all the food groups daily?
- Explain the importance of eating a variety of food on a daily basis to meet vitamin and nutrient requirements.

Homework

The students bring pictures of various foods, cut out of magazines.

Evaluation

Students will be able to

- Identify foods in each group in the pyramid.
- Identify foods they commonly eat.
- Identify the foods groups they usually eat from and those they omit.
- Explain the importance of eating from all of the food groups regularly.
- Describe how they can change their diet to include foods from each group.

Learning Experience 3-14

Planning a Healthy Meal

Grade Level

3–4

Primary Discipline

Health

Learning Objectives

Following this activity, students will be able to construct a balanced meal by choosing appropriate foods.

Time Required

30 minutes

Materials

Pictures of various foods representing all of the food groups, dinner plate

Description of Activity

Each student plans a nutritious meal for breakfast, lunch, or dinner. The student chooses from the pictures of food and arranges them on the plate.

1. Each student plans a nutritious meal for breakfast, lunch, or dinner. The student chooses from the pictures of food and arranges them on the plate.
2. In groups of five or six, students plan a full day's menu. They explain their choices.

Questions for Discussion

- Why is this a healthy meal?
- Does it include various foods from the Food Guide Pyramid?

Homework

The students find pictures of various foods in magazines and bring them to school.

Evaluation

Students are able to identify foods for breakfast, lunch, and dinner that ensure a healthy diet according to the food categories in the pyramid.

Learning Experience 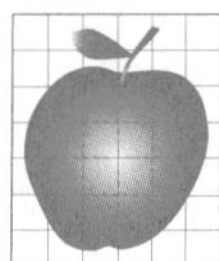 3-15

Energy Experiments

Grade Level

5–6

Primary Discipline

Science

Learning Objectives

Following this activity, students will be able to identify the specific energy-yielding nutrient, fat, and carbohydrate.

Time Required

1 hour

Materials

Small amounts of bread, cheese, cracker, potato chips, carrot, walnut, macaroni, cooking oil, box of toothpicks (or cotton swabs), several brown paper towels or bags cut into 3" × 4" squares, two eyedroppers, a vial of iodine.

Description of Activity

Introduction

Six nutrients are vital to health: fat, carbohydrate, protein, vitamins, minerals, and water. Three of these nutrients—fat, carbohydrate, and protein—provide the energy we need to live, move, and grow. Protein is used primarily for growth and repair, and our bodies rely mainly on fat and carbohydrate as the main sources of energy.

Activity

The class is divided into four groups of six or seven students each. Two groups will do a test to determine whether food samples contain fat. The other two groups will test food samples for carbohydrate. Each group sets up a workstation to conduct their experiment.

Focus on Fat

1. The students label a sheet of paper to match Energy Experiment diagram (on page 112) on which to record their findings.
2. Each student labels paper squares with the names of the foods to be tested.
3. They take turns dipping a toothpick or cotton swab in cooking oil and touching it to the square of brown paper or paper toweling labeled "cooking oil."
4. After waiting 2 or 3 minutes, they hold up the paper to a light and observe and record the results.
5. The students test the remaining food samples by rubbing each one on the paper square labeled with the name of the food. They need to let the paper dry before recording the results because water will evaporate but fat will leave a spot.
6. The students think of other foods that might also leave a fat spot. Although many high fat foods are easy to identify, the fat content of some other foods is hidden. Foods with hidden fat include whole milk, whole milk products, luncheon meats, and many highly processed snack foods and desserts.

Focus on Carbohydrates

Explain that iodine is a chemical that tests for the presence of starch in foods. If starch is present, the iodine changes from red-brown to blue-black. Stress that they must work carefully because iodine is a poison and can stain hands and clothing.

1. The students label a sheet of paper to record their findings, as indicated in the diagram.
2. The students place two drops of iodine on each food sample and record the results. (Emphasize that the greater the color change, the more starch is present. Have students think of other foods that might yield

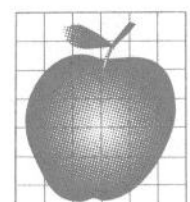

Learning Experience 3-15 continued

positive results when tested with iodine. Breads, cereals, macaroni products, and foods made with flour are high in starch.)

3. Sugar (sucrose) is another form of carbohydrate. The iodine test does not work for this form of carbohydrate. Students name foods that contain sugar. They may think of sweets, soda, and candy. (Tell them that fruits also contain sugar in the form of fructose. Both fructose and sucrose are carbohydrates.)

Homework

Students will bring in three food labels from foods containing fat and three labels from foods containing carbohydrates.

Evaluation

Students from the two groups share their results with the entire class and are able to explain why they occurred. In addition, they can do the following:

- Identify each of the nutrients vital to health.
- Explain what purpose each nutrient plays in healthy body functioning.
- Identify foods that provide each of the nutrients.
- Perform simple tests on foods to determine the presence of fats and carbohydrates.
- Identify and explain nutrients from food labels.

Energy Experiment

Fat

Food	Spot	No Spot

Carbohydrates

Food	Changed Color	Did Not Change Color

Learning Experience 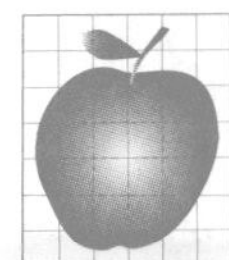 3-16

Food Across America

Grade Level

5–6

Primary Discipline

Social Studies

Learning Objectives

Following this activity, students will be able to identify foods that are indigenous to various states across the country.

Time Required

Variable

Materials

Large map of the United States

Description of Activity

1. Assign one state to each student.
2. Have students prepare a report to present to the class, including information about agriculture and foods for which the state is known (Idaho potatoes, for example) and the food group the particular food falls into.
3. Have the student identify the state on the map.

Homework

Research of assigned state in reference books or on computer, with any appropriate illustrations.

Evaluation

Students will be able to

- Identify one food product from five separate states.
- Locate the mentioned states on a map.
- Identify the food group that the food product belongs to.

Learning Experience 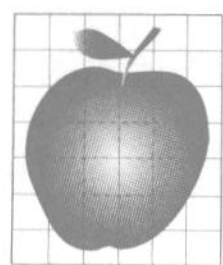 3-17

Sugar Is Sweet and . . .

Grade Level

5–6

Primary Discipline

Science

Learning Objectives

Following this activity, students will be able to identify the various forms of sugar in food.

Time Required

30–45 minutes

Materials

12-ounce can of soda, sugar (12 teaspoons)

Description of Activity

Introduction

Mary Poppins sang a song that goes, "A spoonful of sugar helps the medicine go down." She seems to have convinced the food and drug industries, because sugar pops up as an "added ingredient" in the most unlikely places: soda crackers, spaghetti sauce, soups, ketchup, salad dressings, and toothpaste.

When you start looking for sugar on the food labels, you may not see the word "sugar" in the ingredient list even if you know it is there. That's because sugar comes in many disguises. The word "sugar" on a label refers only to cane or beet sugar, but other sugars are often added to foods.

Activity

1. Write this ingredient list (from a cereal package) on the board or give as a handout:

   Oat Flour
   Sugar
   Defatted Wheat Germ
   Wheat Starch
   Honey
   Brown Sugar Syrup
   Salt
   Almonds
   Trisodium Phosphate
   Sodium Ascorbate
   Calcium Carbonate
   Niacin
   Iron
   Vitamin A Palmitate
   Pyridoxin Hydrochloride
   Riboflavin
   Thiamin Mononitrate
   Vitamin B_{12}
   Vitamin D

2. Have the class point out the "sugars" in the list.
3. Ask the class to guess how many teaspoons of sugar are in one 12-ounce can of soda.
4. Measure out 12 teaspoons of sugar into a glass to show them the amount of sugar one can of soda contains.
5. Point out the possible health problems associated with too much sugar (tooth decay, diabetes, empty calories that replace nutrients).

Homework

Students will bring in two food labels, and they will circle the forms of sugar listed on the label.

Evaluation

Students will be able to

- List three forms of sugar found in foods (for example, sucrose, honey, corn syrup).
- Describe how much sugar content is in each of the more common foods and drinks they consume.
- Describe some illnesses related to sugar.

Learning Experience 3-18

Water, Water, Everywhere

Grade Level

5–6

Primary Disciplines

Math, Science

Learning Objectives

Following this activity, students will be able to identify the function and importance of water in living things.

Time Required

1 hour

Materials

Table salt, filter paper, funnel, water, pocket mirrors

Description of Activity

Introduction

Give a background of this nutrient:

> Our bodies depend on water. Water accounts for almost two-thirds of the body's weight. That means a 90-pound child would weigh a mere 30 pounds if all the water in his or her body were drained off. That wouldn't be possible, of course, because water is hidden inside each cell. None of the other nutrients would be much good to us without water, because water is what takes those nutrients where they have to go. Blood is 90 percent water, and blood carries nutrients to the cells. It transports waste products away to the liver, kidneys, and skin for disposal. Water also helps regulate body temperature by evaporating and cooling the skin when people perspire.

Activity

1. Illustrate for the class how water dissolves and transports nutrients by placing some dry table salt on filter paper. The salt will not be able to pass through the paper. Now put some filter paper inside a funnel and sprinkle salt into the funnel, then pour water through it into a jar.
2. Have a student taste the water before and after pouring it over the salt.
3. Have students exhale on a mirror or windowpane to see the moisture in their breath. Explain that the water the body loses has to be replaced, including water lost through respiration.
4. List the following foods and beverages on the board: milk, orange juice, grapes, watermelon, banana, potato chips, peanuts, bread, hamburger, eggs, cheese. Ask the students to pick the ones that contain water.
5. Explain that all these foods contain water. In an average day we might consume as much as a quart of water in "dry" foods alone, not to mention beverages.

Homework

None

Evaluation

Students will be able to

- Explain how the body uses water.
- Identify three ways the body loses water daily.
- Identify three foods that contain a large percentage of water.

Source: *Nutrition Comes Alive*, Level 4, Division of Nutritional Sciences, Cornell University, 1986. Reprinted with permission.

4

Keeping Kids Active, Keeping Kids Healthy

Linda D. Zwiren and Gayle E. Hutchinson

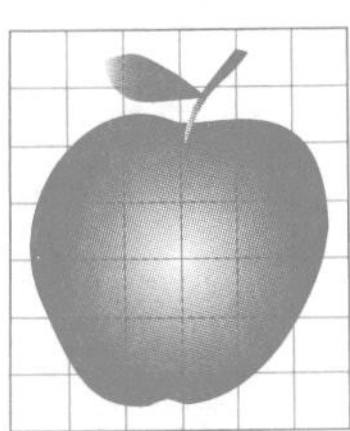

Chapter Outline

Objectives

- Understand how classroom teachers can incorporate movement and activity into classroom learning experiences in content areas
- Recognize the roles of parent, school, and community in increasing the activity level of children and decreasing the time children are sitting down
- Understand how developing an active lifestyle is preventive medicine
- Understand the role of the physical educator in improving physical fitness and in developing skill proficiency in children
- Document the association of lack of physical activity with chronic physical conditions and problems: cardiovascular diseases, obesity, osteoporosis, cancer, immune function, and emotional/mental state
- Learn how to involve parents in their child's physical activity program

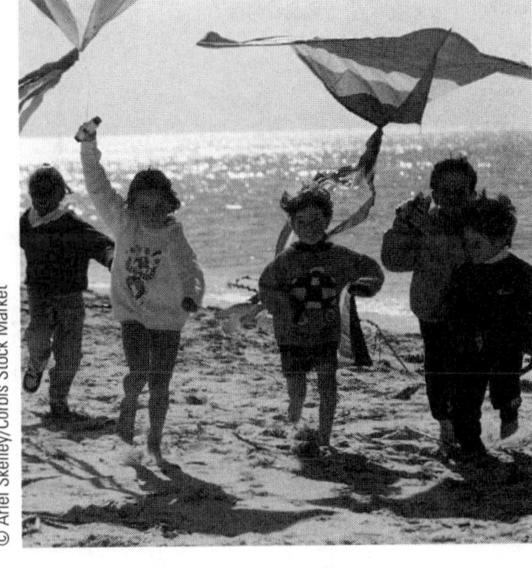

The fifth-grade students were talking in small groups with great excitement. They were sharing information they had collected the night before when they interviewed family members about their own health and the health of other relatives. Each student in class wrote down the information on a family tree chart. The findings were amazing. Farhad discovered that his grandmother had high blood pressure. Andrea shared that her great grandfather, grandmother, and aunt on her father's side were all insulin-dependent diabetics like her younger brother. Antoine revealed that his father and his grandfather suffered heart attacks at the same age, 42. Several students reported fairly good health among all family relatives. Other students stated that they and their family members did not know much about their health history.

Finally, the teacher brought the groups together for a class discussion about risk factors to health and the development of chronic diseases. She asked the class for questions and was thrilled with the depth of the questions. Students asked:

- Why do people develop chronic diseases such as diabetes?
- Why do people have heart attacks?
- What does high blood pressure mean? Why is it bad?
- Why do some people stay healthy and others get sick?
- How can I stay healthy?

• • •

Mr. Kaufman likes to integrate physical activity with reading and language arts. He often has students practice making letters with their bodies, and movement sentences using a collection of locomotor skills as verbs and punctuation marks. One day while the class was creating movement sentences, Juanita stopped what she was doing, walked over to Mr. Kaufman, and asked: "Why do we have to move our bodies to make a sentence?" Using this teaching opportunity, Mr. Kaufman asked the children to gather so they could discuss Juanita's question. Mr. Kaufman guided the discussion and helped children realize the health benefits of moving one's body. The students were so curious about the benefits of moving their bodies that they bombarded Mr. Kaufman with lots of questions. He wrote down these questions so he could address them throughout the year. Here are a few of the questions the students asked:

- Why do I need to move my body to practice letters and words?
- Why do we need to move our bodies at all?
- I'm too tired to move. Do we have to?
- Why do we feel good when we play and move around?

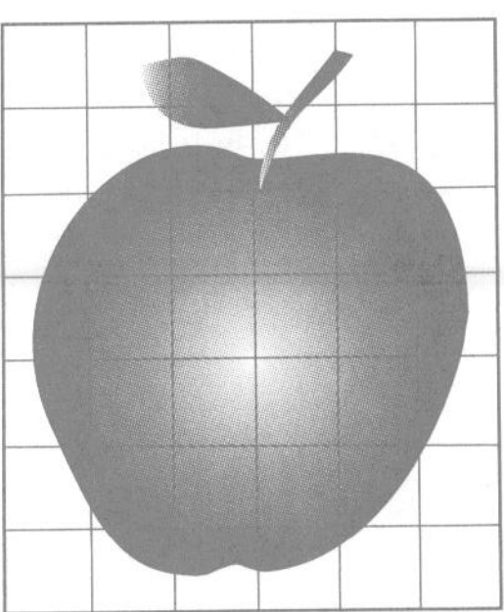

Keeping children active and physically fit is important to their health status. Improving a child's physical fitness requires improving the child's cardiovascular fitness, muscular strength, muscular endurance, and flexibility.

Keeping children active is essential to keeping children healthy. Classroom teachers can integrate developmentally appropriate physical activity into their curriculum. They can intertwine information about the health benefits of staying active into their daily lesson plans.

Physical activity affects many of the body's systems and provides numerous health benefits for adults. Because physical activity confers significant protection from chronic diseases (such as cardiovascular diseases and non-insulin -dependent diabetes mellitus) and because it appears to reduce risk of osteoporosis and some cancers, there is substantial interest in beginning the prevention of these adult diseases during the first two decades of life through regular physical activity. In addition to these disease-prevention benefits, physical activity contributes to quality of life, psychological health, and the ability to meet physical work demands and engage in leisure activities. Regular physical activity improves functional status and limits disability during middle and later years.[1]

This statement makes it clear why the Surgeon General and the U. S. Department of Health and Human Services,[2] the National Institutes of Health,[3] and the Centers for Disease Control and Prevention[4] have made increasing physical activity a primary health goal. Sedentary adults have higher risk for various diseases including cardiovascular conditions (such as atherosclerosis and coronary heart disease), adult-onset diabetes, colon cancer, osteoporosis, and hypertension (high blood pressure).[5] Individuals who have a physically active lifestyle are more likely to have healthier blood cholesterol levels, lower blood pressure, better use of glucose as a fuel by the cells, less depression, better cognitive function, and more efficient immune system functioning.[6]

Childhood experiences, habits, and support systems contribute to the activity levels of adults. Active adults are more likely to have been active children—they are often competent movers (that is, they can do many skilled movements) who enjoy activity, understand the connection between being active and lowering the risk for disease, and have role models (peers, teachers, parents) who are active. Establishing activity as a necessary and regular component of children's daily habits, then, is essential.

Are children becoming less active? Although children are naturally active, debates arise as to whether children are currently active enough to ensure good health. What is clear is that children and adults are getting fatter[7] and that TVs, computers, and video games are major contributors to children developing sedentary lifestyles.[8]

Definitions

People often use the terms *physical activity*, *exercise*, *physical fitness*, and *sports* interchangeably. Actually, each term has a unique meaning. Physical activity is any bodily movement that increases energy expenditure above rest. Therefore, physical activity can consist of walking, gardening, chopping wood, swimming, vacuuming, climbing stairs, playing golf, or riding a bicycle to work or school. Physical activity can be performed at various intensities. To increase children's physical activity level means to decrease the time children are sitting or lying down and to increase the time they are moving.

When physical activity is performed as a structured, repetitive regime, it is called exercise or training. People who regularly attend aerobic classes, or who regularly ride a bicycle, or who do 30 sit-ups a day, or who weight-train three times a week are all engaging in regular exercise.

Physical fitness consists of a group of physical attributes, shown in Figure 4.1—all of which can be improved by engaging in the appropriate exercise program. Children improve their cardiorespiratory endurance by doing large-muscle activities such as running, jogging, swimming, or cross-country skiing. Other physical activities appropriate for children include weight training to increase muscular strength and muscular endurance (the ability to repeatedly do a muscular contraction or to maintain a muscular contraction) and muscular flexibility (including stretching) to improve the range of motion around a joint. Physical fitness is tied to attaining and maintaining recommended body composition. This is achieved through energy expenditure (which expends calories) and proper nutrition (see Chapter 3).

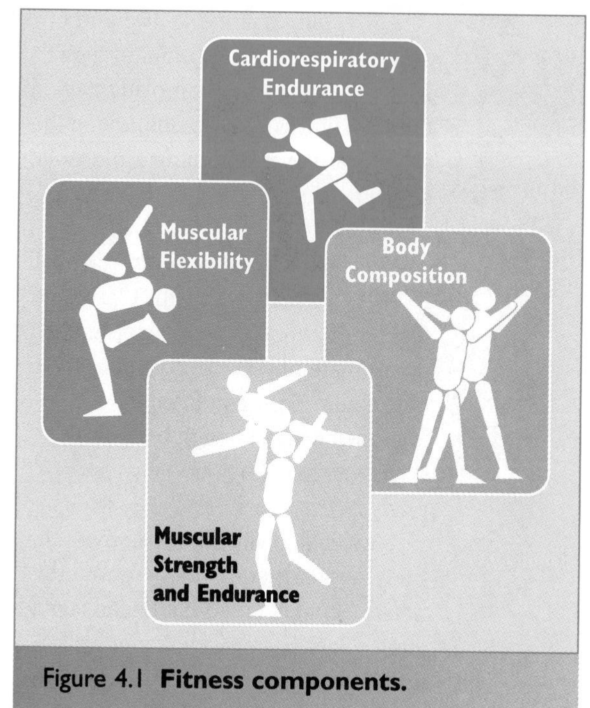

Figure 4.1 **Fitness components.**

Sports are activities that require specific skilled movements and are performed in organized game situations. To participate in sports, children need a certain level of motor fitness (speed, agility, coordination, balance, power, and quick reaction time). Here, the physical educator's role is to help children gain enough skill and confidence for them to participate in and enjoy many activities, not just a few traditional team sports, and to avoid the abysmal sense of failure and embarrassment that often results from a total lack of skill.[9]

To become fully functional adults, children need many opportunities to participate in well-constructed, well-taught learning experiences in physical education.[10] Adults who never learn how to be efficient movers and who lack motor skills will avoid engaging in many physical activities because of embarrassment and inability to perform at a level where they can enjoy the activity. A quality physical education program removes the barrier to movement proficiency and can help prevent children from becoming couch potatoes as adults.

Helping our children develop active lifestyles has become imperative to reduce their chances of developing chronic illness. One way to help children develop active lifestyles is to make developmentally appropriate physical activities an integral part of their daily lives. Physical education classes provide many opportunities for students to learn and develop fundamental movement skills and concepts. As children become skillful, they learn to combine movements so they can participate in a number of physical activities and sports.

How can classroom teachers contribute to increasing children's health status? Whenever possible, make learning a physically active process (i.e., have children move while they are learning). The Learning Experiences at the end of this chapter can be incorporated into social studies, English or language arts, math, or science lessons that involve movement as a part of the learning process. In addition, classroom teachers can focus on the connection between physical activity and increased health, decreased depression, and increased self-esteem.

Children's physiological attributes are, of course, related to their activity preferences. The emphasis of this chapter is on classroom teachers' helping students gain information about the connection between physical activity and health. Children's developmental abilities by grade level and physiological attributes as related to their activity preferences are included.

Physical Activity and Chronic Diseases

Participating in regular physical activity has been found to reduce the risk for cardiovascular diseases, adult-onset diabetes, and some cancers (especially colon); to increase bone density; and to maintain weight loss. Physical activity also has been shown to improve mental health and reduce depression.[11]

Cardiovascular Disease

Strong evidence links the risk of coronary heart disease and stroke with a sedentary lifestyle.[12] Coronary heart disease results from fatty deposits on the walls of the blood vessels (atherosclerosis) that restrict the amount of blood and oxygen carried to the heart. This narrowing of the heart's blood vessels reduces the heart's ability to meet the body's increased energy demands and predisposes the heart to a heart attack (see Chapter 5).

When a person works hard or increases his or her activity level, the heart has to increase the amount of blood circulating through the body. If the vessels supplying the heart muscle with oxygen and fuel are constricted, the heart may not be able to meet this increased energy demand. If a blood clot forms and the body does not dissolve the clot, the clot may start to travel around the body and become stuck in the narrowed blood vessels. This would cut off the blood flow to part of the heart, resulting in a heart attack. If a clot becomes lodged in a cerebral vessel, it may cause a stroke. Several studies have established that a sedentary lifestyle can double a person's risk for coronary heart disease and stroke.[13]

Engaging in regular physical activity has been shown to slow the rate at which fatty plaque is deposited on the inside of blood vessels by improving several physiological factors, including hypertension (high blood pressure), poor blood lipid (fat) profile, and obesity (especially excessive abdominal fat).

Hypertension

Hypertension is defined as having a systolic blood pressure (the top blood pressure number) greater than 140 mmHg or a diastolic blood pressure (the bottom number) over 90 mmHg. Increased systolic and/or diastolic blood pressure doubles a person's risk of developing coronary heart disease.[14] Sedentary and unfit individuals have a 20 to 50 percent greater risk for developing hypertension.[15] Regular, low-to-moderate intensity, large-muscle movement is effective in lowering blood pressure in children with hypertension.[16] Research has established a strong enough link between regular physical activity and hypertension so that several organizations recommend lifestyle modifications, including regular aerobic physical activity, as an effective therapeutic method of treating hypertension.[17]

Blood Lipid Profile and Activity

The amount and type of lipids (fats) in the blood have a strong and proven relationship to the development of atherosclerosis and heart disease. The blood level of cholesterol, and in particular the cholesterol carried in low-density lipoproteins (**LDLs**), is directly related to coronary heart disease. Higher levels of blood cholesterol found in high-density lipoproteins (**HDLs**) have been found to be protective. A high level of triglycerides in the blood also indicates a risk for coronary heart disease, especially in females. Many factors contribute to the levels of LDL, HDL, and triglycerides in the blood, including genetics, obesity, diet, and activity levels.

Studies of adults show that engaging in dynamic continuous exercise results in desirable changes in blood lipids, such as lowering cholesterol and LDLs and increasing HDLs. Children do not have atherosclerosis or die of coronary heart disease; however, streaks of fatty plaque have been seen in the blood of children as young as 10 years old.[18]

Favorable blood cholesterol and triglyceride levels are more often found in active children. Increasing activity levels has positive effects on blood lipid levels in obese and sedentary children and in adolescents with diabetes mellitus.[19]

Obesity

Obesity is defined as having excess body fat. Some body fat is necessary for protection, insulation, and storage of energy. The weight on a standard scale is not an accurate method of determining excessive body fat because weight is a combination of fat, tissue, and lean muscle mass (which weighs more than fat). To determine body composition, the measurement must identify how much of the body weight is fat. Three ways to measure body composition are

1. Underwater or hydrostatic weighing to determine body density
2. Skinfold measurements, which assesses total body fat from measurements of subcutaneous fat
3. Bioelectrical impedance analysis, which is based on resistance to electrical conductivity of fatty tissue

Body mass index (BMI), a popular measure of obesity, is calculated using an individual's height and weight: BMI = body weight (in kg) ÷ height squared (in meters). High BMI in some cases may reflect muscle mass rather than excessive body fat.[20] Many experts do not consider BMI a valid measure of fatness in children.

The health implications of childhood obesity are significant. Obesity is the main cause of high blood pressure in children; additional effects are psychosocial and orthopedic secondary medical complications. If obesity persists into adulthood, the risk increases significantly for developing adult-onset diabetes, coronary heart disease (especially as a result of abdominal obesity), and early death.

Continuum, of Moderate Amounts of Activity

Less vigorous, more time

Washing and waxing a car for 45–60 minutes
Washing windows or floors, for 45–60 minutes
Playing volleyball for 45 minutes
Playing touch football for 30–45 minutes
Gardening for 30–45 minutes
Wheeling self in wheelchair for 30–40 minutes
Walking 1¾ miles in 35 minutes (20 min/mile)
Basketball (shooting baskets) for 30 minutes
Bicycling 5 miles in 30 minutes
Dancing fast (social) for 30 minutes
Pushing a stroller 1½ miles in 30 minutes
Raking leaves for 30 minutes
Walking 2 miles in 30 minutes (15 min/mile)
Water aerobics for 30 minutes
Swimming laps for 20 minutes
Wheelchair basketball for 20 minutes
Basketball (playing a game) for 15–20 minutes
Bicycling 4 miles in 15 minutes
Jumping rope for 15 minutes
Running 1½ miles in 15 minutes (10 min/mile)
Shoveling snow for 15 minutes
Stairwalking for 15 minutes

More vigorous, less time

Note. A moderate amount of physical activity is roughly equivalent to physical activity that uses 150 calories of energy per day, or 1,000 calories per week. Some activities can be performed at various intensities; the suggested durations correspond to expected intensity of effort.

Source: Data from *Surgeon General's Report on Physical Activity and Health.* Surgeon General's Report on Physical Activity and Health, U.S. Dept. of Health and Human services, Centers for Disease Control and Prevention, National Center for Chronic Disease Prevention and Health Promotion, Atlanta, GA 1999.

Most physical fitness test batteries that physical educators administer include a determination of body composition using skinfold measurements. The fat content of male children should be approximately 10 to 15 percent, females 20 to 25 percent, of body weight. An excessively low level of body fat is also a health risk, especially if children are not getting sufficient nutrients.

Factors contributing to obesity include environment (excessive eating, too little activity) and heredity in some debatable mix. In any case, about 1 in 4 children is obese.[21] Many experts attribute increasing childhood obesity to decreased activity levels resulting from more television watching, using computers, and playing video games and to the increased intake of high-fat foods.[22]

To lose body fat, a person has to decrease caloric intake, increase the amount of energy expended, or both. The most efficient way for adults to lose moderate amounts of body fat is to modestly decrease food intake and to increase physical activity. Very obese children and adults require the attention of medical professionals, but most children can derive benefits from the following adjustments in lifestyle.

Improving Nutrition

For children, the emphasis should be on lifestyle habits, i.e., increasing physical movement and decreasing the intake of foods that are high-calorie, high-sugar, high-fat, and full of low-nutrient dense calories. The emphasis should *not* be on weight loss; children should not be placed on diets that have severe caloric restriction. Prevention is the key, because the cure is much more difficult.

Increasing Physical Activity

Substantial evidence shows that low activity level (a sedentary lifestyle) is a significant factor in the development of childhood obesity.[23] The most efficient way to increase physical activity is to change the lifestyle. For children, this might mean walking to and from school.[24] Regimented physical training is not the answer, because repetitive exercises will probably have minimal appeal at this stage in children's emotional and physiological development. (However, some evidence indicates that overweight/obese children find success with strength training programs. These weight training programs need to be supervised by trained personnel and consist of those strength-training protocols that research has shown to be best suited for pre-adolescents.[25])

Teachers should encourage children to keep moving whenever possible and engage students in recreational and fun activities. Research indicates that children are motivated to move by engaging in fun-providing activities and cooperative games and that competition should not be introduced too early.[26] Children want age-appropriate, challenging, cooperative activities that provide energy release. Letting students make some choices by involving them in the decision-making process may help maintain children's interest.[27] Teachers can also be role models by being active with the children—and by being enthusiastic about being active.

Even though the increase in obesity in children and adolescents is the major weight problem in children, a subset of children and young adults are susceptible to eating disorders.[28] Adolescent females, in particular, are preoccupied with body size and weight. Therefore, teachers should be vigilant in identifying children and adolescents who seem susceptible to disordered eating.

There has been an increase in **diabetes mellitus** (also called diabetes type II or NIDDM, non-insulin dependent diabetes mellitus, and formerly known as adult onset diabetes) in children. Diabetes type II occurs when the cells of the body become resistant to insulin secreted into the blood. Individuals with type II diabetes therefore have glucose intolerance because of insulin resistance (in contrast to diabetes type I, wherein the cells of the pancreas are unable to secrete insulin). The main reason for increased incidence of this type of diabetes in children is the increase in childhood obesity and sedentary lifestyle habits.[29]

Osteoporosis

In advanced osteoporosis, the mineral matrix of bone has been lost to such an extent that even minor impact to the bone may cause it to break or crush. Though most of the consequences arise in women age 50 and older and men age 70 years and older, prevention of osteoporosis begins during the periods of major bone growth.

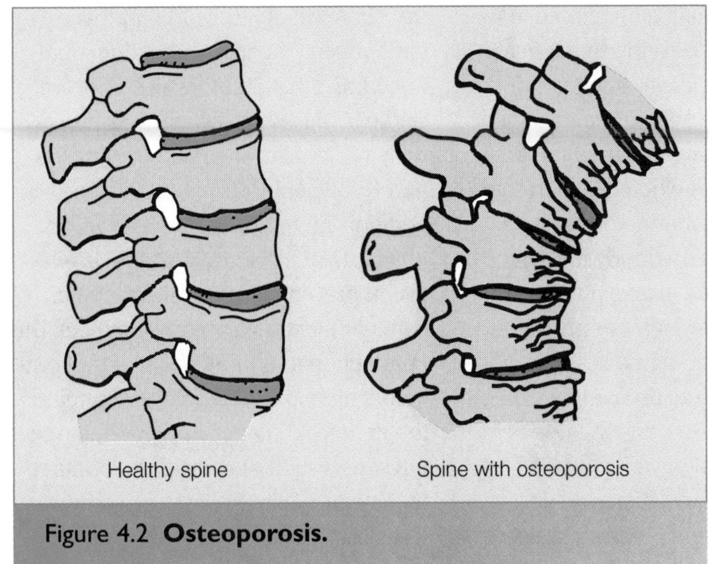

Figure 4.2 **Osteoporosis.**

The thickness of bone is determined by diet, activity, gender, and heredity. Bone tissue is forming constantly and being broken down at all ages. Bone formation proceeds faster than bone breakdown until about ages 25 to 30. After about age 30, bone breakdown proceeds at a slightly faster rate than bone formation. Because of lowered production of estrogen, women lose bone at an accelerated rate after menopause (see Figure 4.2).

Bone has many functions. Besides forming the basic structure of the body, protecting organs, enabling movement, and producing red blood cells, bone provides the body's calcium reserve. Calcium is needed for blood clotting, muscle contraction, conducting nerve impulses, and maintaining osmotic pressure balance. If blood levels of calcium drop too low (either because of not having enough calcium in the diet or not absorbing enough calcium from the digestive system), the bone matrix breaks down, releasing calcium into the blood.

When bone loss is so great that minor trauma will break the brittle, thin bone, the person is diagnosed as having osteoporosis. Once bone mass is lost, regaining it is difficult. At present, treatments merely slow the rate of bone loss. Prevention, which emphasizes maximizing the thickness of the bone at ages 25–30 years, is the best way to reduce this health risk. Therefore, consuming enough calories with sufficient absorbable calcium is important in maintaining bone growth and minimizing bone loss. In addition, bone becomes thicker when forces are placed upon it. Bone *loss* is accelerated during bed rest and during the weightlessness of space. Bone *growth* is accelerated when appropriate force is applied regularly. Therefore, weight-bearing activity is a critical component in bone growth.

In girls, abnormal delay of menarche and chronic irregular menstruation are problematic. Chronic amenorrhea (two or fewer menstrual periods per year) leads to severe bone loss because of the depressed estrogen levels. Food intake inadequate for a person's energy needs (disordered eating) is a primary culprit in amenorrhea. In boys, delayed puberty with low serum testosterone levels reduces bone mineral density.

The term "female athlete triad" has recently gained attention in the health field. The triad refers to three conditions—disordered eating, amenorrhea, and osteoporosis—that are often seen in female athletes who engage in sports accompanied by undue pressure to maintain a particular body physique. Although the triad affects primarily female athletes in "style" sports (gymnastics, diving, and figure skating, for example), many children and adolescents are ingesting too few calories for the amount of energy they expend or are over-exercising to try to achieve an "ideal," yet unattainable, body weight. Young girls and boys with eating disorders, adolescents who are constantly on a diet, and female athletes who restrict caloric intake to maintain unhealthy minimal body weight are all at risk for developing osteoporosis at an early age.[30]

Following are ways to maximize the genetic potential for peak bone mineral density:

1. Eat a well-balanced diet that meets the recommended dietary allowance for calcium.
2. Do not substitute soft drinks for milk.
3. Eat enough calories to meet daily energy needs.
4. Avoid cigarette smoking, because smoking works against the beneficial effects of nutrients such as vitamin C, which aids bone strength and could decrease maximal bone growth.
5. Make a lifetime commitment to physical activity and exercise. Include weight training to improve muscular strength.

Cancer and Immune Function

The major factors in preventing cancer focus on not smoking, using alcohol moderately, if at all, avoiding proven carcinogenic agents, and eating a balanced diet that includes five to seven servings of fresh fruits and vegetables daily (emphasizing intake of vitamins C and E, folic acid, and beta-carotene). In addition, increasing evidence indicates that a physically active lifestyle is effective in preventing some site-specific cancers, most notably colon cancer. The connection to colon cancer is that participating in physical activity decreases the time fecal matter stays in the large intestine, which decreases the contact time with the lining of the large intestine and thereby potentially decreases absorption of carcinogenic agents contained in fecal material.

Attention also has been directed to the role of the immune system in preventing cancer. Exercise of low-to-moderate intensity increases the number of natural killer T cells and the number of circulating **lymphocytes**—a type of white blood cell found in lymph nodes. Natural killer cells are specific lymphocytes that can provide an immediate first line of defense against cancer cells. Excessively high-intensity exercise, however, may have negative effects on the immune system.[31]

Neuropsychiatric Concerns

In recent years, research has been directed toward a possible association between physical activity and mental/emotional health.

Cognitive Function and Classroom Behavior

Some evidence suggests that regular exercise may enhance cognitive function in children and adolescents, may reduce loss of cognitive function in people over 31 years of age, and may preserve full mental function well into old age. Specifically, the research has demonstrated that increased levels of physical activity produces small but reliable improvements in reaction time, math performance, and acuity, with more pronounced results in females.[32]

Research studies have shown a positive relationship between physical activity and self-esteem in children. Enhanced self-esteem may result in better classroom behavior and a greater desire to learn. A review of studies reported significant improvements in students' attitudes, discipline, behavior, and creativity following implementation of physical activity programs.[33]

Depression and Anxiety

Most of the research on the relationship between exercise and the mind has focused on physical activity and depression. Depression is often precipitated by stressful life events (see Chapter 8, "Childhood Stress"). Depression may occur in conjunction with other chronic diseases, is strongly associated with aging, and occurs frequently with other mental disorders (see Chapter 6, "Mental Health"). Research supports that engaging in regular activity can do the following:

- help reduce anxiety
- decrease mild to moderate depression
- reduce various types of stress
- have a beneficial emotional effect
- contribute to improvement in self-concept and self-esteem[34]

Severe depression and clinically diagnosed depression require professional treatment. Improvement in self-esteem and self-concept may have the highest payoff for children with disabilities and for girls.[35]

Promotion of Activity to Enhance Health Benefits

The exercise prescription promoted by the fitness industry and by the media is to exercise three to five times a week for 15 to 60 minutes, keeping the heart rate in a range of 70 to 85 percent of the maximal heart rate. However, to achieve the health benefits cited in this chapter, the emphasis is better placed on keeping children active and moving. Children should be physically active daily as part of play, games, learning, transportation, recreation, physical education, or planned activity, in the context of family, school, and community activities. Integral in this prescription is to have children *enjoy* moving and keeping active and to give children the skill, confidence, and knowledge they need to develop the incentive and behavior pattern to stay active throughout the lifespan.

Promotion of activity levels that will maximize health benefits associated with reduced disease risk and a better quality of life requires the following:

1. Keeping students active throughout the day
2. Reducing the amount of time spent in sedentary activities
3. Giving students the opportunity to develop movement skills and to develop an adequate level of fitness
4. Providing a supportive environment outside of school for children to keep active and moving

The gymnasium is not the only place where activity should take place. In school, opportunities for increasing movement can be provided in the classroom, the lunchroom, the playground, as well as the gymnasium. Children can move while learning. Incorporating movement into classroom lessons should not negatively affect learning and may even enhance acquisition of knowledge. Furthermore, the school community can provide incentives for children to move by promoting fundraising activities such as Jump Rope for Heart, AIDS Walkathon, and Biking for Multiple Sclerosis.

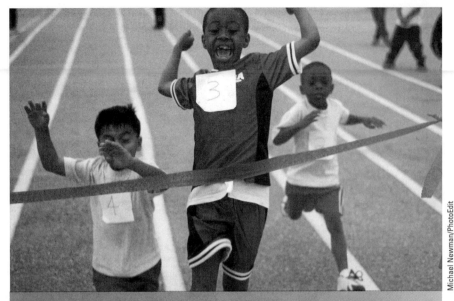

Michael Newman/PhotoEdit

Physical education can provide enjoyable opportunities to develop cardiovascular endurance.

The younger the child, the more influential parents' behaviors are. Parents who participate in activities with their children, who organize activities, who promote walking or biking to school, who transport children to places where they can be active, and who serve as active role models can help children be active and stay active. Many environments outside of school, unfortunately, present unsafe environments and unattractive areas to play. As environments outside of school become more restrictive, it becomes even more important to keep children active throughout the school day.

Success is most probable when adults and children alike accept that the benefits of activity are equal to or greater than the amount of effort they expend. Providing students with the knowledge that activity is an essential component of their health status and communicating how an active lifestyle can reduce their risk for disease will help them understand the risk of being sedentary.

Children need intrinsic as well as extrinsic rewards. Children who are highly skilled will evaluate their own competence by favorable comparison with peers. Children who are not as physically competent, however, feel inferior when having to strive for nationally established norms or compare themselves to their classmates' achievements. Sedentary, obese, and unfit students need realistic goals that are challenging but attainable.[36] Goal setting for acquiring skill (mastery) directs children's attention to physical activity and fitness and rewards learning, improving, and hard work. Mastery involves *self*-comparison, so students see improvement in small steps based on their own abilities. Personal performance is more important than winning or losing and enhances these students' enjoyment.[37]

Schools should foster a cooperative environment in which students achieve their own goals while working in cooperation with others. Boys and girls alike should participate in sports to have fun, to improve their skills, and to be with friends. The emphasis on a cooperative learning environment may help to enhance self-concept and contribute to children being active throughout their lives.

Physiological Considerations

The combination of a poorer sweating capacity than adults and an immature cardiovascular system results in children having less tolerance for exercise in heat and a greater susceptibility to heat stress.[38] Children tend not to drink water, even when it is made available, thus putting themselves at some risk for dehydration. Teachers should make sure that children drink plenty of fluids (flavored water with minimal sugar and salt content might increase fluid intake) and reduce the activity level or intersperse more rest periods on hot, humid days. Children, too, lose heat more rapidly than adults do when active in water. Children do not perceive that they are too hot or too cold. Obese children have a lower tolerance for heat and therefore will experience more problems in hot weather. All children have to be closely supervised to ensure that they are not having trouble dealing with temperatures that are either too hot or too cold.

Children spontaneously prefer short-term, intermittent activities with a high recreational component and variety rather than monotonous, prolonged activities. And children seem best suited for brief repeated activities with short rest periods. The Learning Experiences that follow offer activities that meet these criteria.

Summary

Children should enjoy moving and activity as play, not exercise, so they will make physical activity a habit. Classroom teachers can integrate movement into their teaching of academic disciplines and can contribute to students' knowledge base regarding the importance of an active lifestyle to the maintenance of health.

Inactivity is associated with numerous chronic conditions, including cardiovascular diseases (high blood pressure, heart attacks, strokes), some types of cancer, weak immune system, osteoporosis, and obesity, as well as depression and other emotional and mental problems. Physical activity during childhood can prevent the onset of, or alleviate, the conditions that may become a serious health threat in adulthood. Positive behaviors are promoted when individuals perceive that benefits are greater than the effort expended. Classroom teachers can help to reduce sedentary behavior by teaching students how an active lifestyle can help reduce their (and their parents') risk for disease.

Classroom teachers can incorporate developmentally appropriate movement within subject-matter learning. Learning activities can be created so that parents will be active with their children. Publications are available that list effective policies for school, community, and industry programs to help young people to become active and stay active so that they enhance their health and quality of life.

Web Sites

Centers for Disease Control and Prevention (CDC)
http://www.cdc.gov

Nutrition & Physical Activity

KidsWalk-To-School
http://www.cdc.gov
A guide that encourages individuals and organizations to work together to identify and create safe walking routes to school.

Physical Activity and Health: A Report of The Surgeon General
http://www.cdc.gov
The Surgeon General's first report that specifically addresses physical activity and health. July 1996.

Physical Activity Campaign: Ready. Set. It's Everywhere You Go
http://www.cdc.gov

Promoting Physical Activity: A Guide For Community Action
http://www.cdc.gov
A step-by-step guide to community wide behavior change.

International Walk to School Day
http://www.iwalktoschool.org

Human Kinetics Inc. Publishers
1-800-747-4457: www.humankinetics.com

PE-News
http://www.pelinks4u.org
This site provides information about publications and Web sites that encourage physical activity in youth and families.

President's Council on Physical Fitness Research Digest
http://www.fitness.gov

Resources

R. Clement, ed. *Elementary School Recess: Selected Readings, Games, and Activities for Teachers.* Boston: American Press, 2000.

T. P. Cone; P. Werner; S. L. Cone, and A. M. Woods. *Interdisciplinary Teaching Through Physical Education.* Human Kinetics Inc., Publ. 1988. ISBN 0-88011-502-5.

This reference, for elementary and early childhood classroom teachers, includes 20 complete ready-to-use learning experiences and ideas for integrating activity and health knowledge with mathematics, science, language arts, social studies, and the creative arts.

G. Graham, S. A. Holt-Hale, and M. Parker. *Children Moving: A Reflective Approach to Teaching Physical Education.* Mountain View, CA: Mayfield, 2001.

Human Kindetics Video: Fit Kids Classroom Workout. Champaign, IL: Human Kinetics Inc., Publ., 2001. Videocassette. ISBN 0-7360-3790-X. This videotape provides a resource for K–9 classroom teachers and physical education specialists. It includes 5- and 10-minute movement segments that can be used to invigorate and motivate students during their daily routine or to warm them up in preparation for physical activity.

M. Lee and R. Clements. *Moving to Discover the USA: 142 Action Rhymes, Songs and Games.* Champaign, IL: Human Kinetics Inc., Publ. 1999.

C. Summerford. *PE-4-Me.* Champaign, IL: Human Kinetics, Inc., Publ. 2000. ISBN 0-7360-0165-4.

This reference is for elementary, middle and high school classroom and physical education teachers; administrators, and directors. It includes a blueprint for a K–12 program that integrates physical activity with movement concepts, social skills, stress reduction, nutrition, school safety, and drug resistance education.

Notes

1. J. F. Sallis, K. Patrick, and B. J. Long, "Overview of the International Consensus Conference on Physical Activity Guidelines for Adolescents," *Pediatric Exercise Science* 6 (1994): 301.
2. *Healthy People 2000: National Health Promotion and Disease Prevention Objectives* (DHHS Pub.# PHS 91-50212 (Washington, DC: Government Printing Office, 1991); *Physical Activity and Health: A Report to the Surgeon General* (Atlanta: Centers for Disease Control and Prevention, National Center for Chronic Disease Prevention and Health Promotion, 1996.)
3. "Physical Activity and Cardiovascular Health," *NIH Consensus Statement* 13, no. 3 (1995).
4. "Prevalence of Sedentary Lifestyle: Behavior Risk Factor Surveillance System," *Morbidity and Mortality Weekly* 42, (1993): 576–579.
5. C. Bouchard and J. P. Despres, "Physical Activity and Health: Atherosclerotic, Metabolic, and Hypertensive Diseases," *Research Quarterly for Exercise and Sports* (Special Issue on Physical Activity, Health, and Wellbeing; An International Scientific Consensus Conference) 66, no. 4 (1995): 268–275.
6. E. A. Newsholme and M. Parry-Billings, "Effect of Exercise on the Immune System," in *Physical Activity, Fitness, and Health: International Proceedings and Consensus Statement,* edited by C. Bouchard, R. J. Shephard, and T. Stephens (Champaign, IL: Human Kinetics, 1994); R. S. Paffenbarger, "Physical Activity, Health and Fitness," in *American College of Sports Medicine: 40th Anniversary Lectures* (Indianapolis: American College of Sports Medicine, 1994); World Hypertension League (WHL), "Physical Exercise in the Management of Hypertension: A Consensus Statement by the World Hypertension League," *Journal of Hypertension* 9 (1991): 283–287; J. F. Sallis, K. Patrick, and B. J. Long, Overview of the International Consensus Conference on physical activity guidelines for adolescents. *Pediatric Exercise Science* 6, 299–301.
7. R. P. Troiano, K. M. Flegal, R. J. Kuczmarshi, S. M. Campbell, and C. L. Johnson, "Overweight Prevalence and Trends for Children and Adolescents: The National Health and Examination Surveys: 1963–1991," *Archives of Pediatric Adolescent Medicine* 149 (1995): 1085–1091.
8. W. H. Dietz and V. C. Strasburger, "Children, Adolescents, and Television," *Current Problems in Pediatrics* 1 (1991): 8.
9. G. Graham, S. A. Holt-Hale, and M. Parker, *Children Moving: A Reflective Approach to Teaching Physical Education* (Mountain View, CA: Mayfield, 1992): 21.
10. National Association for Sport and Physical Education (NASPE), *Guidelines for Elementary School Physical Education* (Reston, VA: American Alliance for Health, Physical Education, Recreation and Dance [AAHPERD] 1994); *Checklist for Elementary School Physical Education* (Reston, VA: AAHPERD, 1994).
11. *Healthy People 2000: National Health Promotion and Disease Prevention Objectives* (DHHS Pub.# PHS 91-50212 (Washington, DC: Government Printing Office, 1991); "Physical Activity and Cardiovascular Health," *NIH Consensus Statement* 13, no. 3 (1995).
12. R. S. Paffenbarger, "Physical Activity, Health and Fitness," in *American College of Sports Medicine: 40th Anniversary Lectures* (Indianapolis: American College of Sports Medicine, 1994).
13. C. J. Casperson, "Physical Inactivity and Coronary Heart Disease," *Physician and Sports Medicine* 15, no. 11 (1987): 43–44; S. N. Blair, E. E. Powell, and T. L. Bazarre, "Physical Inactivity (Workshop)," *Journal of Circulation* 88 (1993): 1402–1405; N. K. Wenger, "40 Years of Progress: Physical Activity in the Primary and Secondary Prevention of Heart Disease," in *American College of Sports Medicine: 40th Anniversary Lectures* (Indianapolis: American College of Sports Medicine, 1994), 43–54.

14. C. J. Casperson, "Physical Inactivity and Coronary Heart Disease," *Physician and Sports Medicine* 15, no. 11 (1987): 43–44; S. N. Blair, E. E. Powell, and T. L. Bazarre, "Physical Inactivity (Workshop)," *Journal of Circulation* 88 (1993): 1402–1405.

15. N. K. Wenger, "40 Years of Progress: Physical Activity in the Primary and Secondary Prevention of Heart Disease," in *American College of Sports Medicine: 40th Anniversary Lectures* (Indianapolis: American College of Sports Medicine, 1994), 43–54.

16. American College of Sports Medicine (ACSM), "Position Stand: Physical Activity, Physical Fitness and Hypertension," *Medicine and Science in Sport and Exercise* 25 (1993): i, x.

17. See note 16.

18. N. Armstrong and B. Simons-Morton, "Physical Activity and Blood Lipids in Adolescents," *Pediatric Exercise Science* 6 (1994): 381–405.

19. T. W. Rowland, *Exercise and Children's Health* (Champaign, IL: Human Kinetics, 1990).

20. See note 19.

21. See note 7.

22. T. W. Rowland, *Exercise and Children's Health* (Champaign, IL: Human Kinetics, 1990); W. H. Dietz and V. C. Strasburger, "Children, Adolescents, and Television," *Current Problems in Pediatrics* 1 (1991); L. D. Zwiren, "Exercise in Childhood and Youth," in *Exercise and the Heart in Health and Disease,* ed. R. J. Shephard and H. Miller (New York: Marcel Dekker, 1998): 99–138.

23. M. I. Goran and E. T. Poehlman, "The Role of Physical Activity in the Development of Childhood Obesity," in *Exercise and Disease,* ed. R. R. Watson and M. Eisinger (Boca Raton, FL: CRC Press, 1992), 2–10; C. Bouchard, "Can Obesity be Prevented?" *Nutrition Reviews* (1996): S125–S130.

24. Center for Disease Control (CDC)," Kids Walk-To-School." Available online: http://www.cdc.gov/nccdphp/dnpa/publicat.html

25. W. Westcott and S. Ramsden, *Specialized Strength Training* (Monterey, CA: Exercise Science Publishers, 2001).

26. See note 24.

27. M.R. Weiss, "Motivating Kids in Physical Activity" *President's Council on Physical Fitness and Sports Research Digest* 3, no. 11 (2000): 1–8.

28. O. Bar-Or, and T. Baronowski, "Physical Activity, Adiposity, and Obesity Among Adolescents," *Pediatric Exercise Science* 6, no. 4 (1994): 348–360; A. Must, "Morbidity and Mortality Associated with Elevated Body Weight in Children and Adolescents," *American Journal of Clinical Nutrition* (1996): 445S–457S.

29. American Diabetes Association (ADA), "Position Statement on Diabetes Mellitus and Exercise," *Diabetes Care* 18, no. 1 (1997): 30–37.

30. S. Dhuper, M. Warren, J. Brooks-Gunn, and R. Fox, "Effect of Hormonal Status on Bone Density in Adolescent Girls," *Journal of Clinical Endocrinological Metabolism* 71 (1990): 1083–1088.

31. L. K. Bunker, "Psycho-Physiological Contributions of Physical Activity and Sports for Girls," *Research Digest of the President's Council on Physical Fitness and Sport* Series 3, #1. Washington, DC: PCPFS, 1998.

32. W. J. Chodzko-Zajko, "Physical Fitness, Cognitive Performance, and Aging," *Medicine and Science in Sport and Exercise* 23 (1991): 868–872; J. R. Thomas, D. M. Landers, W. Salazar, and J. Ethnier, "Exercise and Cognitive Function," in *Physical Activity, Fitness, and Health: International Proceedings and Consensus Statement*, ed. C. Bouchard, R. J. Shephard, and T. Stephens (Champaign, IL: Human Kinetics, 1994), 521–529; R. S. Paffenbarger, "Physical Activity, Health and Fitness," in *American College of Sports Medicine: 40th Anniversary Lectures* (Indianapolis: American College of Sports Medicine, 1994).

33. J. J. Keayes and K. R. Allison. "The Effects of Regular to Moderate Vigorous Physical Activity on Student Outcomes: A Review" *Canadian Journal of Public Health* 86 (1995): 62–65.

34. K. J. Calfas and W. C. Taylor, "Effect of Physical Activity on Psychological Variables in Adolescents," *Pediatric Exercise Science* 6, 4 (1994): 406–423; D. Wiese-Bjornstal, "Psychological Dimensions," in the President's Council on Physical Fitness and Sport Report, *Physical Activity and Sport in the Lives of Girls* (Washington, DC: PCPFS, 1997), 46–49; L. K. Bunker, "Psycho-Physiological Contributions of Physical Activity and Sports for Girls," *Research Digest of the President's Council on Physical Fitness and Sport* Series 3, #1. Washington, DC: PCPFS, 1998; R. S. Paffenbarger, "Physical Activity, Health and Fitness," in *American College of Sports Medicine: 40th Anniversary Lectures* (Indianapolis: American College of Sports Medicine, 1994).

35. J. J. Gruber, "Physical Activity and Self-Esteem Development in Children: A Meta-analysis," in *Effects of Physical Activity on Children, American Academy of Physical Education Papers,* ed. G. A. Stull and H. M. Eckerts (Champaign, IL: Human Kinetics, 1986), 30–48; K. J. Calfas and W. C. Taylor, "Effect of Physical Activity on Psychological Variables in Adolescents," *Pediatric Exercise Science* 6, 4 (1994): 406–423.

36. K. R. Fox, "Motivating Children for Physical Activity: Towards a Healthier Future," *Journal of Physical Education, Recreation and Dance* 62, no. 7 (1991): 34–38.

37. G. L. Stein, B. Keeler, and P. J. Carpenter, "Helping Children Enjoy Physical Activity Experiences," *Journal of Physical Education, Recreation and Dance* 62, no. 8 (1991): 17–19.

38. American Academy of Pediatrics (AAP), "Climatic Heat Stress and the Exercising Child and Adolescent" (RF9845). *Pediatrics* 106, no. 01 (2000): 158–159.

Learning Experiences

Below are the various psychological, social interactive, and movement skills children should have developed at various grade levels. Each level also includes the choice of activity and learner expectancies relative to the areas of motor skill, movement knowledge, social development, self-image, and personal development.* You can use these competencies as guidelines to modify the Learning Experience that follow for grade levels K–6 and to develop new interdisciplinary learning activities.

Kindergarten

Emphasis: How I move in my environment

Learner: Children at this age tend to be solo learners.

Motor skill and movement knowledge:

1. Children in kindergarten enjoy exploring space and controlling their bodies.
2. Locomotor skills include balancing, bending, stretching, twisting, and so on. Appropriate activities include opportunities to manipulate soft, light balls, bean bags, ribbons, hoops, sock balls, and so on.

Social development: Kindergarten-age children tend to play alone. Teach them to recognize the concept of self and shared space.

Self-image and personal development: Provide as many opportunities as possible for children to experience personal success.

Grade One

Emphasis: Moving through space and time

Learner: Children are ready to develop the concepts of space, time, and effort.

Motor skill and movement knowledge:

1. Children still need to practice locomotor skills such as running, skipping, leaping, jumping, walking, and so on.
2. In addition, teachers may include concepts such as symmetrical and asymmetrical balances and starting/stopping.
3. or activities such as throwing/catching.

Social development: These children participate in parallel play with other students; they tend to be more involved in individual activities than in interaction with others.

Self-image and personal development: Children can learn that the body undergoes marked changes in height and weight and that those changes influence the movement and coordination of body parts.

Grade Two

Emphasis: My partner and I—How we move in space

Learner: Students are ready to work with a partner. Children may make up their own rules as they play together.

Motor skills and movement knowledge: Children begin to look at movement as it relates to others. Appropriate activities will emphasize

- working with a partner;
- dodging while moving, pantomiming, and mirror moving;
- catching and throwing with a partner or kicking a stationary ball.

---

* Adapted from the *Physical Education Framework of the California Public Schools: K–12*, California Department of Education, Sacramento, CA, 1994.

Social development: Children's awareness of others can help promote a positive appreciation for the differences that exist among children and cultures. Children begin to appreciate the successes of others.

Self-image and personal development: Children see themselves in relation to others. They begin to understand and appreciate the feelings, both positive and negative, they have for others.

Grade Three

Emphasis: Continuity and change in movement

Learner: Reacting and responding to others take precedence.

Motor skill and motivation knowledge: Children gain greater control of movement abilities. They begin to determine appropriate movements for certain situations.

Social development: Students begin to gain respect for classmates and for the property of others. They also understand different types of play and assist each other by practicing, with a partner, the rules of fair play.

Self-image and personal development: Children begin to express themselves through their own creation of movement. Find activities that contribute to joy through active play.

Grade Four

Emphasis: Manipulating objects in and through space

Learner: Children at this age tend to become more skillful. They are likely to test the rules of game play and are capable of creating games.

Motor skill and movement knowledge: Students can work to refine the use of space, effort, force and accuracy. Begin combining complex movement patterns. For example, they learn to hand- or foot-dribble while moving within a group of people.

Social development: Students at this age are able to demonstrate initiative and take on leadership roles. They are able to cooperate.

Self-image and personal development: Grade-four children appreciate different styles of movement and are ready to cope with success and failure.

Grade Five

Emphasis: Manipulating objects with speed and accuracy

Learner: Students may be willing to change rules in order to achieve fairness for all.

Motor skill and movement knowledge: Children continue to improve motor skills and apply them in more diversified situations such as small games.

Social development: They thrive in small-group activity in which three to five students interact in cooperative play. They begin to develop an awareness of individual differences related to gender, cultural, heritage, ethnicity, and physical ability.

Self-image and personal development: Youngsters are able to establish their own goals and determine the appropriate strategies for achieving them.

Grade Six

Emphasis: Work cooperatively to achieve a common goal

Learner: Youngsters are more independent in thought and action than their younger peers.

Motor skill and movement knowledge: They combine skills for practice in lead-up games or small-game situations.

Social development: They recognize the need for rules and adhere to them consistently.

Self-image and personal development: They recognize stylistic differences. They begin to value looking good as they become aware of the varying levels of physical development within their peer group.

All evaluations may be conducted using a 3-point rubric wherein the number 1 represents the lowest level of understanding and demonstrating skills and concepts; the number 3, the highest level. Teachers will use this rubric to evaluate performance on each learning objective. The rubric may be placed with the Learning Objectives on a worksheet like the following example:

Learning Objective 1. Students will demonstrate understanding of self-space by remaining still and moving only as far as they can reach with their arms while standing and lying down.

Name	*Level 1*	*Level 2*	*Level 3*
Ian			
Danielle			
Michael			
Samantha			

Avoid placing children in one single line and evaluating them one at a time. It is less stressful for a child to be evaluated while the whole class is practicing skills.

For other suggestions on creating a rubric with which to evaluate student performance of Learning Experiences, see page 13.

Learning Experience 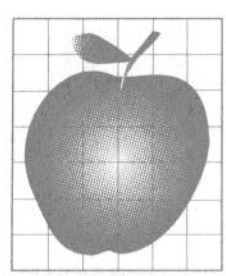 4-1

Making Shapes and Letters in Self-Space

Grade Level

K–2

Primary Disciplines

Fundamental Movement and Spatial Awareness; Language Arts

Time Required

Two sessions, 20 to 25 minutes each (conduct each lesson twice)

Materials

Large pieces of construction paper with letters of the alphabet on them, poly-spots or carpet squares

Learning Objectives

Students will

- Demonstrate understanding of self-space by remaining still and moving only as far as they can reach with their arms while standing and lying down.
- Recognize letters of the alphabet by creating them with their bodies and saying aloud the letter they have created.
- Spell their names by using their bodies to make the letters.
- Make shapes with their bodies while staying in self-space.

Description of Activity

Introduction

- Tell students that self-space is a location; it is that space that surrounds us. It is as big or small as we are.
- First explore self-space by standing still. Self-space will be the space around you; it is as far as you can reach with your arms and legs while standing or lying down.
- You may refer to self-space as an imaginary bubble that surrounds each child.
- Locomotor skills are the fundamental movements that carry us through space, such as walking, running, jogging, skipping, galloping, sliding, hopping, and jumping.
- Non-manipulative skills refer to fundamental movements that do not require manipulating an object or moving the body through general space, such as balance, twisting, and stretching.

Session 1: Exploring Self-Space

Have children spread out and stand in their own self-space. Mark spaces with poly-dots or carpet squares to help children recognize their own self-space area. Say to the children:

1. "Pretend that you are in a place all by yourself. No one can reach you, and you can't reach or touch others. Now move your arms and hands all around you. Stretch and curl into places around your body that you think may be difficult."
2. "Now move your legs and feet all around you. Let me see all of you explore those hard-to-reach places with your feet and legs."
3. "Pretend this place is your very own island. Without traveling through space, staying right where you are, explore your very own island. How many of you can walk around your island? How many of you can walk around your island while keeping your body low? How about while keeping your body in a high level (tiptoes)?"

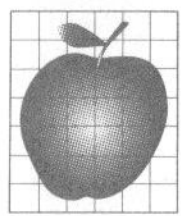

Learning Experience 4-1 continued

4. "Your island is your self-space. When I talk about your self-space, I mean that space around you that is yours without touching other people. It stretches as far as you can reach with your arms and legs while standing or lying down."

Session 2: Making Letters and Shapes in Your Own Self-Space

Say to the children:

1. "Standing in your own self-space, shape your body into the letter I announce and show on the poster." Announce (and show) one letter of the alphabet.
2. Encourage many interpretations of the letter.
3. Encourage children to spell their names.
4. Have the children make shapes with their bodies. Review with the children the concepts of self-space.

Homework

None

Evaluation

See above.

Learning Experience 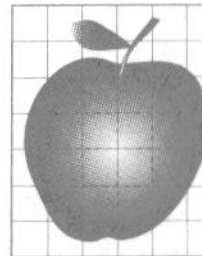 4-2

Moving Through General Space and Creating Shapes

Grade Level

K–2

Primary Disciplines

Fundamental Movement and Spatial Awareness; Math

Time Required

20 to 25 minutes (conduct the lesson twice)

Materials

Large pieces of construction paper with simple words on them; poly-spots or carpet squares; cones

Learning Objectives

Students will make a series of shapes after moving through general space.

Description of Activity

Introduction

1. General space is a location.
2. General space is that space through which we travel, and it is typically marked by boundaries (classroom, a basketball court, a soccer field, a space marked by cones).
3. Safely means not touching or bumping other children.

Activity

1. Have the children, in a single-file line, walk the boundary lines (marked by cones) of the space you are working in.
2. Next have the children walk through general space (anywhere inside the boundaries) and "freeze" on the teacher's signal. Make sure children are moving safely.
3. Now when the children freeze on your signal, have them make a shape with their bodies.
4. Encourage the children to freeze and make shapes at different levels, twisting, turning, and curling.
5. Now when children freeze, call out a number representing the number of body parts the children should have on the ground. For instance, if you call the number three, children may choose to balance on two knees and one hand.

Homework

None

Evaluation

See above.

Learning Experience 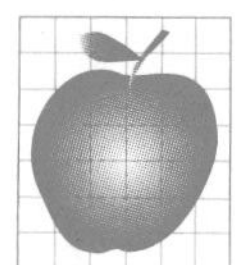 4-3

Movement Sentences and Spatial Awareness

Grade Level

K–2

Primary Disciplines

Fundamental Movement and Spatial Awareness; Language Arts

Time Required

20 to 25 minutes (conduct each of the two lessons twice)

Materials

Index cards, music on tape or CD, poly-spots or carpet squares

Learning Objectives

Students will:

- Create movement sentences and practice the meaning of punctuation marks using movement skills.
- Move safely through general space using various locomotor skills.

Description of Activity

Introduction

Establish a clear start and stop signal. Discuss with the class the meaning of the period, comma, and exclamation point before doing this activity.

Session 1: Shrinking Space (works well with music)

1. Clearly establish the boundaries. In this activity, children may not go out of bounds.
2. Explain that the general space where the children are traveling will shrink. Children must continue to move safely in this shrinking space.
3. Stand at one end of the general space area. Explain that you (the teacher) are a wall extending from one sideline to the next. As you move forward, the general space shrinks. The children must stay in front of you and in bounds.
4. When the space gets too small, have children freeze and check to see that everyone is in his or her own self-space.

Session 2: Movement Sentences

Grades K–1: Have the children act out punctuation marks in general space. For instance, while children move through general space, call out "comma." The children are to pause until the count of five, then continue their movement through general space. If you call out "period," the children freeze where they are and wait for the teacher's signal to continue. If you call out "exclamation point," the children freeze with strong force and await your signal to continue. Children may use a variety of locomotor skills during this activity.

Grades 1–2:

- If children are reading, have them construct movement sentences. All sentences must have a beginning, a middle, and an end. The teacher or the children may list several locomotor skills on an index card or a piece of paper. Each locomotor movement is separated by a comma, and each sentence must end with a period or an exclamation point. For example, a movement sentence may read: "I will walk, gallop, slide, hop, and run!" The child who reads this card then performs these motions safely in general space.
- Create a number of movement sentences on index cards and spread those cards around the movement area. Children select a card and perform the movement. When they are finished, they replace the card and select another.

Homework

None

Evaluation

See above.

Learning Experience 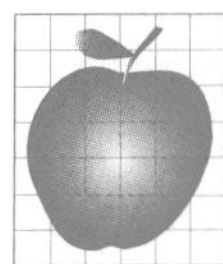 4-4

Food as Fuel

Grade Level

3–4

Primary Disciplines

Physical Education; Science

Time Required

Two sessions, 20–40 minutes each, 2–3 days/week, 3 weeks

Materials

Poster board, markers

Learning Objectives

Students will

- Be able to describe the relationship between food and physical activity.
- Demonstrate, through physical expression, an understanding of the metaphor "food as fuel."

Description of Activity

Session 1: Food as Fuel: A Discussion

Introduction: Discuss the idea that food is fuel our bodies use to get energy needed to perform daily activities.

1. Draw a parallel to nonliving things that use fuel, such as gasoline, coal, and electricity.
2. Ask students to brainstorm nonliving things that use fuel. They may say things such as cars, trains, boats, airplanes, furnace, lamps.
3. Write this list on poster board or chalkboard.
4. Brainstorm the types of fuel living things need for energy. For example, plants need water, sunlight, and minerals from the soil; animals need food and water.
5. Once living and nonliving fuel lists are complete, ask, "What happens when living and nonliving things run out of fuel?" (A: Nonliving things slow down, stop, grow dim, etc. For living things, plants get dry and wilt, animals slow down, people and animals may feel tired, etc.)
6. Now stress the importance of food as fuel and that the body needs nutritious foods to maintain a positive energy level.

Session 2: Food as Fuel: A Demonstration

1. In a gym, multipurpose room, or outside, ask students to imitate an airplane, sports car, train, and other fuel-operated nonliving things.
2. Ask the students to demonstrate what happens to these things as they run out of fuel.
3. As students demonstrate their understanding of the importance of fuel, ask them to show you what happens to people and animals when they don't eat and maintain their fuel level.
4. Review the point that food is fuel. People need food and water to live, grow, play, and do schoolwork.
5. Explain that when we play and exercise, we use up the food we eat. Food and activity go hand and hand. Too much food will make us gain weight and limit our physical activity. Too little food will make us lose weight and too tired to play and exercise.

Homework

None

Evaluation

See above.

Learning Experience 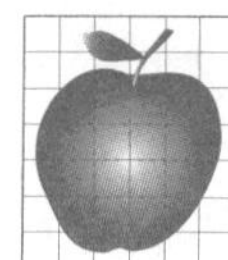 4-5

Digestive System

Grade Level

3–4

Primary Disciplines

Physical Education, Science

Time Required

25–40 minutes for each lesson, 2–3 days/week, 3 weeks

Materials

Resources on digestive system, poster board, markers, jump ropes, mats, hula hoops, handout

Learning Objectives

Students will be able to

- Identify the parts of the digestive system.
- Draw and explain the functions of the digestive system.
- Act out the functions of the digestive system.

Description of Activity

Session 1: Digestive Digest

Identify the key parts of the digestive system, using the information provided in Chapter 2.

1. Use a handout for students to identify the parts of the digestive system, or have students draw the digestive system and label the parts on a plain piece of paper.
2. Post student work around the room.

Session 2: A Zone Tag Game

Divide the gym, multipurpose room, or outdoor area into three sections. Clearly mark the boundaries. Label the sections with signs: (1) mouth and esophagus, (2) stomach, and (3) small intestine.

Zone 1: Students enter the mouth and pick up jump ropes lying about the area. Students jump for 1 minute (stimulating food being ground by teeth). After jumping, students do log rolls across one of four mats. Log rolls represent food passing down the esophagus and into the stomach.

Zone 2: In the stomach, students are faced with four digestive juices (students) placed in each hula hoop spread across the stomach. Students must run, twist, and turn as they churn through the stomach to the small intestine. Students who are tagged by a digestive juice are immediately absorbed into the bloodstream and must exit to the sideline and begin the process again. All other students enter the small intestine.

Zone 3: Four free-floating digestive juices (students) occupy the small intestine. The digestive juices strive to tag as many students as possible. Once tagged, students are absorbed into the bloodstream, exit to the side, and begin the process again. Students who make it to the end without being tagged return to the first section and begin the process again. Switch taggers in hula hoops every 2 or 3 minutes. At the end of the activity, ask students what they learned about the digestive system and its importance to "food as fuel."

Note: In this session, be sure to modify the set-up so you do not have long lines of children waiting to be active.

Homework

None

Evaluation

See above.

Name ____________________ Date ____________________

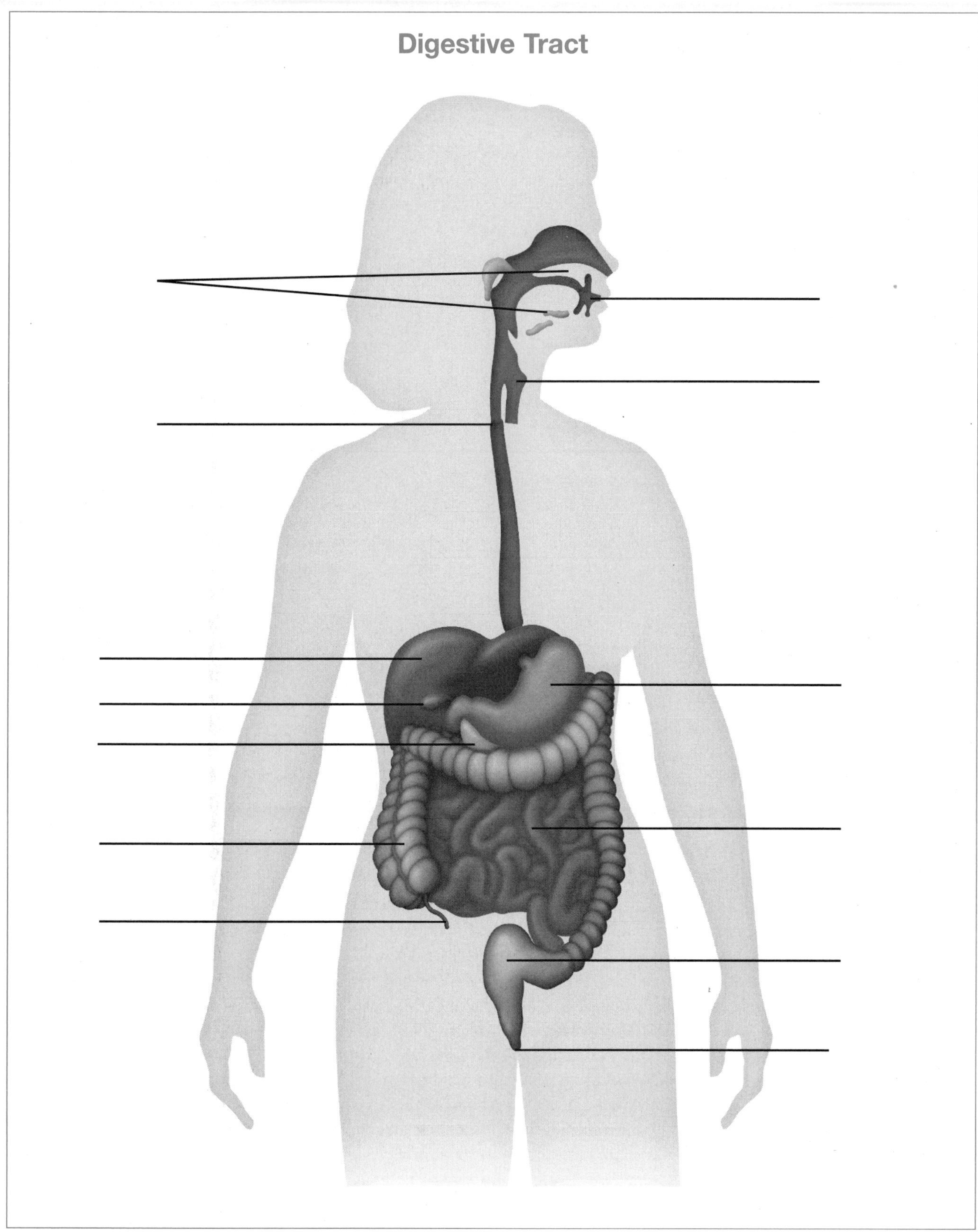

Learning Experience 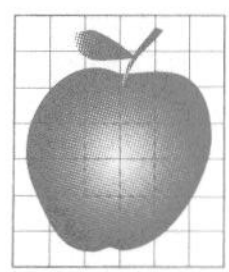 *4-6*

The Heart

Grade Level

3–4

Primary Disciplines

Physical Education, Science, Visual Art

Time Required

25–40 minutes for each lesson, 2–3 days/week, 3 weeks

Materials

Resources on cardiorespiratory system, poster board, markers, music taped or on CD, fabric, handout

Learning Objectives

The students will be able to

- Identify the parts of the heart.
- Explain the function of the heart.
- State the parts and function of blood.

Description of Activity

Session 1: Word Splash for the Heart

Introduction: Discuss the parts and functions of the heart using information in Chapter 2.

1. Each day spend time exploring one concept from the Introduction. For Session 1 it is the whole heart. For Session 2 it may be the chambers of the heart, and so on.
2. Begin each discussion with a word splash about the heart. In a word splash, the teacher writes words to be examined on the board.
3. Students use resources to determine meanings for the words.
4. They write a sentence for each word listed.
5. They group their sentences together to form a paragraph describing the major concept.

Example: List several of the following words for the heart on the board: heart, cardiac muscle; fist; 4 chambers, right atrium, left atrium, right ventricle, left ventricle, strong muscle, septum.

Students may work on the word splash independently or in small groups.

Session 2: Moving to Raise Your Beat

Using music that the students enjoy, have small groups of three create a fun movement to do while standing next to their desk or in a large open area.

1. While the music plays, direct one group at a time to demonstrate their moves for the class.
2. The class joins the group by doing the movements with them.
3. After a few minutes, shift attention to another group, who then leads the class with its own movements.
4. Before the music begins and immediately after it is over, ask students to feel and notice the rate at which their heart is beating. They place a hand over their heart to feel its beat.

Emphasize the importance of raising the heart rate as a way to help keep the heart in good physical shape. Physical activity keeps the cardiac muscle strong.

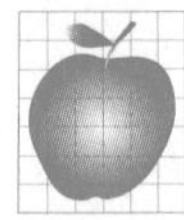

Learning Experience 4-6 continued

Session 3: Heart Healthy Quilt: A Community Project

Using collected fabric, each child will design and create a "healthy heart" square for a class quilt. Each student may work on her or his square during designated class time. This project may be integrated with art. Once finished, the class may want to donate it to a community health facility such as a cardiac rehab program, cardiac unit, or elders home.

Homework

Have the students bring a fabric scrap from home to contribute to a quilt.

Evaluation

See above.

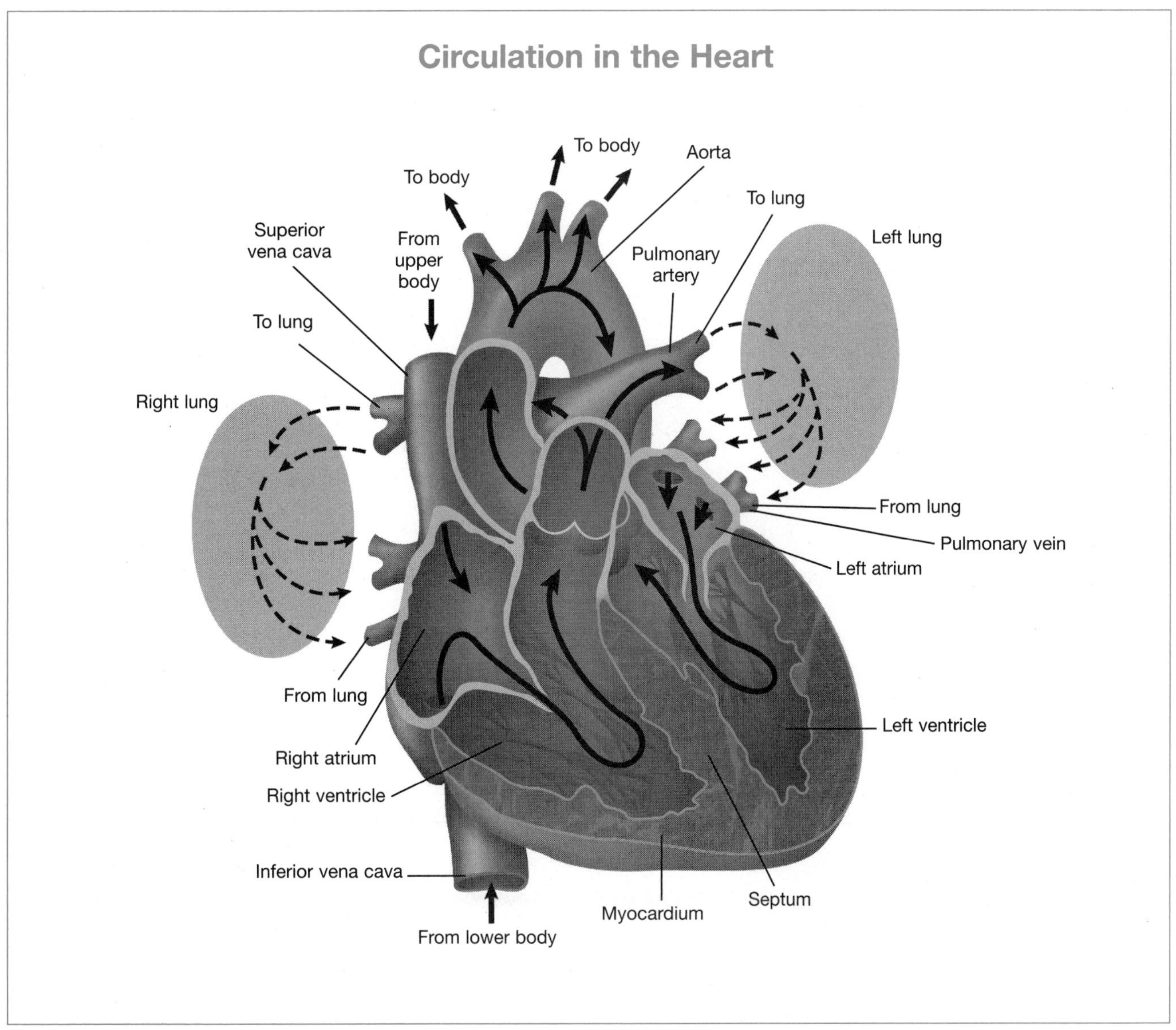
Circulation in the Heart
To body
Aorta
To body
To lung
Left lung
Superior vena cava
From upper body
Pulmonary artery
To lung
Right lung
From lung
Pulmonary vein
Left atrium
From lung
Left ventricle
Right atrium
Right ventricle
Inferior vena cava
Myocardium
Septum
From lower body

Learning Experience 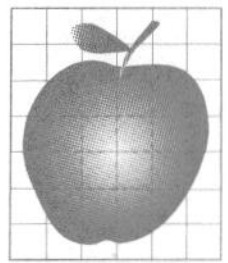 4-7

Great Oxygen Exchange

Grade Level

3–4

Primary Disciplines

Physical Education; Science

Time Required

25–40 minutes for each lesson, 2–3 days/week, 3 weeks

Materials

Resources on respiratory and circulatory systems, poster board, markers, masking tape, parachute or tarp, balls, beanbags, handouts

Learning Objectives

Students will be able to

- Recognize the mutual workings of the circulatory and respiratory systems.
- Demonstrate the process of oxygen exchange.

Description of Activity

Session 1: Introduction

Discuss the heart, blood, and the process of oxygen exchange using information from Chapter 2. Have students together create a poster depicting this body system.

Session 2: Obstacle Course

1. Create a giant replica of the cardiorespiratory system by setting up a heart, lung, and body cell maze in a gym, multipurpose room, or outdoors.
2. Starting at one end of the area, outline the lungs (with masking tape), the heart (including the four chambers) in the middle, and the body cells at the other end of the area. Make the replica large enough for a child to travel through.
3. Drape a parachute or tarp over chairs to create the lung area (tunnel).
4. Create four pathways—one to represent the pulmonary artery (heart to lungs), another representing the pulmonary vein (lungs to heart), the third leading to the body cells area, the fourth leaving the body cells area and returning to the heart via the right atrium.
5. Position two students between the atria and ventricles in the heart. Their job will be to let the blood cells (students) pass through each chamber of the heart one at a time. Position one student between the left and right lung and another in the body cells area. The student in the lungs area will trade a ball (oxygen atom) that each blood cell (other students) carry from the body cell area. The student stationed in the body cell area will trade beanbags for balls.

   Note: You or a student will have to be a runner between the two exchange points, to keep each supplied with balls and beanbags.
6. Vary the locomotor skills students use to travel through the Great Oxygen Exchange.

Homework

None

Evaluation

See above.

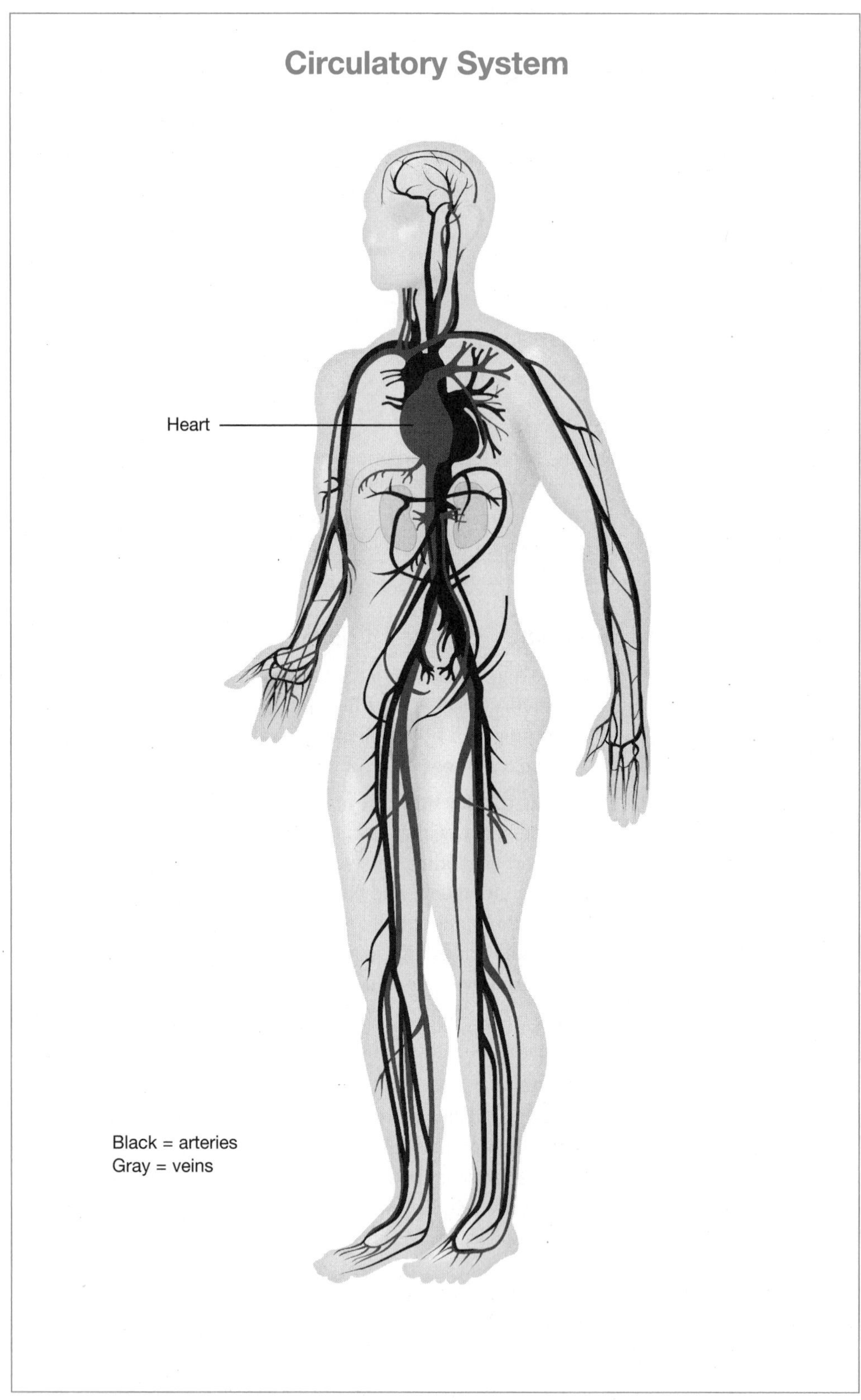
Circulatory System
Heart
Black = arteries
Gray = veins

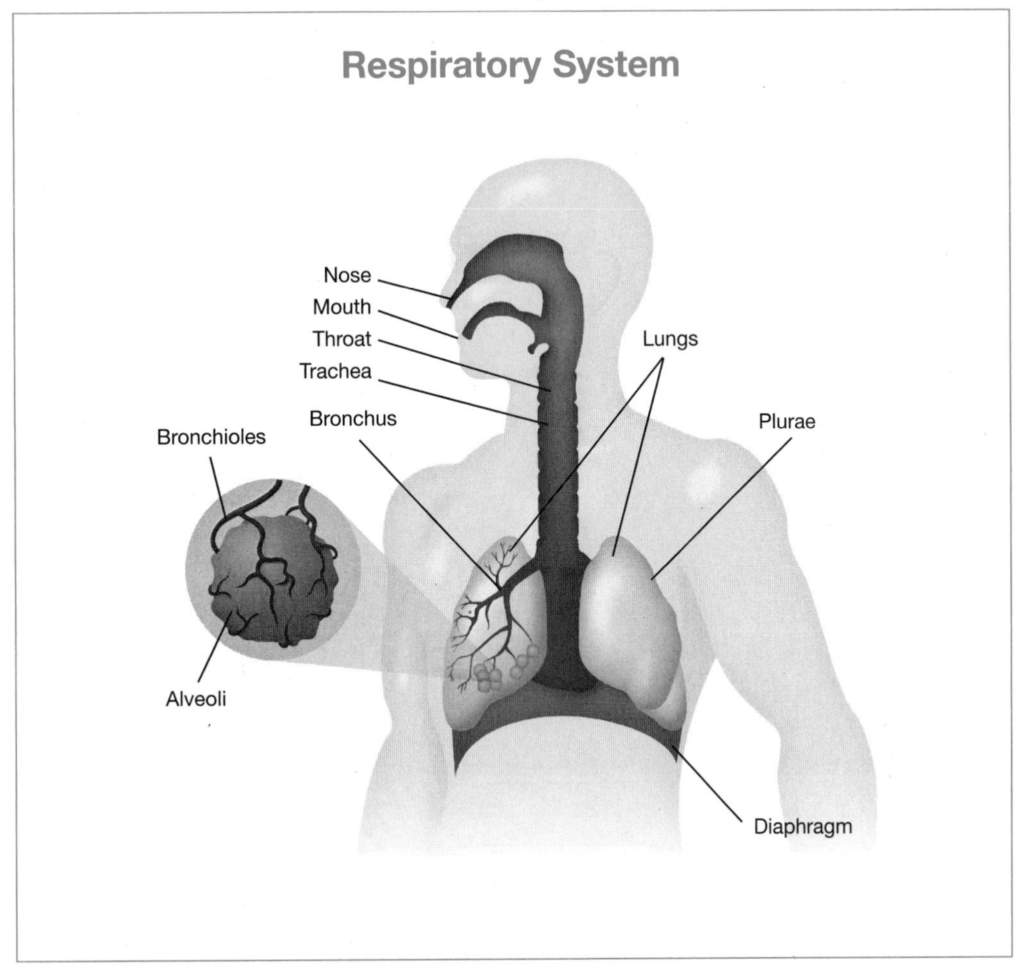
Respiratory System
Nose
Mouth
Throat
Trachea
Bronchus
Bronchioles
Lungs
Plurae
Alveoli
Diaphragm

Learning Experience 4-8

Introduction to the Donner Family: Donner Party Pioneer Expedition

Grade Level

5–6

Primary Disciplines

U.S. History, Geography, Physical Education

Time Required

40 minutes; 2–3 days/week, 3 weeks

Materials

Map of Donner route, documentary film of Donner Party, if possible.

Learning Objectives

Students will:

1. investigate the Donner Party pioneer expedition;
2. explain the difficulties associated with pioneer travel;
3. plan a reenactment of the Donner Party pioneer expedition.

Key Information for Teacher

Collect accurate information about the Donner Party expedition.

Description of Activity

The teacher proceeds as follows:

1. Tell the story of the Donner Party pioneer expedition.
2. Brainstorm why the journey was so difficult.
    a. Difficulty finding food and shelter.
    b. Unfamiliar terrain (deserts, mountains).
    c. Unfamiliar weather (extreme heat, cold, snow, rain).
    d. Isolation from people who can help in times of need.
    e. Unfamiliar illnesses and diseases.
    f. Unfamiliar natural risks, such as wildlife.
    g. Confrontations with American Indians such as the Pawnee and the Sioux.
3. Discuss ways to prepare for travel.
    a. Gather information about where you are going, including: availability of food, water, shelter, terrain, weather, natural risks.
    b. Collect the necessary supplies, food, water, wagon, livestock.
    c. Plan your route, including rest stops and receiving new supplies.
    d. Prepare yourself, exercise, eat well, plenty of sleep.
4. In groups of four or five, students will plan their trip to California using the same route the Donner Party described.
    a. Decide when to leave.
    b. Plan what to bring on the trip.
    c. Decide where to rest and resupply.
    d. Determine what to do in case of emergency.
    e. Estimate date of arrival.
    f. Determine how to get in shape for the trip.

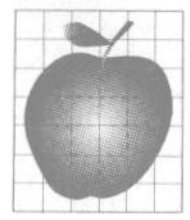

Learning Experience 4-8 continued

Homework

Students interview parents about how they would plan to take a trip. Write down the interview and bring it to share in class discussion.

Evaluation

Evaluation will be conducted using a 3-point rubric. The number 1 of the rubric will be the lowest level of understanding and demonstrating skills and concepts. The number 3 will be the highest level. Teachers will use this rubric to evaluate performance on learning objectives. Teachers may list each lesson objective at the top of a rubric worksheet and evaluate children accordingly. The rubric may be placed on a worksheet like the following example:

Learning Objective

Explain the difficulties associated with pioneer travel.

Name:	Level 1	Level 2	Level 3
Ian	X		
Danielle		X	
Michael	X		
Samantha			X

Learning Experience 4-9

Planning Reenactment of Donner Party Expedition

Grade Level

5–6

Primary Disciplines

U. S. History, Geography, Physical Education

Time Required

40 minutes; 2–3 days/week, 3 weeks

Materials

Map of Donner route, map of United States, construction paper and markers

Learning Objectives

Students will

- Plan a walk/run program to reenact the Donner Party expedition.
- Learn how to mark their daily distances traveled on a map showing the Donner route.

Description of Activity

Introduction

Measure a distance in the schoolyard that is equal to 1/4 mile (440 yards).

1. Inform students that each 1/4 mile walked is equal to 25 miles of the Donner Party expedition.
2. Create or display a map of the United States for groups to record their mileage with cut-out wagons.

Activity

Using information from prior discussion about the Donner Party, develop the in-class walk/run program and scale walks to match distances covered by the Donner Party. Have students design and cut out their own wagon to mark the distance covered on the map.

Homework

Students will be encouraged to walk or run by themselves or with their families.

Evaluation

See above.

Learning Experience 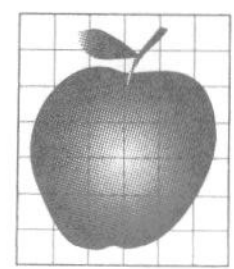 4-10

Reenacting Donner Party Expedition

Grade Level

5–6

Primary Disciplines

U. S. History, Geography, Physical Education

Time Required

40 minutes; 2–3 days/week, 3 weeks

Materials

Map of Donner route, resources on states the Donner Party passed through

Learning Objectives

Students will

- Briskly walk/run in small groups for 20 minutes.
- Record distance walked/ran on the Donner Party map.
- Work in small groups to collect information about one state that the Donner Party passed through.

Description of Activity

Introduction

Make available to students information on the following states: Illinois, Missouri, Kansas, Colorado, Utah, Nevada, and California. Discuss with students that they must walk/run as a group, because they are walking together as a wagon train. Downplay competition between groups; encourage cooperation. Encourage students to dress for the period.

Activity

1. Have groups of students briskly walk/run for 20 minutes around marked area. When done, students mark the distance covered on the map.
2. Assign each small group a state included in the Donner Party expedition. Have students gather information about the state as it existed at the time of the Donner Party expedition, including information about the terrain and weather during all four seasons.
3. Have groups present their state reports to the class. After the presentations, the small groups discuss any adjustments they should make to their travel plans.

Homework

Students continue to walk/run by themselves or with their families at home.

Evaluation

See above.

5

Communicable and Chronic Diseases

Rhona Feigenbaum and Andrina Veit

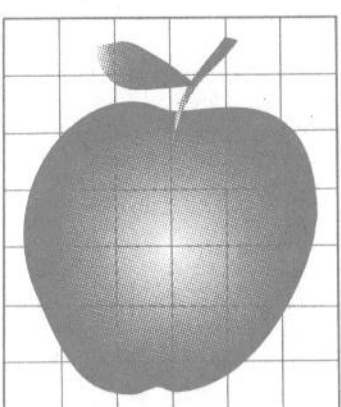

Chapter Outline

Diseases
Communicable Diseases
Chronic Diseases
Some Genetic Disorders
Seizure Disorders In Children
Physical Disabilities

Objectives

- Differentiate communicable and noncommunicable diseases
- Delineate the classes of pathogens and how they transmit disease
- Name the factors that increase susceptibility to disease
- Describe how the immune system fights disease
- Define allergies and autoimmune diseases
- List the stages in communicable diseases
- Explain how sexually transmitted diseases, including HIV, are transmitted and their manifestations
- Define chronic diseases and describe the most prevalent of these: diabetes, cancer, cardiovascular diseases, and asthma
- Describe the process by which genetically inherited diseases are transmitted and give some examples of these conditions

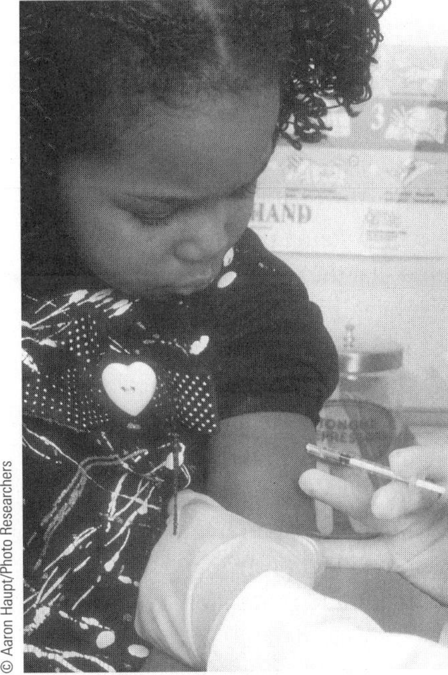

Just last year Ilene found out that her 12-year-old sister, Sherry, has a disease called diabetes. The disease has changed her family life. Her sister doesn't look sick, but her parents are always talking about the disease and how worried they are. Ilene watches as her sister gives herself injections and tests her blood from a prick on the finger several times a day. The entire family now eats different foods at specific times.

Sherry is not the only one in the family who has diabetes. Her grandfather does, too. Ilene sometimes worries that she can get diabetes.

• • •

Alonso's brother just died of AIDS. The second-grade class wrote cards to Alonso and his family telling him how sorry they are about his brother dying. The children are afraid that Alonso has AIDS also and that they can catch it from him. The parents came to school one night to talk to the gym teacher. Some of them do not want their children to be in the same class as Alonso. Amy's mother told Amy that she does not have to worry about getting AIDS from Alonso even if he has it (which he probably doesn't). You don't get AIDS from playing with someone, but you do want to be careful around all children and get help, if they are bleeding. Some of the children are confused and afraid.

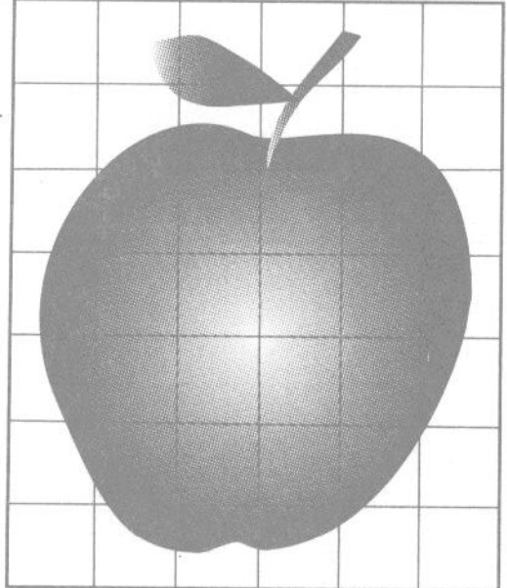

Friends of Ilene and Alonso wonder—can you catch diabetes or AIDS? If your grandfather and your sister have it, will you or your parents get it? Can you die from it? I know that when I have a cold or the flu, I am supposed to stay away from my baby brother. Is he going to die also? How come Alonso's brother didn't get better? Didn't the doctor know what to do?

Educators are faced with answering these and other questions about chronic and infectious diseases, including sexually transmitted diseases (STDs) and HIV/AIDS. The challenge is to provide age-appropriate, accurate information and to help children process and use this information to make responsible decisions that protect their health and possibly the health of others. The goal is to help young people develop a sense that they can have control over their health and that, by choosing behaviors that support their health, they can prevent many communicable diseases and manage the chronic ones.

This chapter differentiates infectious and noninfectious diseases, describes the immune system, and presents information about transmission, symptoms, treatment, and prevention of diseases including common STDs and HIV/AIDS. It also describes the more common diseases of childhood, both chronic and communicable, and focuses on their **etiology** (that is, their causes); the factors that contribute to the causes; how the disease affects the body; and ways in which children, parents, and community can take responsibility for primary prevention. Helpful Learning Experiences for students, by grade level, appear at the end of the chapter and are integrated into other subjects of the curriculum.

Diseases

Human diseases represent changes in the normal structure or function of the human body. Diseases may present generalized or specific symptoms. Sometimes diseases are asymptomatic until they have progressed enough to be detected by some type of abnormal finding in a medical screening test. Crowley considers disease to occur on a continuum that ranges from physical and emotional well-being to severe and life-threatening illness. He explains that between the two extremes is a range of conditions—spanning from mild or short-term illness to moderate good health—that "fall short of the ideal state." He claims that most of us live somewhere between the mid-point or "neutral" position and the ideal state.[1]

Diseases have always threatened the human condition. The types of diseases our ancestors faced, however, are no longer the main causes of illness and death. Today, the major health problems are the non-contagious or chronic diseases that are related to living styles or stress (further discussed in Chapter 8). Heart disease and cancer are prime examples. These are **noncommunicable diseases**; they are not passed from one person to another by pathogens. Some are chronic and **degenerative** diseases. Examples of these are arthritis, diabetes, multiple sclerosis, muscular dystrophy, cerebral palsy, Tay-Sachs disease, and sickle cell anemia. These develop before birth (congenital) or sometimes after birth (developmental).

By way of comparison, congenital heart defects are accidents of embryonic development, whereas lung cancer —thought to be caused by smoking and exposure to pollutants, among other factors—is a chronic disease that usually develops later in life. The diseases influenced by lifestyle are thought to begin early, leading to erosion of health later in life, when their recognizable symptoms appear. For example, a collection of plaque in the arteries that ultimately results in arteriosclerosis later in life is thought to be a result of years and years of eating foods high in saturated fats.

Susceptibility

Why is it that, during a flu epidemic, some children get sick, and others stay well? Why do some children react to pollen or grasses by sneezing or coughing, and others don't? These variations in susceptibility to disease, whether communicable or chronic, indicate that several factors determine who will be affected and who won't. Knowing what these factors are and either eliminating them or controlling their effects can go a long way toward limiting the dangers of these diseases.

The following is a brief summary of factors that contribute to or complicate susceptibility to disease. These include heredity, environment, socioeconomic factors, living styles, diet, drugs and medications, and disabilities.

Heredity

Diseases such as hemophilia, sickle cell anemia, fibrosis, muscular dystrophy, phenylketonuria, and Tay-Sachs disease are passed down from parents to children through their genes. These require that a parent or both parents have, in their gametes (sperm or eggs), the gene **mutations**—changes in the chemical make-up of their **DNA**—responsible for the disease. Many gene mutations are not fatal and do not contribute to disease; they present no problem. Others cause an error in development that may result in a spontaneous abortion (miscarriage) or stillbirth or cause a **birth defect**—an inherited disease that begins during embryonic development and is present at birth. Examples are hemophilia and phenylketonuria. In other cases, such as muscular dystrophy, the results of a gene mutation appear later in life. In yet another case, the gene for the disease may be present, but the disease itself may skip a generation without symptoms to the **carrier** (the person who has the gene mutation). In some cases, such as Down syndrome, a whole **chromosome** (a set of genes), rather than a gene itself, is passed along.

Diseases for which no specific gene has yet been identified seem to run in families. These include heart disease, adult-onset diabetes, and cancer. Genes may play some role in predisposing people to these diseases or to other factors that will result in their occurrence. When a disease appears in more than one family member, it may be a result of habits in common or environmental factors rather than genes. Family members may be smokers, eat foods high in saturated fat, or live under high stress. These factors have been implicated in health problems such as cardiovascular diseases, cancer, and asthma, and often are controllable.

Environment

The environments in which people live can greatly influence their risk of getting certain diseases (see Chapter 13). Pollutants in the air have been linked to lung diseases, such as asthma and chronic bronchitis. Other environmental chemicals are associated with allergies and contact dermatitis. The chemicals in polluted water have been associated with certain birth defects. Other components of the physical environment that contribute to disease include ultraviolet radiation, which can produce cancers from sunburns, and noise, which can produce hearing loss or deafness. Stressors from the environment are implicated in hypertension, cardiovascular disease, ulcers, and asthma (see Chapter 8).

Socioeconomic Factors

The health of family members can be affected by their economic and social standing in the community. An economically disadvantaged or poor family may not be able to afford the foods required for a healthy diet, thereby compromising the health of its members. Inadequate access to medical care may cause a family to put off treating early symptoms, creating the potential for major illness. An inability to access information about health—available through magazines, newspaper, TV, radio, and the Internet—could result in poor health habits which, in turn, weaken the immune system and thereby invite disease. At the other end of the socioeconomic spectrum is affluence—which does not guarantee good health either. Economically advantaged families may overindulge in foods rich in fat, sugar, and salt; lead a sedentary lifestyle; and have other poor health habits that increase their susceptibility to diseases.

Living Styles

Beyond socioeconomic status or driven by it, people make personal decisions about how they live that have serious consequences for their health. What are their daily activities? Do they exercise regularly? Do they smoke cigarettes, drink alcohol, use drugs? Do they skip meals, grab fast food, and eat too much or too quickly? Is their indigestion controlled by popping antacids? Are their jobs or relationships unrewarding or stressful? Do they visit a physician routinely for prevention and screening examinations? Only recently has the medical community recognized the strong relationship between these living styles and the prevention of disease.

The fast-paced life that many people are accustomed to has all too often resulted in ill-advised fads, such as smoking and using recreational drugs, quick weight-reducing diets, unprotected sexual promiscuity, and other health-compromising behaviors. Frequently, people lack understanding of the relationship between these behaviors and health. Sound education about health can result in healthy behaviors and give children an opportunity to examine their health habits, which can have a positive impact on their long-term health status.

Diet

The relationship of nutrition to disease is rapidly becoming of interest to the conventional medical community and lay persons alike. Eating a well-balanced diet can defer the onset, reduce the intensity, and help to prevent the recurrence of disease. Too many people eat too much and are overweight, and too many don't eat enough or eat the wrong foods (see Chapter 3). Being overweight has been linked to medical conditions including infertility, cardiovascular disease, diabetes, and cancer. Eating too little has been associated with vitamin deficiencies that can produce abnormal growth.

Drugs

Medicines and other drugs, whether prescription or over-the-counter, have been developed to treat and possibly cure diseases. If they are misused or abused, however, these chemicals can be harmful and, in some cases, cause death. Medications can be misused by taking more than the recommended dose, taking old medicines that have expired, taking more than one drug at the same time without knowledge of their interaction, or borrowing prescription drugs from a friend (see Chapter 10). Antibiotics are the "miracle drugs" that provide effective and efficient treatment of bacterial diseases. Yet, they have been over-prescribed, inhibiting the body from coming to its own defense or losing their effectiveness. The overuse of antibiotics has also been implicated in the development of specific drug-resistant strains of pathogens, such as the new strains of tuberculosis and syphilis. Thus, medications that were developed to fight disease can end up having the opposite effect.

Disabilities

Congenital defects and accidents may be accompanied by, or result in, physical disabilities. The most common types of disabilities are related to impaired vision, hearing, and mobility. In some cases, such as arthritis, emphysema, and muscular dystrophy, the body degenerates or weakens over time. Damage to the brain, nervous system, skeleton, or muscles may impair functioning. Cerebral palsy, a disability found in young children (characterized by a lack of muscular coordination and possible speech impairment) develops during pregnancy. Developmental anomalies include spina bifida and cystic fibrosis.

In many cases, people with disabilities are more susceptible to diseases and must take extra precautions to prevent them. Because most of us will experience a disability of one sort or another in ourselves or in a significant person in our lives, learning about and becoming sensitive to disabilities is important.

Communicable Diseases

Communicable diseases, also called contagious or infectious diseases, are transmitted by germs or pathogenic organisms from an infected animal or person to an uninfected person, directly or indirectly. Some communicable diseases, such as polio, smallpox, and cholera, are almost nonexistent today

For Your Health

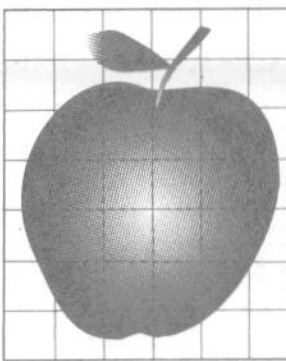

How to Avoid Colds and Cope with Colds

- Wash your hands, especially after contact with someone who has a cold.
- Keep your hands away from your eyes, nose, and mouth.
- Avoid crowds when you can.
- Drink a lot of fluids (at least 8 ounces every 2 hours). Fluids, especially if hot, soothe the throat and help relieve congestion.
- Gargle with salt water. One teaspoon of salt in warm water every 4 hours will help to reduce swelling in the throat.
- Get plenty of rest. Rest helps heal and restore.
- Use disposable tissues instead of handkerchiefs. Handkerchiefs can harbor germs for up to several hours.
- Inhale warm, moist air (steam) from a vaporizer or humidifier or pan of water on the stove. Take moderately warm baths to soothe inflamed mucous membranes.

Source: American Medical Society.

because of widespread public health immunization programs. Others, including AIDS and other sexually transmitted diseases, are serious concerns. Much can be done to reduce their spread and, in some cases, prevent them entirely.

Epidemiology

Infectious diseases can be understood in terms of their cause, their method of spreading throughout a population, and their effects. This information can be applied to prolong life by delaying the onset of diseases or preventing and treating diseases. Epidemiologists constantly advance the knowledge about specific diseases through study of disease patterns and collection of information about similarities and differences between diseases: how they affect populations, who gets them, and who doesn't. Using the data collected about diseases and applying statistics, these scientists try to establish cause-and-effect relationships, then control them through prevention and treatment interventions.

Infectious Agents

Infectious diseases are caused by pathogens that reproduce somewhere inside a person, even if symptoms are not present. Pathogenic organisms, or pathogens, are of five types: viruses, bacteria, fungi, protozoa, and metazoa (see Table 5.1). Each pathogen produces distinct symptoms, often making it easy for a medical professional to diagnose and treat the resulting problem. For some common communicable diseases—such as chicken pox, mumps, and measles, and rubella—vaccinations have been developed that produce lifelong immunity. In most cases, these so-called childhood diseases do not threaten life, although a bout with them can have serious side effects. For example, mumps can leave a male child permanently sterile, and German measles, if contracted during early pregnancy, can damage the fetus. Body lice, ticks, and fleas are also contagious but rarely cause damage. However, they may also carry infectious agents. Therefore, they need to be treated.

From time to time, a new strain of a disease-causing agent appears posing a serious threat to the population. This mobilizes the epidemiological and health community to find ways to control it. An example is Legionnaires' disease, which seems to be spread by pathogens that collect in the condensation of air-conditioning systems.

Table 5.1 **Classes of Pathogens**

CLASS	EXAMPLES (And the Diseases They Cause)
Viruses Poliovirus	Common cold Influenza Poliomyelitis Hepatitis B Hepatitis C Herpes HIV (AIDS) Chicken pox Mononucleosis (Epstein-Barr)
Bacteria Tuberculosis bacilli Syphilis spirochetes	Tuberculosis Strep throat Gonorrhea Syphilis E. coli (food poisoning)
Fungi Yeast Mold	Candidiasis (yeast infection) Ringworm Athlete's foot
Protozoa Trichomonas Amoeba	Trichomoniasis (an STD)
Metazoa (various parasites) Tapeworm	Pubic lice Tapeworm

Table 5.2 shows the route of transmission for some common infectious diseases. Through health education, we can provide information that will delay the onset, minimize the severity, and (in some cases) entirely prevent communicable diseases from infecting children, families, and communities.

The Body's Defenses Against Disease

The body has an elaborate defense system against a wide variety of pathogens and chemicals that may damage or destroy it. Normally, this system is effective in keeping out unwanted foreign matter and often keeps people from getting the associated diseases.

First Line of Defense

In the first barrier, hair follicles in the nose trap dust and other particles, preventing them from getting into the respiratory system. Small cilia in the nasal passages and trachea direct debris outward and trap it in mucous secretions that are expelled by coughing, blowing the nose, or swallowing (in which case, foreign matter is destroyed or eliminated by the digestive process). By keeping out most potential invaders, skin (when unbroken) and mucous membranes constitute the first line of defense.

Second Line of Defense

If foreign matter gets past the skin and mucous membranes, chemical barriers go to work. These consist of digestive enzymes and acids in the stomach that kill bacteria and break down unwanted chemicals. Tears, sweat, skin oils, saliva, and mucus also contain enzymes that can kill pathogens. In addition, the kidneys are continually washing out bacteria that are killed by the acidity of urine and eliminating metabolized chemicals.

The Third Line of Defense: The Immune System

When pathogens get past the first and second lines of defense, the immune system comes into play. It is on constant alert for foreign substances that might threaten the body and swings into action when needed. More than a dozen different types of white blood cells are concentrated in the organs of the lymphatic system. By way of blood and lymph vessels, these white blood cells patrol the entire body (see Chapter 2).

The immune response has four stages:

1. Recognition of the invading pathogen. Specialized white blood cells called **phagocytes** and **macrophages** confront the foreign substances, called **antigens**, and attempt to engulf them. At the same time, they call upon helper **T cells** (a type of white blood cell that originates in the thymus gland) to identify the antigens.
2. Rapid replication of T cells and B cells. The helper T cells alert the **B cells** (a white blood cell that originates in the bone marrow), which are transformed into cells that produce **antibodies** capable of destroying a specific organism.

Table 5.2
Routes of Transmission for Selected Infectious Diseases

	Organism				
Transmission Route	Virus	Bacteria	Fungus	Protozoa	Metazoa
Airborne or droplet	Flu, measles, mumps, smallpox,* cold,* chicken pox*	Impetigo,* whooping cough, TB			
Saliva	Mononucleosis				
Direct contact or touching an infected person	Chicken pox,*	Strep throat, impetigo,* diphtheria	Ringworm,* athlete's foot*		Lice
Surfaces	Common cold,* smallpox,* German measles	Pink-eye, impetigo*	Ringworm,* athlete's foot*		
Oral/Fecal	Hepatitis A			Amoebic dysentery	
Dirt/Feces into blood		Tetanus			
Bloodborne	AIDS,* Hepatitis B,* Hepatitis C				
Sexual activity	AIDS,* Hepatitis B, Hepatitis C, Herpes (type II)				
Infected food		Salmonella, botulism		Tapeworm	
Animal bite	Rabies			Malaria	

*Transmitted by more than one route

3. Attack by killer T cells and macrophages. Alerted by the helper T cells, the killer T cells and macrophages can now search out the targeted organisms and kill them.
4. Memory and suppression of the immune response. Two other white blood cells, **memory T cells** and suppressor T cells, become activated. The memory T cells "remember" the specific antigen and, if ever that antigen gains entry into the body again, the memory T cells will respond more quickly by alerting the immune system to the presence of the antigen. This is called **acquired immunity** (see Figure 5.1), because the body has developed an antibody system against that specific antigen. Once the battle against any foreign substance is won, the suppressor T cells halt the production of antibodies by B cells, and the body returns to homeostasis.

Acquired immunity also can be conferred through vaccination, in which an injection of killed or weakened pathogens that cause a specific disease stimulate the body to build antibodies specific to it. For example, people are vaccinated against the polio virus with killed pathogens. This has nearly eliminated polio. Vaccination programs and their large-scale availability are important in containing and eliminating serious infectious diseases. Table 5.3 (on page 160) shows the standard

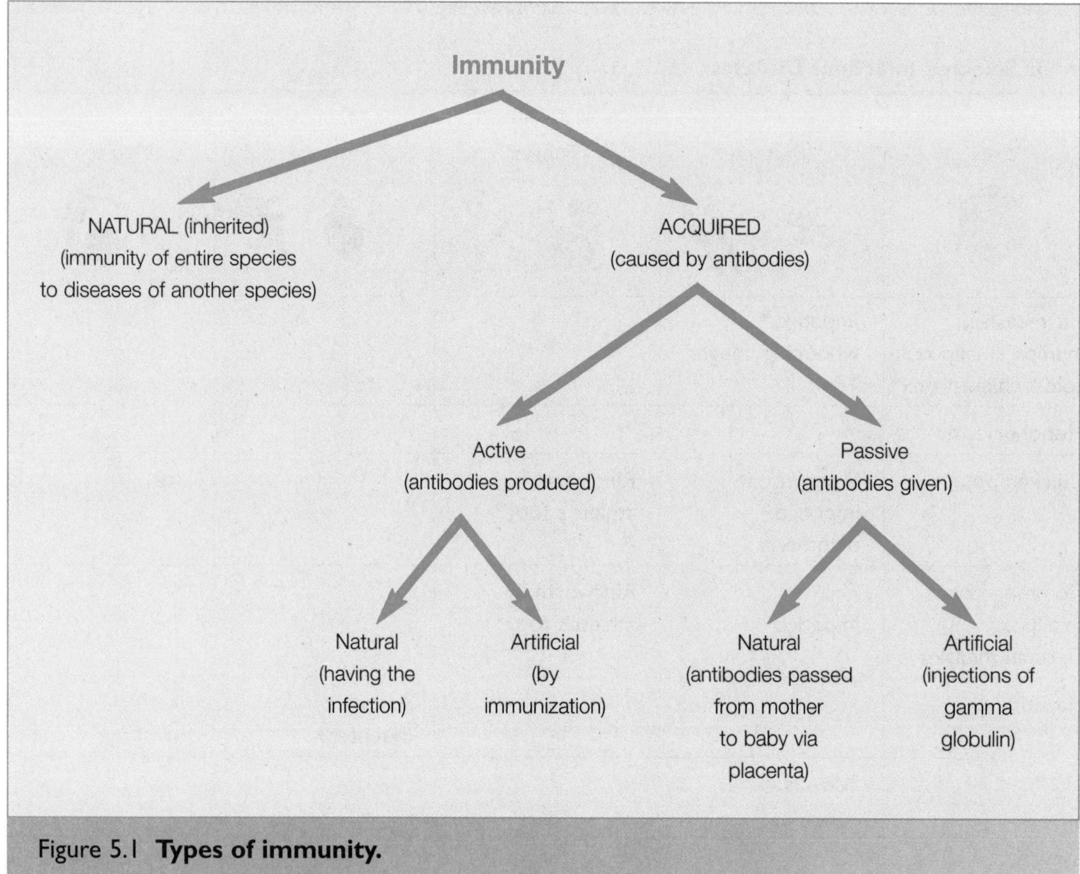

Figure 5.1 **Types of immunity.**

immunization program now recommended for infants and young children.

Sometimes the body is unsuccessful in developing antibody markers for certain pathogens and, in those cases, a person can get the disease again and again. Also, even though the immune system can usually defend the body from foreign organisms, some, like the HIV virus responsible for AIDS, can overpower it and halt its effectiveness. When the immune system is overpowered, the person can no longer defend himself or herself against disease.

Allergic Reactions

Sometimes, the immune system overreacts to a substance in the environment. This reaction is called an **allergy**. Typical symptoms are runny nose, watery eyes, itching, rashes, and swelling. The sources of allergies can be almost anything: dust, foods, insect bites, medicines, perfumes, chemical sprays, plants, and so on. Probably the most common allergy is hay fever, a reaction to hay, pollen, or grasses. Poison ivy, oak, and sumac produce allergic reactions in the form of a skin rash resulting from contact with these plants. Hives—swollen, red, itchy blotches on the skin—are allergic reactions to insects, chemicals, and certain foods. When they occur in the respiratory tract, hives can shut off air passages, which can be dangerous. **Asthma** is a severe chronic allergic reaction affecting the bronchial tubes and lungs.

The most dangerous allergic reaction is **anaphylactic shock**, in which the reaction is so swift and severe that the person can die if not treated immediately. He or she has difficulty breathing because the air passages constrict and blood vessels dilate (expand), producing an extreme drop in blood pressure. Anaphylactic shock can be precipitated by an insect bite, a food (such as shrimp, clams, or peanuts), a drug, or an anesthetic administered during surgery. Allergies not only can pose a serious threat to health but, in some cases, they also impair people's ability to function effectively in their day-to-day activities. Children with allergies often cannot concentrate well in school, and their performance suffers.

Autoimmune Diseases

For some unknown reason, the immune system sometimes fails to discriminate between foreign substances and those normal to the body. In these **autoimmune** diseases the body begins to attack itself, causing progressive degeneration of tissue. Three examples of autoimmune diseases are rheumatoid arthritis, a crippling inflammation of the joints; multiple sclerosis, in which the cells of the immune system attack the cells of the brain and spinal cord; and

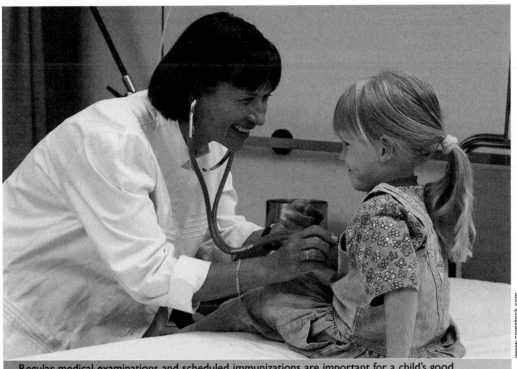
Regular medical examinations and scheduled immunizations are important for a child's good health.

www.comstock.com

myasthenia gravis, resulting in a weakening of the muscles and double vision (muscles of the eyes).

Stages of Disease

Students can be taught to protect themselves against infection and to notice signs and symptoms as they appear in themselves or friends. Moreover, teachers can stay alert to the manifestations of diseases so students who appear with symptoms can be isolated from other students and school personnel, and families and physicians quickly notified.

When they occur, communicable diseases follow several distinct stages:

1. Incubation: from invasion of the pathogen to initial observation of general symptoms. This may take from several hours to several years.
2. Prodromal: early symptoms of the body's reactions, such as headache, fever, malaise, and irritability. In this stage the disease is highly contagious but, because the distinctive symptoms have not yet appeared, the diagnosis is not made easily.
3. Clinical: appearance of the distinct symptoms specific to the disease. The disease is still communicable during this stage.
4. Convalescence: subsiding of the symptoms. Although the person may feel well, the body is still weak. The disease is usually no longer communicable.
5. Recovery: disappearance of symptoms. The person may recover with full immunity, no immunity, or with immunity but still be a carrier.

Communicable Diseases Common in Children

Several communicable diseases are common in children, especially if the children have not been vaccinated. Diseases for which vaccinations have been developed are shown in Table 5.3. A vaccination schedule for many of these diseases is shown in Table 5.4.

Among the most common childhood diseases are chicken pox (for which there is a new vaccine), the common cold (caused by a variety of viruses), intestinal diseases (caused by bacteria or viruses), German measles, meningitis, mumps, measles, whooping cough (pertussis), streptococcal infections (including scarlet fever), influenza, infectious mononucleosis, tuberculosis (for which there is a new strain co-existing with AIDS), hepatitis C (often occurring in conjunction with HIV), diphtheria (now rare in the United States), hepatitis, conjunctivitis (pinkeye), head lice (pediculosis), impetigo, ringworm, scabies and, most recently, AIDS. As children reach adolescence and become sexually active, the incidence of sexually transmitted diseases (STDs) increases.

Viral Hepatitis C

Scientists have presently identified hepatitis A, B, C, D, and E. Hepatitis C deserves special mention because more than half of infected people may

Table 5.3
Communicable Childhood Diseases for Which Vaccinations Are Available

Disease	Characteristics	Dangers
Diphtheria	Bacterial disease usually affecting the throat and sometimes other mucous membranes and the skin. Sore throat, fever, and chills are the main manifestations.	Can make a child choke so badly that all breathing stops. Sometimes causes heart failure or pneumonia.
Hepatitis B and Hepatitis C	Viral diseases of the liver that are transmitted from one infected person to another. Can be passed from mother to infant during birth.	Greatest danger is meningitis and also can cause pneumonia. Potential chronic and progressive liver disease.
Hib disease or H-flu	Form of influenza. Children between 6 months and 1 year old are particularly susceptible.	Serious potential complication is meningitis.
Mumps	Swelling of salivary glands on one or both sides of the face, preceded by fever, headache, and vomiting.	Can cause deafness, diabetes, meningitis, encephalitis, and brain damage. In adult men, can cause sterility.
Rubella (German measles)	Tends to be mild in children; greatest threat is to fetus during early pregnancy, when risk of deformed baby is up to 80%; miscarriage also common. Children usually receive vaccination together with rubeola and mumps vaccines (MMR).	In a pregnant woman, can cause miscarriage or lead to birth defects in the baby.
Rubeola (red measles)	Symptoms similar to cold plus fever; affects respiratory system, skin, and eyes. Overt indication is the characteristic rash—small, red spots on the body.	Can lead to pneumonia, blindness, ear infections and deafness, encephalitis, and brain damage.
Pertussis (whooping cough)	Bacterial disease affecting mucous membranes lining the air passages. Cough for which it is named is a persistent, paroxysmal whooping that is the primary characteristic.	Can cause convulsions and brain damage. Pneumonia is a common complication.
Polio	Virus affecting central nervous system. Depending on the form, symptoms are flu-like, affect respiration, involve muscle stiffness, weakness, and (in one variation,) paralysis. No treatment is available, but development of vaccine in 1955 reduced incidence to near zero.	Often cripples and sometimes kills. If a child gets polio, little can be done.
Tetanus (lockjaw)	Enters the body when something sharp, like a nail, punctures or cuts the skin or from abrasions or insect stings. Main characteristic is spasmodic contraction of muscles, first in the jaw and neck and later at other sites throughout the body.	High fever, convulsions, and pain are common. Can kill.

Table 5.4
Childhood Immunization Schedule

	DTP[1]	Polio	MMR	Option 1[2] Influenza	Option 2[2] Influenza	Option 1[2] Hepatitis B	Option 2[2] Hepatitis B	Chicken Pox
Birth						✗		
2 months	✗	✗		✗	✗	✗	✗	
4 months	✗	✗		✗	✗		✗	
6 months	✗			✗		✗[3]	✗[3]	
12 months					✗			✗[4]
15 months	✗[4]	✗[4]	✗	✗				
4–6 years	✗	✗	✗					

[1] For the 4th and 5th doses, the cellular DTaP pertussis vaccine may be substituted.
[2] Alternate schedules are available. Check with your doctor or county health department.
[3] Many experts recommend these at 18 months of age.
[4] Many experts recommend these at 6–18 months of age.

show no symptoms for years. Those who do show symptoms may have loss of appetite, fatigue, nausea, fever, dark-yellow urine, or jaundice. The long-term danger can be chronic liver disease (cirrhosis, which is irreversible and potentially fatal liver scarring, often requiring a liver transplant).

Transmission occurs when a person comes in contact with blood or other body fluids from an infected person. This can happen from piercing the skin with a contaminated needle; injecting drugs from a shared needle; or sharing razors, toothbrushes, or body-piercing implements with an infected person. Sometimes hepatitis C can be passed from an infected mother to her newborn child. Sexual transmission is also possible, but not considered a high risk—nonetheless, condoms should always be used for protection. Because of shared routes of transmission, co-infection with HIV and hepatitis C is common.

At the present time there is no vaccine against hepatitis C. The treatment of choice is alpha interferon alone or in combination with the anti-viral agent ribavirin. This helps about 40 percent of patients treated. Drinking alcohol can make the liver disease worse.

Sexually Transmitted Diseases

Sexually transmitted diseases are communicated from an infected person to an uninfected person during intimate contact. The organisms that cause STDs all have an affinity for mucous membranes, such as those that line the reproductive organs. Transmission usually requires direct contact between genital areas and other areas (including the mouth, eyes, and throat) that have moist, mucoid linings. Mucous membranes provide an ideal environment for these organisms to grow and multiply. Some also grow and multiply in the bloodstream.

The incidence of STDs has been increasing steadily—in some cases, to epidemic proportions. Common STDs are candidiasis, trichomoniasis, chlamydia, gonorrhea, syphilis, pubic lice (crabs), genital herpes, hepatitis B, genital warts, and HIV/AIDS. Young people who are sexually active are contracting these diseases with great frequency and for many reasons (see Chapter 7), not the least of which is because they do not believe that they are susceptible.

These diseases and their symptoms, diagnosis, and treatment are summarized in Table 5.5. We single out one of them, HIV/AIDS, for further discussion because it often is included in the grade-school curriculum. Once again, educating children about prevention is the first step in giving them control over their health and susceptibility. The second step is their ability to make decisions and choices about behaviors that will keep them healthy. Knowledge about treatments is the third step in the process of protecting children and adults against these diseases.

Table 5.5
Common Sexually Transmitted Diseases

Name	Pathogen type	Distinguishing sign or symptom	Method of diagnosis	Treatment
Candidiasis (yeast infection)	Fungus	*Female*: Cottage cheese-like discharge, strawberry-red color of vagina and labia, pain in genital area *Male*: Usually asymptomatic	Analysis of discharge	Prescription or over-the-counter OTC fungicide, such as miconazole (cure)
Chlamydia	Bacterium	*Male*: Watery discharge from urethra; pains when urinating *Female*: Usually asymptomatic; sometimes a similar discharge; leading cause of PID[1]; can cause prostatitis in men	Culture of discharge	Antibiotics other than penicillin (cure)
Genital herpes	Virus	Blisters in genital and rectal areas	Presence of blisters and laboratory identification of virus in fluid of blister	Zovirax (acyclovir) (not a cure)
Genital warts (venereal warts)	Virus (HPV)	Cauliflowerlike growths in genital and rectal areas; itching and irritation; sometimes no symptoms	Presence of lesions or Pap smear	Removal of lesions by laser surgery, freezing, or chemicals (not a cure)
Gonorrhea (clap)	Bacterium	*Male:* Pus discharge from urethra, burning during urination *Female:* Usually asymptomatic; can lead to PID*; May cause sterility in both	culture of discharge	antibiotics (ceftriaxone) sodium (cure)
Hepatitis B and C	Virus	Jaundice, abdominal discomfort, discoloration in the urine or bowel movements, or feelings of weakness or nausea may represent early signs of viral hepatitis. Most people with acute hepatitis have no symptoms and remain unaware.	During first few weeks: Blood tests that detect hepatitis antigens. During recovery: Blood tests that detect antibodies.	No cure exists for viral hepatitis, although sometimes gamma globulin given immediately after contact may provide some protection to newborns. Hepatitis B vaccine is available; provides protection against Hepatitis D (Hepatitis D can only occur if Hepatitis B is present). No vaccine is available for Hepatitis C.
HIV/AIDS	Virus	Asymptomatic at first; opportunistic infections initial stages	Blood test; usually none in initial stages ORA-SURE (oral specimen collection device)	AZT, ddl protease inhibitors, ddC (not a cure)
Pubic lice	Metazoan	Intense itching of areas covered with pubic hair	Presence of lice and nits (eggs) on pubic hair	Prescription or OTC pediculocide shampoo (cure)
Syphilis	Bacterium (spirochete)	*Primary*: Chancre *Secondary*: Rash *Latent*: Asymptomatic *Late*: Irreversible damage to central nervous system, cardiovascular system	Specific blood test	Penicillin or other antibiotic (cure)
Trichomoniasis	Protozoan	*Female*: Frothy, foul odor, vaginal discharge, itching of genital area; *Male*: Usually asymptomatic	Identification of trichomonad in vaginal discharge	Flagyl (metronidazole) (cure)

*PID = Pelvic inflammatory disease, a term describing inflammation of upper reproductive tract of females

Acquired Immune Deficiency Syndrome (AIDS)

Tragically, some children are born with AIDS. Most often, though, it can be avoided! Many states have mandated that AIDS education be included in K–12 curricula, thus, classroom teachers often are responsible for delivering HIV/AIDS education.

AIDS, acquired immune deficiency syndrome, is caused by the human immunodeficiency virus (HIV). This virus breaks down the body's immune system, exposing the infected person to a variety of life-threatening diseases collectively called opportunistic diseases. People with an intact immune system would not contract these diseases, even though they are prevalent in the environment.

Viruses are a protein-coated package of genes (DNA) that invade healthy body cells (host cells) and alter the host's normal genetic apparatus, causing them to produce more virus cells. This process often kills the host cell. HIV is one of a group of retroviruses that are unique because (1) their genetic code is carried in the form of RNA instead of the usual DNA, and (2) they attack immune system cells. Retroviruses also carry a special enzyme called reverse transcriptase. When HIV attacks a cell, it uses this special enzyme and the host cell's machinery to manufacture new virus particles within the host cell. This process continues until many new viruses are produced. Then it may stop for a long time, or it may continue until the viruses rupture the host cell's membrane and escape into the bloodstream, attacking new host cells and thereby continuing to reproduce.

When the HIV virus enters the bloodstream, it targets the body's immune system cells—macrophages and T4 cells (one type of helper T cell)—because these cells have, on their surface, a protein that the virus recognizes. It then bores into these cells, hides there, and repeats the reproductive process described above. In an uninfected person, the T4 cells mobilize the immune system to fight infection.

Normally, the blood system contains about 1,000 T4 cells per cubic millimeter of blood. The number of T4 cells may remain at about 1,000 per cubic millimeter for several years following infection with HIV, and many people show no symptoms of AIDS while it remains at this level. Then the number of T4 cells declines (because of viral destruction) and still, many people show no symptoms of disease for several more years. People become most vulnerable to diseases when the level of T4 cells falls below 200 per cubic millimeter.[2]

The result is an immune system deficient in T4 cells and therefore unable to combat other opportunistic infections. The person becomes ill and eventually dies from these infections, most commonly Kaposi's sarcoma (a form of cancer), pneumocystis carinii pneumonia (a lung disease), or a variety of others (including tuberculosis and hepatitis C) that the weakened immune system cannot overcome.

At this time, research suggests that the vast majority of HIV-positive people eventually do develop AIDS. A person whose immune system is compromised in some way before infection with HIV probably will progress from infection to AIDS more quickly than someone whose immune system is healthy. A seemingly healthy person, showing no outward symptoms, is as contagious as an infected person who is symptomatic and even severely ill. People cannot tell who has the HIV virus and who does not. Although the time frame varies from person to person, the pattern for the course of HIV infection to AIDS generally is as follows:

Stage I: Primary HIV Infection. Soon after contracting HIV, some people develop a fever, swollen glands, fatigue, and perhaps a rash. These early symptoms usually disappear within a few weeks.

Stage II: Chronic Asymptomatic Infection. This stage is marked by a gradual decline in T4 cells but no particular disease symptoms. At the same time, there is often evidence of chronically swollen lymph nodes and an increasing vulnerability to opportunistic infections.

Stage III: Chronic Symptomatic Infection. At this stage, thrush (a fungus infection in the mouth) may appear. Infections of the skin and moist inner membranes of the body may appear, along with general feelings of discomfort, weakness, night sweats, weight loss, and frequent diarrhea.

Stage IV: Clinical AIDS. This diagnosis is made after one or more of 26 opportunistic diseases have been manifested in an HIV-infected person.

Why HIV infection can take more than 10 years to progress to AIDS is still not entirely clear. In some cases, the person has been exposed and HIV infection is not present. Are these individuals naturally immune? More research is being done on these few cases in an attempt to discover why certain people seem to be protected from getting HIV.

When people are infected with the HIV virus, their bodies combat the infection by activating T cells and producing antibodies. The presence of these antibodies in the blood is what indicates that a person is carrying HIV (is HIV-positive). In most cases, 3 to 12 months after exposure to the virus is sufficient time for the antibodies to show up in the commonly used blood test, called ELISA (enzyme-linked immunosorbent assay). If insufficient time has elapsed for production of antibodies, the test will be negative even though the person is infected. Sometimes the ELISA test is positive even though no antibodies are present (a false positive). Then a second test is done.

When the ELISA test results are positive for both tests, the Western Blot (immunoblot) test is administered for confirmation. Although it is more accurate than the ELISA, the Western Blot is expensive and, therefore, not used as the primary test for HIV. Pharmaceutical companies are continually working on new and better testing methods that can test for the presence of the actual virus rather than for its antibodies.

Contracting HIV is not easy to do. HIV is not circulating in the air or water or living on toilet seats, drinking glasses, combs, brushes; it is not in foods that infected people touch. Because it is a virus, it does not know a gay person from a straight person, an African-American person from a white person, or a woman from a man. It can be transmitted from any infected person to any other person without discrimination. The body fluids that best support the transmission of the virus are blood, semen, breast milk, and vaginal secretions. A person must choose to participate in specific behaviors that give the virus access to his or her bloodstream, where it can get into the cells needed to multiply itself. The modes of transmission are as follows:

1. Having unprotected sexual intercourse, anal or vaginal, with an infected person. The vagina and anus have accessible blood vessels through which the virus, deposited by the semen or vaginal fluid of the infected person, can enter the bloodstream. Although oral sex may be a mode of transmission, the virus must find entrance into the bloodstream through a cut or sore in the mouth, or digestion will destroy it. Cases of transmission from oral sex are difficult to document because most people who participate in it also participate in other sexual behaviors that could transmit the virus.
2. Sharing contaminated drug needles or syringes from an infected person. When people use intravenous drugs, they often share needles, with little concern for sterilization. The blood of the infected person is drawn into the vial that contains the drug, mixes with it, and then is left as residue that mixes with the next user's drug.
3. Women infected with HIV transmitting the virus to their babies during pregnancy, childbirth, or breast feeding. HIV can be transmitted through the placenta and infect the fetus. Some fetuses however, receive only antibodies from infected mothers. During childbirth, the blood vessels of mother and baby may rupture, allowing the virus to be transmitted through the blood.

Prior to 1985, when blood screening began, some people became infected by receiving blood transfusions. Now that the blood supply is tested, however, donating blood is not a mode of transmission. Because the equipment for giving blood is new or sterile for each user, one cannot get HIV from donating blood either.

Health care workers including dentists, physicians, and nurses have not been known to transmit the HIV virus in their work. The case of the dentist who treated Kimberly Bergalis in 1991 is the only known case of HIV transmission from a health care worker to a patient. Tests on more than 15,000 patients and physicians have not uncovered one case of health care provider-to-patient transmission.[3]

As of January 1996, according to the Centers for Disease Control and Prevention, there has not been a documented case of HIV transmission from bites of any kind. Also, though the virus is known to appear in saliva and tears, the quantity and the environment do not seem to support its transmission.

Armed with information and an ability to make informed decisions about risky behaviors, people can protect themselves from becoming infected. Because HIV/AIDS has no realistic cure in the immediate future, prevention is the first, and probably the only, line of defense in stopping this disease. Accurate information should be disseminated through education, as early and as comprehensively as possible. Because the primary sources of transmission involve sexual behaviors, the question is how much to teach students, and at what point in their development. In any case, education must begin in the earliest grades and continue in developmentally appropriate stages throughout a child's education.

Chronic Diseases

Noninfectious or chronic diseases are even more troubling than communicable diseases because their causes are more difficult to pinpoint. They encompass a wide variety of disorders—from diabetes, cancer, and heart disease to backaches and tooth decay. Although some have genetic causes, many are thought to be caused by a combination of risk factors over time. Sometimes they stem from infectious diseases, and the severity of symptoms progresses over time.

Because most chronic diseases are thought to be an outcome of lifestyle behaviors that begin in childhood and generally first appear in adulthood, prevention must begin early. Also, because people are living longer, the likelihood of experiencing the symptoms of chronic diseases is increasing. What follows is a brief description of some of the major chronic diseases of which students tend to be aware because of contact with someone who has one of these conditions.

Diabetes

Diabetes mellitus is a disease in which the body cannot metabolize carbohydrates adequately. The pancreas either cannot produce insulin at all (called Type I or insulin-dependent diabetes) or (in Type II or adult-onset diabetes) it produces amounts of insulin insufficient for the metabolism of carbohydrates. Type I diabetes is often referred to as juvenile diabetes because it commonly occurs in children or early adolescents. However, Type I diabetes *can* occur in adults. Type II diabetes usually occurs in mid- to later life.

Children with Type I diabetes require daily injections of insulin and have to modify their lives so they eat regularly and understand their diet in relation to their medication. Upon diagnosis, some children find the adjustment difficult, and others adjust easily. A feeling of being different from their friends is common as they struggle to adjust. If teachers and health professionals are aware of these concerns, they can make the adjustment easier. Considerable community agency support is available for juvenile diabetics, their families, and their teachers.

In healthy people, the body breaks down carbohydrates into glucose, the primary form of sugar, which provides the body with necessary energy. Insulin is needed to move the glucose into the body's cells and convert it into energy. When the insulin is not available, the sugar cannot get into the cells and the kidneys excrete it in urine. The body begins to digest proteins and fats for energy. This causes the production of acids called ketones, an accumulation of which can lead to abdominal pain, nausea, vomiting, drowsiness, coma, and possibly death.

A viral infection of the insulin-producing cells of the pancreas or their destruction by the immune system may be causal factors in some cases of diabetes. It is also highly correlated with family history, suggesting a hereditary origin. Adult-onset diabetes is thought to be preventable, or at least delayable, so that the onset occurs late enough in life to avoid the serious complications associated with having the disease for a long time.

People with diabetes need to modify their diet and increase their exercise so they gain a sense of control over their own health and can live a fairly normal life. With the necessary accommodations, they can play sports, travel, work, and do most things that healthy people do.

Risk Factors for Diabetes

- A family history of diabetes
- Obesity, especially more than 30% over recommended body weight
- Age above 45 (although Hispanics over age 30 are at high risk)
- Lack of exercise
- Ethnic background: Hispanic Americans, African Americans, and Native Americans are more likely to develop diabetes and run a greater risk of complications
- Women: Having a baby that weighed more than 9 pounds at birth

Cancer

Just the mention of cancer brings shudders to most people because of the debilitating nature of the disease and its associated treatments. As a result of our ability to control communicable diseases and other chronic disorders so people live long enough to develop it, cancer is often considered a disease of old age. Also, as we become more efficient at treating cancer, people are living longer with the disease in remission. Although cancer occurs less often in children, most of them will have experience with it at some time or another in relatives, parents, grandparents, neighbors, or friends. Therefore, students need to be aware of the forms of cancer and their symptoms. To lessen students' fears, teachers should stress that cancer is not communicable. Also, they need to understand and be sensitive to people living with this disease.

Cancer is actually a set of diseases, all of which are caused by the rapid, uncontrolled growth and reproduction of abnormal cells. Clusters of these cells are called tumors.

Tumors may or may not be cancerous. Non-cancerous tumors are called benign; they stay encapsulated in the original site. The cancerous type is called **malignant**; the mass of cells does not remain enclosed and eventually invades neighboring tissues or organs. When malignant cells break off from the main tumor and travel to other parts of the body, they produce secondary-site tumors. This spread of cancer is called **metastasis**.

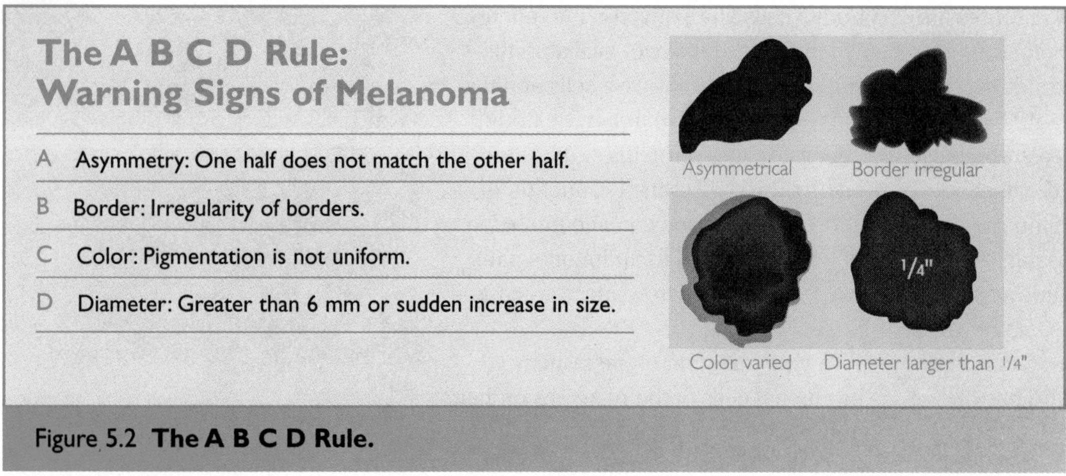

The A B C D Rule:
Warning Signs of Melanoma
A Asymmetry: One half does not match the other half.
B Border: Irregularity of borders.
C Color: Pigmentation is not uniform.
D Diameter: Greater than 6 mm or sudden increase in size.
Asymmetrical
Border irregular
1/4"
Color varied
Diameter larger than 1/4"

Figure 5.2 **The A B C D Rule.**

Types of Cancerous Tumors

Tumors are of several types:

1. **Carcinomas**: tumors that develop in secretory organs—in the skin, glands, or membranes
2. **Sarcomas**: tumors of the connective tissues, including muscles, ligaments, tendons, bones, nerves, and blood vessels
3. **Lymphomas**: tumors of the lymph glands or nodes in the throat or armpits
4. **Leukemias**: tumors of the bone marrow and blood-forming cells

Cancer has no single cause, because it appears in so many different forms. Some seem to be caused by chemical, physical, or biological irritants called **carcinogens**. Examples of chemical carcinogens are the tars of tobacco, asbestos, coal tars, and some food additives. Physical agents include radiation, such as x-rays and ultraviolet (UV) rays from prolonged exposure to the sun.[5] Several viruses also have been implicated as biological causes.

The earlier cancer is discovered, the sooner it can be treated, life prolonged, and an early death prevented. The American Cancer Society published a list of the seven early warning signs of cancer organized by the mnemonic CAUTION:[4]

C Change in bowel or bladder habits
A A sore that does not heal
U Unusual bleeding or discharge
T Thickening or lump in the breast, testicles or elsewhere
I Indigestion or difficulty in swallowing
O Obvious changes in warts or moles
N Nagging cough or hoarseness

Common Cancer Sites

Common sites of cancer are the skin, lungs, mouth, breast, testicle, colon, prostate, and female reproductive organs. Other cancers occur in the blood, bone marrow, and lymph.

1. **Skin** The most common forms of skin cancer—basal or squamous-cell carcinomas—are slow-growing and relatively easy to treat. A rarer form, **melanoma**, usually begins as a mole-like growth and spreads rapidly, making it dangerous. Cancers of the skin are most common in people who are exposed to the sun. A severe sunburn early in life can result in a skin cancer many years later. This is one of the cancers that individuals can prevent by avoiding excessive exposure to the sun. However, there are some cases of melanoma that no amount of risk reduction behavior can prevent. (Scientists believe this may be caused by a genetic predisposition.) Nevertheless, consistent skin self-examinations are recommended for early detection (see Figure 5.2). A simple way to stay safe in the sun is to remember SLIP, SLOP, SLAP, and WRAP:

   SLIP on a shirt

   SLOP on sunscreen of 15+

   SLAP on a hat

   WRAP on sunglasses

   Also, find shade in the middle of the day
2. **Lung** This is the most common form of cancer and is the leading cause of cancer-related deaths in the United States. It is difficult to identify because symptoms do not appear until the cancer has spread. Early detection through regular screening examinations, though, can sometimes reverse its course. Tobacco use has been identified as the primary cause of lung cancer. Young people should be discouraged from starting to smoke in the first place.

3. **Mouth** Oral cancers occur in locations from the lips to the throat. More common in males than females, it is detected easily by a doctor or dentist and is generally associated with cigarette smoking, chewing tobacco, and alcohol abuse.
4. **Breast** Breast cancer is a major threat to women. In most cases, breast cancer produces no pain but is experienced most frequently as a lump in the outer quarter of the breast. Early diagnosis by monthly breast self-examinations (BSE) and mammograms can result in effective treatment. Yet, the research indicates that too many women do not do BSE regularly or get mammograms as suggested by the American Cancer Society. Although breast cancer is not usually found in young women, regular BSE should begin in adolescence. Though much less common, breast cancer also occurs in men.
5. **Testicular** Cancer of the testicles is not common, but it is found in men aged 20–34 for the most part. Self-examination will reveal a lump on the side of the testicle or a change in testicle shape. A dull ache in the groin or scrotum may be another symptom. If detected early, it is easily treated.
6. **Colorectal** Cancer of the colon and rectum is the second most fatal type, after lung cancer. Evidence suggests that a diet high in fat or low in fiber increases the risk. Symptoms include bloody stool, bleeding from the rectum, and a change in bowel habits.
7. **Prostate** This is the third most common cancer in males and is also associated with a high-fat diet. The prostate is a gland at the base of the male's urethra, just below the bladder. Difficulty urinating, blood in the urine, and low-back pain are common symptoms.
8. **Ovaries, Cervix, and Uterus** These cancers are responsible for about 9 percent of women's deaths each year. Cancer of the ovaries can produce vaginal bleeding and sterility. Most cancers of the uterus affect the inner lining (the endometrium) or the cervix. These types produce unusual vaginal discharge or bleeding between menstrual cycles.
9. **Leukemia and Hodgkin's disease** These are cancers of the blood, bone marrow, or lymph tissues. Leukemia produces millions of abnormal, nonfunctioning white blood cells, which weaken the immune system. This results in weight loss, repeated infections, and anemia. Hodgkin's disease is characterized by a painless swelling of the lymph nodes, fever, and weight loss. The cure rate for these cancers has risen dramatically. Leukemia is the type of cancer most commonly found in children and young adults.

Many cancers can be prevented or the onset delayed by reducing the risk factors, as follows:

Do not use tobacco.

Avoid drinking alcohol.

Avoid the sun's ultraviolet rays or use a sunscreen.

Avoid environmental carcinogens when possible.

Eat high-fiber foods.

Reduce the fat content in your diet.

Eat foods rich in vitamins A and C.

Exercise regularly and maintain recommended weight.

Avoid unnecessary x-rays.

Do regular self-examinations.

Cardiovascular Diseases

Diseases of the heart and blood vessels constitute the leading causes of death in the United States. Substantial evidence indicates that cardiovascular diseases begin in childhood. Research on the remains of young war veterans revealed the start of plaque build-up in the arteries of a sizeable percentage of them.

Five manifestations are

1. Hypertension, or high blood pressure;
2. Coronary heart disease, which may lead to a heart attack;
3. Stroke, the bursting of a blood vessel in the brain;
4. Rheumatic and congenital heart disease;
5. Other heart problems, including congestive heart failure, irregular heartbeat, and defects of the heart valves (such as a murmur).

Hypertension, rheumatic heart disease, and heart defects are the most common forms in children.

Hypertension

Hypertension is of two types: primary and secondary. Primary or essential hypertension has no known cause and can be controlled by proper diet, weight, exercise, and skills for controlling stress. Secondary hypertension is triggered by other diseases, such as diabetes and **arteriosclerosis** (hardening of the blood vessels).

Coronary Heart Disease

Coronary heart disease involves damage to the blood vessels of the heart itself. This is usually attributable to a build-up of fatty deposits on the walls of the tiny blood vessels of the heart. As the build-up continues, the channels for blood movement narrow, resulting in a decrease in the supply of nutrients to the heart tissues. Complete blockage results in angina (heart pain) or a heart attack (death of heart muscle). Immediate medical attention has saved many lives.

Stroke

Stroke is caused by the blockage of a blood vessel in the brain—caused by a blood clot that formed there or formed elsewhere and traveled to the brain. This causes the vessel wall to weaken, leak, or rupture.

Rheumatic Heart Disease

Rheumatic heart disease develops as a result of repeated acute bacterial infections of the throat or of rheumatic fever, which damages the heart valves. It occurs mainly in children ages 5 to 15. Rapid medical attention can prevent severe damage.

Congenital Heart Disorders

Congenital heart disorders are defects in the heart that arise during embryonic development. They can be caused by German measles, chemicals the mother uses during pregnancy, or genetic factors.

Some heart diseases cannot be prevented entirely, but a healthy lifestyle can delay their onset and reduce their intensity, thereby preserving life. Diet, smoking, weight, exercise, and stress all play a role. Public participation in physical activity and healthier diets (lower in fats and salts) over the last two decades have reduced the incidence of heart disease. Not much progress has been made, however, in controlling stress—also considered a causative agent (see Chapter 8 for a discussion of stress). Students should recognize that their early decisions and behaviors influence the likelihood of their developing heart conditions later.

Asthma

A disease that affects more than 2 million children, asthma sometimes is seen in the first months of life. Although it is highly correlated with families, no genetic cause has been identified as yet. Asthma is the most frequent contributor to absenteeism from school.

Asthma attacks are periodic episodes of difficulty with breathing, wheezing, and shortness of breath. These symptoms result from swelling of the membranes, spasms, or a build-up of mucus in and around the bronchial tubes. An attack can last anywhere from several minutes to several days, and its severity can differ with each incident. Frequently, people become stressed and anxious about their inability to breathe comfortably and react by contracting their chest muscles, which further constricts their breathing.

Factors that contribute to the condition and trigger attacks include allergic reactions of all kinds (accounting for 75 percent of the cases), bacterial or viral respiratory infections, emotional stress, and environmental pollutants. Sometimes a change in the weather or even exercise can trigger an attack. Asthma attacks that are triggered by changes in the weather or allergic reactions to pollen and grasses often occur during late spring, early summer, or the beginning of winter.

When children who have asthma feel breathing distress, they are unable to concentrate on schoolwork or perform tasks efficiently. Sometimes they are unable to attend school at all. When the asthma is not acute, however, they can be expected to participate in activities like the other students. Teachers should be aware of the effects of this condition on motivation, performance, and the accuracy of test measurements as children progress through school.

New thinking and new drugs to treat asthma have changed the etiology of this disease considerably. The treatment protocol is individualized. Some asthmatics are treated symptomatically, and others are regularly maintained on medications that control or prevent the disease from flaring up into dangerous, severe attacks. Also, an asthmatic child can be helped to relax and breathe slowly by sensitive and empathetic teachers and classmates, thereby curbing the anxiety during an attack.

Some Genetic Disorders

Over the past several years, scientists have discovered more than 300 different kinds of genetic disorders, and still more are being discovered. Genetic disorders are passed from parents to children. At least one parent must have the defective gene. If only one recessive gene is passed, the recipient is known as a carrier and usually does not show symptoms of the disease. Some genetic disorders, such as Huntington's disease, are passed on by dominant genes and can be passed by only one parent. Figure 5.3 shows how sickle cell trait is passed along. Some of the most common genetic disorders are briefly described below and are summarized in Table 5.6.

Down syndrome is caused by a chromosomal defect and characterized by abnormal facial characteristics and other physical deformities, cardiovascular problems, and varying degrees of mental retardation. Most individuals with Down syndrome require constant care and supervision.

Sickle cell anemia is a blood disease wherein the red blood cells take

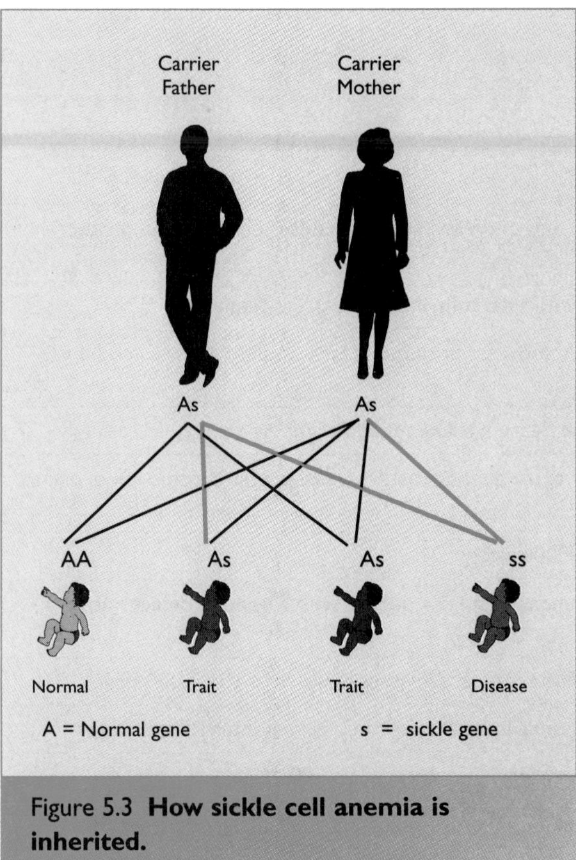

Figure 5.3 **How sickle cell anemia is inherited.**

on a sickle shape and are less able to transport oxygen. Having only one gene produces the milder, sickle cell trait (and creates a carrier); having both produces full-blown sickle cell disease. This disease appears in about 10 percent of African Americans. It is characterized by weakness, fatigue, irritability, shortness of breath, and severe pain because the deformed red blood cells do not pass through the blood vessels easily and are unable to transport sufficient oxygen to vital organs. The sickling (shown in Figure 5.4) typically appears after exertion or stress and results in repeated hospitalizations and treatment. Many individuals born with sickle cell disease die before age 20.

Cystic fibrosis affects the respiratory system and the sweat and mucous glands; it produces serious respiratory and digestive problems. A sticky mucus can clog the lungs and lead to chronic infections. Twelve million Americans are thought to be carriers, and those with the disease have an average life span of 26 years.

Phenylketonuria (PKU) is caused by the absence of an essential amino acid: tyrosine, used to break down phenylalanine and commonly found in food. The result is severe mental retardation. Fortunately, the symptoms can be totally prevented if its presence is detected immediately after birth by a simple blood test and the infant is put on a strict diet that contains tyrosine.

Seizure Disorders in Children

Classification of **seizure** disorders have evolved considerably over time. The use of such terms as "grand mal" or "petit mal" epilepsy has largely been supplanted by more detailed classifications based on specific clinical manifestations, mode of onset (for instance, focal or generalized), and discrete clinical syndromes.

At present, the **epilepsy** of childhood is most frequently classified using variations of the International Classification of Epileptic Seizures. This nomenclature delineates seizures in three general categories: generalized, partial (focal), and special epileptic syndromes.

The etiologies that underlie the development of epilepsy in childhood vary in an age-dependent fashion. Seizures in neonates, infants, and toddlers most frequently result from perinatal brain injury, congenital central nervous system infection, genetic epilepsy, and neuro-degenerative disorders that are more likely to present with seizures beginning in later childhood. These causes stand in stark contrast to the adult population, where traumatic brain injury, cerebrovascular disease, and neoplasms represent the most frequent causes of seizures.

Treatment for a child with epilepsy must be individualized based on the specific type(s) of seizure, the child's age, and likelihood of significant side effects. Medications include barbiturates, phenytoin, valproic acid, and ethosuximide.[6]

Physical Disabilities

In addition to the diseases and disorders described already, a variety of conditions, including impaired vision

Table 5.6
Some Genetic Disorders that May Affect Children

Disease	Comments
Alcoholism	At least some alcoholism is genetic.
"Bubble-boy" disease (ADA deficiency)	The child lacks a working immune system and must live in a bubble-like enclosure to protect against infection.
Colon cancer	Researchers have discovered one major gene that contributes to this disease.
Coronary atherosclerosis, premature	Hardening of the arteries normally doesn't show up until much later in life.
Cystic fibrosis	Mucus in the lungs is so thick it cannot be cleared, killing most victims by age 27.
Down syndrome	This inherited condition, characterized by extra genetic material in the 21st chromosome, occurs in 1 of 650 births.
Duchene muscular dystrophy	This muscle-wasting disease affects 1 in 5,000 males.
Emphysema, premature	Usually associated with smoking, emphysema also strikes people with a genetic defect known as alpha 1-antitripsin deficiency.
Fragile-X syndrome	This is a common genetic form of mental retardation, affecting more than 1 in 1,000 males.
Hemophilia	In this disorder, blood fails to clot, and the individual experiences painful internal bleeding.
Huntington's chorea	This lethal, degenerative brain disease strikes between ages 15 and 80.
Lesch Nyan syndrome	This disorder causes spasticity and self-mutilation and affects 1 in 100,000.
Neurofibromatosis	This hereditary disease of the nervous system produces birthmarks, tumors of the skin and nerve cells, and learning disabilities in about 100,000 Americans.
Phenylketonuria (PKU)	This genetic disorder occurs when a crucial liver amino acid, phenylalanine, is absent. It produces severe mental retardation if not treated.
Polycystic kidney	This genetic disease causes kidney disease cysts, leading to kidney failure; it affects 1 in 1,000.
Retinoblastoma	Eye cancer.
Sickle cell anemia	This is a severe form of anemia brought about by abnormal hemoglobin, the molecule that carries oxygen to the blood. It affects 8–10% of African Americans.
Tay-Sach's disease	This fatal enzyme deficiency affects 1 in 3,600 Ashkenazi Jews.
Thalassemia	This form of blood disease (a type of anemia) is found in people of Mediterranean, African, and Southeast Asian descent.

Source: B. K. Williams, and S. M. Knight, *Healthy for Life: Wellness and the Art of Living*. Copyright © 1994 Brooks/Cole Publishing Company, Pacific Grove, CA 93950, a division of International Thomson Publishing Inc. Reprinted with permission.

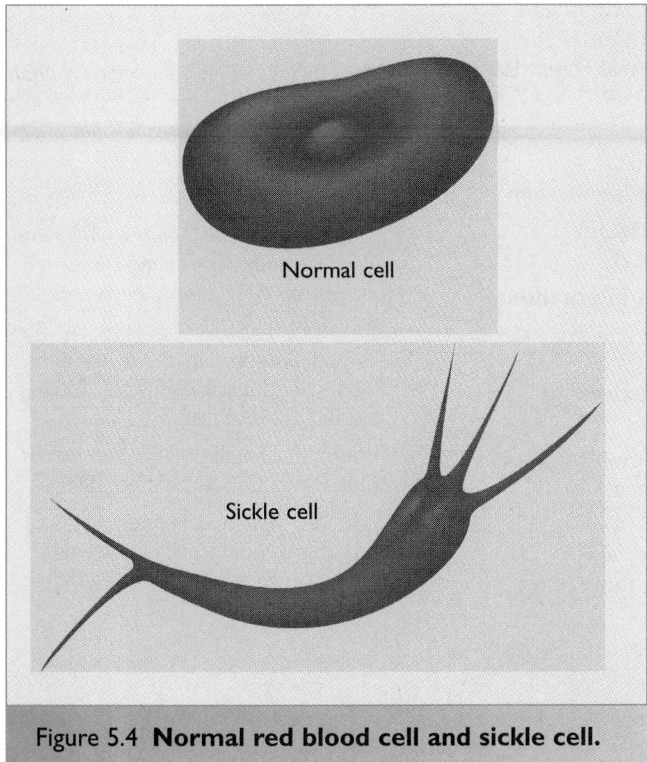

Figure 5.4 **Normal red blood cell and sickle cell.**

or hearing, reduce or prevent total physical functioning. Sometimes developmental abnormalities, such as cerebral palsy or accidents and injuries result in partial or complete paralysis of body parts, loss of sensation, coordination problems, and impaired mobility. People with physical disabilities, if treated properly by health-care professionals, can adapt to their physical limitations and lead productive lives.

Summary

In the early 1900s, the major causes of death in the United States were infectious or communicable diseases that wiped out entire communities. They included such ominous-sounding diseases as tuberculosis, scarlet fever, and polio. With scientific advances in antibacterial prevention and treatments over the century, the health problems shifted to chronic or noncommunicable diseases. Still ominous in their names, cancer, cardiovascular diseases, and stroke remain the primary causes of death and disability today. Different from communicable diseases, these chronic diseases occur over time, and their prognoses are considered to be influenced by lifestyle behaviors. More recently, we are beginning again to hear about some communicable diseases whose causative agents have strengthened themselves so as to survive antibiotics and others that are caused by viruses over which we have little defense. Even in the case of viral infections such as hepatitis B and C, HIV, and so on, the patient's lifestyle component requires attention. Hence, the health education/health promotion system remains a major player in the control of disease.

Education about communicable and chronic diseases centers on several primary themes:

- Instilling and increasing students' sense of control over diseases through information-giving
- Encouraging the adoption of lifestyle behaviors that will prevent a disease from occurring or delay its onset and minimize the symptoms of disease when one does occur
- Orienting students in the direction of sensitivity toward friends, family members, and others with whom they interact who are living with a disease
- Helping students to recognize their own susceptibility to disease and be able to make adjustments when a disease is contracted
- Encouraging students and their parents to maintain access to the health care system for screening and treatment

Among these, education must focus on prevention of those diseases, both chronic and communicable, that now claim most lives through promoting lifestyle habits that ward off or delay disease with particular emphasis on increasing exercise and activity, avoidance of smoking, adopting good eating habits, and minimizing potential exposure through sexual and other bodily contacts. What better time than to begin this education than in early childhood—before sedentary and other poor health habits are established?

Web Sites

American Academy of Asthma, Allergies, and Immunology
www.execpc.com/-edi/aaaai.html

American Cancer Society
1-800-ACS-2345
www.cancer.org.

American College of Sports Medicine
www.al.com/sportsmed/

American Heart Association
www.amhrt.org/

American Lung Association
www.lungusa.org/

American Liver Foundation
1-800-891-0707

American School Health Association
1-800-783-9877
www.ashastd.org

American Society for Clinical Nutrition
www.faseb.org/ascn

Arthritis Foundation
www.arthritis.org/

Body Health: A Multimedia AIDS and HIV Information Resource
www.thebody.com

Resources

Chris Jennings, *AIDS: A Book for Everyone*: Health Alert Press, 1993.

Breast Cancer Roundtable
www.seas.gwu.edu/student/tlooms/
www.MGT243/breast_cancer_round-table.html

Cancer Net of the National Cancer Institute
www.cancernet.nci.nih.gov

Centers for Disease Control and Prevention, National STD Hotline
(800) 227-8922 or (800) 342-2437
www.cdc.gov/std/

The Heart: An Online Exploration
www.fiedu/biosci/heart.html

Centers for Disease Control and Prevention, National Center for Infectious Diseases Viral Hepatitis C
(888) 4-HEP-CDC, (888) 443-7232

Food Safety and Nutrition Information
www.ificinfo.health.org/fdsninfo.htm

Forum on Women's Health
www.women's health.org/

Hepatitis Foundation International
1-800-891-0707
www.hepfi.org;

Hotline (Hearing Impaired)
www.heptt.org

JAMA HIV/AIDS Information Center
www.ama-assn.org/special/hiv/hivhome.htm

Master Anti-Smoking Page
www.autonomyu.com/smoke.htm

Men's Health Issues
www.vix.com/pub/men/health/health.html

National AIDS Hotline
800/342-AIDS (24 hours)

National HPV and Cervical Cancer Hotline
(919) 361-4848
Resource Center
www.ashastd.org/hpvccrv/

National Cancer Institute
www.nci.hih.gov

National Herpes Hotline
(919) 361-8488

National STD Hotline
800/227-8922 (M–F, 8:00 A.M.–2:00 P.M. EST)

National STD Hotline (in Spanish)
800/344-7432
(7 days, 8:00 A.M.–2:00 P.M. EST)

National TTY/TDD AIDS
800/243-7889 (M–F, 10:00 A.M.-10:00 P.M. EST)

Testicular Cancer
www.vax2.jmu.edu/-taylorbw/

The National Institute of Diabetes and Digestive and Kidney Diseases of the National Institute of Health
www.niddk.nih.gov/

The Online Allergy Center
www.sig.net/-allergy/welcome.html

Notes

1. L.V. Crowley, *An Introduction to Human Disease: Pathology and Pathophysiology Correlation*, 5 ed. (Boston: Jones & Bartlett, 1999), 4–6.
2. See note 1.
3. J. Nevid, *A Students' Guide to AIDS and Other Sexually Transmitted Diseases* (Needham Heights, MA: Allyn and Bacon, 1993), 27.
4. J. Nevid, *Choices: Sex in the Age of STD's* (Needham Heights, MA: Allyn and Bacon, 1995), 27.
5. American Cancer Society, *Sun Basics* (Skin Protection Federation, 1993).
6. T. Hoban, "Seizure Disorders In Children," Loyola University Medical Education Network August 11, 1996.

Learning Experiences

Young students will not be able to understand the scientific and technical details of disease. They need to begin their study slowly, first learning the basics of personal cleanliness and its impact on health, then understanding the difference between wellness and illness and ways to avoid certain illnesses, and finally, understanding the differences between communicable and noncommunicable diseases and how people get them.

The emphasis should be on developing an internal locus of control so students begin to accept that what they do and how they live can affect their health. They can come to understand that, through sound health practices, they will be less susceptible to disease and, if they become ill, they will be likely to recover more quickly. Even children with chronic diseases can improve if they adopt healthy behaviors within the limitations imposed by the disease.

Children at all ages are exposed to a wide variety of diseases at home and in school and the larger community. They know how they feel when they are sick and how they feel when they "get better." These personal experiences become the basis for teaching about diseases, what causes them, how to deal with them, and how to prevent them.

Grades K-2

In these early grades, students should learn about the relationship between disease and modes of prevention—for example, relating germs to cold symptoms, such as a sore throat and sneezing. They need to recognize the importance of simple routine behaviors that can keep them healthy, such as how to drink from a water fountain, not to share utensils or to drink from the same cup as another person, to cover the mouth when coughing, wash their hands before eating and after going to the bathroom, and so on. They also need to learn when and how to report symptoms to a teacher or a parent and when and why they stay home when they are ill. They also should begin to know what to do when they have serious symptoms and who can help them (see Chapter 15). By the end of second grade, students will be able to:

1. Understand the difference between illness and wellness.
2. Define "germ."
3. Recognize that germs can make people sick.

4. Recognize that there are different kinds of germs.
5. Understand the facts about HIV/AIDS.
6. Explain common modes of transmission of germs, such as coughing and sneezing.
7. Explain how the body fights germs.
8. Describe some ways to prevent diseases and stay healthy.
9. Explain the importance of physical examinations.

Grades 3-4

By third grade, a discussion of immunizations is important. These students are also interested in common childhood diseases such as chicken pox and measles. By the end of fourth grade, children should understand locus of control—that they can take responsibility for their health by behaving in ways that promote wellness. They can begin to understand some of the scientific knowledge about the immune system and how certain behaviors are helpful, whereas others are harmful. They can begin to learn elementary concepts about the different types of germs, such as bacteria and viruses. By the end of fourth grade, in addition to the mastering the objectives from grades K–2, students will be able to:

1. Describe behaviors that can speed recovery from disease.
2. Distinguish between infectious, noninfectious, and chronic diseases.
3. Understand the function of the immune system, types of immunity, and how immunizations prevent disease.
4. Recognize that many illnesses and HIV/AIDS are caused by bacteria and viruses.
5. List the several ways that HIV/AIDS is usually acquired. Understand that a person cannot become infected with HIV by simply being around or touching someone with AIDS.
6. Explain how diseases can be avoided by preventive behavior.
7. Understand that any illness can affect an entire family.
8. Identify places to go when feeling sick.

Grades 5-6

By now, students are ready to study specific diseases and to discuss their experiences. They are ready to discuss more abstract disease agents, such as environmental pollutants, and the impact of diseases on certain populations (for example, sickle cell anemia). After studying about diseases, students in grades 5 and 6 will be able to:

1. Differentiate diseases as contagious, noncontagious, and chronic.
2. Identify the factors that can cause disease and ways of preventing them.
3. Name the classes of pathogenic organisms.
4. Understand how the immune system works.
5. Name the common sexually transmitted diseases, including AIDS, and know how they are transmitted.
6. Recognize the difference between safe and unsafe sexual behaviors.
7. Explain the effects of diseases on individuals, family, community and society.

For suggestions on creating a rubric with which to evaluate student performance of Learning Experiences, see page 13.

Learning Experience 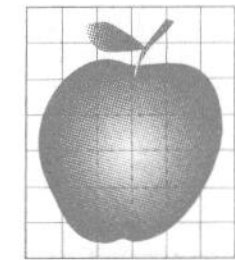 5-1

Gloves to Keep Me Germ-Free

Grade Level

K–4

Primary Disciplines

Science, Language Arts

Learning Objectives

Following this activity, students will be able to

- Define what germs are.
- Describe how germs get into the body.
- Describe how cleanliness helps prevent germs from getting into the body.

Time Required

One session

Materials

Latex gloves, broad-tip marker

Description of Activity

Put on a latex glove and make a number of marks across the palm of the glove with the marker. Show the students the glove and tell them that you are pretending to be a dentist and that the lines represent germs that came from a patient's mouth—from saliva or blood. Then remove the glove and ask the students if they see any lines (germs) on his/her hand.

Questions for Discussion

- Why is wearing a glove important for dentists?
- In what other professions do people wear gloves?
- What are germs?
- How do they get into the body?
- What would happen if the glove was torn and you had a cut on your hand?

Homework

Have the students think of ways germs can get into the body and professionals who wear gloves.

Evaluation

Students will be able to

- Explain what a germ is and what germs do when they get into the body.
- Describe ways in which germs enter the body.
- Describe simple hygiene measures that can prevent them from getting sick.

Learning Experience 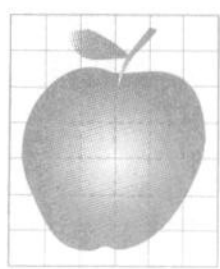 5-2

Understanding Germs

Grade Level

K–4

Primary Disciplines

Science, Language Arts

Learning Objectives

After this activity, students will be able to

- Define what germs are.
- Describe how germs get into the body.
- Describe how cleanliness helps prevent germs from getting into the body.

Time Required

One session

Materials

Attached handouts

Description of Activity

Discuss the following with the class and read the content aloud with the class.

- Thousands of germs enter your body every day, but your immune system can fight most of them. You are more likely to get sick, however, if you have not been eating or sleeping well or are under a lot of stress. Fever during illness is a sign that your immune system is working hard; an elevated body temperature helps your white blood cells and antibodies fight illness. The body must make a different antibody to fight each type of bacteria or virus that enters. Once a germ invades the body, your immune system "remembers" it and is always ready to make more antibodies, in case that germ enters your body again. That is why we generally get illnesses such as chicken pox just once.

What happens when you catch a cold virus?

You might have a stuffy nose and a sore throat. Maybe you'll get a headache. A few days later, your nose may start to run. A few days after that, you start to feel better.

Your body has been able to fight the cold, thanks to your immune system.

Your immune system fights most of the germs that enter your body before they make you sick. If you do get sick, your immune system works hard to kill the germs so you'll get better faster.

Complete these sentences:

______________________________ make the ____________________ that fight germs such as viruses. Together, they are the key parts of your body's ________________ ________________.

Just what is your immune system?

Even though your blood looks red because of all its red blood cells, there are many white blood cells in it, too. Some white blood cells make antibodies, your body's germ-fighting chemicals. Together, white blood cells and antibodies are the key parts of your immune system.

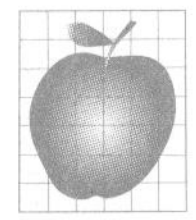

Learning Experience 5-2 continued

Invite students to come up with other ideas for good hygiene that help prevent germs from spreading. Discuss what personal items can be shared and what should not be shared. Tell students that germs are all around us and that we can't eliminate them, but we can help keep them out of our bodies by practicing good hygiene. Explain:

Germs pass through the air when people talk, cough, or sneeze. You can pick up germs by touching doorknobs or telephones, shaking hands, or picking up garbage. Germs will get into your body if you put your fingers, pencils, and other objects in your mouth or if you rub your eyes or nose.

Homework

None

Evaluation

Students will be able to

- Explain what a germ is and what germs do when they get into the body.
- Describe ways in which germs enter the body.
- Describe simple hygiene measures that can prevent them from getting sick.

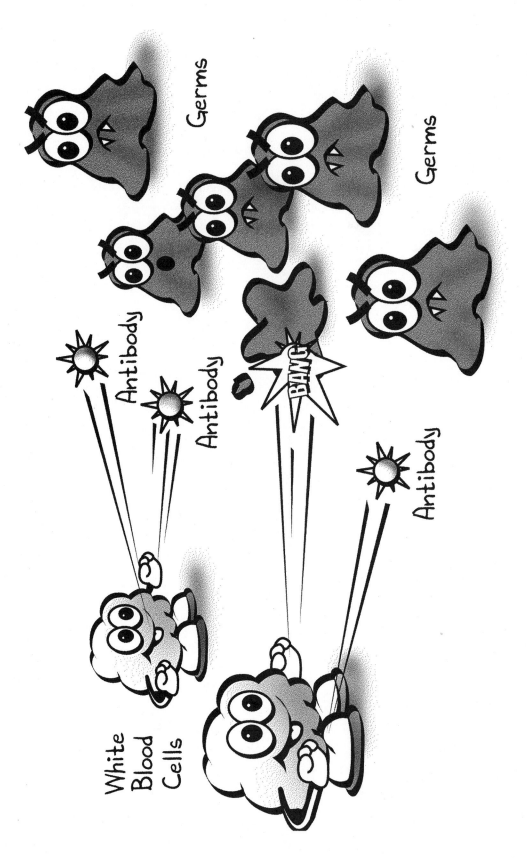

The immune system of a healthy person works like this: If germs get into your body, white blood cells will rush over. They make antibodies to fight the germs.

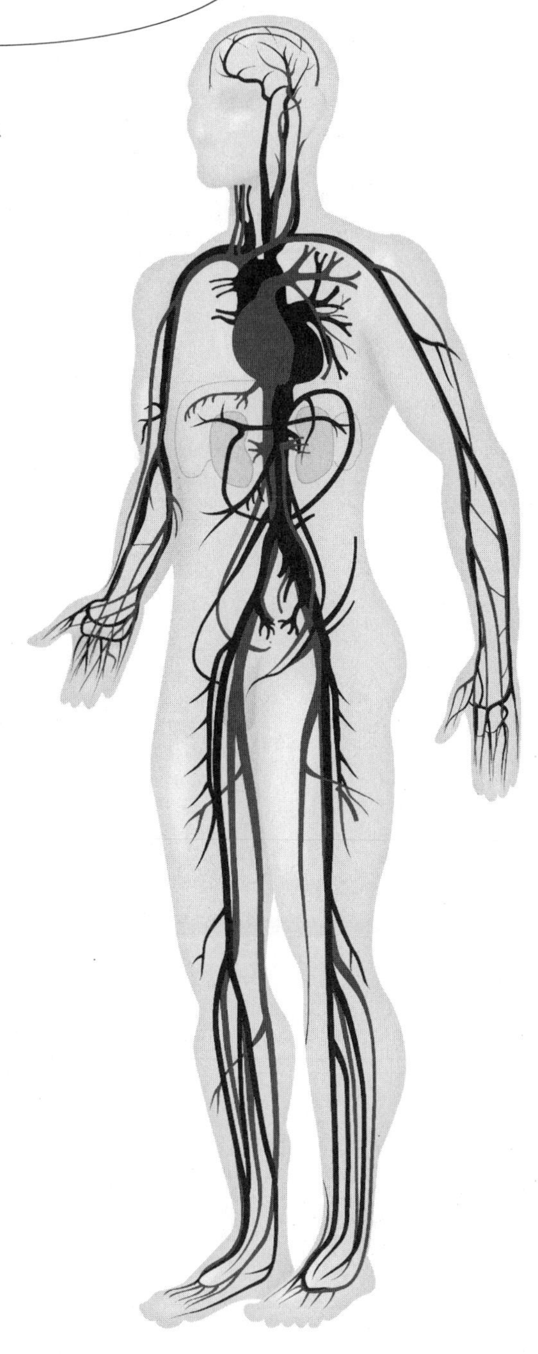
White blood cells that fight germs travel to all parts of the body.

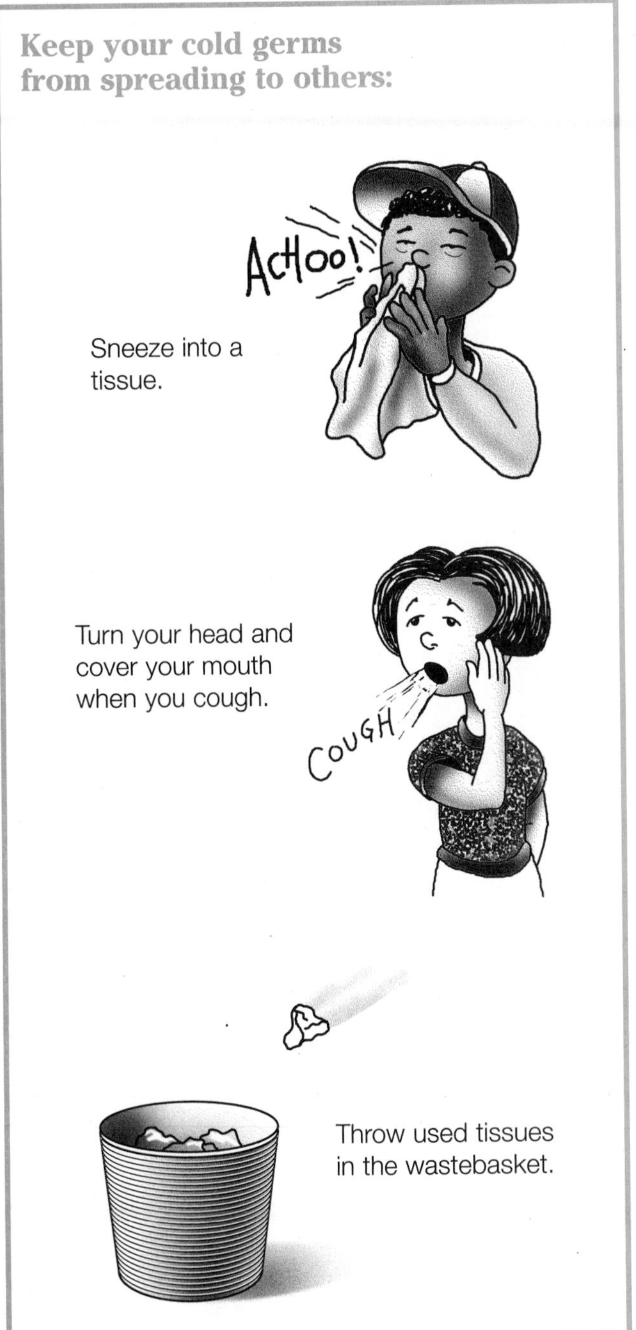

Sneeze into a tissue.

Throw used tissues in the wastebasket.

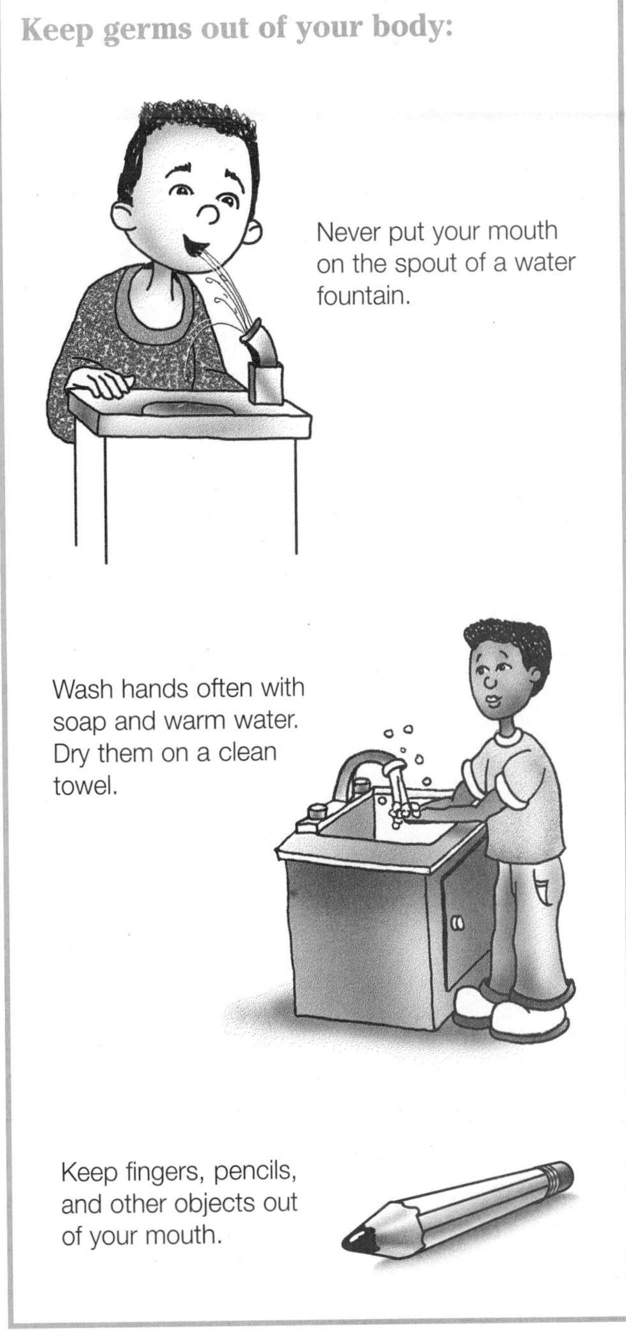
Keep germs out of your body:
Never put your mouth on the spout of a water fountain.
Wash hands often with soap and warm water. Dry them on a clean towel.
Keep fingers, pencils, and other objects out of your mouth.

Can you think of other ways to keep germs from spreading? List them here:

____

____

____

____

____

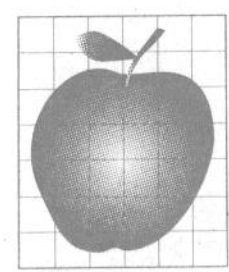

Learning Experience 5-3

Invisible Germs in the Air

Grade Level

K–2

Primary Disciplines

Science

Learning Objectives

After this activity, students will be able to

- List the important reasons for not spreading germs.
- Describe how to get rid of germs.
- Describe how the first line of defense works.

Time Required

One session

Materials

Plastic bottle with a spray nozzle and a tissue

Description of Activity

Use a plastic bottle with a spray nozzle to demonstrate how germs get into the air when we talk, sneeze, or cough. Then cover the nozzle with the tissue. Demonstrate how the tissue blocks the spray, and how the germs are invisible.

Homework

None

Evaluation

Students will be able to

- Explain why they must practice behaviors that prevent the spreading of germs.
- Describe how to get rid of germs.
- Explain how the body's immune system begins to work.

Learning Experience 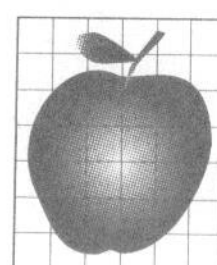 5-4

Caring About Myself And Others

Grade Level

4–6

Primary Disciplines

Social Studies, Language Arts

Learning Objectives

After this activity, students will be able to

- Identify unhealthy behaviors.
- Identify healthy behaviors.
- Understand how one person's behavior affects another.

Time Required

Two sessions

Materials

Chalkboard and chalk; attached handout

Description of Activity

Session 1

On the chalkboard, write the following three headings: High-Risk, Low-Risk, No Risk. Ask the students to state behaviors that fit into each category, relevant to the transmissions of germs. Write students' responses in lists on the chalkboard or on an overhead, follow this with discussion of various risky behaviors as they pertain to communicable infections.

Session 2

Have the students individually respond in writing to the attached handouts. Then, in their groups, have them read their responses to each other and summarize the group responses before sharing one list with the entire class.

Homework

None

Evaluation

Students will be able to

- Spell the new vocabulary words correctly.
- Effectively use writing skills to distinguish high-risk from low-risk behaviors.
- Effectively use writing skills to describe feelings about themselves and others in regard to illness and wellness.
- Differentiate between healthy and unhealthy behaviors.

Source: Adapted, in part, from *HIV/AIDS, Instructional Guide, Grades K–12*, State University of New York, Albany, April 1996.

Name:____

- I can help myself make healthy decisions when I:

- I can help my family, friends and others make healthy decisions:

- I show I care about myself when I:

- I show I care about others when I:

Keep Germs Away!

You can help keep germs out of your body. You can help stop your germs from spreading to other people.

Use a tissue when you sneeze.

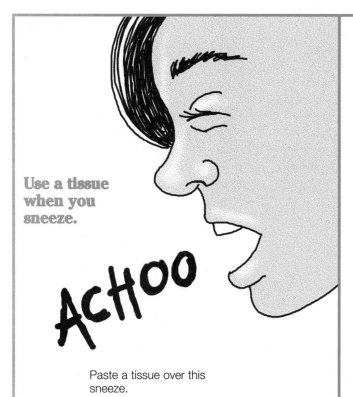

Paste a tissue over this sneeze.

Cover your mouth when you cough.

Cut out a picture of a hand. Paste it over this mouth.

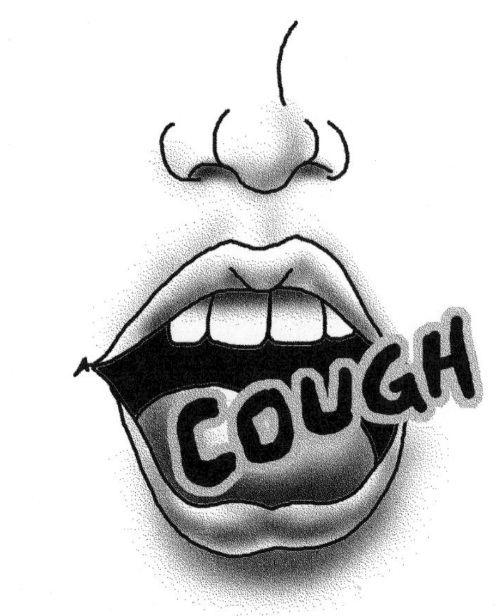

Wash your hands before you eat.

Wash your hands after you go to the bathroom. Use soap and warm water.

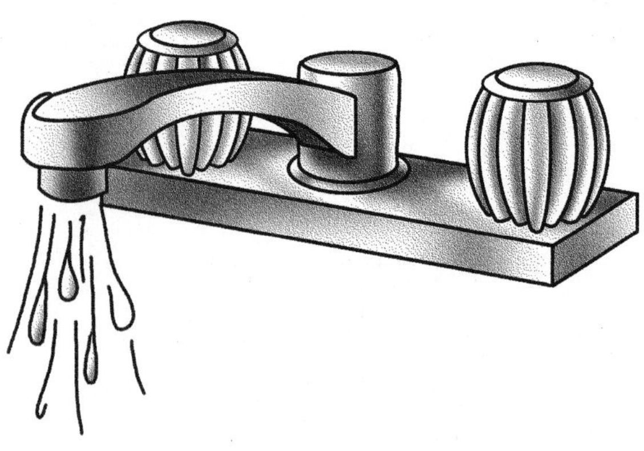

Cut out a picture of soap.
Paste it here.

Don't drink out of someone's glass.

Don't share forks or spoons.

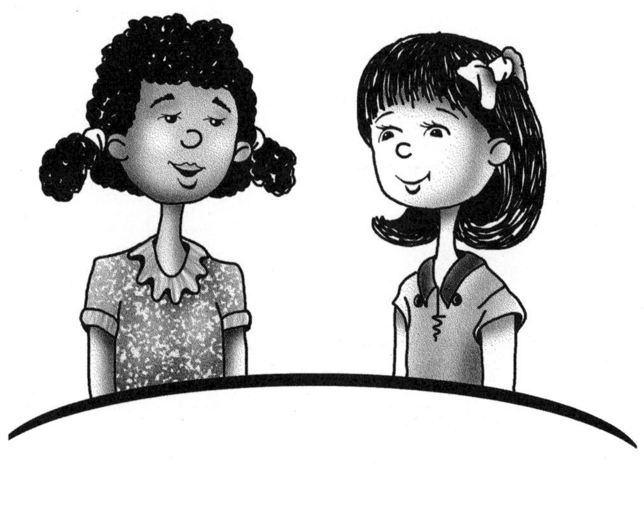

Draw a glass for each child.

Some of these children are spreading germs! Put a circle around them.

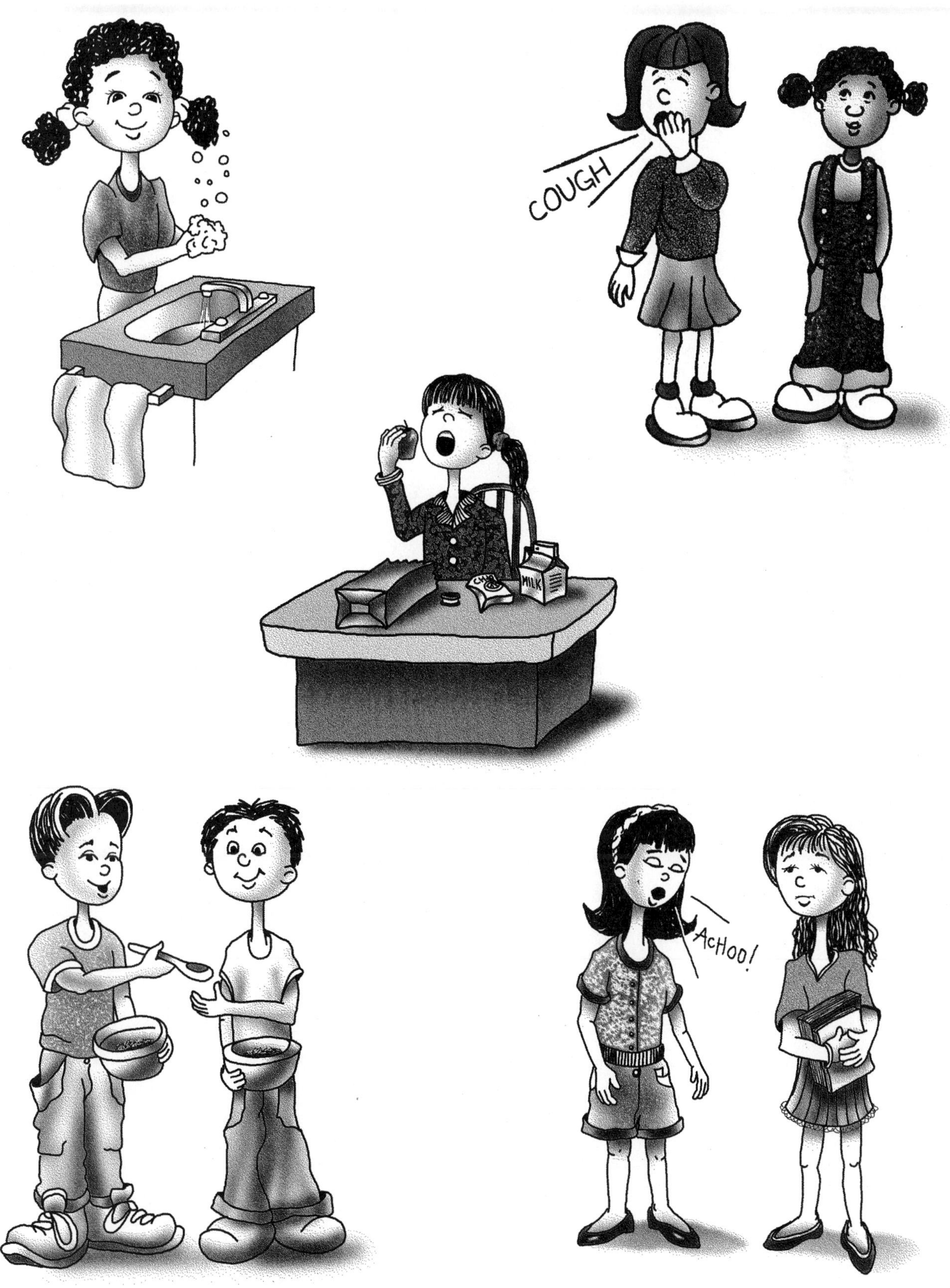

Learning Experience 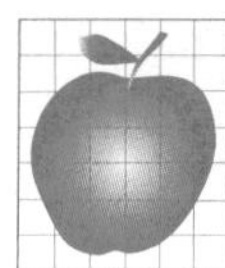 5-5

Making Healthy Choices

Grade Level

3–6

Primary Disciplines

Social Sciences, Language Arts

Learning Objectives

After this activity, students will be able to

- Understand the concept of making choices.
- Define the concept of healthy choices.
- Understand the importance of "thinking about" choices.

Time Required

Two sessions

Materials

Chalkboard and chalk; attached handout

Description of Activity

Session 1

Ask students to respond to the following:

Would you rather be ...

1. a parent or a child?

2. a student or a teacher?

3. a Jeep or a sports car?

4. a Volkswagen or a Jeep?

5. a Mercedes or a Jeep?

6. a human being or an animal?

...and so on.

Ask the students to think about how and why they made the choices they did and to think about examples of any healthy and unhealthy choices. Write the choices on the chalkboard and discuss the concepts with the students.

Session 2

Review the session on healthy choices versus unhealthy choices and then ask the students to respond (individually and in writing) to the Top Three Hopes handout on next page. Place the students in small groups and ask them to read and discuss their responses. Process as a class. Help the students to make the connection between healthy choices and healthy lives.

Homework

None

Evaluation

Students will be able to

- Use writing skills to describe how they prioritize choices in their own lives.
- Explain the concept of choices and how it applies to healthy choices.
- Recognize their own ability to make choices and the consequences of their choices.

Source: Adapted, in part, from *HIV/AIDS*, State University of New York, Albany, April 1996.

Name:____

- My top best three hopes are:

  1. ____
  2. ____
  3. ____

- I can turn my best hopes into reality when I respect myself and others, evaluate risks to make healthy choices, abstain from unhealthy behaviors, care about myself and others, and help make healthy choices for myself and others.

- Today's date is:

____

Learning Experience 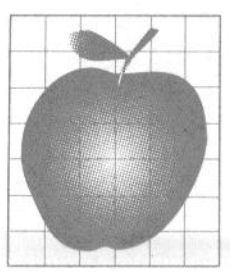 5-6

Understanding Infections and Noninfectious Diseases

Grade Level

5–6

Primary Disciplines

Science, Language Arts

Learning Objectives

After this activity students will be able to

- Recognize the difference between communicable and noncommunicable diseases.
- Explain how they can protect themselves from becoming infected.

Time Required

One session

Materials

Written role-play on index cards and chalkboard

Description of Activity

Write a list of six diseases on the chalkboard and choose different pairs of students to role-play a friend visiting another friend who doesn't feel well. Give students who are playing the sick person roles the name of a specific infection, together with a list of typical symptoms to act out. As a result of watching the various role-plays, the remainder of the class writes down the following:

1. the name of the infection
2. whether the infection is communicable
3. if it is communicable, how they can protect themselves from getting sick

Homework

None

Evaluation

Students will be able to

- Differentiate between communicable and noncommunicable diseases.
- Describe how they can prevent themselves from becoming infected.
- Describe how they can prevent the spread of disease.

Learning Experience 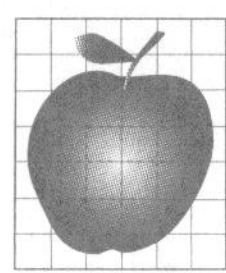 5-7

Reading a Thermometer

Grade Level

3–4

Primary Discipline

Arithmetic

Learning Objectives

Following this activity, students will be able to

- Describe how a thermometer works.
- Explain what a fever is and what causes it.
- Describe the symptoms associated with having a fever.

Time Required

One session

Materials

One or more thermometers

Description of Activity

Explain the purpose of a thermometer and how it is used.

Homework

Using room thermometers, students record various temperatures at home—room temperature, outdoor temperature. With this list of temperatures, demonstrate how to get an average.

Evaluation

Students will be able to

- Explain the concept of body temperature as it relates to health.
- Describe how a thermometer is used and how to read it.
- Explain how symptoms of illness relate to body temperature.

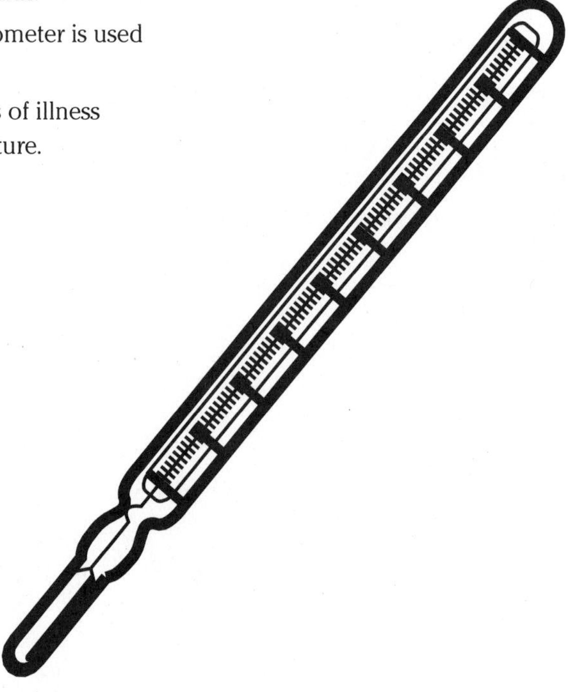

Learning Experience 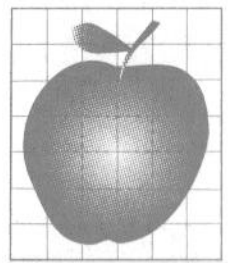 5-8

AIDS—Facts and Myths

Grade Level

5–6

Primary Disciplines

Science, Social Studies, Creative Arts

Learning Objectives

Following this activity, students will be able to understand the differences between HIV and AIDS.

Time Required

Two or three sessions

Materials

Guidelines on myths and facts, oak tag, markers, magazines, index cards

Description of Activity

Sessions 1 and 2

Use the information in Guidelines for Teachers, page 194, to discuss myths about AIDS.

1. After teaching relevant information, put the students in groups of four.
2. Provide each group with index cards on which are written all myths or all facts about HIV/AIDS.

Session 3

Have each group create a poster without a title on the index cards. Each group decides whether their poster depicts myths or facts, but does not tell their choice to the rest of the class. Each group hangs its poster on the wall. The students must decide if the poster represents myths or facts and gives reasons. At the end, the groups put a title on their poster.

Homework

None

Evaluation

Students will be able to

- Work cooperatively in a group to effectively complete an assignment.
- Produce a creative project (poster) that describes the facts and myths about HIV/AIDS.
- Differentiate facts and myths about HIV/AIDS.

Guidelines for Teachers: Myths About AIDS

When a major crisis threatens a group of people, a lot of myths and rumors start circulating. Below are listed some myths that have been started about AIDS. Think about why each of these myths perhaps got started. Then after each one, write down the truth.

- AIDS affects only gay men. AIDS can be spread only through homosexual activities. Homosexuals are to blame for the AIDS epidemic.

- AIDS can be spread by infected people coughing, sneezing, or breathing on another person.

- AIDS can be spread by infected people using the same telephone, water fountain, or bathroom as others.

- The spread of AIDS in the United States is part of an evil plot by our enemies.

- If you feel healthy, you don't have the virus that causes AIDS.

- Mosquitoes and other insects can spread AIDS.

- You can get AIDS by donating blood.

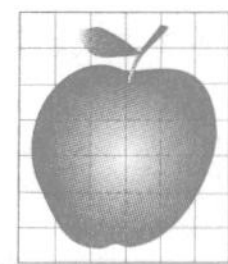

Learning Experience 5-9

A Public Service Announcement

Grade Level

6

Learning Objectives

The students will be able to

- Express the importance of advocating for family and community health.
- Describe how HIV is transmitted.
- Identify the behaviors that reduce risk for HIV infection.
- Identify the risk factors for HIV infection.

Time Required

11 hours

Materials

Paper, pencils, class notes, computer access, phone book, resource materials

Description of Activity

1. Have the students design an informational pamphlet, public service announcement, or lesson that would help their peers resist pressure that might make them contract HIV. Tell them that you will use the criteria in the table on the following page to evaluate their work. Consider the following:
   a. How HIV and AIDS are transmitted
   b. How HIV and AIDS are not transmitted
   c. What HIV and AIDS are
   d. HIV/AIDS risk behaviors
   e. Non-HIV risk behaviors
   f. Treatment
   g. Testing
   h. Health strategies that build the immune system
2. Tell students that the pamphlet, PSA, or lesson should be sensitive to the age group of the target audience—in this case, their own peers.
3. Students may use the class notes, the phone book, or the Internet sites listed below as resources.
   - www.westnet.com/~cgi-bin/body.cgi
   - www.plannedparenthood.com
   - www.thebody.com

Homework

None

Evaluation

See above.

Source: Patrick A. Veltri, *HIV/AIDS Project, Task 3*, NY. Reprinted with permission.

HIV/AIDS Pamphlet, PSA, or Lesson Criteria

Criteria	4	3	2	1
Content	Information is accurate. The pamphlet, PSA, or lesson includes a clear message about the dangers of HIV/AIDS infection. The pamphlet, PSA, or lesson includes all of the key facts about HIV/AIDS.	Information is accurate. The pamphlet, PSA, or lesson includes a clear message about the dangers of HIV/AIDS infection. Graphics and information is logical. The pamphlet, PSA, or lesson includes at least eight important facts about HIV/AIDS.	Information is accurate, but the message about HIV/AIDS is unclear. The pamphlet, PSA, or lesson includes at least seven important facts about HIV/AIDS.	Content is vague and/or inaccurate. The pamphlet includes at least six important facts about HIV/AIDS.
Design	Graphics are visually appealing and complement the information. Information is logical and effectively communicated.	Graphics are visually appealing and complement the information. Information is logical and effectively communicated.	Information is logical and effectively communicated.	Placement of the graphics or poor design does not communicate information effectively.
Communication	The grammar is correct and conveys information clearly and effectively.	The grammar is correct and conveys information clearly and effectively. Project submitted late.	The grammar is correct and conveys information clearly and effectively. Project submitted late.	The grammar is poor or incorrect.

NS — No work submitted or assignment is incomplete.

6

Mental Health

Robert Lazow

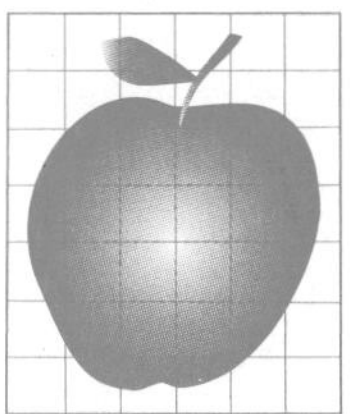

Chapter Outline

The Mental Health of Children
Some Definitions
Shapers of Personality
Forms of Mental Illness
Developing Emotional Health: The Teacher's Role

Objectives

- Explain the importance of mental health in learning
- Define and describe mental illness
- Define personality and theories underlying it
- Describe Maslow's hierarchy of needs
- Explain Erikson's eight stages of development
- Name and explain the shapers of personality: awareness of death, freedom, emotional separateness, meaning, self-worth, self-love, authenticity, self-consciousness, values, feelings, and social skills
- Explain two forms of mood disorder: major depressive disorder and dysrythmic disorder
- Define anxiety disorders: separation anxiety, panic attack, acrophobia, social phobia, obsessive/compulsive disorder, post-traumatic stress disorder, avoidant disorder
- Describe the teacher's role in developing students' emotional health

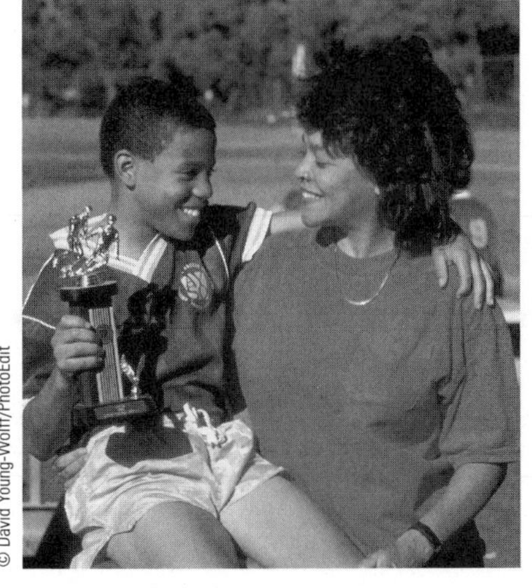

Many of us know this homeless woman who wanders around on the streets in our neighborhood. She is very messy and scary to look at. She wears lots of clothing at the same time and pushes a cart with all kinds of garbage in it. Most of the kids in the neighborhood make fun of her, tease her, and even throw things at her. Sometimes she shouts at people for no apparent reason. She often walks around talking to herself, and at other times she just stares into space. I heard my dad telling his friend that when he was a teenager, she used to work in the bank. He said he thinks she doesn't have any family or friends at all. He feels sad when he sees her and wishes he knew what to do. His friend says he thinks she is just a drunk or a drug addict or maybe just "mentally deranged" and that she ought to be locked up in a mental institution.

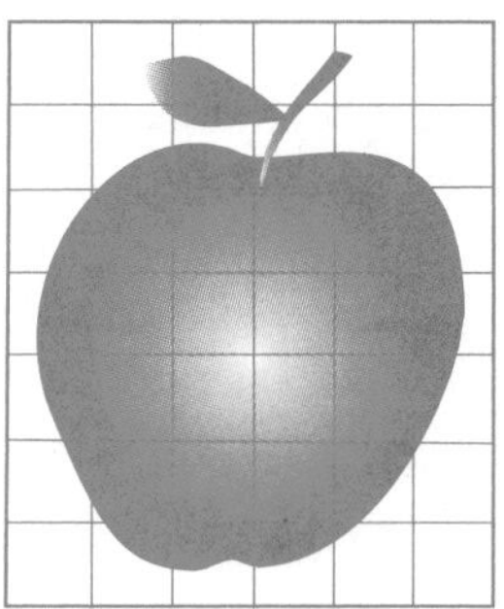

Children are familiar with words such as "insane," "anxious," "nervous," "depressed." They hear these words in everyday conversation. They have heard the expressions, "People who are crazy should be 'put away,'" or "They'd better get some help." They wonder, "What kind of help? How do you get like that? Could that happen to me? Where do people get put away?"

The Mental Health of Children

Mental health is intrinsic to the overall health and well-being of children and adults alike. Mentally healthy children and adults thrive at play, in schoolwork, and in relationships with other people. They do not seem to get as many colds or other illnesses or have many absences from school or work. To the contrary, evidence is ample that negative general health consequences accrue from poor mental health.

Research over the past 25 years has demonstrated the strong relationship between high levels of stress and cardiovascular disease, chronic lung disease, the common cold, and a number of other illnesses.[1] We know that poor self-esteem and depression in children are risk factors for substance abuse, adolescent injury, and suicide. Poor mental health also influences a child's ability to learn, which, in turn, will negatively affect that child's ability to make healthy life choices in adulthood in areas such as sex, diet, exercise, and decisions to seek timely medical care. Accordingly, mental health must be a part of any consideration for achieving a healthy lifestyle.

Some Definitions

Defining mental health is not a simple task. The wide array of definitions reflects the complexity of mental health. In its most basic definition, mental health can be considered the absence of mental illness. By **mental illness** we mean problems or disorders related to the psychological processes or organic functions of the brain. This is a limited view, though. More than the lack of illness, mental health is a combination of neurological, cognitive, social, and (most significantly) emotional elements that contribute to a state of mental well-being.

This chapter will focus primarily on emotional aspects of mental health because emotional states, particularly in childhood, are influenced greatly by the input of parents, other significant adults, peers, and the community (including school, television, music, computers, and so on). Emotional health does not mean the absence of conflicts, challenges, disappointments, and troubles. Rather, it refers to the capacity to recognize and constructively respond to conflicts, challenges, disappointments, and troubles. Most people, at one time or another, experience some confusion or discomfort about who they are or what their life means. They may not be satisfied with their relationships. They may question the worth of a marriage, a friendship, or a job. They may even choose to end or change these situations. They may lose sleep or their appetite for a while and feel nervous or "down" when they are under pressure from work or school.

Although these experiences are emotionally uncomfortable and confusing, they do not, in themselves, constitute emotional or mental illness. The person facing these situations is experiencing the expected problems that come in the course of living. Children, too, have some of these experiences. They experience rejection by or loss of a friend, poor grades in school, separation of parents, and other mentally taxing situations.

Some people find it difficult or impossible to respond constructively or effectively to life. They may be confused about who they are because they lack a self-identity. They may feel bad about themselves and feel so nervous and hopeless that they have trouble succeeding in school, having rewarding relationships, working steadily, or caring for themselves on a long-term basis. They may be fearful of their inability to cope with real or imagined life events and challenges. Their attitudes and behaviors may become irrational, unpredictable, and even self-destructive. They may be verbally abusive to family, friends, and co-workers. They may abuse alcohol and drugs as a way of avoiding uncomfortable situations. Their emotional condition can be described as unhealthy or ill.

A number of social and environmental factors can hamper emotional development or give rise to emotional illness. In addition, a wide variety of mental illnesses and developmental and learning disabilities can foster emotional problems. Mental illness has signs and symptoms such as:

- irrational or confused thought patterns
- perceptual distortions (hearing or seeing things that do not exist)
- extremes of emotions (going from emotional highs to emotional lows)
- distorted beliefs (incorrectly believing that one is being monitored by beings from outer space or thinking that all people are out to hurt you)
- bizarre or irrational behavior (wearing strange or inappropriate clothes or not changing clothes for extended periods, perhaps for months).

Problems with intellect, thought processes, or perception can impede children's emotional development by, for example, limiting their ability to accurately perceive and understand themselves and their environment, negatively affecting their emotional state or sense of self-worth, or significantly interfering with the development of social skills and the ability to have positive relationships.

Not all behaviors that appear different or bizarre are signs of mental illness or an emotional problem. All children have some behaviors or mannerisms that are unique to them, but are not necessarily signs of mental illness. A child may be boisterous, excitable, loud, and wear "funny" clothes. Another may be extremely quiet because he or she is shy. Teachers should take care not to label children mentally ill.

The social customs and behaviors of a recently arrived immigrant may not fit norms in the United States. For example, people sometimes extend friendship by putting an arm around a person they are meeting for the first time. The immigrant may come from a culture in which people are more restrained in their approach with strangers. They may view hugging a stranger as brazen or bad manners. In their country, a simple bow or a nod of the head may be an appropriate greeting. Moving away from a friendly hand on the shoulder does not mean the child is fearful or unnecessarily suspicious. It may simply be a matter of custom.

In the classroom, teachers have the opportunity to provide a support for emotional health from which children can be boosted in a lifelong process. This chapter provides teachers with a framework from which to develop the knowledge and skills that are helpful in promoting emotional health.

Personality

Personality can be defined as the sum of a person's feelings, beliefs, perceptions, attitudes, communication style, and behaviors. These attributes are a manifestation of a person's emotional, intellectual, and social functioning in this world. The extent to which these attributes contribute to an individual's ability to function well is a guide to an individual's mental health. The patterns these attributes take on—personality traits—allow us to identify and recognize an individual or a group of individuals who have a number of similar traits. Thus, when a child is described as being shy, that child is assigned to a similar group of children who talk quietly, don't raise their hand in class, and do not want to participate in large-group activities. That same child, however, has other aspects of his or her personality. He or she may be hard-working, responsible, and loyal—perhaps someone who stays after school to help the teacher, always completes homework, and gets it in on time. Often, one or more traits dominate in a personality. We tend to describe people by those dominant traits.

When we describe people as emotionally healthy, we are ascribing to them the following attributes of emotional health:

- A sense of autonomy or independence in thought and action
- An ability to accept the thoughts, ideas, and guidance of others without a loss of identity or autonomy
- A unity of personality
- A positive feeling and view of themselves and an accurate perception of themselves and the world around them
- An openness to knowing and accepting themselves and the world around them
- A willingness to learn about and participate in the world, although not always being fully accepting
- Being flexible when facing life's challenges, disappointments, and limitations

The Personality Core

The core of human personality is formed before birth and is the basis of our **self-concept**. This core is a product of the genetic and overall structure and functioning of the brain, as well as overall development of the human body. Humans could not learn or acquire the traits of personality from their environment without the biological ability to do so.

Cognition

Cognitive functioning, one of the brain's inborn attributes, plays a major role in personality development. Cognitive functioning includes abilities such as short- and long-term memory, attention, focus, judgment, and problem solving. These functions provide humans with the ability to retain, process, store, and use information. The capacity to be influenced by one's environment, through interactions with that environment, depends on cognitive ability. Humans would not be able to learn new behaviors—such as dressing appropriately, mastering reading and writing, or acquiring appropriate social skills—without attention and problem-solving abilities.

The Survival Need

Instincts dictate many of the behaviors that humans exhibit, as exemplified by an infant's preoccupation with eating and seeking attention. Supporting the need for survival is the **fight-or-flight** response to situations perceived as dangerous or a threat to survival. Behaviors through which the flight-or-fight response is expressed include fear, caution, avoidance, or aggression (see Chapter 8). In addition, survival is ensured by humans' inborn capacity to define what they like and do not like, what is pleasurable and not pleasurable. Infants not only know when they are hungry, they also know which specific foods are gratifying.

Inborn Attributes

Certain personality attributes seem to be developed before birth. Some students, for example, are fascinated by working on math or physics problems, whereas others are artistically inclined. In addition, how students react to situations and people around them may be related to inborn attributes. Some students are consistently more sensitive to stressful situations, such as the separation from parents at the beginning of the school year or the prospect of a class test. Some students are more assertive than their classmates or may more easily take on the role of leader when in a group activity. These preferences, as part of a person's personality, are probably inborn, not learned.

Our Complex Brain

Unlike other living things, humans have a complex mental process that intercedes or negotiates between neuro-biological functioning and the environment. This process is human consciousness. Although many living species have cognitive ability, feelings, and a repertoire of behaviors, humans have a more developed and complex brain.

The segment of our brain that makes it uniquely human in its mental and emotional capacities is the cerebral cortex. This structure provides humans with self-consciousness or a conscious awareness of themselves—what they feel, what they believe, and what they think. Consciousness takes place within the context of a person's awareness of time (memories of the recent and distant past, awareness of the present, and thoughts of the future plus the person's awareness, thoughts, and feelings about the universe—parents, friends, mate, children, people in general, school, work, community, country).

Personality Theorists and Their Theories

Erikson	Stages of Psychosocial Development
Freud	Psychoanalysis
Kohlberg	Development of Moral Reasoning
Maslow	Hierarchy of Needs and Self-Actualization
Piaget	Development of Thought (Cognition)
Skinner	Behaviorism

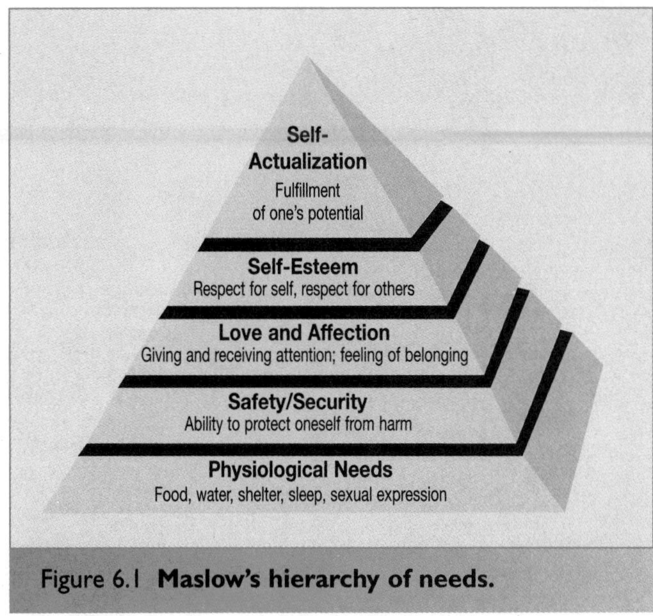

Figure 6.1 **Maslow's hierarchy of needs.**

Accordingly, individual human awareness, feelings, and thoughts are at the core of personality and give us our individual beliefs, attitudes, perceptions, emotions, and behaviors. Human beings are similar to each other in many areas of their awareness, feelings, thoughts, and biological brain processes (that is, mental activity). The consciousness that the cerebral cortex gives human beings, however, also gives us our uniqueness, our individuality. No two person's thumbprints, facial features, or (especially) DNA are the same. In the same way, no two brain structures or brain processes are exactly alike. Consequently, no two humans experience, think about, or react to the surrounding world in the same way. No two personalities are exactly alike.

The Role of Experience in Personality

The core of personality is enhanced and further individualized by the attributes, knowledge, and skills humans acquire through a lifetime of fulfilling needs, acquiring learning, and gaining experiences. Accordingly, personality development is a combination of nature and nurture.

Human awareness, cognitive perceptions, feelings, beliefs, attitudes, values, and behaviors are influenced and shaped by interactions with parents, siblings, significant adults, and peers. All humans have the capacity to feel. The direction these feelings take toward themselves and others and their ability to identify these feelings in what are called emotions (love, hate, anger, sadness, fear, and others) are dependent on childhood needs and how they are dealt with or fulfilled by parents and other significant adults, as well as what a child learns from these adults.

Maslow's Hierarchy of Needs

According to Abraham Maslow, in the process of seeking and receiving fulfillment of our needs, we form the social or experiential aspects of personality.[2] Maslow identified the most basic physiological needs as air, food, water, warmth, shelter, sleep, and sexual expression. These needs ideally are met by the infant's parents or other significant adults. Beyond the birth process itself, the infant's fulfillment of basic needs and the parents' ability to meet those needs is the basis for bonding between parent and child. These needs form the foundation of Maslow's pyramid, shown in Figure 6.1

When basic needs are met, individuals seek fulfillment of their needs of safety, then love and belonging, identity, and self-esteem, and, finally, self-actualization—all located higher on the pyramid. These needs are at first met by parental figures, but as the child enters the toddler period and later childhood stages, teachers, other significant adults, and friends increasingly meet these needs.

Eventually, human beings meet these needs for themselves by providing for their own security and responsibility, self-respect, self-love, self-identity, and the ability to care and love others, as well as creativity and self-sufficiency. Once all these needs are met, the individual can turn to the more satisfying "self-actualized" needs of meaningfulness, authenticity, self-sufficiency, creativity, vitality, and finally, knowledge, insight, wisdom, synergy, integration, and beauty.

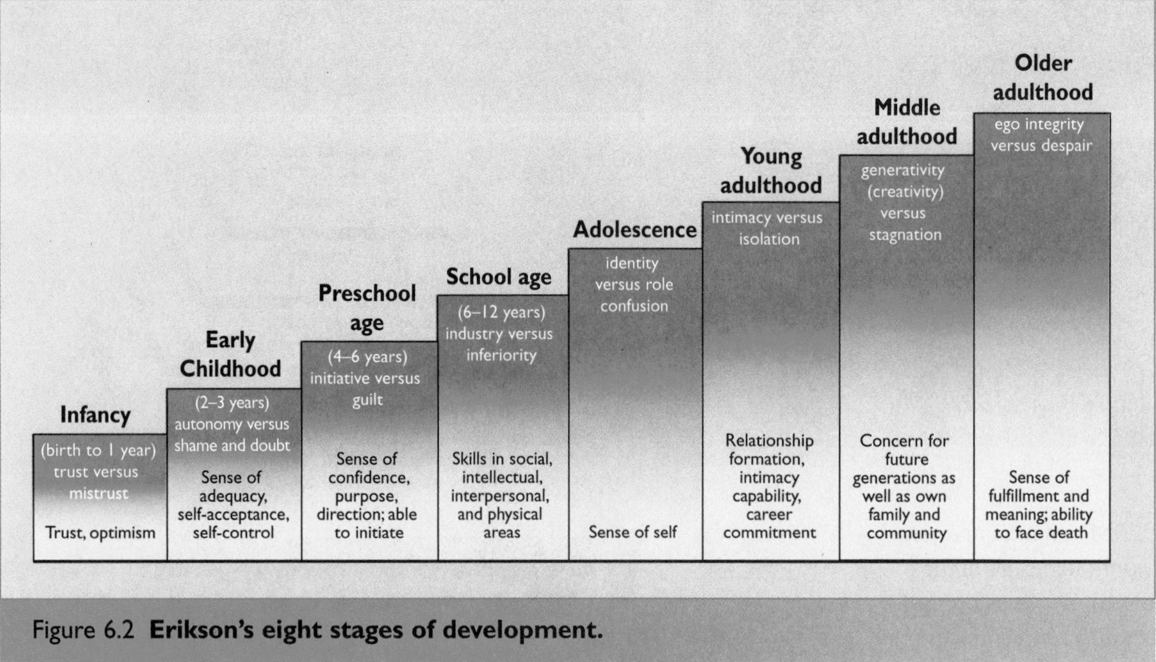

Figure 6.2 **Erikson's eight stages of development.**

Although Maslow proposed that human beings fulfill their self-actualized needs in an orderly progression after they have fulfilled their basic needs, human beings more likely begin to experience self-actualization in the process of obtaining more basic needs. Young people probably attain self-actualization when, as children, they receive attention from parents or teachers or when they successfully complete a house chore or a school project, or when they play with other children, or when, as young adults, they care for themselves or others.

Erikson and Personality Development

In terms of human development, Maslow's hierarchical structure is a good framework in which to view how the self and, therefore, personality develop. In many ways this framework closely parallels the stages of ego development theorized by Erik Erikson. Erikson not only described how fulfillment of needs is directly related to specific facets of personality development, but also indicated that emotional problems would develop if these needs were not met.[3] As in Maslow's hierarchy, Erikson's theory of needs is based on neurophysical and experiential growth and development.

Whereas Maslow appears to have placed self-esteem farther along in the process of personality development (after basic needs are meet), Erikson theorized that the building of self-esteem occurs at each stage of life—starting in infancy in the process of basic needs fulfillment. The extent to which a child's needs are met or not met will have a direct influence on the development of self and, therefore, self-esteem. Erikson divided the lifespan into eight stages, given in Figure 6.2

Stage I: Infancy to about the first year: Trust versus mistrust. These traits develop out of the infant's certainty that the basic needs of life will consistently be provided for. If parents or significant adults do not provide the infant with water, food, warmth, shelter, and a safe, comfortable place to sleep, he or she can become distrustful and lose faith. Further, according to Erikson, it is not enough to have the basic needs met; it is the way in which these components are given—ideally, with warmth, love, and caring, communicating a sense of belonging. Children who do not have these needs met—or whose needs are met in an unloving way—may become distrustful and feel unloved and think something is basically wrong with them.

Stage II: Early childhood, second and third years: Autonomy versus shame/doubt. Children begin to feel an identity separate from parents and a sense of self-control and self-determination. Children test the waters around them. The security, love, and sense of belonging achieved in infancy enable the child to risk establishing an independent sense of self. Children who are prevented from, or made to feel badly about, seeking autonomy may feel what Erikson calls "shame" or doubt themselves as autonomous people. A prevailing feeling of dread or feeling badly about themselves may permeate their lives from childhood through adulthood.

Stage III: Later preschool years: Initiative versus guilt. During this time, the child gains a sense of direction and purpose through initiative shown at play. If a child is made to feel badly about this show of initiative because of the disapproval of significant adults, the child may begin to think of himself or herself as bad and grow into an adult inhibited from pursuing freedom and initiative because of feelings of guilt.

Stage IV: School age: Industry versus inferiority. In school, the child's universe expands beyond family. The student learns that creating and producing things and starting and completing tasks gain positive attention (and the pleasure associated with it) from persons other than immediate family members. If children succeed at this, they will gain a sense of self-assurance and confidence. If the children believe they cannot perform or, indeed, cannot actually perform up to the standards required of them in the classroom, they may develop feelings of failure and inferiority.

Stage V: Adolescence: Identity versus role confusion. During adolescence, humans develop a stable, integrated perception of self that is grounded in the reality of the perception others have of them. During this stage, humans evaluate themselves in terms of social choices such as career, significant friendships, romantic relationships, values, and political views. This period is filled with questions of identity and choices. As a result, the adolescent develops the ability to make commitments toward specific life decisions such as marriage, college, an occupation, a certain religious belief, or a worldview. People who do not fully complete this stage experience identity confusion and may have difficulty committing to anything.

Erikson's last three stages of emotional growth take place in adulthood. Although they are not pertinent to the discussion here, they do put general human development in context and, therefore, warrant review. These stages are as follows.

Stage VI: Young adulthood: Intimacy versus isolation. Love is the ability to emotionally commit to and develop a significant relationship with another human. This is, in part, dependent on having established an identity earlier.

Stage VII: Adulthood: Generativity versus stagnation. People immerse themselves in a career, a vocation, or a significant life in a selfless manner.

Stage VIII: Ego integrity versus despair. People in this stage have the opportunity to make sense out of their lives through an inventory of and insight into their past. They have a more immediate sense of life's ultimate end in death.

Shapers of Personality

Significantly, four themes or "ultimate concerns of life" run through both Maslow's and Erikson's theories of personality. Yalom identified these as death, freedom, emotional separateness or isolation, and meaning.[4] These are overriding issues that color or shape the way human beings, from childhood through adulthood, interact with their world. These concerns are uniquely human and are a product of the higher brain functioning of humans that results in the uniquely human quality of self-awareness or consciousness.

Awareness of Death

Although all animals have an awareness of, fear of, and resistance to the threat of death, humans have an immediate fear of death as a result of human consciousness and the resulting awareness of oneself in the context of time (past, present, and future). Humans also are aware of their own gradual decline through the process of aging as an indication of eventual and undeniable death. No human really wants to die because it is in direct opposition to the human instinct to survive. Because dying is out of human control, some humans develop defense mechanisms or coping skills to deal with this uncomfortable reality.

One common mechanism is **denial**, placing the thought of death out of sight and out of mind. Other humans believe in an afterlife. Still others place themselves in at-risk situations, such as sky diving or automobile racing. Even very young children have an awareness and fear of death. Childhood responses to death often take forms such as preoccupation with ghost stories and monsters. Chapter 12 provides an in-depth discussion of children in relation to death and loss.

Freedom

Freedom can be equated to the neurobiological need for survival, autonomy, and independence. How individuals pursue these needs depend on the interactions they have had with parents and other significant adults, such as teachers, as well as their own intellectual capacity to plan and make life choices.

Having the need to survive or to achieve autonomy is not enough to ensure that these needs will be met. Humans must be educated about how to make choices and use them responsibly and productively. Individuals who have not been educated to make wise choices or to act responsibly are often unmotivated to fulfill their own or others' needs. These are the children who are talked into experimenting with drugs because they do not know how to say "no" to peer pressure or are more concerned with fulfilling another's expectations, even when they know that this could be destructive. They also are the children who do not complete their homework when it becomes too challenging or when they would rather do something more pleasurable, such as playing games on the computer or watching TV. As adults, these children usually depend on others to help them survive, by seeking financial support or having others do their tasks on the job or at home. Adults who do not take responsibility are frequently seen as lazy.

Emotional Separateness

The uniqueness of humans and the autonomy we strive for also have the effect of creating a separateness from other human beings. This separateness creates a dilemma: Humans are also social beings who desire and need human contact and support. Most humans experience this dilemma as a feeling of loneliness—which is not the same as being physically alone. An individual may spend a good deal of time alone and not feel lonely. Conversely, people can be surrounded by family and friends and still have deep feelings of loneliness. Much of a lifetime is spent trying to achieve a balance between separateness and social interaction. For many people, loneliness is uncomfortable or even frightening. People who have not fully developed a sense of an independent self or who cannot bear being alone sometimes overreact by immersing themselves in social contact.

As Erikson postulated, younger children are dependent on parents or significant others for emotional support and identity. Even young children, however, have a desire for emotional separateness. The young child also has a desire to feel that what he/she thinks is all right. A child's feelings and beliefs, however, are not yet developed. Children, thus, are dependent on parents to help them develop those feelings and beliefs. Children feel loneliness when parents do not approve of them or are not around to approve of their emotions. In older children and adolescents, as well as adults, avoiding aloneness hampers their personality development because time spent with oneself is necessary to fully integrate things learned from one's environment with one's own feelings, thoughts, and perceptions.

Meaning

The ability to question where humans came from and where we are going in our lives and to solve problems, imagine, and plan from the present into the future enables us to search for and define the meaning of our lives. With freedom, humans may question the purpose of their lives. In addition, through responsible thought and actions, we may define for ourselves what that purpose is. This definition can take place in the areas of relationships, work, education, recreation, retirement, and so on. When children are not encouraged to define what is significant for them or taught how to pursue what is significant, they become adults who depend on others to define life's meaning for them. Because meaning is central to how we identify ourselves, lack of meaning obscures who we are from ourselves.

Self-Worth/Self-Esteem

Maslow's and Erikson's theories of personality development have demonstrated that the uniquely human factor of self-awareness, or self-concept, is largely shaped by experiences of childhood and adolescence. People's self-concept is made up of perceptions and feelings and the judgments made about the self. These perceptions, feelings, and judgments are used to self-evaluate the self. Synonymous terms are **self-worth** and **self-esteem**.

Self-esteem plays a central role in emotional health. Three of the attributes of emotional health are essentially descriptions of good self-esteem: having a positive feeling and view of self and the world, being open to knowing and accepting oneself and the surrounding world, and having a sense of autonomy or independence in thought or action.

Two other emotional attributes cited previously—unity of personality[5] and an accurate perception of oneself and world—are prerequisites to achieving self-esteem. The remaining attributes cited—ability to accept the thoughts, ideas, and guidance of others without a loss of identity or autonomy;[6] openness to knowing and accepting oneself and the surrounding world; and willingness to learn about and participate in the world—can be fully obtained only as a result of having self-esteem.

The attributes of self-esteem form a foundation made up of our positive perceptions and feelings about self, as well as awareness, knowledge, and honesty about who we are. As noted previously, how people feel about and see themselves is based largely upon the feelings their parents had for them and how these feelings were displayed, combined with the extent to which their parents were able to care for their basic needs. Accordingly, it may be said that children learn about having feelings for themselves by the example their parents set. When children and adolescents feel and perceive that parents love, accept, respect, and care for them in a consistent, supportive manner, they gain the perception that they themselves are lovable, worth caring about, and of value. Their parents are validating them.

Because parenting is, at best, imperfect—parents are only human—children cannot have all of their needs met, all of the time, in all of the ways they want. Consequently, no human has perfect self-esteem. Sometimes people's self-esteem is high; they feel good about themselves and confident about their school or job performance and personal relationships. At other times they have self-doubt, believing they lack the ability to obtain a goal in life or perceiving themselves to be unattractive to others. People with generally good self-esteem are able to help themselves through the more vulnerable times when they are questioning their self-worth. They are able to recognize their inner strength—which is really a recognition of their own value and abilities. When questioning their self-worth after experiencing the loss of a relationship or something else they value, the same people may be able to remember that they have also experienced successes and that they have been able to function effectively on a consistent basis. Consequently, they are better able to accept disappointment as part of life's experiences and less likely to judge their self-worth negatively.

Having good self-esteem on a consistent basis is necessary for emotional health. Children need this to thrive at school and to have satisfying relationships. They need to have a sense of self-worth to derive pleasure from themselves and their accomplishments. They need a sense of self-worth in order to meet life's unknown challenges.

In extreme cases, children suffer from outright emotional or physical neglect or abuse. These children experience significant damage to their self-esteem and are at risk for emotional or mental illness.

People with continued low self-esteem are not likely to function to their full potential and may even harm themselves. Young children with poor self-esteem may refuse to engage in competitive play when they fear they might lose. They may act aggressively toward other children or seek attention, such as being the class clown. Or they may avoid unstructured activities, such as drawing and painting, where there is a chance that they will expose themselves emotionally. Teenagers who see themselves as losers or as ugly may isolate themselves from classmates. Young people who never feel good enough have a consistent fear of social rejection and may succumb to drinking or taking drugs to fend off these feelings and thoughts.

Lack of self-esteem does not mean that a person will automatically fail in life. It means that a person goes through periods of poor self-esteem more often, and times of high self-worth less often, than peers with higher self-esteem. In times of crisis, people with low self-esteem have a harder time perceiving their own qualities, abilities, or emotional strength. Children who have esteem problems may experience successes in some areas and still feel uncomfortable about themselves. A child may be a gifted student, a talented musician, or a highly creative artist and at the same time have higher anxiety and self-doubt.

Adults with poor self-esteem can have successful college performance, career, and marriage—yet their poor self-esteem can interfere with their ability to recognize their strengths and enjoy their accomplishments. They may even sabotage themselves by setting themselves up for failure in relationships or at work because they are convinced that they will fail anyway. They can be extremely harsh on themselves when they make a human error, telling themselves that they are "no good" or "stupid." They may be confused about what they believe in or how they feel and, as a result, see themselves as "crazy" or "insane." They may not recognize their feelings at all, which leads to more serious problems such as being out of touch with reality or highly paranoid and fearful.

Self-Love

Self-love itself is at the core of positive feelings about oneself. Self-love can be defined as a strong positive attachment to oneself. People usually express self-love in the same way their parents did for them, through a set of actions or behaviors that strive to fulfill the basic needs of sleep, food, shelter, safety, comfort, and care given in a supportive, consistent manner. In addition, good parents give frequent verbal and physical demonstrations of love such as telling the child "I love you" and kissing and hugging them. In the absence of these positive expressions of love, children may have a difficult time identifying the fulfillment of needs with love. In fulfilling their own needs, they are also imparting the message to themselves that they are of value.

Authenticity

The feelings of love and value that people have for themselves are interwoven with their feelings and self-perception of being authentic or real human beings. Authenticity means feeling autonomous and separate. Authenticity is also at the center of people knowing who they are and accepting themselves for what they are. If people do not know themselves and see themselves as separate human beings, they have difficulty feeling good about self and life.

Humans are helped to develop authenticity at first in childhood. Initially their parents validate them through the acts of love, care, and attention. In addition parents foster authenticity by encouraging their children to develop a sense of individuality. Authenticity is facilitated by teachers who assist and support the development of students' knowledge, thoughts, ideas, beliefs, creativity, skills, and abilities that are unique to them.

Self-Consciousness

Self-consciousness is cognizance of the meaning people place on their own feelings, values, and social skills. It is also a consciousness of the actions they take as a result. Consequently, what individuals perceive and feel about themselves influences how they will interact with the environment around them. Self-consciousness is at first shaped or socialized by what children learn from their parents, then it expands to include what they learn from other family members, then teachers, and then from the larger community of media, work, and other influences. Self-consciousness is gained from interactions with the social environment.

Values

All cultures live by a set of social codes or norms to guide people in their behaviors and actions toward each other. The judgments that people make about themselves and others are based in part on a set of **values**. Some values are universal: They are accepted by all cultures. Two of these are

> Do unto others as you would have them do unto you. (The Golden Rule)
>
> "If I am not for myself, who am I? But if I'm only for myself, what am I? And if not now, when?" (attributed to Hillel, a biblical scholar)

Both of these values stress respect for and responsibility to self and to others.[7] They therefore provide a foundation and reference point for nearly all other values and behaviors. These include, among others, justice, liberty, truthfulness and honesty, altruism, faith, and courage.

Values stem from a person's family and the larger culture. Some cultures place a higher value on the individual in terms of individual rights, freedom, ability, and success. Other cultures place more of an emphasis on community over the individual. People who move too far outside the cultural norms face pressure to conform and ridicule for not conforming.

The concept that values are an integral part of who people are as human beings is reinforced throughout life in school, church, literature, movies, and so on. Consequently, values are used as a measure of a person's self-worth. People who do not have a code of values they live by have diminished self-respect and self-esteem.

Values aren't always positive. We might place value on attributes such as appearance. An example is the value that being tall and thin with blonde hair and blue eyes is preferable. This value diminishes people who have the attributes of being shorter, heavier, and having dark eyes and hair. These are the messages expounded through television and in magazine advertisements.

Demonstrating values inconsistently can confuse a child. For example, parents may act honestly some of the time and at other times lie or rationalize a dishonest deed. Children usually are aware of their parents' actions and inconsistencies. At the extreme are people who never were taught values and act mostly in ways that are antisocial and damaging to themselves and others. A valueless childhood can lead to an adult who engages in a career of crime without remorse. A person who lacks a sense of right and wrong and acts in antisocial ways is called a **sociopath**.

Feelings

People learn to recognize, identify, and differentiate feelings in relation to their experiences. Emotions include love, hate, fear, anger, happiness, and others. Humans usually place subjective values on feelings, calling them "good" or "bad." In dysfunctional families, children may become confused about their feelings. The result is that the children may evaluate their feelings as being bad or good. When people do this, they, in turn, judge themselves to be bad or unworthy. The boy who is taught "Don't feel afraid—boys who have courage aren't afraid" on the first day of school or camp is being taught to deny his feelings. He is being given the message that the natural and necessary feeling of fear is bad. Such messages are particularly damaging if done on a continuous basis.

For example, children may think that if they are afraid, something is wrong with them or they are less of a person; they feel ashamed of themselves. Children who come to recognize and understand fear and other feelings will accept them as a natural part of the human experience.

Social Skills

Social skills are the means by which an individual can attain confidence and motivation. In their most basic form, social skills are necessary to survive. The ability to communicate and the ability to work cooperatively has enabled the human species to survive numerous trials.

In an educational setting, goal setting, flexibility in setting goals, and task completion are necessary for successful social interaction. Teachers can facilitate the development of social skills through the Learning Experiences at the end of this chapter.

Forms of Mental Illness

Criteria for mental or emotional illness have been developed by the American Psychiatric Association.[8] These criteria help professionals diagnose a problem so it can be treated. The most common psychiatric problems in children are mood disorders and anxiety disorders.

Causes

Whereas the risks or causes for mental illness have been debated for over 200 years, it is certain that psychiatric problems are related to a combination of both biological and psychosocial factors. The degree to which a psychiatric problem is brought on by either a biological or a psychosocial factor is not fully known. However, it is generally accepted by mental health professionals that persons with major mental illnesses—such as schizophrenia or major depressive disorder as well as the more moderate but long-term problems of dysthymia (moderate depression) and anxiety—have some predisposed neurobiological risk factors contributing to illness onset. These biological risks, it is postulated, are either genetic (inherited) or are due to illness or physical trauma that has caused damage to the neurochemical processes of the brain. Additionally, it is hypothesized that major traumatic life events, such as the ongoing abuse of a child, can permanently and negatively alter the neuro-chemistry of the brain and lead to lifelong problems of anxiety and depression. Pychosocial factors—such as how a child is parented, what experiences he or she has with other significant adults or peers, or how early a child gets mental health and educational services—can contribute to lessening or increasing the severity of these illnesses.

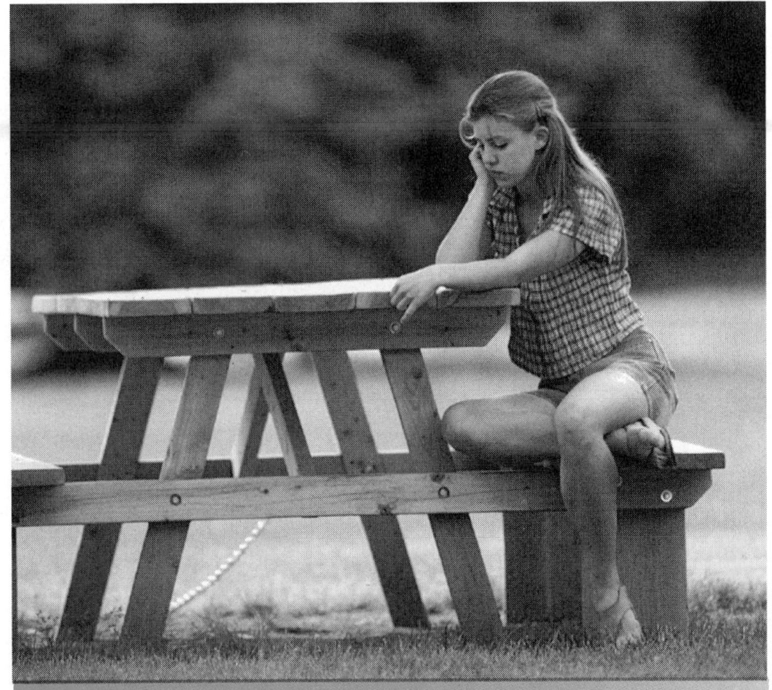

© Fitness & Wellness, Inc.

A depressed person lacks energy and interest in life.

Mental illness, whether biological or psychosocial in origin, ultimately can be devastating to the well-being of a child not only because the symptoms are painful but also, as noted earlier, because these illnesses can affect the process of normal emotional and educational development.

Diagnosis of Psychiatric Problems

The diagnosis of psychiatric problems can be difficult and confusing. Presently, the technology does not exist to conclusively diagnose such problems. There are no laboratory tests or x-rays that can identify a specific psychiatric disorder. Diagnosis is based on the observation of mental health professionals, who use categories and descriptions found in the American Psychiatric Association's *Diagnostic and Statistics Manual IV* along with oral and written psychiatric tests or screening scales. The manual, tests, and scales are ultimately the results of compilations of human observations. Whereas observations based on professional training and experience can approach some accuracy, observations can never be as rigorous as the diagnostic technology used for physical illnesses. Consequently, there is a greater potential for misdiagnosis with psychiatric illnesses. What can appear to be a psychiatric problem can be a developmental problem. Behaviors and emotions that appear in depressed children may also be seen in children with attention deficit/hyperactivity disorder. Additionally, a child who is accused of being a discipline problem may actually have attention deficit/hyperactivity disorder.

Mood Disorders

The two forms of mood disorder most relevant to school-age children are major depressive disorder and dysrhythmic disorder.

For Your Health

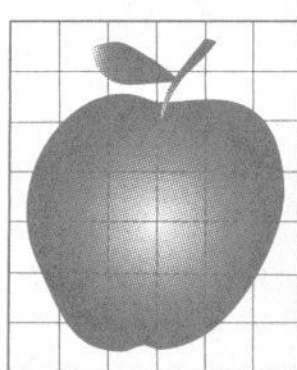

Suicide Prevention

Most people who threaten suicide are really asking for help, and they usually respond positively when they receive human contact and support. Some of the following suggestions may help.

- Ask the person if he or she is really thinking about suicide.
- Reassure the person of his or her strong qualities, attributes, and importance, but do not try to analyze the person's behavior.
- Listen to the person and show genuine interest. Show strength, stability, and firmness.
- Reassure the person that you are going to do everything possible to help him or her remain alive.
- Seek professional help as quickly as possible.
- Never make challenging statements such as, "You won't kill yourself!" or "Go ahead—I don't believe you'll do it." This person needs support.

Many institutions, agencies, and organizations are prepared and equipped to help people who are at "wit's end." Counseling centers, health services centers, private mental health organizations, and religious support services are just a few of the possible services in your area.

Major Depressive Disorder

Major depressive disorder symptoms are marked by a depressed mood and loss of interest or pleasure. The depressed mood is present for most of the day, with feelings of sadness or emptiness nearly every day, as indicated by self-report or by others' observations. The person exhibits a marked loss of interest and pleasure in life's activities most of the day, nearly every day. This may be accompanied by significant weight loss or weight gain (a change of more than 5 percent in 1 month). Another sign may be **insomnia** or **hypersomnia** (sleeping too much). The person may be either hyperactive or lethargic to the extreme, accompanied by feelings and expressions of worthlessness or guilt. Diminished ability to think or concentrate, and indecisiveness, is common. Recurring thoughts of death and suicide pose a serious problem in the school-age population.

Dysrythmic Disorder

Dysrythmic disorder is the preferred name for the condition better known as neurotic depression. It occurs in about 3 percent of the general population, according to the American Psychiatric Association. Individuals with this disorder describe their mood as sad or "down in the dumps." A child's mood may be irritable rather than depressed. This condition differs from major depressive disorder mainly in the severity of symptoms. It is more chronic than acute, and the person may function at a somewhat higher level.

Anxiety Disorders

School-age children may have a variety of anxiety disorders. These include separation anxiety (most often in kindergarten students), panic attacks, acrophobia, social phobia, obsessive/compulsive disorder, post-traumatic stress disorder, and generalized anxiety disorder. When a teacher observes symptoms of anxiety or depression it is best to seek the consultation of school guidance counselors, psychologists, or supervisors for direction.

Separation Anxiety Disorder

Separation anxiety disorder is characterized by inappropriate and excessive anxiety when separated from a person to whom the child is emotionally attached. It is found in about 4 percent of children and young adolescents. Worrying excessively about leaving home or a significant adult, children may refuse to go to school. The child also may worry that some harm may come to the significant adult. On school days the child may complain of physical symptoms (nausea, stomach aches, headaches) in the form of tantrums, crying, or pleading with the parent not to leave. Separation anxiety disorder may develop after some life stress as, for example, the death of a relative or a pet, an illness of the child or a relative, a change in school, a move to a new neighborhood, and the like.[9]

Panic Attack

Panic attack is the sudden onset of intense apprehension, fearfulness, or terror often associated with feelings of impending doom. It is seen in adolescents (as well as adults), but not in younger children.

Agoraphobia

Agoraphobia is anxiety about or avoidance of places or situations from which escape may be difficult or embarrassing and from which help may be unavailable. It is seen in school-age children, as well as adults.

Social Phobia

Social phobia is brought about by exposure to certain social or performance situations, often leading to an avoidance of the situation, as in school phobia. In young children, anxiety from the social phobia may be expressed by crying, tantrums, "freezing," and clinging. Predisposing factors for children with this disorder may be events such as being locked in a closet or witnessing accidents.

Obsessive/Compulsive Disorder

Obsessive/compulsive disorder is characterized by obsessions that increase anxiety or distress, such as a child's recurring fear of being contaminated by germs or compulsive behavior such as repetitive hand-washing. It is most often experienced by children of substance abusing and abusive parents and also may be a symptom of sexual abuse.

Post-Traumatic Stress Disorder

Post-traumatic stress disorder is characterized by frequent re-experiencing of an extremely traumatic event, such as sexual or physical abuse, or witnessing or being injured in an accident. This disorder is accompanied by anxiety and depression and avoidance of stimuli associated with the trauma.

Avoidant Disorder

Avoidant disorder is identified by persistent and excessive shrinking from contact with strangers, constant desire for affection from family members or other significant persons, and avoiding others to the extent that it interferes with social functioning and peer relationships.

Attention Deficit/Hyperactivity Disorder

Attention deficit/hyperactivity disorder, or ADHD, is characterized by an ongoing pattern of inattention and/or hyperactivity and impulsivity. Whereas the behaviors are ongoing, they are not necessarily continuous but more likely episodic, with intensity and duration of episodes varying in different settings and in different children. The behaviors in children are usually more graphically displayed in school and/or home settings as opposed to the playground or athletic field.

Attention deficits in children can take the form of an inability to give attention to details or the making of careless mistakes with schoolwork, work, play, or other tasks. Additionally, children with this problem often seem to have a difficult time organizing, following through, and finishing tasks. Children may lose things or become distracted and forgetful. They often seem not to listen when spoken to, but rather their attention is diverted elsewhere.

Hyperactive children often can't seem to sit still in their seats. They may fidget or squirm, frequently attempt to leave the classroom, run around excessively (regardless of whether it is appropriate to the situation). They may talk excessively or blurt answers before the question is completed or another student is through responding. They may not wait their turn in lines or intrude into others' conversations or activities. They can be in constant motion and find it difficult to sit quietly.

Children may have either or both problems of attention deficit and hyperactivity disorder. Diagnosing a child as having both attention deficit and hyperactivity disorder is based on having at least six symptoms in each category. Children may have only one of these problems, in which case six symptoms would be found in only one of the categories, attention deficit or hyperactivity. Additionally, for the child to be diagnosed with this problem, the symptoms/behaviors must have been evident for at least six months, have started to occur before the child was 7 years old, and be inappropriate to the child's age (for example, a given behavior is inappropriate for 10-year-old but normal for a young toddler).

Developing Emotional Health: The Teacher's Role

Children spend 30 to 35 hours a week in school under the guidance and authority of teachers. Consequently, teachers have a unique opportunity to have a positive influence on the emotional and mental well-being of children. Ample evidence shows that children who are helped to develop good self-esteem stand a stronger chance of thriving as adults. Children do not develop self-esteem solely within the classroom, of course. Self-esteem is an extremely complex human dimension tied most tightly to the relationship between parent (or surrogate) and child. The parent/child relationship cannot be substituted for, or replicated, within a classroom environment; there it can only be supported and complemented. Accordingly, the classroom teacher can only help to enhance and build upon the self-esteem a child has developed in the home. This does not diminish the role of classroom teachers. Enhancing a child's self-worth is a major contribution to that child's well-being.

Children who have suffered neglect or abuse with obvious damage to their personality development are beyond the purview of the classroom teacher. These problems require psychotherapy for the child and the child's family. The child, however, can be helped by the teacher. These children need the extra attention, care, and guidance of healthy adults. People who have survived an emotionally or physically deprived childhood and have gone on to productive and satisfying adulthood usually can name a mentor or significant adult who made a difference in their lives. This mentor—whether a health educator, teacher, member of the clergy, relative, or friend—provided the emotional support and guidance that sent a message that the person mattered, that he or she had self-worth.

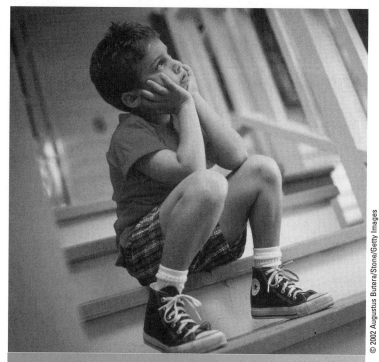

Reflecting on positive reinforcement builds self-esteem.

Summary

Mental health is intrinsic to overall health and to students' learning in school. Its opposite, mental illness, is defined as problems or disorders related to the psychological processes or organic functions of the brain. Personality attributes that contribute to mental health are autonomy, emotional separateness, meaning in life, self-worth, self-love, authenticity, self-consciousness, values, and social skills.

Among the relevant theories is Abraham Maslow's hierarchy of needs. At the bottom of his pyramid are the needs related to basic survival, then safety and security, followed by love and belonging, identity and self-esteem, and finally, self-actualization. These needs are met first by the parents, then the school, expanding eventually to the broader community.

Another theorist, Erik Erikson, proposed eight stages of human development and outlined the conflicts at each stage. Teachers are involved mainly with individuals in Stages III (initiative versus guilt), IV (industry versus inferiority), and Stage V (identity versus role confusion). These are preceded by stages in which the family has set the stage for trust versus mistrust and autonomy versus self-doubt—both of which the student carries into school.

To aid professionals in diagnosis and treatment, the American Psychiatric Association has developed criteria for identifying various forms of mental illness. Of most relevance to teachers and school personnel are the depressive mood disorders and anxiety disorders: separation anxiety, panic attack, agoraphobia, social phobia, obsessive/compulsive disorder, post-traumatic stress disorder, and avoidant disorder.

Although teachers usually are not the primary influences in children's lives, they can do much to foster mental health by affirming students' self-worth, giving praise for achievements, supporting universal values, and promoting social skills.

Resources and Web Sites

American Academy of Child and Adolescent Psychiatry. *Facts for Families: Helping Children After a Disaster* (Fact Sheet No. 36). Washington, DC: Author, 1998.

Copeland, E., and V. Love. *Attention Without Tension: A Teacher's Handbook on Attention Disorders*. Atlanta: 3 C's of Childhood, 1992.

Elias, M. J., J. E. Zins, R. P. Weissberg, K. S. Frey, M. T. Greenberg, N. M. Haynes, R. Kessler, M. E. Schwab-Stone, and T. P. Shriver. *Promoting Social and Emotional Learning: Guidelines for Educators.* Alexandria, VA: Association for Supervision and Curriculum Development, 1997.

Elias, M. J., S. E. Tobias, and B. S. Friedlander. *Emotionally Intelligent Parenting: How to Raise a Self-disciplined, Responsible, and Socially Skilled Child.* New York: Harmony Books, 1999.

Goleman, D. *Emotional Intelligence: Why It Can Matter More than IQ*. New York: Bantam Books, 1995.

Grover, P. L. *Preventing Substance Abuse Among Children And Adolescents: Family-Centered Approaches: Prevention Enhancement Protocols System Reference Guide*. Rockville, MD: Center for Substance Abuse Prevention, 1998.

Harris, K., and S. Graham. *Helping Young Writers Master the Craft*. Cambridge, MA: Brookline Books, 1992.

Johnson, D. *I Can't Sit Still—Educating and Affirming Inattentive and Hyperactive Children: Suggestions for Parents, Teachers, and Other Care Providers of Children to Age 10*. Santa Cruz, CA: ETR Associates, 1992.

LaGreca, A. M., E. M. Vernberg, W. K. Silverman, A. L. Vogel, and M. J. Prinstein. *Helping Children Prepare For and Cope with Natural Disaster: A Manual for Professionals Working with Elementary School Children*. Coral Gables, FL: The BellSouth Foundation and the University of Miami, 1994.

Markway, B.G., et al. *Dying of Embarrassment: Help for Social Anxiety and Phobias.* Oakland, CA: New Harbinger Publications, 1992.

Miller, Alice. *For Your Own Good: Hidden Cruelty in Child-Rearing and the Roots of Violence.* NY: Fassar, Straus & Giroux, 1992.

Monahon, C. *Children and Trauma: A Parent's Guide to Helping Children Heal.* New York: Lexington Books, 1993.

Parker, H. *The ADD Hyperactivity Handbook for Schools*. Plantation, FL: Impact Publications, 1992.

Rapoport, J. L. *The Boy Who Couldn't Stop Washing.* New York: E. P. Dutton, 1989.

Terr, L. *Too Scared to Cry: Psychic Trauma in Childhood*. New York: Harper & Row, 1990.

Strock, Margaret. *Plain Talk About Depression*. Information Resources and Inquiries Branch, Office of Communications and Public Liaison, National Institute of Mental Health (NIH Publication No. 00-3561), Rockville, MD: NMIH, 2001.

U. S. Dept. of Health and Human Services. *Children's and Adolescent's Mental Health.* Washington, DC: Government Printing Office, 2000.

The American Academy of Child and Adolescent Psychiatry
3615 Wisconsin Ave. NW,
Washington, DC 20016-3007
Tel: 202-966-7300; Fax: 202-966-2891
http://www.aacap.org

The American Academy of Pediatrics
141 Northwest Point Blvd.
Elk Grove Village, IL 60007-1098
847-434-4000; Fax: 847-434-8000
http://www.aap.org

American Association of Psychiatric Services for Children
Child Mental Health Division
440 First St. NW, 3rd floor
Washington, DC 20001-2085
Tel: 202-638-2952
http://www.cwla.org/default.html

American Foundation for Suicide Prevention
120 Wall St., 22nd Floor
New York, NY 10005
Tel: 888-333-AFSP (toll free) or 212-363-3500

American Orthopsychiatric Association
330 7th Ave., 18th Floor
New York, NY 10001
Tel: 212-564-5930
http://www.amerortho.org/

Anxiety Disorders Association of America
11900 Parklawn Dr., Suite 100
Rockville, MD 20852
Tel: 301-231-9350 or -9259
http://www.adaa.org

The Center for Child Health and Mental Health Policy
Georgetown University
Child Development Center
3307 M St. NW
Washington, DC 20007
Tel: 202-687-8635
http://gucdc.georgetown.edu

Center for the Prevention of School Violence
313 Chapanoke Rd.,
Suite 140
Raleigh, NC 27603
Tel: 800-299-6054
http://www.ncsu.edu/cpsv

Child and Adolescent Bipolar Foundation
Child & Adolescent Bipolar Foundation
1187 Wilmette Ave.
P. M. B. #331
Wilmette, IL 60091
www.bpkids.org

Children and Adults with Attention-Deficit/Hyperactivity Disorder (CHADD)
8181 Professional Pl., Suite 201
Landover, MD 20785
Tel: 800-233-4050 or 301-306-7070

The Collaborative for Academic, Social and Emotional Learning (CASEL)
Department of Psychology (MC 285)
University of Illinois at Chicago
1007 West Harrison St.
Chicago, IL 60607-7137
Tel: 312-413-1008
http://www.casel.org

Families for Depression Awareness
118 Waltham St., Second Floor
Watertown, MA 02472-4808
Tel: 617-924-9383

Federation of Families for Children's Mental Health
1021 Prince St.
Alexandria, VA 22314-2971
Tel: 703-684-7710
http://www.ffcmh.org

Join Together; Boston University School of Public Health
441 Stuart St.
Boston, MA 02116
Tel: 617-437-1500

Mental Health Net
www.cmhc.com

National Alliance for the Mentally Ill
Colonial Place Three
2107 Wilson Blvd., Suite 300
Arlington, VA 22201-3042
Tel: 703-524-7600 or 800-950-6264
http://www.nami.org

National Association of Anorexia Nervosa and Associated Disorders
P.O. Box 7
Highland Park, IL 60035
Tel: 847-831-3438
http://www.anad.org

National Association for Children of Alcoholics
11426 Rockville Pike, Suite 100
Rockville, MD 20852-3007
Tel: 301-468-0985
http://192.131.22.19/health/nhic/data/hr2000/hr2080.html

National Association of School Psychologists
4330 East West Highway
Suite 402
Bethesda, MD 20814
Tel: 301-657-0207; Fax: 301-657-0275
http://www.nasponline.org

National Clearinghouse on Child Abuse and Neglect Information
330 C Street SW
Washington, DC 20447
Tel: 800-394-3366
http://www.calib.com/cbexpress

National Information Center for Children and Youth with Disabilities
P.O. Box 1492
Washington, DC 20013-1492
Tel: 800-695-0285 (V/TTY)
or 202-884-8200 (V/TTY)
www.nichcy.org

National Institute of Mental Health
5600 Fishers Lane, Room 7C-02
MSC 8030
Rockville, MD 20892-8030
Tel: 301-443-3675 or -4513
http://www.nimh.nih.gov

National Association of Psychiatric Treatment Centers for Children
1025 Connecticut Ave. NW, Suite 1012
Washington, DC 20036
Tel: 202-857-9735

School Social Worker Association of America
P.O. Box 2072
Northlake, IL 60164
Tel: 847-289-4527

Substance Abuse and Mental Health Services Administration (SAMHSA); Center for Mental Health Services (CMHS)
5600 Fishers Lane
Rockville, MD 20857
Tel: 301-443-0001; Fax: 301-443-1563

University of California Los Angeles/ Center for Mental Health in Schools; School Mental Health Project
Department of Psychology
P.O. Box 951563
Los Angeles, CA 90095-1563
Tel: 310-825-3634

Notes

1. R. H. Rosenman, "The Role of Behavior Patterns and Neurogenic Factors in Pathogenesis of Coronary Heart Disease," chap. 5 in *Stress and the Heart,* ed. R. S. Eliot (New York: Futurea, 1974); D. A. McKay, R. L. Blake, and J. M. Colwill, "Social Support and Stress as Predictors of Illness" *Journal of Family Practice* 20 (1985): 575–581.
2. A. Maslow, *Toward a Psychology of Being,* 2d ed. (Princeton, NJ: Van Nostrand Reinhold, 1968).
3. E. K. Erikson, *Identity and the Life Cycle* (London: W. W. Norton, 1994).
4. I. D. Yalom, *Existential Psychotherapy* (New York: Basic Books, 1980).
5. R. H. Jahoda, "Toward a Social Psychology of Mental Health," in *Symposium on the Healthy Personality. Supplement II. Problems of Infancy and Childhood,* ed. J. E. Senn (New York: Josiah Macy, Jr. Foundation, 1950).
6. See note 5.
7. *Diagnostic and Statistical Manual,* 4th ed. (Washington, DC: American Psychiatric Association, 1994).
8. See note 7.
9. C. G. Last, "Anxiety Disorders in Children," in *Internalizing Disorders in Children and Adolescents,* ed. W. M. Reynolds (New York: John Wiley and Sons, 1992).
10. See note 3.

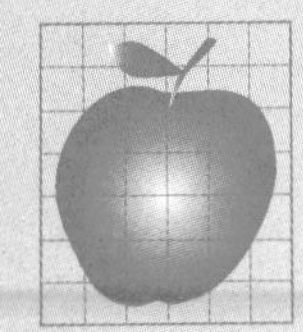

Learning Experiences

Activities can promote emotional health by enhancing children's social skills and self-concept. Activities that give students messages that they are good or special without connecting this to mastery of a skill or accomplishment of a project or task will not build self-esteem; such activities become cheerleading sessions or pep rallies. Self-esteem can be enhanced only by helping children to recognize their unique attributes, perceptions, and feelings; reinforce the development of values; learn social skills; develop and experience their autonomy, separateness, and self-control; and develop awareness, knowledge, skills, and abilities by completing actual educational tasks.

The teacher might view the activities presented here as templates or starting points for the teacher's further development of emotional health–promoting activities. In developing activities for classes, the teacher should keep in mind the observations of Erik Erikson.

The growing child must, at the very least, derive a vitalizing sense of reality from the awareness that her or his individual way of mastering experience is a successful variant of the way other people master experience and recognize such mastery. In this, children cannot be fooled by empty praise and condescending encouragement. They may have to accept artificial bolstering of their self-esteem in lieu of something better, but what I call their accruing ego identity gains real strength only from wholehearted and consistent recognition of real accomplishment—that is, achievement that has meaning in their culture.[10]

Emotional health will be enhanced in the classroom through the teacher's awareness of the child's emotional needs and the teacher's recognition, support, and encouragement of each child's unique abilities and successes as applied to actual learning and development of skills.

For suggestions on creating a rubric with which to evaluate student performance of Learning Experiences, see page 13.

Learning Experience 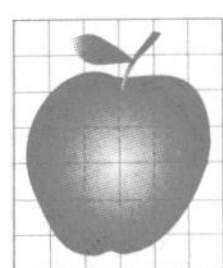 6-1

The Me Poster

Grade Level

K–2

Primary Discipline

Art

Learning Objectives

Following this activity, students should be able to

- List their interests.
- State their feelings.
- Describe people, places, or things that have meaning for them.

Time Required

Two 1-hour sessions

Materials

Posterboard or drawing paper, scissors, glue, magazines, family photographs

Description of Activity

Have each child make a poster using pictures cut from magazines, personal pictures, and their own drawings. The pictures should show people, places, or things that are important to the child; people, places, or things that the child likes or makes him/her happy, sad, glad, angry, and so on.

When the posters are completed, ask the children to describe their poster and to share what they like; what makes them happy, glad, sad, and so on; what are important people, places, and things in the poster; and why they are important.

Homework

None

Evaluation

Grade Levels K–1

(a) Students will identify pictures in the poster that are important to the student.

Excellent	Good	Fair	Poor
3 pictures	2 pictures	1 picture	0 pictures

(b) Students will identify the feelings they have in relation to the pictures in the poster.

Excellent	Good	Fair	Poor
3 feelings	2 feelings	1 feeling	0 feelings

Grade Level 2

(a) Students will identify pictures in the poster that are important to the student.

Excellent	Good	Fair	Poor
3 pictures	2 pictures	1 picture	0 pictures

(b) Students will identify why the pictures in the poster are important to them.

Excellent	Good	Fair	Poor
Closely	Loosely	Vaguely	Cannot identify

(c) Students will identify the feelings they have in relation to the pictures in the poster.

Excellent	Good	Fair	Poor
3 feelings	2 feelings	1 feeling	0 feelings

Learning Experience 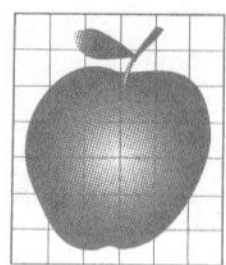 6-2

The Me Box

Grade Level

3–4

Primary Discipline

Art

Learning Objectives

Following this activity, students will be able to describe their own identity, meaning, feelings, creativity, mastery, and responsibility.

Time Required

Three 1-hour sessions

Materials

Shoebox, magazines, small photographs, pictures, and other mementos or objects that can fit inside shoebox, crayons, drawing paper

Description of Activity

Ask each student to design the inside of a shoebox so it represents themselves in terms of their identity; the things they care about; the things that they love or that make them sad, happy, glad, or angry. The designs will be created from pictures from magazines, photographs, mementos, and the students' own drawings.

Homework

Students will collect objects for the Me Box that they feel are representative of their identity. These objects may be clipped photos or pictures from newspapers or magazines, as well as *borrowed* family photos or mementos. In addition, students should be required to do at least one small identity drawing for the box.

Evaluation

(a) Students will be able to identify feelings from the objects in the box.

Excellent	Good	Fair	Poor
5 feelings	3 feelings	2 feelings	1 feeling

(b) Students will be able to describe reasons why the represented objects in the box are important to them.

Excellent	Good	Fair	Poor
3 reasons	2 reasons	1 reason	0 reasons

Learning Experience 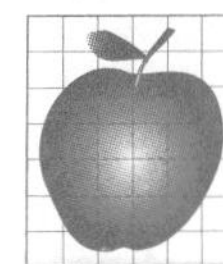 6-3

The Story's Lesson

Grade Level

3–4

Primary Discipline

Reading

Learning Objectives

Following this activity, students will be able to

- Identify emotions.
- Describe their values.

Time Required

1/2 hour to 1 hour

Materials

Story from *The Children's Book of Virtues* (William Bennett, New York: Simon & Schuster, 1993), *Aesop's Fables*, or other books with moral lessons at appropriate reading levels

Description of Activity

Have students take turns reading to the class. At the end of the story, ask the students to identify and discuss the emotions they have in relation to characters in the story and the story itself. Students will try to identify the moral lessons in the story.

Homework

None

Evaluation

(a) Students will be able to identify emotions and be able to discuss emotions as they are related to the story.

Excellent	Good	Fair	Poor
3 emotions	2 emotions	1 emotion	0 emotions

(b) Students will be able to identify and be able to discuss moral lessons from the story.

Excellent	Good	Fair	Poor
3 lessons	2 lessons	1 lesson	0 lessons

Learning Experience 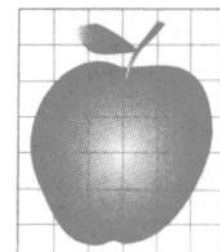 6-4

Storytelling Picture Game

Grade Level

K–2

Primary Disciplines

Language Arts

Learning Objectives

Following this activity, students should be able to

- Differentiate feelings of sadness, anger, happiness, fear.
- Express feelings.
- Appropriately express feelings of anger.

Time Required

1-hour sessions (each session emphasizing a different emotion)

Materials

Magazines, posters, posterboard, glue, scissors

Description of Activity

Cut out large pictures of people's faces from magazines, posters, and other sources; paste each picture on a separate sheet of posterboard, creating an individual poster. Each face should have an expression representing a different emotion: happy, sad, glad, angry, and so on. Have each child make up a story about the person in the poster, including an explanation of why the person in the poster is feeling the way he or she appears. Ask each child to share his or her story with the class.

If a picture is of a sad person, ask the class for suggestions on how they might help that person. The children can also be asked about the times they feel sad and how they can express their own sadness. If a picture is of an angry person, ask the class how they can respond to this person and how they can act when they get angry. Allow time for the children to describe times when they felt happy or good, and support this activity with assurances and suggestions on appropriate ways to express sadness and anger.

Homework

None

Evaluation

Students will be able to create an explanation of the emotion they identified in the photo.

Excellent	Good	Fair	Poor
Clearly	Loosely	Vaguely	Not defined

Learning Experience 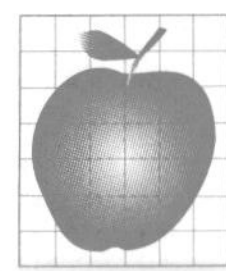 6-5

What Is The Moral of the Story?

Grade Level

3–6

Primary Disciplines

Language Arts: Writing, Drama

Learning Objectives

Following this activity, students should be able to

- Differentiate the values of respect, responsibility, freedom, helpfulness, and honesty.
- Work in teams.
- Demonstrate leadership qualities.

Time Required

Grades 1–3

10 minutes creating the play, 5 minutes acting for each group, 5 minute follow-up discussion for each play.

Grades 4–6

30 minutes writing the play, 10 minutes acting for each group, 10 minute follow-up discussion for each play.

Materials

Large sheet of paper for writing the play

Description of Activity

1. Divide the class into small groups.
2. Ask each group to develop a short play with a moral lesson (honesty, cheating, stealing, responsibility, helping, freedom, and so on). Allow each group time to work on their play.

In grades 4 through 6, have each group write out its play and then assign roles to each student in the small group. Have each small group choose one of its members as a recorder or a team leader, who will write the play on a large sheet of paper so all group members can see it.

After the play has been presented, ask the students what moral lessons they can learn from the play. Have the students describe any experiences they have had like those in the play and what they learned from their experiences. Support this discussion by encouraging responses from the students and by making his/her own observations and suggestions on values.

Homework

None

Evaluation

(a) Students are able to identify moral lessons from the activity.

Excellent	Good	Fair	Poor
3 lessons	2 lessons	1 lesson	0 lessons

(b) Students are able to identify experiences they have had that are similar to the experiences presented in the play.

Excellent	Good	Fair	Poor
3 lessons	2 lessons	1 lesson	0 lessons

(c) Students are able to identify what moral lessons they learned from their own experiences.

Excellent	Good	Fair	Poor
3 lessons	2 lessons	1 lesson	0 lessons

Learning Experience 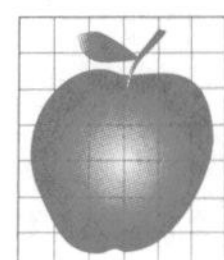 6-6

Storytelling

Grade Level

K–6

Primary Disciplines

History, Biography, Literature

Learning Objectives

Following this activity, students should be able to

- Identify and describe the values of caring, loyalty, honesty, and responsibility.
- Work as part of a team.
- Explain the concept of uniqueness or individuality.

Time Required

15 minutes to 1 hour, depending on grade level

Materials

The Children's Book of Virtues (William Bennett New York: Simon & Schuster, 1993) or other book with moral lessons.

Description of Activity

Storytelling is one of the oldest teaching methods. You can either read a story or tell a story from memory. It can be a story of fiction, history, or biography. It should present an ethical or moral dilemma or human struggle. After reading or telling the story, bring up values, human struggles, and challenges the story raised. Ask the students to describe any similar experiences and the values attached to those experiences.

Homework

None

Evaluation

(a) Students are able to identify experiences from their own lives that are similar to those experiences presented the story.

Excellent	Good	Fair	Poor
Clearly	Loosely	Vaguely	Cannot define

(b) Students are able to identify values in relation to their own experiences that are similar to those in the story.

Excellent	Good	Fair	Poor
3 values	2 values	1 value	0 values

Learning Experience 6-7

Affirmations

Grade Level

5–6

Primary Disciplines

Language Arts: Writing

Learning Objectives

Following this activity, students should be able to

- Describe their self-worth and the worth of others.
- Recognize the uniqueness of themselves and others through the contributions they make.

Time Required

1/2 to 1 hour

Materials

Paper and pen

Description of Activity

Have each student write a brief essay on a contribution he/she makes in school, at home, or in the community. The contribution may be cleaning up at home, doing dishes, cleaning the classroom board, being an altar boy or girl, taking care of a pet, helping a friend with schoolwork, and so on. Lend your support to each student in finding what contribution the child has made. Students who are particularly shy or have a difficult time being accepted by other children may need extra help in discovering this part of themselves. Ask students to read their report in class.

Homework

None

Evaluation

The student is able to clearly define, in his or her essay, the contributions he or she makes in school, at home, or in the community.

Excellent	Good	Fair	Poor
Clearly	Loosely	Vaguely	Cannot define

Source: T. Lickona, *Educating for Character: How Our Schools Can Teach Respect and Responsibility* (Bantam Books, a division of Bantam, Doubleday, Dell Publishing Group, Inc., 1992). Reprinted with permission.

Learning Experience 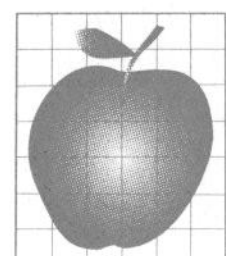 6-8

Caring for Needs, Part 1

Grade Level

K–3

Primary Discipline

Biology

Learning Objectives

Following this activity, students should be able to

- Express concern for something.
- Demonstrate that they value respect and responsibility.

Time Required

5 to 10 minutes a day of plant care plus three 45-minute discussions

Materials

Houseplants, planters or pots, watering cans, plant food, shelving paper

Description of Activity

Introduction

Begin this activity with a discussion about the needs of living things. This can be related to having one's own needs met.

Activity

Give each child a cutting of a house plant. The child is responsible for potting the cutting and caring for the plant throughout the school year: watering it, giving it plant food, and so on. Students are given their plants to take home at the end of the school year.

Homework

Students might be asked to bring a plant cutting or other materials from home.

Evaluation

Students care for their individual plants on a daily basis.

Excellent	Good	Fair	Poor
Every weekday	4 days per week	2 or 3 days per week	0 or 1 day per week

Learning Experience 6-9

Caring for Needs, Part 2

Grade Level

4–6

Primary Disciplines

Biology, Writing

Learning Objectives

Following this activity, students should be able to

- Identify the needs of other living things.
- Demonstrate that they value respect and responsibility.
- Cooperate.

Time Required

10 minutes a day, 45-minute initial discussion, 15-minute group or individual presentations

Materials

One or more fish tanks and corresponding equipment, tropical fish, fish food; cages, cage feeders, cage liner, animal food, Guinea pigs, hamsters, or birds; poster board, crayons

Description of Activity

Divide the class into small groups and give each group one animal or fish tank to care for throughout the school year. Assign a task to each child in each group for care of the animal or fish. Tasks are rotated every month. For each group draw a check-off grid on poster board, listing each child and his or her assigned task. Each group is assigned a new leader each month. Under close supervision, the leader makes sure each task is completed daily and checks off the completed task on the grid.

Three separate discussions are held:

1. At the beginning of the project, introduce a discussion about the needs of living things and what these needs are (food, shelter, water, comfort, affection, and so on) and the importance of having those needs fulfilled. Students are asked to identify their own needs and how they are met. Students then are made aware of the importance of not only being cared for but also caring for others.
2. Discuss expressing needs in an appropriate manner and on coping with unmet needs.
3. This activity emphasizes the importance of cooperation and teamwork; make the connection with the small groups caring for the animals.

Homework

Assign each student a book to read about the animal or fish he or she is caring for; have students write a report on their books.

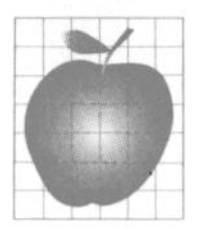

Learning Experience 6-9 continued

Evaluation

Grade Levels 4–5

(a) Students carry out their assigned tasks on a daily basis.

Excellent	Good	Fair	Poor
Every day	4 days	2 or 3 days	0 or 1 day

(b) Students are able to identify the needs of living things.

Excellent	Good	Fair	Poor
3 needs	2 needs	1 need	0 needs

(c) Students are able to identify appropriate ways to express needs.

Excellent	Good	Fair	Poor
3 ways	2 ways	1 way	0 ways

(d) Students are able to identify ways to cope with unmet needs.

Excellent	Good	Fair	Poor
3 ways	2 ways	1 way	0 ways

Grade Level 6

(a) Students carry out their assigned tasks on a daily basis.

Excellent	Good	Fair	Poor
Every day	4 days	2 or 3 days	0 or 1 day

(b) Students are able to identify the needs of living things.

Excellent	Good	Fair	Poor
4 needs	3 needs	2 needs	0 or 1 needs

(c) Students are able to identify appropriate ways to express needs.

Excellent	Good	Fair	Poor
4 ways	3 ways	2 ways	0 or 1 way

(d) Students are able to identify ways to cope with unmet needs.

Excellent	Good	Fair	Poor
4 ways	3 ways	2 ways	0 or 1 way

7

Sexual Health, Family Life, and Relationships

Estelle Weinstein

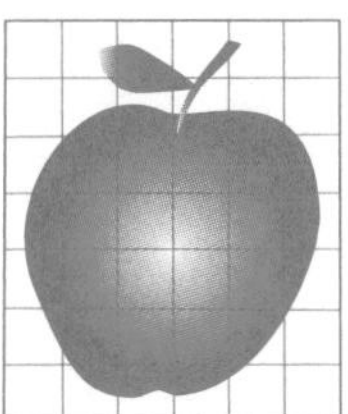

Chapter Outline

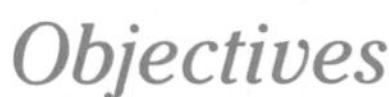

Objectives

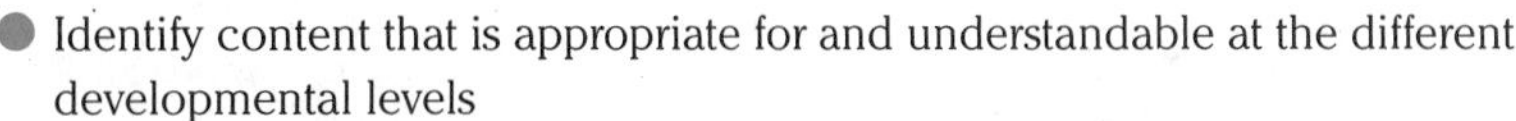

- Identify content that is appropriate for and understandable at the different developmental levels
- Begin a gender-neutral dialogue on sexuality and sexual orientation and introduce the concept of self-exploration
- Identify appropriate terms and definitions for sexuality and anatomical parts
- Promote a healthy body image and respect for self to give students a foundation for decision-making regarding their sexual behavior and protecting their health
- Integrate discussions of feelings and emotions with the physiological aspects of sexuality
- Describe the progression of relationships beginning with the family, extending to friendships, and progressing to dating and choosing a mate
- Describe the interaction between love and sex; delineate the types of love and intimacy
- Explain the relationship issues of boundaries, jealousy, and ending a relationship, including separation and divorce
- Identify bodily changes during puberty
- Explain the basic physical processes of menstruation, sexual response, pregnancy, and childbirth
- Describe sexually transmitted diseases, with emphasis on HIV/AIDS prevention and transmission and on acceptance of people who have AIDS
- Expand knowledge about different family configurations, family roles and responsibilities, and cultural/religious influences on sexuality

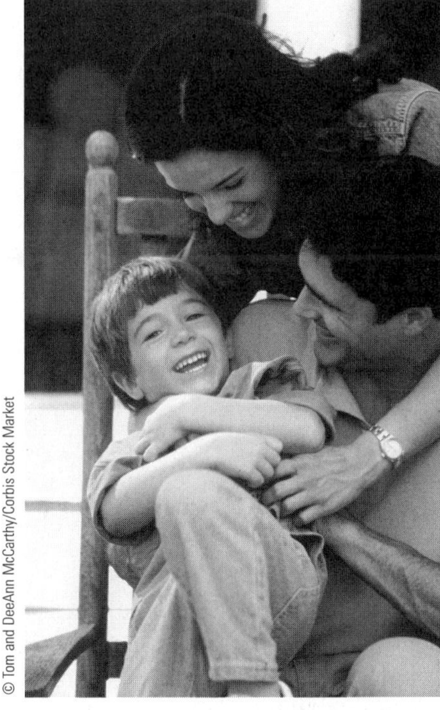

A school district in the suburbs of upstate New York that had believed its safe little community was far enough from "the big city" to protect its students from the problems of nearby communities has recently acknowledged that "times have changed." This started 10 years ago with the first unmarried teenager, pregnant during her sophomore year in high school and not wanting to drop out of school. Her family fought hard to keep her in school to ensure that she did not lose her chance for a better life. The school district lost the court case to expel her, and the pregnant teen completed her education during her pregnancy and returned after the baby was born. The district knew about other pregnant teens, but they usually disappeared for a while, if not permanently.

• • •

About 5 years ago, one high-school girl accused some of the school "jocks" of attempted rape, which she said happened after a school football party. Since then, rumors about other assaults have emerged. To add to the district's problems, several high school students were openly accused of being gay. The district's position had been that "sexual preference" is not its business and is not an issue that deserves attention.

• • •

In the past few years the community has had to deal with a family that returned "home" from the "big city" because one of the children had been diagnosed with AIDS. The state mandates that HIV/AIDS education occur in every district K–12, but there is room for local interpretation of how this mandate would be achieved. The local school board decided that the district should do its part in educating children K–12 against the growing sexuality-related problems of its students. Classroom teachers would have to indicate where, in their curriculum, they have incorporated topics associated with human sexuality, family life, and HIV/AIDS.

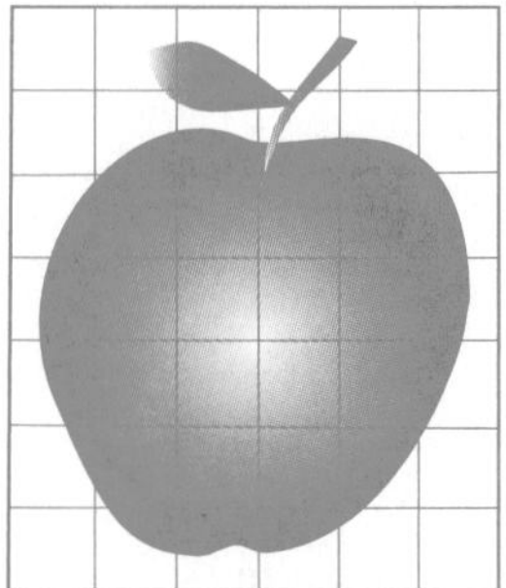

What is appropriate to teach in elementary school? If the above scenarios were to happen in your school district, how would they affect your curriculum? Is the elementary school level appropriate to prepare students for these experiences? What are the children in your elementary school thinking about that relates to sex and AIDS, and what kinds of questions might they begin to ask at this level?

Imagine for a moment that your school is asking you to include information about human sexuality in your curriculum beginning this semester. Some teachers feel this is a reasonable request, because they see this subject as an integral and healthy part of their life's experiences and, therefore, support its place in an educational setting. For others, the subject is ridden with values and morals and belongs exclusively within the educational purview of parents and religious institutions. For still others, regardless of their opinion about the mandate, the mere thought of being required to teach about human sexuality sends them into a dither. Whichever category one falls into, most classroom teachers have had no professional education and brief, if any, in-service training with which to execute such a mandate.

The social and health problems—teen pregnancy, STDs including AIDS, date rape, and more—associated with sexuality and with separating or divorcing families do not seem to be waning. By including aspects of human sexuality and family life education in their curricula, school districts can participate with families and communities in providing students with information and resources for enriching their lives and avoiding problems. The combination of sexuality and family life education "brings together knowledge about individuals as sexual beings and as family members and addresses the relationships between the family and the rest of a society's institutions."[1]

Thus, this chapter is aimed at providing classroom teachers with enough information to determine which areas are appropriate for inclusion in their curriculum and which should be left to "the specialists." Moreover, the information presented here is intended to help teachers become more comfortable with the philosophy of sexuality and family life education.

Teachers could begin an educational dialogue with their students about sexuality early in their students' psychosexual development. The dialogue can help students begin to see their sexuality as a healthy, normal part of their personality and lifestyle, and their sexual behaviors as choices that emerge from their personal values, attitudes, and decisions. Moreover, when sexuality and family life education are integrated into K–12 school curricula within interdisciplinary contexts (science, art, literature, and so on), it resembles the way people experience their sexuality in the many facets of their lives.

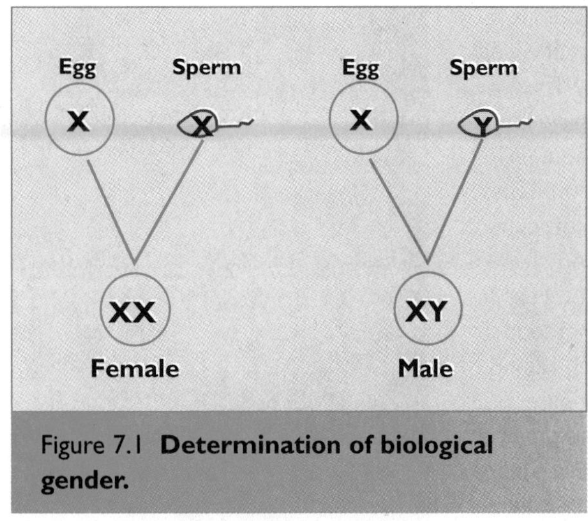

Figure 7.1 **Determination of biological gender.**

Sexuality and family life are part of life even before birth. Boys have erections and girls' vaginas lubricate within the first days of life. Infants explore their bodies, including their genitals, and derive pleasure from that exploration without thinking that something is wrong with it. They derive pleasure from sucking at their mother's breast.

At home, children are bombarded by the media and the actions of family members, friends, and religious leaders with powerful sociocultural and religious messages that overtly or covertly teach about human sexuality and family life. Sexuality education also occurs each and every day in every classroom. The way teachers relate interpersonally, the way they dress, the examples they portray from their personal lives when teaching, and how they express gender-related messages are some of these influential learning experiences.

Definitions

Frequently, the words used in this subject area are slang or they have vague or clinical meanings that produce mixed messages. The following definitions attempt to provide a clear understanding about the ideas being transmitted in this chapter.

In today's language, sex refers to all types of genital behaviors including sexual intercourse, intimacy, and eroticism. **Gender** refers to the biological state of being male or female. Biological gender is determined by inherited factors identified by an X (female) or Y (male) chromosome (see Figure 7.1) and anatomical structures that differentiate females from males (for example, penis, vagina). Gender is assigned at birth by visualizing the genitalia or before birth through **amniocentesis** or fetal sonography (**ultrasound** testing). It is supported later by hormonal secretions that determine the gender-specific anatomical and physiological changes and body shapes.

In contrast, **gender identity**, sometimes called "sexual identity," refers to a person's conviction about being male or female. It includes personal notions about masculinity and femininity. Gender identity is usually established as early as 2 or 3 years of age.[2]

Gender role refers to culturally established norms that determine what roles males and females play. These socially differentiated roles have implications for relationship boundaries, career expectations, and so forth. They begin at birth and continue throughout life. To identify gender roles one has to think of the different behavioral expectations associated with motherhood and fatherhood, or wife and husband.

Gender role stereotypes are behaviors, characteristics, and nuances ascribed to men and women regardless of whether they actually possess them. In most cases they are not inherent in gender identity but, rather, are part of a socialization process. For example, men are said to be less emotional than women. Actually, men do not have fewer emotions than women, but they generally have been socialized to express them less overtly, whereas women generally have been socialized to express emotions overtly. Gender role stereotyping would proclaim women to be exclusive nurturers and men to be exclusive protectors, or wives to be caregivers and husbands to be breadwinners, for example.

Sexuality is the aspect of one's total sense of self that relates to attitudes, values, feelings, and beliefs about gender, body image, expressions of intimacy, love, affection, fears, fantasies, and decisions about sexual behaviors. It also encompasses an understanding of the spiritual, cultural, religious, and personal influences that affect all interpersonal relationships.

Sexual orientation describes an individual's gender-specific interests for participating in sexual activity. These interests in potential partners may be for someone of the same biological gender (these are labeled **homosexual** or **gay/lesbian**), the opposite gender (**heterosexual**), or either gender (**bisexual**). Some researchers are not comfortable with the limitation of sexual activities as the definitions of these terms and prefer a broader notion of homoeroticism or heteroeroticism, which they believe describes the breadth of an "intimate emotional and sexual relationship" with people of the same or opposite gender.[3] It is not yet clear what biological or social forces operate to determine an individual's sexual orientation. Formerly classified as illnesses, orientations are no longer categorized as emotional illness or pathological deviation from "normal" but, rather, simply as differences in the range of human sexual expression.

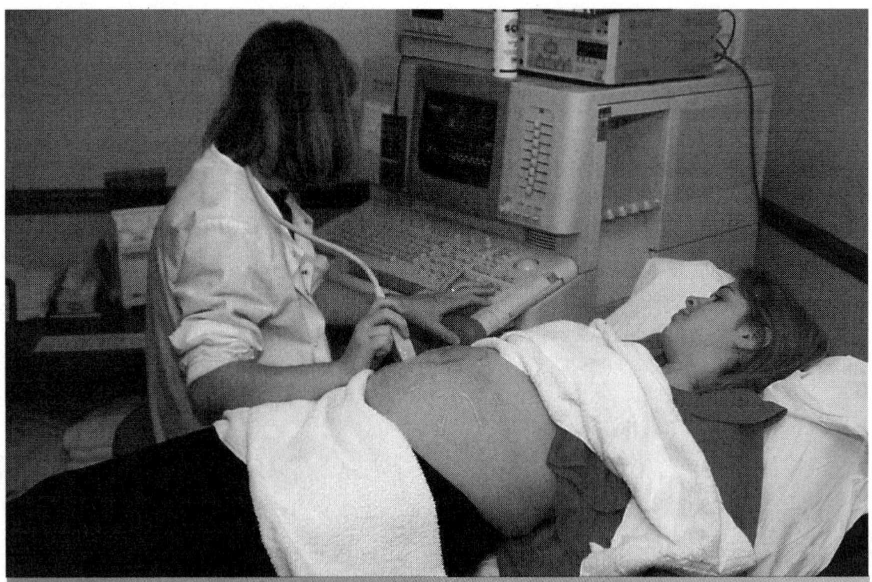

John Crawley

Ultrasound testing can show position of the baby, any abnormalities, and often the gender.

Sexuality education is "the formalization of sexual learning within an educational program, which must explore the biological, emotional, social, spiritual and intellectual variables" that compose the total person.[4] This includes learning about gender identity; family, gender, and social roles; genital and other sexual expressions; sensuality and eroticism; affection, love, intimacy, body image, and relationships. The breadth of experiences, decisions, risks, and of overt and covert messages all contribute to learning about sexuality.

Family life education is learning about the family, including types of families, patterns of partner selection, family love, intimacy, roles and boundaries; dating and courtship styles; marriage and parenthood options; living styles; and separation or divorce.

Why Teach About Human Sexuality and Family Life?

If human sexuality is a "normal" and ongoing part of life, why does education about it create so much conflict? Probably because it is misinterpreted and misunderstood in its parameters, its intent, and even its definitions. It is often thought of as "how-to" education about sexual acts not connected to human expression, human need, or everyday existence. Moreover, some see sex education as indoctrinating values that will undermine the values of the family. Sexuality education is a learning process that can help people become more comfortable with themselves and each other and also mitigate some of the associated problems in people's daily lives that ultimately influence society, including the following:

1. Early sexually intimate behaviors that contribute to the prevalence of STDs/AIDS and teen pregnancy are also associated with a decrease in the ability to sustain meaningful, serious, permanent relationships. Students often exist in an environment of misinformation, poor self-esteem, discomfort with their developing body, mixed messages about appropriate behavior, and a general lack of acceptance of their own sexuality as a natural and healthy part of relationships and life. Providing information that focuses on positive attitudes and encourages developmentally appropriate sexual behaviors—beginning in early childhood and continuing throughout the child's development—contributes to solutions to the problems.
2. The gender gap between men and women persists: Power, control, and respect issues continue to invade relationships, the seeds of which begin in early childhood. The school program can dispel myths and misconceptions about gender differences and counteract the negative messages about gender and sexual behavior that appear in the media—especially television and music videos.
3. The many different family living styles and cultural beliefs existing today can lead to misunderstandings and prejudice. The school setting is an ideal place to develop tolerance for the wide range of family constellations and customs. Teachers can include a cultural and linguistic sensitivity toward and relevancy about these topics in their curriculum.

Learning about sexual and reproductive anatomy and physiology will help students develop a healthy body image, accept their sexual selves throughout the life cycle, and optimize their sexual and reproductive health.

The following overview of human sexuality and family life lends itself to the learning of elementary-school students. These topics lay a foundation for later, more in-depth, developmentally appropriate inquiry in the middle and senior high schools.

Learning About Gender

Every few years we hear about another study that attempts to document physiological or anatomical differences in brain development between genders. Although some studies have successfully documented differences, the relationship between these differences and the behavioral differences between males and females is not clear.[5] A mixture of social, biological, and environmental forces, in some combination, account for differences between the genders, but they do not provide all possible boundaries and defined outcomes. Teaching about gender development should not restrict or determine any individual's behavior or choices but, rather, should open the field of possibilities and understanding for young people to find their own human potential with the utmost respect for each other, regardless of gender.

Learning About Gender in the Family

Before a child is born, people speculate about the child's gender. At birth, the first thing that is communicated is whether the new baby is a boy or a girl. From that moment on, the process of social scripting and socialization around that gender is mobilized, from the gifts for the baby to religious and ethnocultural ceremonies. Some research suggests that nurses, doctors, and parents handle babies in blue blankets different from babies in pink blankets. Later, toys and games that children are encouraged to play with and expectations about their behaviors begin to mold their notions of themselves and their gender. The messages that confirm their understanding of their gender also include things such as dress (rugged versus frilly), assigned chores (taking out the garbage versus washing the dishes), and the general demeanor expected (tough for boys, gentle and sweet for girls).

The roles and behaviors exhibited by significant adults reinforce children's sense of masculinity or femininity. The jobs the adults hold, the tasks they perform at home, and who handles money and other decisions in the family often deliver gender messages. These influence the way children see others of the same or opposite gender and what is expected of them. When they play, one can observe them replicating their family's and teachers' experiences.

In families that ascribe to traditional gender-specific behaviors, male children are likely to be encouraged to be independent, aggressive, and tough and to limit their expression of emotions such as fear and sadness. Female children are encouraged to be dependent, sensitive, and gentle. Crying is acceptable in females. Other families seek more gender-neutral development for their children.

Religious and Cultural Messages About Gender

Each society has different culturally defined views and customs. What may be acceptable or expected behavior in one culture is often unacceptable or different in another. Because the United States has such a variety of cultures, a school child may be exposed to many different conceptualizations of gender roles. This is particularly noticeable among recent immigrants who find themselves immersed in several cultures different from their own. Classroom opportunities for children to share their cultural customs and beliefs regarding gender will encourage understanding of options and alternative ways of behaving.

Learning About Gender in School

The classroom teacher's role is not to systematically counteract the family's religious or cultural messages, whether they are traditional or gender-neutral but, rather, to create an environment wherein children learn about options and alternatives. Teachers should be sensitive to their own gender-stereotypical attitudes and behaviors. A curriculum that exposes students to gender-neutral options promotes independent thinking and attitudes.

Physiological Differences

A newborn with a penis and scrotum is labeled "boy," and one with a vulva is labeled "girl." The **vulva** appears in female infants as two rounded outer folds or lips (labia major) that have within them a thinner set of folds (labia minor), a **clitoris**, and the separate openings to the urethra and the vagina. As physical development continues and puberty nears, the bodies of boys and girls begin to differentiate further. The genitalia of males and females are illustrated in Chapter 2.

Puberty

Puberty is a time of rapid physical changes and psychosexual adjustments that move children rather quickly toward adulthood. Physical maturity may come earlier than emotional maturity. The greatest physical changes that actually prepare both the male and female body for sexual activity and childbearing begin around 9 to 12 years of age and continue until all of the **secondary sex characteristics** are fully developed. This process can take somewhere between 5 and 8 years.

The onset of puberty can be confusing to children who have not been prepared for it. Unexplained changes create doubts that raise the question, "Am I normal?" Some children experience changes earlier than their closest peers; others, much later. These individual differences, at a time when "sameness" and acceptance by friends seems necessary to happiness, are often stressful to students (see Chapter 8). In healthy and physically normal development, children will reach their full growth based on individually inherited factors, internal signals, diet, and health status (see Chapter 2).

The onset of puberty results from a signal by the hypothalamus acting on the pituitary gland to start the production of genital hormones. These hormones—**estrogen** in females and testosterone in males—are in part responsible for growth of the genitals and the secondary sex characteristics that further differentiate boys and girls.

The genitals are the organs responsible for reproduction and, in combination with other parts of the body (known as **erogenous zones**) are also the sources of sexual pleasure. The pleasure center in the hypothalamus of the brain is stimulated when one desires, feels, experiences, or even thinks about sexual activity. During puberty children usually begin to experience and understand these sexually pleasurable thoughts and feelings and recognize them as such. Without these feelings, people would probably not search for a mate they find sexually attractive or one with whom they can ultimately reproduce and continue the human race.

Puberty in Females

Puberty generally begins with an increase in body fat that rounds out the body. At this time a girl first notices the growth of her breasts. Sometimes this change is not symmetrical: At first one breast feels like a bump, and the other feels flat.

Along with continued breast development, the secondary sex characteristics begin to develop. A young woman notices the beginning of hair growth under her arms and in a triangular shape around her external pelvic area. Other changes are in body shape and size, including the widening of her hips, giving the waist a narrower appearance, a fairly rapid growth in height, and the development of soft hair on her arms and legs.

The external genitalia continue to grow and develop throughout puberty, readying the female body for sexual activity and reproduction. The vulva, especially the clitoris and lower third of the vagina, which have nerve endings connected to the pleasure center of the brain, become more sensitive to sexual stimulation. The vagina, a barrel of muscle tissue that is able to expand and contract, also continues to develop and secretes lubrication upon sexual arousal. When the vagina is relaxed, it is only about 3 to 4 inches in depth; when it expands, it can become large enough to comfortably contain an erect penis and allow a newborn baby to pass through it.

Just inside the vagina is the **hymen**, a small membrane that has historical and sometimes religious roots as the

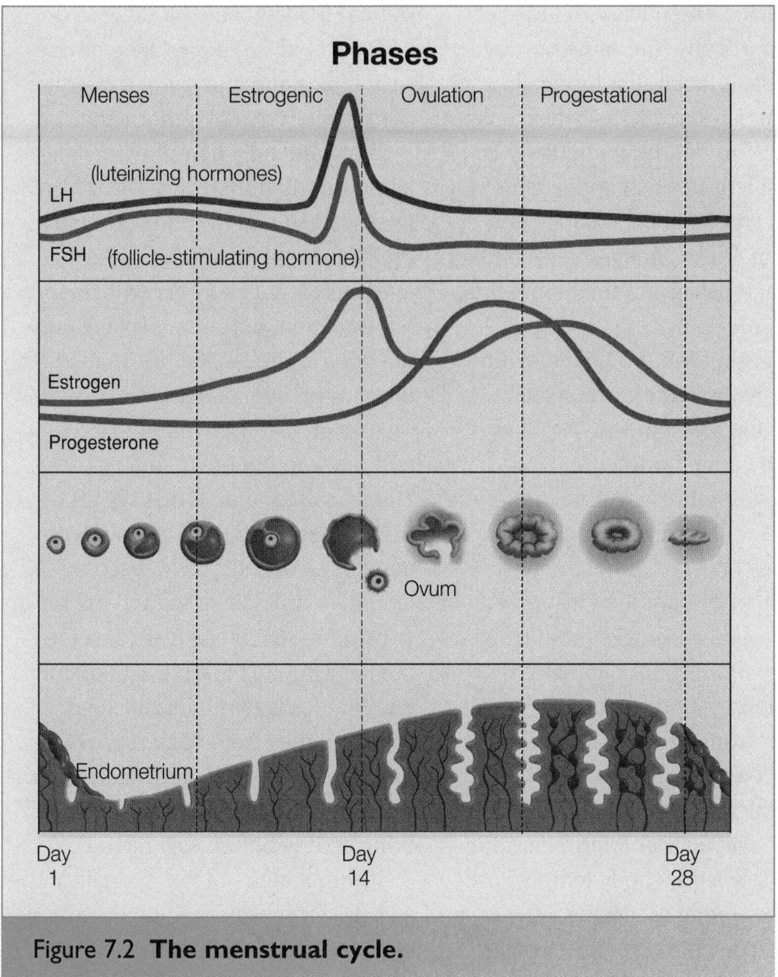

Figure 7.2 **The menstrual cycle.**

marker of female virginity. As a female child develops from infancy to adulthood, this membrane stretches and thins out. In many cases, especially in physically active girls, the membrane breaks before or during puberty. When the hymen breaks, it usually is accompanied by the presence of a small amount of blood. In some cases it remains intact and is torn during first intercourse or, in some rare cases, it must be removed surgically in a simple medical procedure for intercourse to be possible and pleasurable. Thus, virginity is marked not by the presence or absence of the hymen but, rather, from having or not having participated in sexual intercourse.

Menstruation

As growth and change continue on the outside, the ovaries inside the pelvis are readying for participation in reproduction by developing immature ova (the eggs contained within the ovaries from birth to maturity), one each month, in a cycle known as **menstruation**. For young women in the United States, the first menstrual period, known as **menarche**, occurs on the average between their 12th and 13th year, but variations from 8 or 9 to 15 or 16 years old are considered normal. Figure 7.2 depicts the menstrual cycle. Young women are sometimes apprehensive if they begin menstruating before or later than their friends. They need to understand that they are following normal physical development.

During the menstrual cycle, the uterus prepares to receive a fertilized egg (zygote) that, if implanted, will grow there from an embryo to a fetus and ultimately to a newborn baby. If the egg is not fertilized, it disintegrates and the inner uterine lining (endometrium), which was prepared to nurture it, sloughs off. The cycle then begins again. Menstruation continues throughout a woman's childbearing years and ends at menopause.

The first menstrual cycle does not usually contain a mature ovum. As the cycles regulate themselves over the next several months (to an average 28- to 30-day cycle, with the onset of menstrual flow marking the first day), ova will mature and the young woman will become familiar with how the cycle establishes itself for her. Most females discharge only about half a cup of menstrual blood, which mixes with tissue and body fluid in each cycle, making it appear to have much more volume. The discharge is usually more red in color at the beginning of menstruation and then more brown in color toward the end.

Sometimes the menstrual flow is clotty and sometimes smooth. Sometimes menstruation begins with, or is accompanied by, headache, bloating, malaise, mood disturbances, and abdominal cramps, and other times none of these symptoms occurs. These symptoms are common in some women and absent in others. These distressful periods are known as premenstrual syndrome (PMS). Sometimes the symptoms are severe enough to warrant medical intervention. Other times, exercise, a modification of diet, and decrease of stress will be enough to alleviate PMS.

Discussions about menstrual flow protective devices should be included in classes about puberty. A show-and-tell format might be used to demonstrate that some of them are worn outside of the vagina (sanitary pads of all shapes and widths), and some are worn inside (tampons). They come in different thickness and widths to catch and hold the amount of flow that is expected. Both internal and external products are safe for women of all ages, irrespective of whether they have participated in sexual intercourse. Choosing the best product is a matter of personal choice and comfort. Pelvic models are available that show how tampons fit into the vagina. Such discussions and demonstrations often take away the fear and mystery and place menstruation in the realm of other normal physiological processes.

Poorly informed premenstrual girls worry a great deal about things such as, "How will I know when I will get it?" "What will I do if I get my period during a class?" "Can everyone see that I am carrying or wearing a sanitary napkin?" "If I use a tampon, will I be injured or lose my virginity?" Names like "the curse" are not helpful. Men, too, have misconceptions about menstruation. They are confused about the amount of bleeding. They often don't know what to make of PMS and other menstrual symptoms and either take it too seriously or not seriously enough.

Traditionally, when education about menstruation did take place, the lesson was delivered only to girls and consisted of the physiological changes. Personal questions were rarely addressed. Therefore, education should be for both boys and girls and should explain the emotional and social, as well as the physical, aspects.

Puberty in Males

At the first signs of puberty, boy's genitals begin to grow. Hair also begins to grow under their arms and around the genitals. Voice changes begin with a cracking or squeaking and end with a deepened voice. Boys also begin to grow coarse hair on their chest, arms, legs, and face. The release of testosterone or androgens (the same hormones that stimulate facial skin lubrication and facial hair growth) may also create skin acne. This can be particularly distressing at a time when appearance seems so crucial to acceptance and self-esteem. These changes in secondary sex characteristics and the broadening of the shoulders and narrowing of the hips result from the **testosterone** secreted by the **testes**, which are enclosed in the scrotum (the two sacs outside the male body).

The testes are responsible for the production of sperm. In contrast to females—who have inside their ovaries at birth all of the ova they will release until menopause—males produce millions of sperm throughout their lives. Sperm, along with prostate fluid and secretions from the seminal vesicles and the Cowper's gland, makes up the semen, which, spurts out of the urethra during an ejaculation. Sperm must be stored at lower-than-body temperature. Hence, the scrotal sacs hang away from the body to keep the testicles cooler, one sac hanging slightly lower than the other (which sometimes causes young men to think that something is wrong with them).

A typical cause for concern among young men during puberty is the size of their penis. The penis and the testicles grow in size during puberty. Their growth and ultimate size varies from person to person depending on hereditary factors. Penis size has been related to "manliness," and many boys worry about how normal they are and how they will "measure up" to their friends.

Puberty is also a time when erections occur frequently and sometimes unexpectedly. An erection results from expansion of the arteries that fills the tissue inside the penis (corpora cavernosa) with blood. The length of the penis during erection (about 4 to 8 inches) is not necessarily related to the length of the unerect penis (about 1½ to 4 inches). And penis size in the normal healthy male has little to do with his ability to experience or give sexual pleasure and is not a measure of his skill in sexual performance.

Boys generally have their first ejaculation during puberty. Ejaculation is the release of semen in spurts through the urethra out the head of the penis. Ejaculation is usually accompanied by a pleasurable sensation of small contractions in the genital area, called an **orgasm** or "climax." Ejaculation and orgasm are two different phenomena, and one can occur without the other. The ejaculate or fluid that comes out of the penis in the first ejaculations appears clear; later, it will become more cloudy or milky in color and thicker in consistency. Each ejaculate of semen contains about 1 teaspoonful of fluid and hundreds of millions of sperm. Although they both come from the same opening, urine and semen do not mix. A valve normally closes off the urine shortly before ejaculation.

If young men are not sexually active and do not masturbate, the first ejaculation probably will occur during sleep, termed **nocturnal emission**, commonly known as a "wet dream." Sometimes boys do not know what happened to them and think they have urinated in their sleep. Imagine the many concerns they have as a result of this experience: "Will it happen when I sleep over at my friend's house?" "Will my mother or my sister see it?" "Will it happen during school or at some other unexpected time?" Often they are embarrassed at their inability to control it and may refuse to sleep at friends' houses or go to sleep-away camp. They need information and reassurance.

On the average, males begin and complete puberty later than do females. As a result, boys appear less adult-like and are less physically mature than girls in late elementary and middle school.

What Does "Long-Term Relationship" Mean

Following are nine characteristics of a happy marriage/long-term relationship.

1. Spouses/partners are giving people, meeting their emotional needs by doing for others—and they do not keep score.
2. They have a strong sense of commitment, do not take their happiness for granted, and are determined to make their relationship work.
3. They do not lose themselves in the relationship. Although they value their independence—the right to form their own opinions, make their own decisions, and pursue their own goals—marital/relationship harmony is a top priority.
4. They have vigorous sexual drives. Sex plays a central and profoundly important role in the relationship.
5. They like to talk, sharing their thoughts about all sorts of subjects. They are open and direct, not manipulative.
6. They have a positive outlook on life.
7. They express appreciation and are generous with praise.
8. They recognize the needs of others, respect their differences, consider their feelings, and put themselves in the other person's shoes.
9. They are willing to grow, change, and work hard at the relationship. They know that a good relationship requires flexibility and effort to keep it alive.

Source: Adapted from the Ohio State University Extension-Columbus Families Priority-1, Family and Consumer Sciences, 1997.

Psychosocial Issues in Puberty

The onslaught of hormones, the changes to their bodies, and the social context during puberty cause teens to become romantically and sexually interested in one another. The constant search for answers to "Am I normal?" results in their modeling each others' behaviors for acceptance and worrying about their bodies and performance. Puberty is typically a difficult time for young men and young women alike. Receiving constructive, accurate information and knowing which people and places to go to for answers to their questions can alleviate their anxieties.

These natural changes and functions should be discussed in school as just that—natural and healthy occurrences that result in the physical maturity of adulthood. The discussions should not be entirely bio-physiological and technical; they should include feelings and experiences. Open handling of these topics, although at first uncomfortable, will ultimately result in a more open, accepting forum about sexual subjects that were formerly considered too sensitive and secretive to discuss. It will encourage communication about sexuality between parents and children, patients and medical practitioners, and particularly between sexual partners.

Relationships Within the Family

When **Jon** and **Sherry** married, each brought one child to the marriage from prior marriages. They later had two more children and recently adopted another. Jon also had two children who did not come to live with the family permanently but stayed with them off and on. The adopted child was long-awaited, and the adoptive parents went to a foreign country to get him. To get away from inner-city problems, the family recently moved to a suburban setting. Most of their new neighbors have lived in that community a long time. Most of the children live with both parents and a few with just their mothers.

The teacher in the third-grade class told the students they would be preparing a family tree. She asked them "What makes a good family?" Several of the children, including one of Jon and Sherry's children, were in that class. Imagine the variety of answers that emerged! Some of the children explained that a family is a mother and father and children that live in one house and care for each other. Others said families are people with the same last name who live together. Still others said a family is where the mother takes care of the children and the father works. Jon and Sherry's child made a different contribution to the definition of family. He said his family members do not live together all of the time, and some of them have different last names. Some aren't even of the same race.

If you were asked, "What makes a good family?" would your answer differ from when you were a child? What are your underlying values about how families function best?

What defines a family and the functions of a family have changed dramatically over the past century. These changes have been influenced by many socioeconomic and cultural factors. In the past, families lived in one community for most, if not all, of their lives. Today, school, jobs, finances, and other factors dictate where people live.

Blended cultures, religions, educational levels, and social status are present within families and within the community. Moreover, what defines a family—its structure, roles, attitudes, and values—is constantly changing. Students in elementary school are likely to have experienced many of these changes in their own family or witnessed them in the families of their friends and neighbors.

What Is a Family?

Not too long ago most people would have agreed about what constitutes a family. **Marriage**, a legally sanctioned, permanent arrangement between a man and a woman who produced children and shared a residence and finances was called a **nuclear family**. The extended family consisted of their relatives by blood or marriage. But, even then, the family had variations. A widowed adult and his or her children were considered a family, even though there was no longer a marriage. Couples with adopted children and stepchildren, not only biological children, have been considered a family all along, as have married couples with no children.

More recently, the concept of family has grown to encompass groups of people living together in many different constellations.[6] These include

1. The traditional nuclear family consisting of husband, wife, and children.
2. Unmarried and married couples of the same gender with and without children.
3. One-parent families, including never-married–, widowed-, and single-parent households of divorced and separated spouses.
4. Families with adopted children.
5. Reconstituted families, or stepfamilies, consisting of children from multiple marriages and blended families in which either or both partners bring children and may have additional children together.
6. Communal families: a group of families with or without children and single adults living together.

Also, families have blended cultures, ethnicities, and other social and educational experiences that define their uniqueness. Children need to learn about other children's families and begin to recognize the family as a dynamic social institution with many forms. In 1991, 42 percent of families were married couples living together without children, and 36 percent were married couples with children, many consisting of stepfamilies with children from former relationships.[7]

Knowing what family members can be expected to do and how to be an effective family member are important concepts for children to consider. Families perform several roles in society, and individuals perform several roles in families. Among the functions that traditional families have assumed are reproduction, rearing, and socializing of children; economic maintenance and the provision of material resources; provision of affection, belonging, emotional security; and protection of the members through establishing and maintaining family boundaries and standards.

Healthy families can foster satisfaction with life, unconditional love, mutual respect, safety, and belonging in environments that enable personal growth and development. They provide opportunities for fun and celebration.

Families can also be the cause of pain and suffering. Framo describes some the psychological damage that members in dysfunctional families inflict upon one another, including scapegoating; humiliation and shaming; parentification; crazy-making; physical, sexual, and verbal abuse; cruel rejections; lies and deceit; and [in general] outrage against the human spirit.[8]

Assuming Roles Within the Family

The roles that family members take emerge as the family develops and its needs grow and change. These roles are determined by age, position in the family, social and cultural factors, morals, values and attitudes, and the family's management needs. The roles differ by age and developmental stage. Sometimes parental roles are allocated to children. Children's roles in single-parent and dual-working–parent families tend to involve more responsibility. This may be appropriate as children reach adolescence, but is very burdensome for younger children.

Learning about the expected roles of parents and what parenting is all about will help students determine their own readiness—or more appropriately, lack of readiness—for parenthood. Students can develop understanding of their roles in their own families and the roles they can expect to play in the future.

Family Communication

Communication patterns are part of the total family dynamic. How the family disseminates information to its members and whether each member has free access to information that involves him or her is integral to family life. Communication patterns within families are influenced by gender, culture, and social class. Healthy families provide opportunities for children to develop communication skills they can use in other settings. School is a practice field for trying out family-learned styles of relating and communicating.

Healthy families support healthy attitudes toward self and contribute to high self-esteem and confidence. They build up their members. They teach about acceptance, love, and optimism. They influence values and attitudes about sexuality and sexual expression, responsible decision-making, and coping styles.

When studying families in school, students can learn about the various styles and constellations within which families function successfully. Sharing experiences and stories from their own families creates an environment for building understanding of and tolerance for differences and the implications of unique cultural and ethnic factors. Students can begin to reflect on their contribution to the functioning of their own family and the resources available for assisting families that are not functioning well.

Separation and Divorce

Separation and divorce disrupt the family system. Not only does each partner have to find his or her way as a single person, but when children are involved, family patterns change. For example, the family's income often changes and, with that, their lifestyle.

Divorce can create feelings of guilt, failure, fear about the future, and depression in the children. During the first year after a separation, children are likely to have problems with adjustment. This evidences itself in sleeping and eating disruptions, increased anxiety, academic declines, and conduct disorders. If the children do not become the pawns of dissent, these problems begin to decrease when the family approaches a new homeostasis. Children whose parents remain consistently involved in their lives will eventually overcome commonly experienced feelings that they were the cause of the divorce.

The lasting effects of divorce on children may surface later in their own intimate relationships. Sometimes they have difficulty trusting partners and making commitments.

Separation and divorce usually represent the culmination of difficult relationships. Children probably lived with anger, loneliness, and other negative feelings for some time. If the separation brings relief, children may feel guilty about that, too.

Divorce is a complicated issue for families, and volumes have been written about it. Because it is so common among elementary schoolchildren, this subject should be included in the family life curriculum. Children in various stages of divorcing families often help each other, and they find some consolation in knowing that others have survived. The classroom teacher should focus less on individual children's problems (these should be referred to mental health professionals) and more on the process of divorce, common feelings and outcomes, and various ways in which families adjust. Teachers can introduce developmentally appropriate resources for children who are having trouble. For example, young children need family, religious, or school resources, whereas older children may be more amenable to community counseling settings.

Friendships

Friendships are relationships between two people involving mutual trust, support, respect, and intimacy that may or may not be sexual. Meeks, Heit, and Burt outlined several types of intimacy in relationships as follows:[9]

1. Philosophical intimacy in which people share beliefs and philosophies about life.
2. Psychological intimacy in which people share needs, drives, vulnerabilities, strengths, emotional feelings, and problems.
3. Creative intimacy in which people share their work, projects, artistic endeavors, and the like.
4. Physical intimacy wherein people express their affections through sexual and other physical expressions (including, but not restricted to, sexual intercourse).

The boundaries and characteristics of a friendship are specific to the people involved and require that the friends be able to communicate their understandings, needs, and affections. As the needs of the people involved change, so do the friendships. The ability to develop deep and lasting friendships is often a measure of a person's mental health.

In the lower grades, children's relationships are just beginning to extend beyond their family, and their notion of friendship represents an outgrowth of family messages and friendship styles. Although many families encourage and value friendships, they define them and act on them in different ways.

Early Friendships

Preschool and kindergarten children are in the development stage at which they are just learning to share with others. They are still self-centered (egocentric). They may play with each other, but they do not exhibit the bonding associated with later friendships. They may begin to experiment with their sexuality as they negotiate relationships, watch their body changes, and play "doctor" or "I'll let you see if you let me see." Their inquisitiveness about their own and each other's body parts is just that—inquisitiveness.

For Your Health

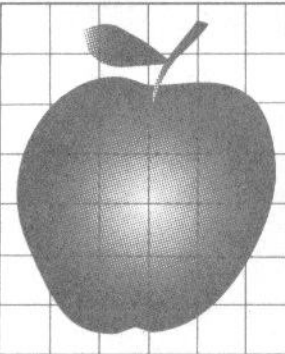

Building Friendships

- Create a tradition. It could be a weekly walk or watching your favorite team's midweek game. Select something you both enjoy.
- Work together. Side-by-side work provides a good opportunity to share thoughts and feelings about what's going on in your lives.
- Help someone heal. Take time to be with a friend who is having problems.
- Say "thanks." Friends show their gratitude for favors and thoughtfulness.
- Ask for help. Both people in a friendship need to know the other will come through for them if needed.
- Learn trust. It's tough to face possible rejection when you let someone in on your deepest secrets, but a true friend will love and accept you regardless of your flaws.
- Be willing to share your most personal thoughts and feelings, as well as your time, your possessions, and other things that are important to you.
- Be a good listener. Your friend needs a confidant, too.

As they approach their seventh year, children begin to develop relationships of give-and-take with classmates and others outside of the family. They also begin to understand and accept the needs of others. They experience trust, acceptance, and a feeling of comfort with some children and not with others as they try out their earliest friendships. The feelings of closeness are associated with a liking for one another that deepens as children get to know each other's characteristics and share interests.

As children proceed through elementary school, they begin to recognize and define the ingredients they value in a friend. Sometimes friends are people with whom they share recreational interests, but the intimate bonding that sustains deep friendship does not develop. In other friendships they become dependent upon one another and do not nourish each other's independence. They say things like, "I couldn't do anything without [him or her]." Sometimes they are pressured into friendships by a need for popularity or acceptance or by the selections of their parents, teachers, or other family members. They may commit to relationships that do not work because of unrealistic expectations and then become reluctant to form deep friendships later on.

True intimacy is thought to develop during the preadolescent period, as "chum" relationships. Chums are friends who validate each other's self-worth and thereby can adjust their needs toward more mutual satisfactions. Preadolescent friendships are most often same-gender relationships. As children mature, opposite-gender relationships develop as well. In either case, as children reach preadolescence, they become more seriously attached to one another. The feelings of closeness that represent a "special person" are difficult for immature young people to discern from the intimacy that comes with maturity, particularly that of commitment, permanency, and dependability.

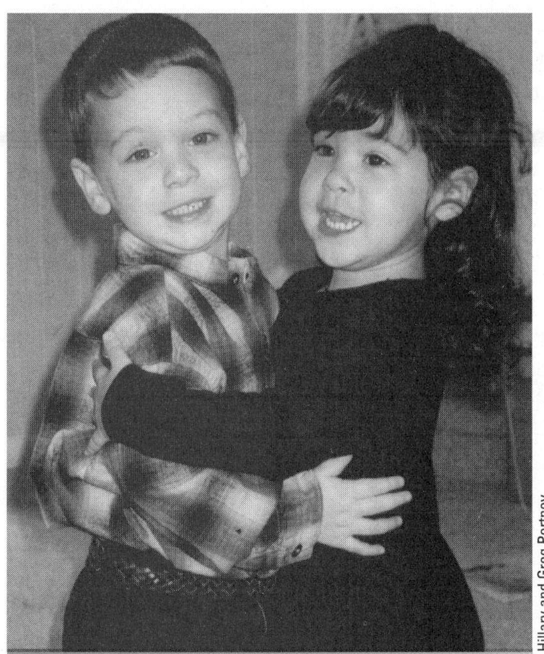
Hillary and Greg Portnoy

In lower grades, friendships are beginning to extend beyond the family.

Friendships in Adolescence

Like preadolescence, early adolescence is characterized by changes in the identification and significance of friendships. At this stage of development, the need for intimacy is risky but is motivated by a need for acceptance and attachment to peers. During middle adolescence, the focus is on the resolution of ego-identity; self-identity is still being assessed and relationships are maturing. In late adolescence, the teen is able to integrate the needs for security, intimacy, and lust into mature relationships. Hence, early experiences with friendships happen somewhat haphazardly, and their outcomes are often a matter of "luck." Later they represent a need for acceptance by the peer group. With maturity, friendships become independent choices. If young people choose healthy relationships that last, are supportive, nourish their sense of self, and in which they feel relaxed and accepted, they learn to trust their ability to make friends.

Learning about the functions of friendships, how to seek out friends who will complement them, how to be a good friend, and how to set boundaries around friendships will help young people to be less vulnerable to peer pressure during adolescence and to develop important relationships throughout their lives. This is fostered by discussing what is valued in friends, how to develop mutually acceptable expectations of friendships, and how to maintain friendships as the individuals grow and change.

Dating Relationships

As children leave elementary school, their social lives tend to change from group friendships to dating that includes expressions of intimacy within the boundaries and norms defined by that generation. Children tend to find their initial romantic interests in people whom they find physically attractive and those that are generally acceptable to their peer group. In late adolescence, personality characteristics such as being outgoing or having a sense of humor as well as interpersonal dynamics such as trust and ability to self-disclose become more important and form the basis for more serious and permanent co-habitational or marital relationships.

Individual notions of physical attractiveness and how to behave on dates are rooted in culture, gender roles, messages from the media, and children's literature (Cinderella and Snow White are examples). Sometimes these manifest themselves in gender-stereotypical behaviors and expectations, especially about sexual behaviors (for instance, boys are interested only in sex, girls are interested only in love and commitment). Class discussions about how to behave in dating relationships can help to decrease these biases.

Also, these influences, especially media messages about physical attractiveness and unrealistic perfectionism, support biases against people with special needs. Physically challenged people often are portrayed as unattractive, infantile, and even nonsexual. Their sense of themselves, especially from preadolescence to early adulthood, is often restricted, as are their peers' notions about them as potential partners. Classroom teachers have the opportunity to counteract some of these harmful biases against those with disabilities.

As dating relationships develop, so do expressions of sexual intimacy. Preadolescents sometimes begin sexual experimentation. Thus, sexuality education should include discussions about how to express intimacy in ways other than sexual and how to make decisions about sexual involvement that represent personal and family values and attitudes. Children need to know how they can show their liking for one another, what factors to consider when choosing dating partners, what sexual behaviors they will participate in, and how to communicate their sexual decisions effectively to a date. They need to learn how to say "No" comfortably and how to accept "No" without feeling rejected. This will help them reject peer pressure at a time when being accepted by the peer group has so much importance to their self-worth.

Sexuality education also includes the "etiquette" of dating. The earliest lessons are an appropriate time to discuss the mechanics of dating: How do I ask someone to go out? How do I accept or refuse without making the other person feel rejected? Where should we go? What should we do? These early discussions should also address the issue of setting boundaries within and around relationships.

Ending Special Relationships

Ending relationships can be painful, and sometimes embarrassing, especially if the decision is not mutual. Therefore, learning how to say "Goodbye" in fair and considerate ways should be another topic of discussion in sexuality curricula at the later elementary level.

As observers of their parents' divorce, some children have experienced the ending of important relationships. These children can learn to recognize the signals of distancing and loss of feelings and apply them to their own relationships. Some of the early signs of a breakdown in relationships are avoidance and unavailability. Communication may break down. Either person may no longer be listening to or willing to hear the other and may become argumentative or verbally abusive. Abuse has no place in a good relationship, and people need to learn not to permit themselves to remain in relationships in which they feel bad most of the time. Love doesn't feel like that! Leaving an abusive situation and seeking professional help are good ideas. A relationship should not continue unless the abuse stops.

Young people move from one relationship to another as their interests, needs, and experiences change. The ending of a relationship is often painful and confusing to the person in the relationship who does not initiate the separation. When a relationship is dying, one or both partners lose interest in the other's life. Young people often confirm the correctness of their decision to break off by gathering their friends into an "army camp" to help them validate their case against their partner. No one likes to be the bad guy! Friends tend to be biased and therefore not always able to offer rational help. Also, they may say cruel and sometimes untruthful things about the former partner, bringing him or her further pain and humiliation.

Non-destructive strategies for dissolving relationships require open communication to minimize the hurt, rejection, and embarrassment a separation brings. Young people need to learn how not to attack each other's basic personality as a means of explaining why their relationship is over. Recognizing changes in the dynamics, feelings, and interests of the partners can lead to agreement that the relationship has changed and should end. If young people learn how to redefine or dissolve relationships and to minimize the pain of rejection as they move through adolescence, they will be better prepared to recognize when their adult relationships are running into trouble. They can build an appreciation for and practice making changes before they choose lifetime mates.

Sexually Intimate Relationships

In a world bombarded by confusing media messages about sex and sexuality, children develop meanings about themselves as sexual beings earlier and earlier in their lives. Driven by a variety of developmental tasks and influenced by multigenerational issues, family systems, and peer groups, they attempt to engage in sexual behaviors.

Self-Pleasuring

Infants first become aware of their sexuality through the sensations of touch, feel, smell, and taste of their own bodies (including their own genitals) and through the touch, feel, smell, and taste of their caregivers. Physically exploring their genitals brings sensual pleasure to the infant, even though this pleasure is not usually described as "sexual" or "erotic." Yet, babies and very young children exhibit a sexual response that is, or closely resembles, orgasm. As childhood continues, curiosity about the genitals and exhibiting genitals to one another become common in play. Hence, sexuality is a part of young children's sensual repertoire.[10] Later in adolescence, that experimentation sometimes increases to include oral-genital behavior and attempts at sexual intercourse.

Early messages about touching one's own genitals can have a profound effect later on body image, sexual behavior, and self-concept. These messages reflect the wide differences in attitudes and values about self-pleasuring. With roots in culture, religion, and family values, exploration of one's own genitals may be discouraged with a parent's slap, harsh word, or embarrassed reaction. Or it may be encouraged with an explanation about privacy and appropriate times and appropriate places for sexual pleasuring. If self-pleasuring is discouraged, children may learn to perceive their genitals as something dirty or bad. When exploratory behaviors are understood as a natural part of growing up, children will be more comfortable with their sexuality and physical self.

When touching one's own genitals is a deliberate attempt to derive sexual pleasure, it is called **masturbation**. It is not uncommon for young children to rub their genitals when they are concentrating or when they are napping. "Tugging on labia or rubbing one's penis seems to relieve stress and tension and may help a child settle into sleep more readily."[11] Many myths and misconceptions about masturbation should be clarified. It does not cause hair to grow on the palms of hands; it does not cause people to go insane; it doesn't stunt growth or make the genitals fall off. Further, masturbation is not a sign of a bad sexual relationship. Yet, if a child's masturbatory activities seem to be compulsive and do not seem to relieve tension, one might consider traumatic issues occurring in the child's life that need attention.[12] Also, on the rare occasions when an adult masturbates to the exclusion of other social and developmentally appropriate sexual activities, it can be considered excessive or problematic.

Masturbation presents a moral dilemma for some people. In these cases a personal decision that supports the person's commitment to a religion also represents a health decision not to participate. What is important is that masturbation be understood as a normal part of sexual development that both men and women can, and usually do, participate in at one time or another.

Sexual Intimacy

We are living in a time when experiences with sexual intimacy and sexual behaviors between people often begin in preadolescence. Even though the link to emotional harm, unwanted pregnancy, illness, and even death is explained to them, adolescents participate widely in sexual activity.

People move through several stages in their development to sexual maturity.[13] The earliest phase constitutes an attempt to understand sexual intimacy and associate it with their search for their own sexual self ("Who am I as a sexual being?"). This means exploring the meaning of the physical changes of puberty. Self-explorations by comparison of their physical self to others, including the size of their genitalia and masturbatory activities, are characteristic of initial sexual behaviors. The next phase is characterized by a sexual interest in others as sexual partners ("Who are you as a sexual being?"). This includes the search for a first partner, and sexual activity is a means of understanding the other's sexual experience and their part in it.

In sexual maturity, sexual intimacy is understood in the context of the self and the other ("Who are we as sexual partners?") in an attempt to successfully merge the two into a meaningful and satisfying sexual relationship.

Sexual Desire

The desire for a sexual experience with someone else is a natural phenomenon, like the desire for food and sleep. It begins noticeably during puberty when the hormones that stimulate physical changes also stimulate the emotional center in the brain. The desire to be sexual is influenced by other emotions. If people feel healthy, happy, attractive, good about themselves, and good about sex, they will have more sexual desire. If, on the other hand, they feel sad, angry, sick, or guilty about sex, they probably will have less sexual desire. People can feel sexy spontaneously or because of interest in, attraction to, or love for another person.

Men and women have the same potential for feeling sexual desire. The desire for sexual activity does not mean one has to act on it. People need to make decisions about who they will be sexual with; what sexual activities they are willing to participate in; and where, how often, and under what circumstances they will be sexual. People also need to consider their parents' or friends' standards, the standards prescribed by their culture or religion, and the commitments they have in their other relationships.

A common belief among young people is that, if they have already been sexually active (even once) with someone they loved in a past relationship, there is little point in refusing sexual activity with the person they now love. Once you have intercourse, that decision is over. To the contrary, each sexual experience should represent a separate decision. When people determine that they can choose sexual experiences freely, without coercion, and be comfortable with each act, the experience is likely to contribute to their lives positively. The notion of sexual activity as a personal decision should be stressed in a curriculum about sexuality and family life.

For sexual experiences to be positive, participants also should learn about how their bodies can be expected to behave or feel. Information about human sexual response and human sexual dysfunction is a necessary part of sexual learning. This information gives sexually active people realistic knowledge about what to expect throughout their sexual lives. Although this specific subject matter is most appropriate later in sexuality education, preparation for talking comfortably about sex and using appropriate language for body parts and functions can begin in elementary school.

Love and Sex

Children's earliest notions about couple relationships are an outgrowth of their family experiences and, later, an outgrowth of their dating experiences as related to popularity, gender roles, media messages, and so on. How their own sexual behavior fits their beliefs about how couples function is also a product of these societal influences. Although the Freudian notion of a latency period of sexuality (ages 6–12) remains to some theorists an accepted phenomenon, it is not without controversy. There is evidence of an intensity of romantic feelings as children approach their 10th and 11th years. Thus, sexuality education during the 5th and 6th grades aims to help young people understand the connection between sex and love in relationships.

Sex between two people can represent nothing more than a physical experience meant to derive physical pleasure for each person individually, or it can represent an expression of love and commitment. When it is a physical experience that does not represent a special relationship, sexual activity is perceived as recreation and should occur only when both participating adults consent to it. When it represents love between two people, it is an expression of their deep caring for one another. In that context, sexual behavior is shared and mutually agreed upon and, again, never coercive. It enhances the couple's feelings about one another. It takes into account the preservation of each partner's health and includes actions that decrease or eliminate the risk of disease or unintended pregnancy.

Individuals' notions of love and the behaviors that represent love are influenced by culture, the media, the arts, and social constructors. Love is a basic human emotion. One way to talk about love is in terms of a "triangle of love":[13]

1. Intimacy involves mutual self-disclosure, having high regard for each other, giving and receiving emotional support, valuing each other, and having a desire to share oneself and possessions with another.
2. Passion involves a feeling of attraction, romance, or longing for a sexual or emotional union.
3. Decision/commitment involves some combination of intimacy and passion (for example, a liking for someone with no passion involved, an infatuation or feeling of passion only, romantic love, companionate love, and so on) in a permanent relationship.

"Romantic love," though it involves intimacy and passion, may or may not involve decision/commitment. "Empty love" that involves decision/commitment does not involve passion. The configuration of the love triangle depends upon the balance of intimacy, passion, and decision/commitment in the relationship.[14]

Another way to teach about love is as five different types:

1. Infatuation or passionate love, the initial "falling in love" feeling
2. Erotic love, which is sexual love
3. Dependent love, which is love that includes a psychological need or that provides security or approval
4. Friendship love, representing a special liking and relaxation with one another
5. Altruistic love, which is an unselfish concern for another person

Another explanation of love is offered by Eric Fromm. In his classic book, *The Art of Loving*, where he describes love as having four parts: labor (representing a willingness of one person to work at or give of himself or herself for the other); responsibility (the process by which people evaluate their behavior as it will affect their loved one and be prepared to help the other when needed); respect (holding the other in high regard and not benefiting at the expense of the other); and understanding (in which each person understands and accents the needs, desires, values, and attitudes of the other).

Love is expressed differently and has different meanings in different cultures. When people determine that romantic love is "real love," they tend to seek to give it permanency in marriage or some other long-term relationship structure.

In U. S. culture, love is a romantic notion expected to be a binding force that determines and cements relationships. Marriage is a statement by two people that they are experiencing the highest form of love and commitment, and it is one of the appropriate places for sexual behavior. The laws in many states do not legally recognize certain love relationships through marriage (for example, homosexual couples or couples too closely related). This only limits their public and legal statement, not their love or commitment.

A person's values and attitudes influence the relationship between love and sex. Thus, one goal of sex education is to help students develop their own personal meaning for love. Another is to help them develop their understanding of appropriate sexual behaviors: how they fit into their relationships, that they occur by choice, and that they enhance their life experiences. Students, as they mature, might reflect on the attributes associated with love and sex and how they fit into their own expectations. Twelve central attributes of love could be discussed in classroom curricula: trust, caring, honesty, friendship, respect, concern for the other's well-being, commitment, loyalty, acceptance of the other the way he or she is, supportiveness, wanting to be with the other, and interest in the other.[15] Attributes associated with sex can be placed into three categories:[16]

1. Emotional attributes: caring, closeness, happiness, communication, love, and so on
2. Physical attributes: intensity, excitement, pleasure, desire, lust, sensuality, and so on
3. Consequential attributes: pregnancy, pain, violence, disease, danger

Jealousy and Boundaries

An aspect of relationships that often arises is jealousy. Young children are familiar with the intensity of jealousy in sibling and friend relationships. Jealousy is a painful emotion associated with self-esteem, interdependence, personal expectations of behavior in relationships and, sometimes, violence. It occurs when boundaries established in a relationship are not maintained and one of the partners is thought to be involved with another person.

The boundaries and behaviors that determine a relationship differ across culture, ethnicity, and gender by factors such as the culture's values and attitudes about things such as possessions, independence/dependence, and exclusivity. The most intense jealousy is probably experienced in a committed romantic relationship when one partner is thought to be sexually involved with another person. This is considered a violation of the expected sexual exclusivity of the relationship.

The underlying behaviors that result in jealousy from misplaced trust can be real or imagined. When they are imagined and boundaries are not actually violated, jealousy often stems from personal feelings of inadequacy. Because jealousy is so difficult to deal with, it tends to eat away at the relationship and develop into insecurities in the suspicious partner. When jealousy results from an actual occurrence, it is just as painful and often causes the relationship to change or dissolve.

Children should learn about how to mutually establish the boundaries of a relationship such that each partner agrees to them and is willing to maintain them or communicate a need to renegotiate when necessary. This kind of commitment and agreement, which can begin in the development of early friendships, increases self-esteem because each person feels secure, heard, understood, and respected. Learning to talk with one another about personal issues and to negotiate and renegotiate boundaries as children mature, grow, and change will prepare them with the skills needed for later, more intense relationships.

Sexual Messages and Sexuality Education

Children receive some early messages about sex, especially from the media, that are often distinctly different from the messages received from their familial, religious, or cultural communities. By late elementary school, children become influenced by the information they get from friends. Some of the messages are positive messages about sex as a means of reproduction, or sex as a way of expressing intimacy in a relationship, or sex as an expression of love in a marriage. Others are negative messages about sex as a thing one can barter for favors, goods, or services. The tasks for students are to separate the positive from the negative messages and set standards for themselves to ensure that (1) they participate in sex only with someone and under circumstances they choose, (2) participation in sex does not represent coercion by either partner (3) sex will not result in an unwanted pregnancy or sexually transmitted disease. These concepts can begin to be developed before completing elementary school in the context of other values clarification and decision-making activities. Later, they can be applied more specifically to their own sexual behavior.

In their classic and timeless book about the facts of love for young people, Alex and Jane Comfort provide some suggestions that could be encouraged in sexuality curricula:[17]

> Don't be in a hurry. Sexual intercourse is for men and women, not children, and there is plenty of time.
>
> Do be considerate, caring, and sensitive to other people's needs and feelings. Never harm people in any way.
>
> Don't ever, on any account, run the risk of producing a baby whose needs you will not be able to meet.
>
> Do learn to value and enjoy your body without fear, but without ever being selfish.

Pregnancy and Childbirth

Young elementary school children are particularly inquisitive about pregnancy and childbirth. Children are likely to have experienced the pregnancy of their mother, an aunt, or a friend's mother. They may have been told many different things regarding where babies come from, how they get in there, and how they get out. They may be told that babies are growing in mommy's "stomach," that "the stork" or "God" brings new babies, or some other such explanation. Better, they should be told, in simple language, about how babies are made, where they grow, and how they develop. In addition, an atmosphere should be created wherein children feel comfortable asking questions. Figure 7.3 depicts the stages of birth.

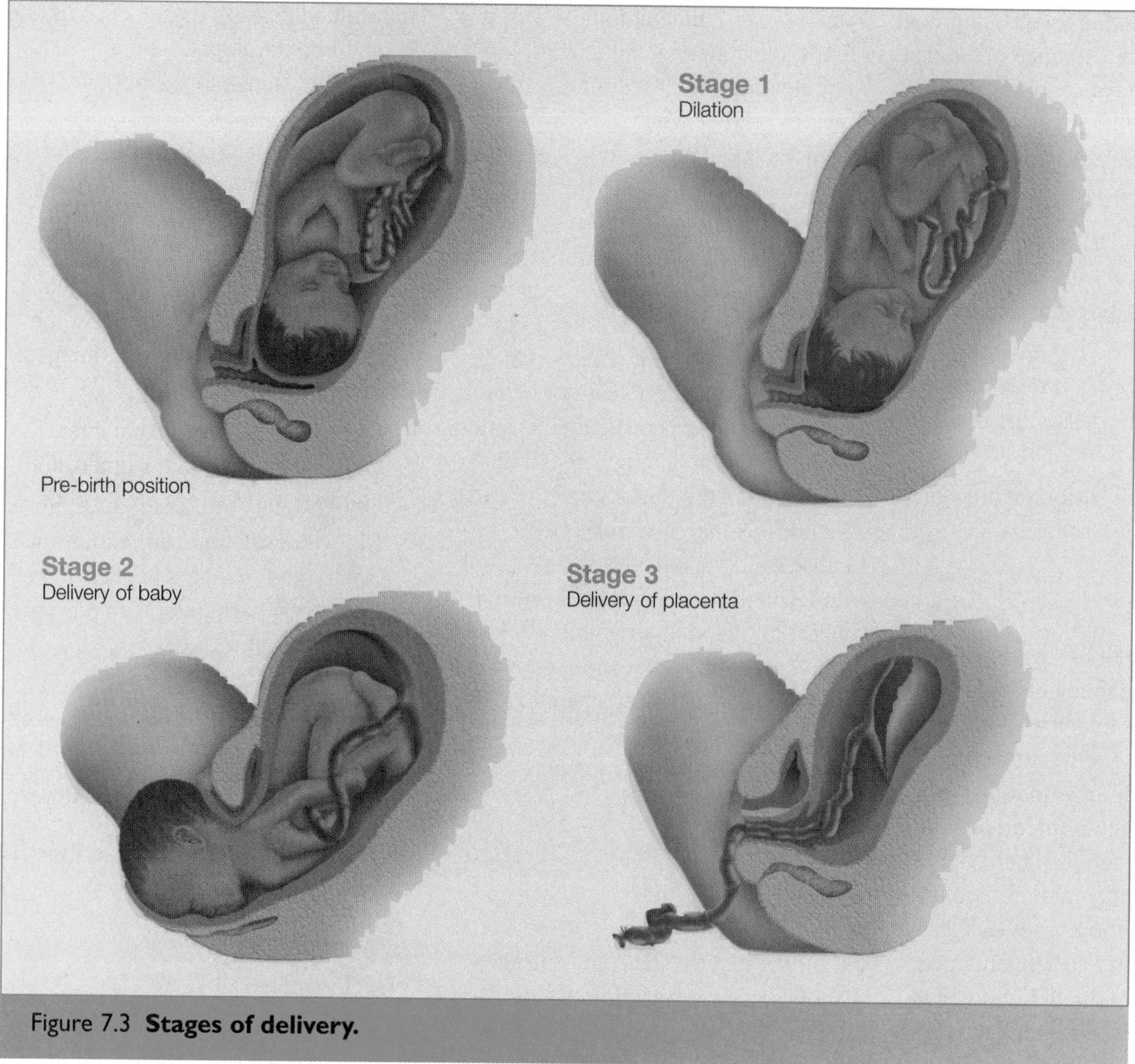

Figure 7.3 **Stages of delivery.**

Children will absorb only what they are developmentally and experientially prepared to understand. The rest will go over their heads until some later query. Pregnancy is a teachable moment or opportunity to create a dialogue between adults and children. It offers an opportunity to begin an educational process that can lead to knowledgeable teens who will become parents only when they want to. The idea is for children to begin to formulate, early in their lives, their understanding of pregnancy, childhood, and parenthood and of the responsibilities and timing associated with being a successful parent. In the context of the realities of caring for a child, the seeds of family planning begin.

Adolescent pregnancy is a major social problem in American society. Although children learn early in childhood that sexual behavior can lead to pregnancy, adolescents seem to participate in sexual activities with the same sense of invulnerability as they do with other things in their lives: "It can't happen to me!" They also deny the responsibilities and their own lack of readiness for parenting sometimes because the concepts are so abstract.

Messages that can be conveyed early in childhood include: Having a baby should be a planned decision. It does not happen by chance; it can be controlled and avoided until a person is ready. These messages should be coupled with actual experiences and anecdotal information about such things as what pregnancy is like; the relationship between good parental health care and the health of newborns; the day-to-day care of infants; and how life changes when people become parents. This learning is an important early component of human sexuality and family life education.

Later in the curriculum, birth control and the specific contraceptives should be discussed in accordance with the students' developmental stage, the values of the community, and the student's previous educational preparation.

Summary

In recent years there has been a change in the political climate that has powerful implications to the delivery of sex education.[18] While researchers and professionals in and associated with the discipline continue to support "comprehensive sex and HIV education", there are federal funds and efforts being diverted to provide "abstinence-only" education. The professional sex education community has identified abstinence-only education as a "fear-based" curriculum that places severe limitations on the ability of educators to provide information about pregnancy and STD/HIV prevention and other health information that young people need to foster their sexual development. At the elementary school level abstinence only curricula do not permit information about human anatomy and human reproduction to be disseminated.

Children need to learn about their body parts and the correct terminology for them. Moreover, they need to know that their body parts belong to them. Parents want help from schools in providing "critical information" about human sexuality.[19] Furthermore, a report by the National Campaign to Prevent Teen Pregnancy reports that abstinence education does not delay initial sexual intercourse.[20]

In an effective human sexuality and family life curriculum, physical and psychosocial components are integrated in a developmentally appropriate way. The education is placed in a context that is sensitive to and shows respect for individual differences and orientations, cultural/religious backgrounds, and differing values of the family of origin. It also points out social problems and threats to health, most prominently sexually transmitted diseases, including HIV/AIDS, as well as teen pregnancy.

In fostering open communication and understanding of family relationships and sexuality, the goal is to give students the tools they need at various levels to protect their health. Also, armed with solid information, students should be better able to engage in emotionally rewarding friendships and, later, satisfying intimate relationships with a sexual component, as well as the means to end a relationship with the least amount of pain.

The curriculum emphasizes respect for one's own and others' bodies, as well as the divergent backgrounds and family constellations of classmates. This is done through discussion of roles and responsibilities of family members and differing values. At the later levels, it incorporates a discussion of teen pregnancy and the importance of self-respect and decision-making.

The discussion of physiology should cover differences and similarities in the physiology of gender. Later, more complex concepts are introduced, related to menstruation and other changes of puberty, the sexual response cycle, reproduction, contraception, pregnancy, and childbirth. The depth of which sexually transmitted diseases including HIV/AIDS is developed as part of the discussion is determined by appropriate developmental levels.

The classroom is an ideal setting to explore the differences in family and cultural backgrounds and values, promote honest and open discussion of sexual issues, and engender respect for and sensitivity toward people who are different from themselves, including students with disabilities.

Web Sites

Abortion Law Homepage
http://www.members.aol.com/_ht_a/abtrbng/index.htm

Alan Guttmacher Institute
http://www.agi-usa.org

American Association for Sex Education, Counseling and Therapy (AASECT)
http://www.aasect.org/

American Board of Sexologists
http://www.esextherapy.com

American Academy of Clinical Sexologists
http://www.esextherapy.com

CDC National AIDS Clearinghouse
http://www.cdcnac.org.

Coalition for Positive Sexuality
http://www.positive.org/cps/Home/index.html

Divorce Online
http://www.divorce-online.com

Gay, Lesbian, Bisexual, and Transgender Links
http://www.indiana.edu/-glbserv/global.html

Go Ask Alice: Columbia Universities Health Education & Wellness Program
http://www.goaskalice.columbia.edu

Infertility Resource
http://www.ihr.com/infertility/index.html

Kids Health Organization Children's Health and Parenting Information
http://www.kidshealth.org/index2.html

Male Infertility
http://www.ivf.com/male.html

Men's Health Resource Guide
http://www.menshealth.com/new/guide/index.html

Menopause Matters
http://www.world.std.com/-susan207

National Gay and Lesbian Task Force
http://www.ngltf.org

National Organization for Women
http://www.now.org

National Abortion & Reproductive Rights Action League
http://www.naral.org/

National Right to Life Committee
http://www/nrlc/org

Planned Parenthood Federation
http://www.ppfa.org/ppfa

Sex & Gender
http://www.bioanth.cam.ac.uk/pip4amod3.html

Sex Information and Education Council of the United States (SIECUS)
http://www.siecus.org

Smart Parent
http://www.smartparent.com

Society for the Scientific Study of Sex (SSSS)
http://www.ssc.wisc.edu/ssss

The Kinsey Institute for Research in Sex, Gender, and Reproduction
http://www.indiana.edu/-kinsey

Women's Studies Resources
http://www.inform.umd.edu/EdRes/Topic/WomensStudies/

Resources

Journals

Adolescence

Archives of Sexual Behavior

Family Life Educator

Family Planning Perspectives

Journal of Homosexuality

Journal of Sex and Marital Therapy

Journal of Sex Education and Therapy

Journal of Sex Research

Journal of Sex Roles

Journal of Sexually Transmitted Diseases

SIECUS Report

Educational Films and Video Distributors

ETR Associates
P.O. Box 1830
Santa Cruz, CA 95061-4284

Fanlight Productions
47 Halifax St.
Boston, MA 02131

Filmmaker's Library
124 E. 40th Street
New York, NY 10016

Films for the Humanities and Sciences, Inc.
P.O. Box 2053
Princeton, NJ 08543

Human Relations Media
175 Tomkins Avenue
Pleasantville, NY 10570

Notes

1. R. Somerville, *Introduction to Family Life and Human Sexuality* (Englewood Cliffs, NJ: Prentice Hall, 1972), 1.
2. J. Turner and L. Rubinson, *Contemporary Human Sexuality* (Englewood Cliffs, NJ: Prentice Hall, 1993).
3. B. Silberman and R. O. Hawkins, Jr., ed., *Lesbian Women and Gay Men: Issues for Counseling* (Pacific Grove, CA: Brooks/Cole, 1998).
4. M. Carrera, *Sex: The Facts, the Acts and Your Feelings* (New York: Crown, 1981), 303.
5. See note 2.
6. C. Mahoney, ed., *Perspectives: Human Sexuality* (Boulder: Coursewise Publ. Inc., 1997).
7. P. Barker, *Basic Family Therapy,* 4th ed. (New York: Oxford University Press, 1992).
8. G. Kelly, *Sexuality Today: The Human Perspective,* 4th ed. (Guilford, MA: Dushkin Publishing Group, 1994).
9. J. Framo, *Family of Origin Therapy: An Intergenerational Approach* (New York: Brunner/Mazel, 1992), 7.
10. L. Meeks, P. Heit, and J. Burt, *Education for Sexuality and HIV/AIDS* (Blacklick, OH: Meeks Heit Publishing, 1993).
11. A. S. Honig, "Sexuality & Young Children," *Child Care Information Exchange* (March, 2000): 27–30.
12. See note 11.
13. E. Weinstein and E. Rosen, "The Development of Adolescent Sexual Intimacy: Implications for Counseling," *Adolescence* 26 (1991): 102.
14. R. Sternberg, *The Triangle of Love* (New York: Basic Books, 1988).
15. R. Sternberg and M. Barnes, "Real and Ideal Others in Romantic Relationships: Is Four a Crowd?" *Journal of Personality & Social Psychology* 49 (1985): 1589–1596.
16. B. Strong and C. DeVault, *Human Sexuality* (Mountain View, CA: Mayfield, 1994).
17. A. Comfort and J. Comfort, *The Facts of Love: Living, Loving and Growing Up* (New York: Mitchell Beazley, 1979), 122.
18. R. Mayer, "1996–97 Trends in Opposition to Comprehensive Sexuality Education in Public Schools in the United States," *SIECUS Report* 25, no. 6 (1998): 20–26.
19. Louis Harris and Associates, *America Speaks: Americans' Opinions on Teenage Pregnancy, Sex Education and Birth Control* (NY: Planned Parenthood Federation of America, 1998).
20. National Campaign to Prevent Teen Pregnancy: Evaluating Abstinence-Only Interventions (2000) (Pamphlet).

Learning Experiences

A comprehensive sex education program that begins early with discussions about relationships, family, love, and commitment can serve as a foundation for young people to make decisions that will protect their health and well-being. The following activities, geared to the developmental level, will reinforce learning and make it applicable to real-life situations.

Grades K–2

By the time children reach kindergarten, they have already been influenced by attitudes and behaviors about their bodies, their sensuality, their notions of the same and opposite gender, and similar things. Children are inquisitive about their own anatomy, especially their genitals and, as their world expands beyond the family, the anatomy of others. Setting the foundation for development of basic concepts of human sexuality and family life is a challenge of the kindergarten teacher. The beginning messages about privacy, nudity, and touching themselves have already been covertly and overtly delivered by family and media.

This is the time when children ask questions about their body parts and functions and often use childhood labels (pee pee or wee wee) or street language (tool or dick) to express themselves. Children at this level can be introduced to more appropriate terminology in nonthreatening, nonjudgmental ways. They can also begin to learn about modesty, privacy, and appropriateness of settings for self-exploration.

From kindergarten through second grade, students are interested in the basics of reproduction, pregnancy, birth, love, and marriage. They sometimes talk about marrying their mother, father, or grandparent. This is an ideal time for students to begin to learn about family life, roles, and responsibilities. Following sessions about human sexuality and family life, students will be able to

1. name their body parts and their locations;
2. describe common feelings and explain how feelings are expressed;
3. describe different kinds of families;
4. identify the roles and responsibilities of family members;
5. describe some nonstereotypical gender options for behavior;
6. report undesirable touches and what to do and where to go for help if they occur;

7. describe prenatal development;
8. give reasons why people decide to have babies.

Grades 3–4

From about third grade on, students become more interested in social relationships outside the family. Learning about friendships, dating, intimacy, and how to discuss sexuality becomes increasingly important. Reflections about relationships, body image, and body functions continue to be of interest. Discussions about masturbation and sexual expressions between people might continue in developmentally appropriate contexts. Because they are not used to talking about these issues with adults, students will often giggle and feel uncomfortable. If they get answers to their questions at a level they can understand, they will become more open with their questions and less uncomfortable. The teacher is an effective resource. By the end of these sessions students will be able to

1. describe their family's values about gender and sexuality;
2. explain pregnancy and childbirth including simplistic explanations of the origins of gender and how multiple births occur;
3. identify different family constellations and family members' roles;
4. describe new responsibilities and life changes when a baby arrives;
5. explain how communities; friends, and other support networks help families;
6. describe their own attitudes and expectations about friendship, love, and intimacy.

Grades 5–6

In grades 5 and 6, students are beginning to undergo puberty. For some, these changes are accompanied by anxiety and fear. Students are concerned about looking different from peers. Teaching them about the changes in their bodies will help them overcome their fears. The goals for these grades also include reviewing and expanding their understanding of menstruation, fertilization, pregnancy, sexually transmitted diseases, and couple and family love. Further, discussions about how to date and select a mate should be included. After these sessions, the students will be able to

1. explain sexual orientations and demonstrate respect for those that are different from their own;
2. name factors that determine a person's readiness to be sexually active;
3. say how they would refuse to participate in sexual activity and feel comfortable saying no;
4. describe their concepts of dating and love relationships;
5. explain alternative expression of feelings in a special relationship other than through sexual activity;
6. give reasons why people delay sexual activity;
7. describe the changes, including secondary sexual characteristics, accompanying puberty;
8. identify the physical and emotional factors surrounding menstruation;
9. identify the emotional changes that can accompany puberty;
10. demonstrate acceptance of sexually related values, attitudes, customs, and behaviors that are different from their own;
11. demonstrate respect for differences in gender, culture, and physical disabilities;
12. identify signs of a declining relationship;
13. explain the concepts of boundaries and jealousy.

For suggestions on creating a rubric with which to evaluate student performance of Learning Experiences, see page 13.

Learning Experience 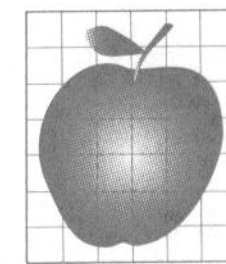 7-1

The New Baby

Grade Level

K–2

Primary Discipline

Social Studies, Language Arts

Learning Objectives

Following this activity, students will be able to

- Describe what a family consists of.
- Explain why babies need families.
- Differentiate biological and social parenting.
- Describe the roles of family members.

Time Required

Two sessions (90 minutes total)

Materials

Collection of pictures of families with babies in diverse ethnic settings, bulletin board

Description of Activity

The children will study the pictures of families and tell a story about a family with a baby. Each student should contribute at least one sentence to the story. The class discusses the differences and similarities among families, including single-parent, dual-parent, and extended families; families with mothers and fathers, two mothers, or two fathers; and families with one child, several children, and children of different ages. The discussion should include families of different ethnic and cultural backgrounds. Ask what role each person in the family (parent, sibling, relatives, others) plays in caring for the baby.

Homework

Children ask their parents to help them select pictures of their family to bring to class and pictures clipped from magazines that represent families that are different from their own.

Evaluation

You can use a rubric or scale that includes the following criteria for measuring learner outcomes.

For a grade of

A, students will

- Identify at least three different family constellations
- Correctly spell all of the new words assigned as part of the activity
- Know the meanings of all of the new words
- Identify at least three cultures or ethnicities different from their own
- Identify at least three roles that family members play in baby care

B, students will

- Identify only two different family constellations
- Correctly spell most of the new words assigned as part of the activity
- Know most of the meanings of the new words
- Identify only two cultures or ethnicities different from their own
- Identify only two roles that family members play in baby care

C, students will

- Identify only one different family constellation
- Correctly spell some of the new words assigned as part of the activity
- Know some of the meanings of the new words
- Identify only one culture or ethnicity different from their own
- Identify only one role that family members play in baby care

D, students will

- Not be able to identify different family constellations
- Spell only a few of the new words assigned as part of the activity
- Not know the meanings of the new words
- Identify only one culture or ethnicity different from their own
- Identify only one of the roles that family members play in baby care

Learning Experience 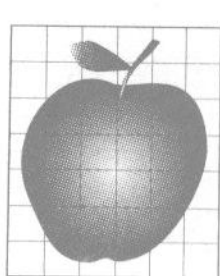 7-2

Where Do Babies Come From?

Grade Level

K–2

Primary Discipline

Science, Language Arts

Learning Objectives

Following this activity, students will be able to

- Describe how different animals reproduce.
- Identify where human babies come from.

Time Required

Two to four sessions.

Materials

Chicken eggs, fish bowl with fish that reproduce (such as guppies), pregnant gerbils, rabbits, rats, or mice

Description of Activity

The class receives a lesson in reproduction. Demonstrate how any one or all of the above animals reproduce. A chick comes from an egg that is laid by the mother hen. Fish come from a fertilized egg that is in their mother's body, for example. Identify similarities in human families.

Questions for Discussion

- How are babies similar to their parents?
- How are they like other species?
- How are they different from other species?

Homework

Children, with parents' help, collect pictures of a variety of animals and human families that resemble each other.

Evaluation

You can use a rubric or scale that includes the following criteria for measuring learner outcomes. For a grade of

A, students will be able to

- Identify at least four ways human babies are similar to their parent(s)
- Identify at least three ways they are similar to rabbits, gerbils, or other animals
- Identify at least two ways they are different from the other species above
- Simply explain that an egg and sperm that meet begin the development of a baby
- Identify where the baby grows
- Correctly spell all of the new words the teacher chooses from the activity

B, students will be able to

- Identify only three ways human babies are similar to their parent(s)
- Identify only two ways they are similar to rabbits, gerbils, or other animals
- Identify only one way they are different from the other species above
- Simply explain that an egg and sperm that meet begin the development of a baby
- Identify where the baby grows
- Correctly spell most of the new words the teacher chooses from the activity

C, students will be able to

- Identify only two ways human babies are similar to their parent(s)
- Identify only one way they are similar to rabbits, gerbils, or other animals
- Identify only one way they are different from the other species above
- Simply explain that an egg and sperm that meet begin the development of a baby and identify where the baby grows
- Correctly spell some of the new words the teacher chooses from the activity

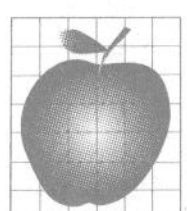

Learning Experience 7-2 continued

D, students will

- Identify only one way human babies are similar to their parent(s)
- Identify only one way they are similar to rabbits, gerbils, or other animals
- Not be able to identify ways they are different from the other species above
- Not be able to simply explain that an egg and sperm that meet begin the development of a baby
- Not be able to identify where the baby grows
- Correctly spell only one or two of the new words the teacher chooses from the activity

Learning Experience 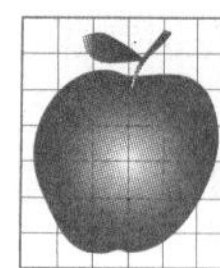 7-3

Two Families

Grade Level

3–4

Primary Disciplines

Math, Social Studies, Spelling

Learning Objectives

Following this activity, students will be able to

- List the different numbers of people in different families.
- Show how family composition can change.

Time Required

One session (45 minutes)

Materials

Posterboard with pictures of families of different sizes, name signs for family members, number cards to mount next to each family

Description of Activity

Read the following story to the class:

I'd like you to meet two families, Family A and Family B. Family A is composed of Grandma A and Grandpa A. Family B is composed of Father B, Mother B, and their daughter, Beverly. How many people are in each family? How many people are in both families together?

One day Grandma A receives a phone call from her daughter Dorothy and son-in-law Sam. They are moving to Grandma A's town, and Grandma A invites them to come and live with her and Grandpa A until they find a home of their own. Sam and Dorothy move in with Grandma A and Grandpa A.

The B family changes, too. Mother B is pregnant; she goes to the hospital and comes home with a new baby brother for Beverly. Soon after that, they move into a new house. How have the families changed?

Beverly recently graduated from college and got a job in her college town. She moved out of Sam and Dorothy's house but, younger brother still lives at home. How many people now live in Sam and Dorothy's house?

Grandma A gets another phone call, this time from a dear friend, Sarah C, whose husband had just died. Sarah C doesn't like living by herself. Grandma A invites Sarah C to come and live with her and Grandpa A. How many people are in Grandma A's family now?

The children identify their own family members. They discuss how the families in the story change with friends and relatives moving in and out. They discuss how families might change.

Homework

The students ask their parents how their families have changed over the years.

Evaluation

You can use a rubric or scale that includes the following criteria for measuring learner outcomes. For a grade of

A, students will

- Know how to describe all of the members of a nuclear family
- Be able to accurately count and add the numbers of family members in Family A, in Family B, and the total of both families by the end of the story
- Be able to identify at least two ways by which families can change in size

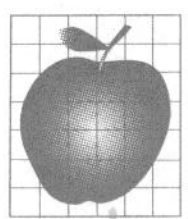

Learning Experience 7-3 continued

- Be able to identify the members of their family
- Correctly spell all of the new words from the exercise (including family titles)

B, students will

- Know how to describe most of the members of a nuclear family
- Be able to accurately count and add the numbers of the family members in Family A, in Family B, and the total of both families by the end of the story
- Be able to identify only one way by which families can change in size
- Correctly spell most of the new words from the exercise (including family titles)

C, students will

- Know how to describe some of the members of a nuclear family
- Be able to accurately count and add the numbers of the family members in Family A and in Family B, but not the total of both families by the end of the story
- Be able to identify only one way by which families can change in size
- Be able to identify the members of their own family
- Correctly spell some of the new words from the exercise (including family titles)

D, students will

- Not know how to describe the members of a nuclear family
- Accurately count and add the numbers of the family members in Family A and in Family B, but not the total of both families by the end of the story
- Identify only one way by which families can change in size
- Be able to identify the members of their own family
- Not be able to spell the new words from the exercise (including family titles)

Learning Experience 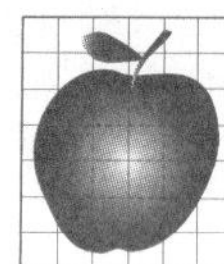 7-4

Qualities of a Friend

Grade Level

3–4

Primary Disciplines

Social Studies, Writing

Learning Objectives

Following this activity, students will be able to

- Explain the importance of friendships.
- List the qualities of a good friend.

Time Required

Two sessions (90 minutes total)

Materials

Pencil and paper

Description of Activity

The students brainstorm the qualities of a good friend; from this, the teacher generates a comprehensive list on the board. The class copies the same list on paper. The class explores the qualities listed in more depth. In small groups they tell a story about a good friend of theirs or their family's that shows the qualities they have identified above.

Homework

The students invite family members to add to the list of qualities of a friend.

Evaluation

You can use a rubric or scale that includes the following criteria for measuring learner outcomes. For a grade of

A, students will be able to

- Identify at least four qualities of a good friend
- Identify at least four qualities they possess that make them a good friend
- Correctly copy the list from the board using good penmanship
- Make up a story that identifies at least four of the qualities of a good friend

B, students will be able to

- Identify only three qualities of a good friend
- Identify only three qualities they possess that make them a good friend
- Correctly copy the list from the board using good penmanship
- Make up a story that identifies a least three of the qualities of a good friend

C, students will be able to

- Identify only two qualities of a good friend
- Identify only two qualities they possess that make them a good friend
- Correctly copy the list from the board using good penmanship
- Make up a story that identifies only two of the qualities of a good friend

D, students will be able to

- Identify only one quality of a good friend
- Identify only one quality they possess that makes them a good friend
- Correctly copy the list from the board with weak penmanship skills
- Make up a story that identifies only one quality of a good friend

Learning Experience 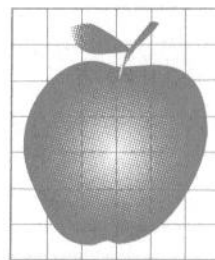 7-5

Family Responsibilities

Grade Level

3–4

Primary Discipline

Social Science, Language Arts

Learning Objectives

Following this activity, students will be able to describe the various responsibilities of each family member.

Time Required

One session

Materials

List of family responsibilities, list of family members, handout

Description of Activity

Distribute the list of family responsibilities shown on page 234.

Questions for Discussion

- Who is the person in your family responsible for you?
- Who has the most responsibility?
- Who has the least responsibility?
- Which responsibilities belong to you?
- How were these responsibilities assigned? Did the same family member always have the same responsibilities?
- Which responsibilities are performed by both men and women, boys and girls?

Homework

Students ask their parent(s) who is responsible for each task. Students ask parents to identify their responsibilities when they were children.

Evaluation

You can use a rubric or scale that includes the following criteria for measuring learner outcomes. For a grade of

A, students will be able to explain/define responsibility by

- Listing at least five responsibilities that family members have to each other and the family
- Describing which family members in their family have each responsibility
- Describing at least three ways by which family responsibilities can change
- Give at least three examples of how families differ from their own in dispersing of their roles
- Consistently show evidence in their writing and verbal assignments of their understanding that, in some families, gender does not necessarily define family responsibility

B, students will be able to explain/define responsibility by

- Making a list of only four responsibilities that family members have to each other and the family
- Describing which members in their family have each responsibility
- Describing only two ways by which family responsibilities can change
- Giving only two examples of how families differ from their own in dispersing of their roles
- Mostly showing evidence in their writing and verbal assignments of their understanding that, in some families, gender does not necessarily define family responsibility

C, students will be able to explain/define responsibility by

- Making a list of a least two responsibilities that family members have to each other and the family
- Being unable to describe how most of the responsibilities in his/her family were dispersed
- Describing only one way by which family responsibilities can change
- Being able to give only one example of how families differ from their own in dispersing of their roles

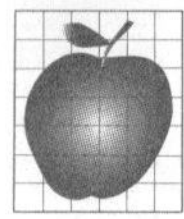

Learning Experience 7-5 continued

- Showing little evidence in their writing and verbal assignments of their developing an understanding that, in some families, gender does not necessarily define family responsibility

D, students will

- Be able to explain/define responsibility by identifying only one responsibility that family members have to each other and the family
- Not be able to describe how most of the responsibilities in his/her family were dispersed
- Be able to explain/define responsibility by describing only one way by which family responsibilities can change
- Not be able to give examples of how families differ from their own in dispersing of their roles
- Not be able to show evidence in their writing and verbal assignments their understanding that, in some families, gender does not describe family responsibility

Family Responsibilities

_________________ Keeps the house clean

_________________ Buys groceries

_________________ Works outside of the home

_________________ Helps with chores

_________________ Does the dishes

_________________ Picks up toys

_________________ Hangs up clothes

_________________ Washes/irons clothes

_________________ Cooks meals

_________________ Mows the lawn

_________________ Takes out trash

_________________ Takes care of children

_________________ Earns money

_________________ Fixes things

_________________ Makes the beds

_________________ Feeds pets

_________________ Weeds the flowers

Learning Experience 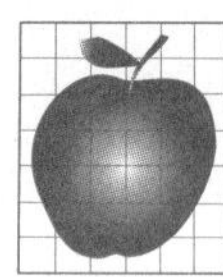 7-6

Benefits of Being in a Family

Grade Level

3–4

Primary Discipline

Social Studies, Language Arts

Learning Objectives

Following this activity, students will be able to describe the benefits of being a family member.

Time Required

One session

Materials

List of family benefits

Description of Activity

In small groups, the students discuss how they benefit from being in a family, using the following list, which is written on the board.

1. Love and affection
2. Security
3. Comfort
4. Belonging
5. Companionship
6. Friendship
7. Food, clothes, shelter
8. Problem solving

Choose a story about a family from the culture the class is studying in Social Studies. The students read the story and describe which of the characteristics could be found in the family in the story.

Homework

Students generate their own list of family benefits.

Evaluation

You can use a rubric or scale that includes the following criteria for measuring learner outcomes. For a grade of

A, students will be able to

- Explain all of the characteristics on the above list
- Describe at least four ways students benefit from being in their own family
- Identify at least four characteristics from the list in the chosen story

B, students will be able to

- Explain most of the characteristics on the list supplied
- Describe only three ways students benefit from being in his/her own family
- Identify only three characteristics from the list in the chosen story

C, students will be able to

- Explain some of the characteristics on the list supplied
- Describe only two ways students benefit from being in his/her own family
- Identify only two characteristics from the list in the chosen story

D, student will not be able to

- Explain one or two of the characteristics on the list supplied
- Describe only one way students benefit from being in his/her own family
- Identify only one characteristic from the list in the chosen story

Learning Experience 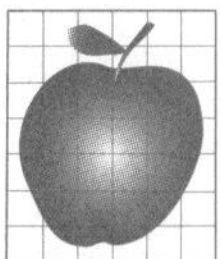 7-7

Growth and Development: Puberty

Grade Level

5–6

Primary Discipline

Science

Learning Objectives

Following this activity, students will be able to

- Describe how the body grows.
- List the changes associated with puberty.
- Identify the gender differences as boys and girls grow.

Time Required

Two sessions (90 minutes total)

Materials

Bulletin board, pictures of student when they were babies or young, slips of paper with each student's name

Description of Activity

Students bring in baby pictures of themselves and a picture of a parent or close relative of the same sex without showing them to others in the class. You (the teacher) number the pictures and place them on the bulletin board. The students try to identify the students from their pictures and their parents. On a piece of paper they write the numbers on the pictures and the names of the students they think are a match.

Place the correct name next to each picture on the bulletin board so the students can see how many they identified correctly. The class discusses how the students have changed since the pictures were taken and how they still must change to look like their parent(s). The class lists the changes involved for girls and boys in growing up.

Homework

Students collect baby pictures several days before this activity.

Evaluation

You can use a rubric or scale that includes the following criteria for measuring learner outcomes. For a grade of

A, students will be able to

- Identify at least five ways parents and children in a family may be alike
- Identify at least five ways parents and children in a family may be different
- Explain at least four changes that occur during puberty for girls and for boys
- Identify at least four similarities between males and females
- Identify at least three differences between males and females

B, students will be able to

- Identify only four ways parents and children in a family may be alike
- Identify only four ways parents and children in a family may be different
- Explain only three changes that occur during puberty for girls and for boys
- Identify only three similarities between males and females
- Identify only two differences between males and females

C, students will be able to

- Identify only three ways parents and children in a family may be alike
- Identify only three ways parents and children in a family may be different
- Explain only two changes that occur during puberty for girls and for boys
- Identify only two similarities between males and females
- Identify only one difference between males and females

D, students will

- Identify only one way parents and children in a family may be alike
- Identify only one way parents and children in a family may be different
- Explain only one change that occurs during puberty for girls and for boys
- Identify only one similarity between males and females
- Identify only one difference between males and females

Learning Experience 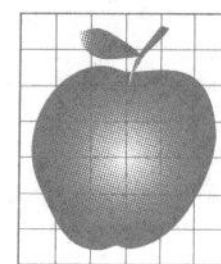 7-8

Whom Can I Ask?

Grade Level

5–6

Primary Disciplines

English, Social Studies

Learning Objectives

Following this activity, students will be able to

- List sources of information on sexuality and family life.
- Evaluate the quality and accuracy of each source.

Time Required

One session

Materials

List of possible sources of information and examples of material from each of these sources

Description of Activity

The students each develop a list of places where they can get information about sexuality. They then prioritize their own list based on how accurate they think the information is.

The students pair off in twos or threes and, from the combined lists, come up with three or four sources they trust the most for accuracy. The students report to class the reasons they think these sources are accurate.

In a full class discussion, have a student from each group report his or her group's reasons; you (the teacher) list the top three sources from each group on the board. If the class has omitted any important sources, add them to the list and ask the students to discuss why they are accurate sources. Some of the following should be included: Internet, movies, TV, magazines, the teacher, priest/rabbi/minister, friends, parents, older brothers or sisters, books from local library, doctor, newspaper columns (Dear Abby and the like), textbooks.

Homework

The students bring in two samples of materials or information about a health topic that they can trust and have them identify why the material is reliable.

Evaluation

Have the students write a brief essay in class about a person who finds out he/she has an illness. They are instructed to include information about where these people went for help; how they selected the services, what information they were able to gather about their illness, where they got the information, and how they knew it was reliable. Before the students submit their essays, they are to develop a rubric or list of criteria, in consultation with the teacher, that will be used to evaluate their essay, indicating the level at which they know where to go for services and how to assess the quality of services and information (for example: How many services should they identify? How many qualities should they identify?).

Learning Experience 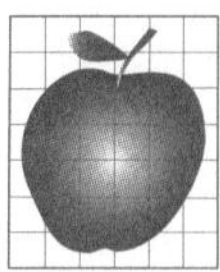 7-9

A Want Ad for a Friend

Grade Level

5–6

Primary Disciplines

Language Arts, Social Studies

Learning Objectives

Following this activity, students will be able to

- List the qualities that make a good friend.
- List qualities they have that make them a good friend.
- Recognize, develop, and maintain healthful relationships.

Time Required

Two sessions (90 minutes total)

Materials

Newspapers and magazines with samples of want ads for "nanny" and "companion for elderly person," pencil and paper

Description of Activity

Review with the class the qualities that the prospective employer desires in a nanny or companion. In pairs or triads, the students select one want ad they think is a good example. They identify the components of the ad that are clearly stated, persuasive, and well-communicated.

The students, in their groups, brainstorm the qualities they think are important in a good friend. Using the want ads they reviewed and selected from the newspapers and magazines as a basis, they construct a similar ad for a friend they believe would be most desirable to them. List, on the board, the qualities that each group identifies as important in a good friend. Suggest qualities the students have omitted, such as a person who likes himself/herself, someone you can trust, someone who speaks well of his/her own family member, someone who has his/her own mindset and is not easily persuaded by others, someone who has goals, someone who does not use alcohol or other drugs, someone who is loyal, and so on.

The students each write a brief response to their own want ads, describing the characteristics they have that would make them eligible for the friendship. The groups share their responses with one another and decide (if they can) which one of them they would choose if they were to receive these responses in the mail.

Looking at the qualities on the board, the students each select the five qualities most important to them. Collect the anonymous lists and tally them, identifying what the class thinks are the most important qualities for a friendship.

Homework

Students collect want ads from newspapers and magazines that are advertising for a nanny or a companion for an elderly person.

Evaluation

You can use a rubric or scale that includes the following criteria for measuring learner outcomes. For a grade of

A, students

- Choose an ad that includes at least three of the criteria that make an ad effective
- Can identify at least five qualities of a good friendship
- Can construct an ad that indicates knowledge of effective criteria of friendship and also includes strong, persuasive statements, clarity of communication, correctly spelled words, creative design, and the like

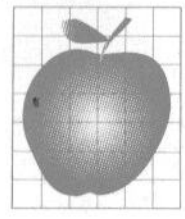

Learning Experience 7-9 continued

- Can explain the criteria that make them a good friend and give an effective example of each

B, students

- Choose an ad that includes only two of the criteria that make an ad effective
- Can identify only four qualities of a good friendship
- Can construct an ad that indicates knowledge of effective criteria of friendship and also includes some persuasive statements, clarity of communication, correctly spelled words, creative design, and the like
- Can identify the criteria that make them a good friend and give an example of or effectively explain only two of the criteria

C, students

- Choose an ad that includes only two of the criteria that make an ad effective
- Can identify only three qualities of a good friendship
- Can construct an ad that indicates knowledge of effective criteria of friendship and includes a few persuasive statements, some clarity of communication, some correctly spelled words, some creative design, and the like
- Can identify the criteria that make them a good friend and give an example of or effectively explain only two of the criteria

D, students

- Choose an ad that includes only one of the criteria that make an ad effective
- Can identify only two qualities of a good friendship
- Construct an ad that indicates knowledge of effective criteria of friendship in which the statements do not clearly communicate and are not persuasive statements, correctly spelled, or creatively designed
- Cannot identify the criteria that make a good friend; can give an example of or effectively explain only one of the criteria

Learning Experience 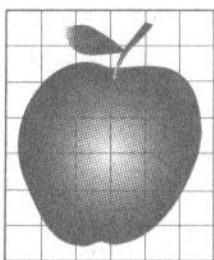 7-10

Gender Roles and Careers

Grade Level

3–4

Primary Disciplines

Spelling, Writing

Learning Objectives

Following this activity, students will be able to

- Identify career options that have no gender bias.
- Describe the limitations of stereotypical gender roles.
- Describe non-gender stereotypical roles and behaviors.

Time Required

1–2 hours

Materials

Magazines of all kinds (men's, women's, children's, careers, and so on), newspapers, scissors, paste, several large poster sheets, crayons or felt-tip pens

Description of Activity

The class is divided into four groups: one group of all boys, one group of all girls, and two groups of boys and girls. Each group is given some magazines, newspapers, scissors, and paste. Each group is given a large poster sheet as follows: the boy group and one boy/girl group gets a picture of a woman at the top; the girl group and the other boy/girl group gets a picture with a man at the top. Pictures include men and women at work, at play, in sports, with musical instruments, with cars, and so on.

The students in each group prepare a collage describing women or men (depending upon their poster sheet). When the collages are finished, the teacher hangs them around the room.

Questions for Discussion

- What are the differences and similarities between the men's and women's pictures?
- Which pictures are not on both poster sheets. Could they be?
- The students develop a list of jobs they think only women can do and jobs only men can do. They discuss what it is about the gender that restricts the opposite gender from doing those jobs. The students share with each other the types of jobs their family members do outside the home and inside the home. Which could the opposite gender do?

Homework

Each child brings at least three magazines to school. After the exercise, each child prepares a small collage with pictures of men and women doing the same jobs, playing the same games, and so on.

Evaluation

You can use a rubric or scale that includes the following criteria for measuring learner outcomes. For a grade of

A, the poster sheets show that students can identify

- at least five jobs, four sports, and four musical instruments that either males or females can do
- at least four characteristics that are different for males and females
- at least four characteristics that are similar for males and females
- at least three jobs done at home by a woman that can be done by a man, and visa versa

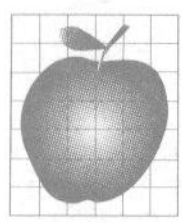

Learning Experience 7-10 continued

B, the poster sheets show that students can identify

- only four jobs, three sports, and three musical instruments that either males or females can do
- only three characteristics that are different for males and females
- only three characteristics that are similar for males and females
- only two jobs done at home by a woman that can be done by a man, and visa versa

C, the poster sheets show that students can identify

- only three jobs, two sports, and two musical instruments that either males or females can do
- only two characteristics that are different for males and females
- only two characteristics that are similar for males and females
- only two jobs done at home by a woman that can be done by a man, and visa versa

D, the poster sheets show that students can identify

- only one job, one sport, and one musical instrument that either males or females can do
- only one characteristic that is different for males and females
- only one characteristic that is similar for males and females
- only one job done at home by a woman that can be done by a man, and visa versa

Learning Experience 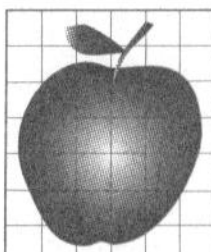 7-11

Changing Friendships

Grade Level

5–6

Primary Disciplines

English/Writing

Learning Objectives

Following this activity, students will be able to

- Describe the qualities of a good relationship and the ways that relationships change.
- List the feelings people have when they are hurt by a relationship that dissolves.
- Describe effective strategies for ending or changing a relationship.

Time Required

1 hour

Materials

Paper and pencil

Description of Activity

Read the following story to the class and then have the students answer the questions:

Scott and Jon were the very best of friends from kindergarten to fifth grade. They played sports together on the same teams. They went to summer camp together and often slept over at each other's houses. They lived around the corner from one another and walked to and from school together on most days.

Some time around fifth grade Scott became friendly with Alex, but Jon and Alex didn't get along too well. Alex was a very popular kid. He was tall and strong, and the girls in school thought he was very handsome. He was a sixth grader and the captain of the baseball team that Scott and Jon played for.

One night Alex asked Scott if he wanted to sleep over, and Scott did. Jon was hurt and angry at Scott because Jon thought they had plans for the same night. Scott thought Jon was sleeping over the following night, and Jon said no.

Scott was interested in girls and wanted to have a girlfriend like Alex did. Scott was particularly interested in Ilene. Jon thought girls were dumb, and he didn't want any part of the parties and other activities that Scott was becoming interested in. Jon kept telling Scott how dumb it was to be interested in hanging out with girls. Scott and Jon were arguing a lot.

Questions for Discussion

- If you had to choose whose behavior you like most, whom would you choose? Why?
- If you had to choose whose behavior you dislike most, whom would you choose? Why?
- What do you think is happening between Jon and Scott?
- What would you do if you were Jon?
- What would you do if you were Scott?
- If you wanted to change this relationship, what would you do?

Homework

Each student writes a story about two friends whose relationship has changed.

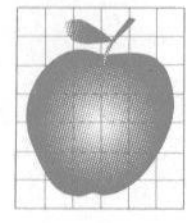

Learning Experience 7-11 continued

Evaluation

The teacher can use a rubric or scale that includes the following criteria for measuring learner outcomes. For a grade of

A, the students can

- Effectively explain why they favor one behavior from the story over another
- Effectively explain why they dislike a certain behavior from the story
- Identify at least four qualities that make for a good relationship
- Describe at least three ways relationships change
- Identify at least three emotions one feels when a relationship dissolves
- Explain at least three things they can do to minimize the hurt when ending a relationship

B, the students can

- Effectively explain why they favor one behavior from the story over another
- Effectively explain why they dislike a certain behavior from the story
- Identify only three qualities that make for a good relationship
- Describe only two ways relationships change
- Identify only two emotions one feels when a relationship dissolves
- Explain only two things they can do to minimize the hurt when ending a relationship

C, the students can

- More or less explain why they favor one behavior from the story over another
- More or less explain, why they dislike a certain behavior from the story
- Identify only two qualities that make for a good relationship
- Describe only one way relationships change
- Identify only one emotion one feels when a relationship dissolves
- Explain only two things they can do to minimize the hurt when ending a relationship

D, the students

- Cannot effectively explain why they dislike a certain behavior from the story
- Can identify only two qualities that make for a good relationship
- Can describe only one way relationships change
- Can identify only one emotion one feels when a relationship dissolves
- Can explain only one thing they can do to minimize the hurt when ending a relationship

Learning Experience 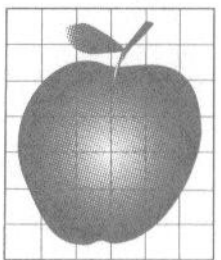 7-12

Egg Babies

Grade Level

3–6

Primary Disciplines

Social Studies, Mathematics, Language Arts

Learning Objectives

Following this activity, students will be able to

- List different cultural customs associated with newborns.
- Describe the tasks associated with caring for a baby.
- Describe how families change when babies are born.
- List the factors people consider when they make a decision to have a baby.

Time Required

3–4 grade level: 1 week total
5–6 grade level: 2 weeks total

Materials

Medium boiled eggs; small cartons from fruit stores (ones that hold berries or tomatoes); cotton or tissue paper, paint; script money; first aid equipment including bandages, glue, splints, poison antidotes, antibacterial ointment, Tylenol, burn spray, and so on

Description of Activity

In grades 3–4, each student receives an egg and pretends it is his/her baby. In grades 5–6, the students are paired and each pair receives an egg.

The students use the materials provided to create and decorate a "crib" or carrying case for their baby. An "egg baby hospital" is set up in one corner of the room. One student is assigned to be the doctor and one to be the nurse for each session devoted to this activity. (Be sure that gender does not influence who is the doctor and who is the nurse.)

Instructions to individual students or pairs of students are as follows:

1. Pretend that this egg is your baby. You will be responsible for the baby at all times. It cannot leave your (or your partner's) side unless you have made other arrangements for someone to take care of it. It must sleep in your room and come to school with you.
2. You must choose a name for the baby. In a brief paper, describe how you chose the name and whom (if anyone) you named the baby for. Ask your parents how their own names were chosen. In class, discuss how different cultural, religious, and ethnic groups choose names and follow traditions surrounding birth and babies.
3. Bring in the list of the things you would have bought for the baby along with the prices of each item and the total price (see Homework).
4. Visit the pretend hospital to check on the baby's health. If an egg is dropped, bring the baby to the hospital for emergency attention. Keep track of the costs for medical care.

At the end of the period allotted for the activity, discuss the list of tasks (done as Homework) that have to be done when a baby comes to live in a home. Discuss how these tasks were (are) done in the student's own family.

Questions for Discussion

- What was your overall reaction to having the responsibility designated in this activity?
- What did you learn from this activity?
- How do families change when a new baby arrives?
- How do families decide who does what tasks in caring for a baby?
- What are some things people need to think about before they have babies?

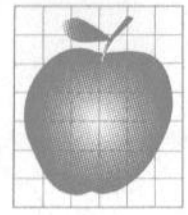

Learning Experience 7-12 continued

Homework

Students will generate a list of things that must be done in any one day to care for a baby (feeding, changing diapers, bathing, playing with, buying things for, washing clothes, and so on). Students go to the supermarket with a parent or other adult and pretend to buy one day's food and diapers, wipes, and other supplies for the baby; they then write up the information (including cost of items) to bring to class.

Evaluation

In a paper and pencil test, ask the students to identify at least five things that have to be done every day in caring for a newborn and three ways families change when a baby comes. In a matching test, have the students match the chores with the approximate amount of time required to do each of them.

After the homework assignment, each student tells a story about how people in his/her family were assigned their names. Evaluate the story based on the students' developmental ability to articulate or communicate their story, including how clear and concise they are, how creative and enthusiastic they are, and the like. When the class is over, have each student describe (in one sentence each) at least three ways families decide on babies' names.

Have the students develop a list of important items that have to be bought for babies and, based upon the homework assignments posted around the classroom, identify approximately how much each item might cost. Grade the students on their ability to correctly spell the items and add the total approximate cost.

Learning Experience 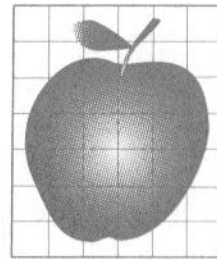 7-13

Babies in Families

Grade Level

5–6

Primary Discipline

Social Studies

Learning Objectives

Following this activity, students will be able to

- Describe baby care from a non-gender-biased perspective.
- Identify several different family constellations.

Time Required

1 hour

Materials

None

Description of Activity

The procedure is as follows:

1. Invite to the classroom a male parent, a female parent, and a parent couple who each have a young baby.
2. In preparation, have the students prepare (or bring from home) questions to ask of these parents (how they decided to have a baby, how having a baby has changed their lives, how having a baby has affected their family, how giving care is arranged in their family, and so on).
3. Send the list to the parents so they will be prepared to address each question.
4. When the parents are on hand, put the questions in a hat and have one student at a time select a question and read it.
5. After the parents have left, ask the students the following questions:
   a. What did you learn about these families?
   b. What are the similarities and differences between these families and your own family?

Homework

The students prepare a list of questions to ask the visiting parents.

Evaluation

After the parents have left, give the students a short quiz, asking that they identify four different family constellations and four roles people in the family play in caring for a baby.

Learning Experience 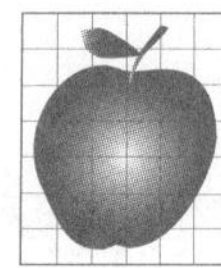 7-14

Role Plays

Grade Level

3–4, 5–6

Primary Disciplines

Reading, Drama

Learning Objectives

Following this activity, students will be able to

- List criteria they value in a "special" relationship.
- Communicate their dating interest in one another.
- Effectively refuse and receive a refusal of a dating request.

Time Required

1 hour

Materials

None

Description of Activity

The students are paired and asked to role-play the scenes listed below. The class discusses the various ways people can respond to each situation. (This activity can be used with all grade levels as long as the subject matter is developed appropriately for that level.) It provides students with opportunities to practice refusing skills.

1. Ask a classmate you like to go skating, rollerblading, or to a movie with you. The partners exchange accepting and refusing roles.
2. Ask a partner if you may kiss him or her. The partners agree or refuse.
3. Tell a partner why you like him or her and ask how he/she feels about you.

The students discuss why doing these things is difficult and what they learned from this activity. Then they develop a list of refusal strategies, which the teacher records on the board.

Homework

The students research dating customs in a foreign country that are different from those in the United States and write a paper about these customs, rules, and regulations.

Evaluation

You can use a rubric or scale that includes the following criteria for measuring learner outcomes. For a grade of

A, the student

- Shows a strong ability to ask for what he or she wants
- Shows a strong ability to accept a refusal
- Can clearly and firmly communicate refusals

B, the student

- Shows some ability to ask for what he or she wants
- Shows some ability to accept a refusal
- Can clearly communicate refusals but is not always firm

C, the student

- Shows a somewhat weak ability to ask for what he or she wants
- Shows a somewhat weak ability to accept a refusal
- Can communicate some refusals but is weak in communicating them

D, the student

- Is unable to clearly ask for what he or she wants
- Is weak in ability to accept a refusal
- Cannot communicate a refusal clearly

8

Childhood Stress

Efrem Rosen

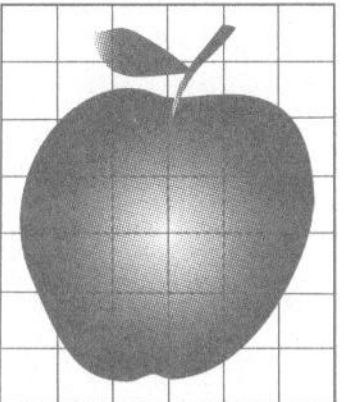

Chapter Outline

Objectives

- Learn about stress and its effects on the body
- Differentiate between eustress and distress
- Name the variables contributing to the individuality of the stress response
- Explain the fight-or-flight syndrome
- Identify the three stages of the general adaptation syndrome
- Describe how chronic stress contributes to disease
- Identify some sources of stress that apply specifically to children
- Describe positive and negative ways children cope with stress
- Differentiate common stressors by developmental level (K–6)
- Name some nutritional factors in stress
- Explain the relaxation response
- Describe the processes of meditation and yoga, progressive relaxation, deep breathing, autogenic training, and biofeedback

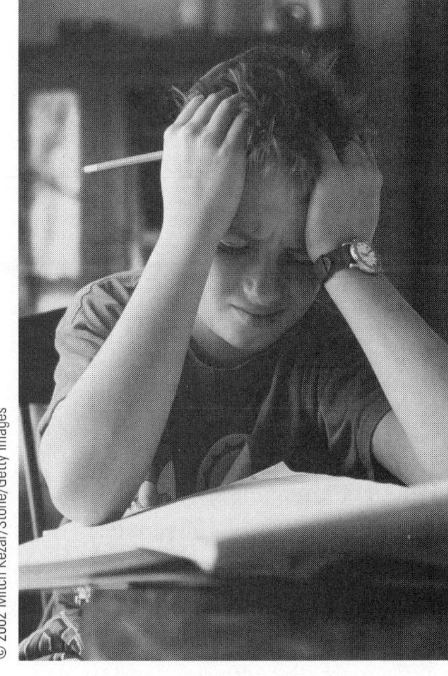

Tom was feeling very proud of himself as he walked into his sixth-grade class one bright Monday morning. He had an exciting weekend because the Little League baseball team on which he plays second base won the division title. Tom hit three for four—a double and two singles—adding significantly to the team's victory.

Shortly after he sat down in his usual seat, his teacher asked the students to put away their books and take out a sheet of paper. She was going to give a surprise test on the homework. The homework! In all the excitement, Tom had forgotten to do it. His vision blurred as he tried to think about the homework topic. His thoughts came quickly, like cars whizzing by on the highway. What was he going to do? How could he fail a test? It would ruin his grade average. His parents probably would not let him play on the baseball team any more.

He broke out in a cold sweat, his hands shaking, his breathing labored, his heart pounding. From the recesses of his brain, he heard the teacher say, "Put your name on the sheet of paper and fold it in half; number the left side from one to ten and the right side from eleven to twenty." He glanced around the room. His classmates were busy filling out the sheet of paper. What was going to happen to him?

The teacher then said, "Now fold the paper in half, and in half again, then in quarters, and throw it in the wastepaper basket." Tom could not believe her words. Why did she trick them into believing that they were going to have a test? Then she said, "Now you know what stress is!" Realizing what had happened and relieved as he threw the paper away, Tom sank into his seat, exhausted.

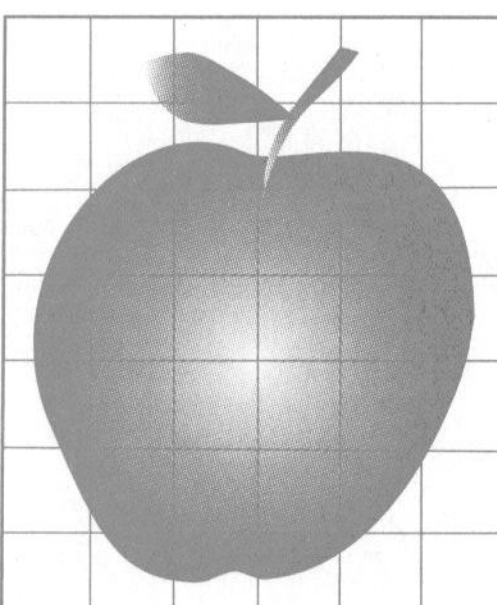

Hans Selye, considered to be the father of stress research, would say that Tom was indeed under stress. Selye defined **stress** as the state of the body that is affected by a wide variety of stimuli that cause a specific set of changes in the body. Stress is the nonspecific response of the body to any demand placed on it. "Nonspecific" means that the stress response is the same no matter what the source. Tom showed some of these changes characteristic of stress: excitement, faster heartbeat, sweating, blurred vision. The stimuli that produce these bodily changes are called **stressors**. (In Tom's case, stimuli came from, first, the excitement of winning the game and then from the prospect of failing a test.) The body is called upon to adjust to maintain its usual or "normal" balanced state, called **homeostasis**. Obviously, children are also vulnerable to stress and show stress responses in a variety of ways. Many adults tend to view children as happy, without a care in the world, and thus stress-free. But, as Tom made clear, children also experience stressors and respond to them.

History of Stress Research

Originally, the term "stress" was used in physics to describe the forces on an object that could bend or break it. Later, primarily because of Selye's research, it became associated with physical arousal and the mechanisms that enhance survival. Now it is more closely associated with the complexities of modern culture and living style that often result in illness and disease and claim the lives of millions of people. "Stress" is frequently used to describe the level of tension resulting from demands of the job, family responsibilities, and the complexities of relationships.

High technology and the living styles it drives have resulted in frequent exposure to stressors and the resulting decline of personal health. Stress is implicated as a factor in several health-related problems, including coronary heart disease, some cancers, the common cold, migraine headaches, ulcers, hypertension, and so on.

What Is Stress?

Who experiences stress? All people do! Stress is not confined to the business executive, the harried mother, or the child who is doing poorly in school. It affects everyone regardless of gender, age, ethnicity, occupation, or activity. Children are certainly not immune to it. Too much stimulation results in stress; the lack of stimulation, called "deprivational stress," can also produce a stress response. The body's response to the intensity, duration, and frequency of stress, not the exposure itself, is the salient feature of stress.

Manifestations of Stress

Common Physical Manifestations

Headache	Eye strain, blurred vision
Burning in the upper abdomen	Chest pain
Lower back pain	Shortness of breath
Knots in the shoulder	Reddening of the skin or face (blushing)
Hives, skin rash	Diarrhea, constipation
Fatigue	Recurring colds
Tightness in the back of the neck	
Stomachache	

Common Emotions and Behaviors

Anger	Anxiety
Boredom	Depression
Fear	Feeling bothered
Forgetfulness	Frustration
Feeling hurried	Indecisiveness
Irritability	Inability to concentrate
Nervous laughter	Lack of motivation
Nail biting	Loss of appetite
Overeating	Nervousness
Poor attention span	Being overly critical
Teeth grinding	Crying
Withdrawal	Feeling upset

The first event in the sequence is the stressor or stimulus, which can come from either external (environmental) or internal (thought processes or perceptions) sources. The second event (the stress) is the set of changes in the body that occurs as a direct consequence of the stressor. The third event is the body's adaptations or changes that attempt to counteract the stress and return the body to a normal state of homeostasis. Included in this stress response are the many behaviors and actions that help the body return to this stable state.

A three-year-old may show anxiety because Mom and Dad are too busy and may not be paying enough attention to satisfy his/her needs. A child's first school experience may be stressful because of the effects of separation. As children get older, social and school pressures (for example, sibling rivalry and peer pressure) create stress. In many cases, the stressors come from parents who have high expectations of their children, who may be unavailable when help is needed, or who punish behaviors without explanation or reason.

Stress manifests itself in a variety of ways. The list in the box above can be used for a diagnosis of stress.

Eustress and Distress

People cannot live without stress, nor should anyone want to. Stress is not necessarily bad or something people would want to eliminate. Good stress arises from situations that are exhilarating, inspiring, or simply enjoyable, such as falling in love, winning a game (as in Tom's case), getting a good grade on a test or feeling the excitement of a good book. This form of stress, called

eustress, can motivate people, especially children, to reach their goals or complete tasks. Negative stress, called **distress**, in contrast, can lead to physical or psychological overload (breakdown) if it occurs chronically and without relief. Distress, usually just called "stress," is potentially harmful, especially if it lingers. In Tom's case, the distress was short-lived.

Both eustress and distress can be acute (one time only) or chronic (repeated over time). A sudden screeching of the brakes of a car nearby and the sirens of fire engines are obvious examples that can result in acute distress. Repeatedly being scolded by a parent or a teacher and just living in a crowded, noisy city are other, less obvious, examples of stressful situations that can result in chronic distress, which can be accompanied by emotional and physical problems. Sometimes, if severe, such distress can create emotional trauma and the potential for suicide. The box on page 271 lists the common exterior manifestations of stress.

Whether the stressor produces eustress or distress, the response of the body is the same and depends on the qualities of the stressor itself. The ability to cope and return to homeostasis, however, tends to be easier with eustress than with distress, because the former requires less energy. Fun or partying can be exhausting, but recovery is quicker and usually produces fond memories.

Stressors

Stressors encompass a wide variety of stimuli that affect the body by producing stress. Some stressors are produced by the physical environment, such as extreme temperature changes of hot or cold or being caught in a snowstorm or thunderstorm. Today, we recognize that a great many stressors are psychological. These can be divided into three categories:

1. A real or actual stressor. A change in the environment that is perceived as stressful. Again, these stressors may be either good or bad. For example, getting a high grade or a low grade on a test might be equally stressful.
2. The anticipation of an event or activity. Simply thinking about it can produce anxiety. Worrying about a test is an example.
3. Events or actions that are totally imagined, as in dreaming or fantasizing, can result in emotional responses. Worrying about what a parent will think about a child's behavior can produce a lot of stress.[1]

Degrees of Stress

The degree of stress produced depends on three characteristics of the stressor: frequency, intensity, and duration. Frequency refers to how often, over time, the stressor repeats. It may happen only once or it may repeat over time. Intensity is the strength of the stressor, how much impact it has, whether real or imagined. The duration of the stressor is how long it lasts. It may be a fleeting thought or a drawn-out nightmare. Also to be considered is the number of stressors occurring at the same time, also called summation.

The Individuality of Stress Response

Children's responses to stress vary widely because of the individualized or variable nature of the stressors and the body's level of responses to them. These variables, which are interrelated, are influenced by the following factors:

1. **Genetics**. With the exception of identical twins, no two people have the same set of genes. Because genes control the basic body plan, including the nervous and endocrine systems, people have individual responses to stressors.
2. **Experience**. A law of physics says that no two objects can occupy the same space at the same time. In the same way, because no two people are in the same position in the world at the same time, they cannot experience stressors in exactly the same way. Past experience with stressors modifies the way a given person mediates and responds to the stressors.
3. **Culture**. People are brought up in different cultures with different values and customs. Culture can categorize stressors as anything from meaningful to insignificant. These cultural differences can affect an individual's responses to stress.
4. **Body senses**. The body receives stressors through the sense receptors (seeing, hearing, smell, taste, touch). Each sense has its own way of getting information from the environment. This ability is controlled by genes and modified by experience and development. The senses are fine-tuned by experience, ability, and interest, resulting in greater sensitivity. Some people are hearing-focused, and others are visually-focused. No two people are alike in the way they process and respond to information from the environment.
5. **Development**. Children grow and age differently. As they mature, they can become limited in their ability to receive information from the outside world. Some of these differences can be modified by applying medicine and technology (for example, eyeglasses, hearing aids, computers).

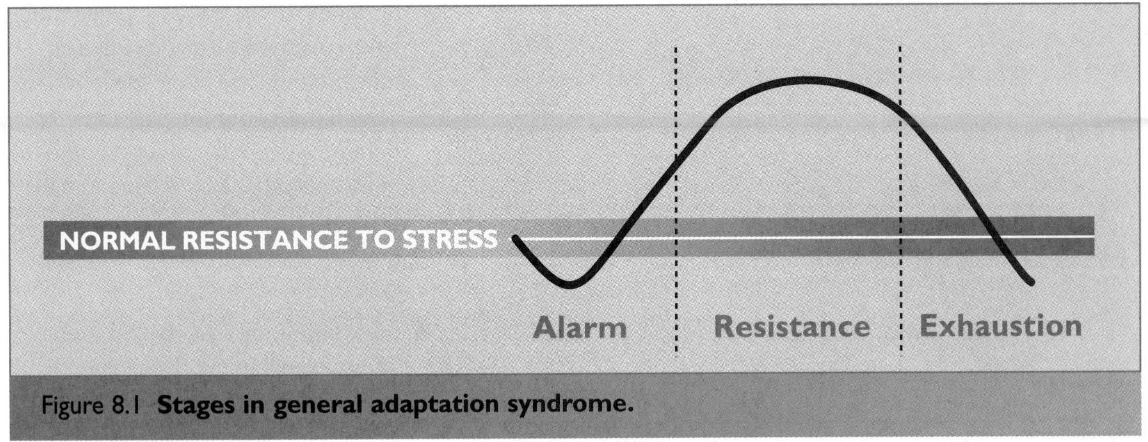

Figure 8.1 **Stages in general adaptation syndrome.**

6. **Brain function**. Children are both physical and psychological beings. The ability of a child's brain to interpret the environment depends on all of the above factors and, in addition, on how the emotions and mental state affect their responses.
7. **Personality**. People have many personality traits (introverted and shy or extroverted and socially confident, insecure or self-assured, leader or follower). One method of classifying personality types uses the categories **Type A** (described as hard-driving, competitive, aggressive, easily angered, unable to relax, and prone to stress-related diseases) and, at the other extreme, **Type B** (described as laid-back, easy-going, relaxed, and rarely angered). Most children fall between these two extremes.

Each of these seven factors interact in complex ways. Thus, predicting or generalizing about how people or children react to stress is difficult. Yet we can note that, for instance, children who are sick are more likely to have experienced stressful life events within the year prior to their illness and, if the stress levels are high, they are more likely to have accidents than healthy or low-stressed children.

Fight or Flight

When presented with a stressor, the body prepares itself for one of two courses of immediate action: to attack and fight to defend oneself, or to withdraw, running and hiding to escape from a real or perceived threat. This is called the fight-or-flight response. The fight response can be triggered by anger or aggression in defense of one's personal space or property and requires the mobilization of energy, both physical and psychological, usually resulting in confrontation or active combat. Conversely, the flight response is triggered by fear, either real or imagined, and usually results in fleeing or hiding. However, regardless of whether the specific response is fight or flight, the physical changes in the body are the same. They occur in three stages, collectively known as the general adaptation syndrome, depicted in Figure 8.1 and described below.

General Adaptation Syndrome (GAS)

By administering high doses of stressors, such as cold temperature shock to experimental rats over long periods, Selye was able to describe for the first time the physiological responses to stress.[2] Some of these changes are subtle physiological adaptations, and others are much more overt, sometimes ending in pathology. Selye called this sequence of bodily changes the **general adaptation syndrome**. These changes occur in three stages: the general alarm reaction, the stage of resistance, and the stage of exhaustion. This sequence helps to explain the relationship between stress and disease.

General Alarm Reaction

Stressors in the form of stimuli from one or more of the five senses (sight, sound, smell, touch, taste) are sent to the brain for processing. If the stressor is interpreted to be a potential threat, the brain activates three body systems —the central nervous, autonomic (or visceral), and endocrine (or hormonal) —to quickly prepare for fight or flight. In the opening vignette, Tom was experiencing these changes. These systems respond in fractions of a second and stay activated until the threat is over or the stressor is removed. The sequence of the alarm stage of the general adaptation syndrome is diagrammed in Figure 8.2.

1. The quickest of the three systems, the central nervous system (the brain and spinal cord) produces fast reflex reactions and awareness of what is happening and is responsible for the rapid activity of the

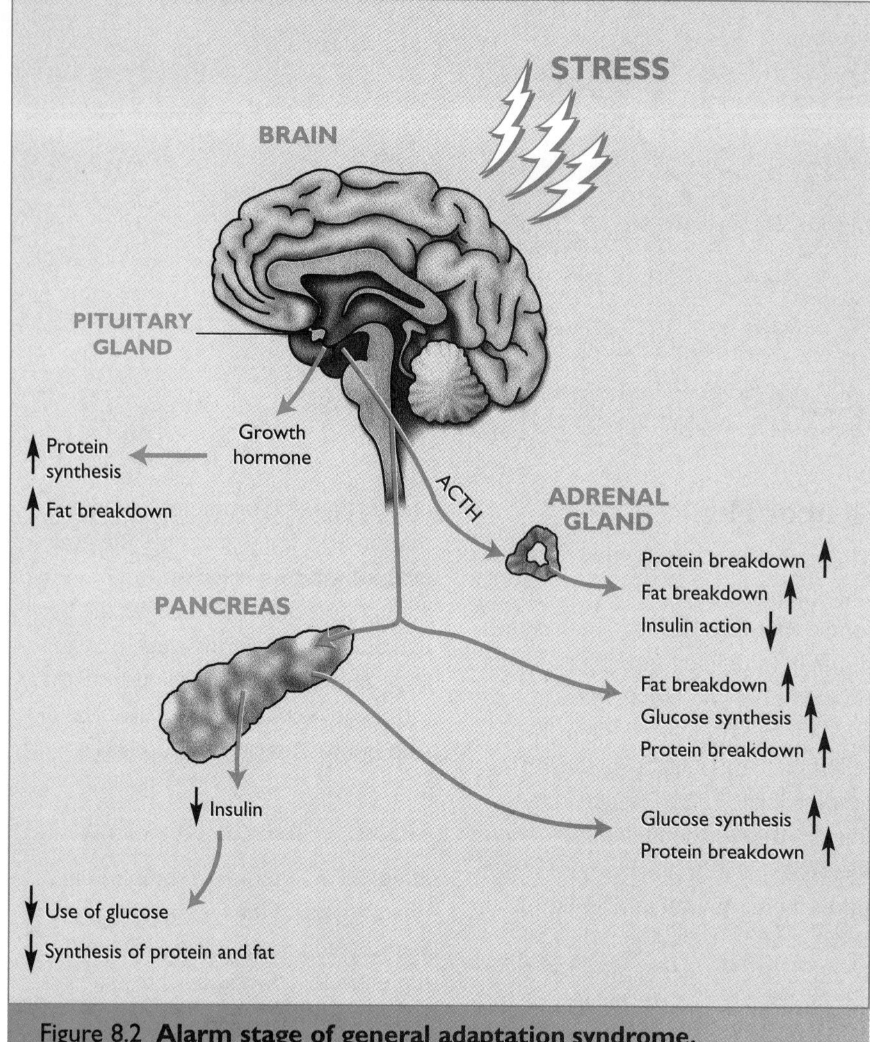

Figure 8.2 **Alarm stage of general adaptation syndrome.**

voluntary muscles resulting in behavioral responses. It also liberates adrenaline, the stress hormone, from nerve endings.

2. The second system, the autonomic nervous system, makes connections between the brain and the internal organs such as the intestine, heart, lungs, kidneys, and glands. These result in increased respiration, elevated blood pressure and heart rate, sweating, pupil dilation, and other physical responses.
3. The **endocrine system**, the slowest to react, is activated by the continued presence of the stressor and releases hormones from the adrenal gland (adrenal steroids and adrenaline) (see Figure 8.2).

In school, children may experience several of these changes on a short-term basis when they are exposed to new and complicated information, when they fight with one another, when they are overloaded with homework, and so on. If they resolve the stress and eliminate the stressor, the effects will be only short-term.

Exposure to chronic stress continuously elicits the general alarm reaction above and causes these characteristic changes in the body:

- Enlargement of the adrenal cortex.
- Constant release of stress hormones.
- Shrinking of the thymus, spleen, and lymph nodes associated with a significant decrease in the white blood cells. If this continues over time, the immune system becomes compromised, resulting in a decline in the body's ability to fight off simple infectious diseases such as viruses and colds.
- Gastrointestinal distress and formation of ulcers in the stomach and intestine, which is evidence of the acidity and poor digestion associated with stress.

Stage of Resistance

During this stage, the body's defenses are activated. The body attempts to overcome the alarm reaction and return to homeostasis, the state of the body prior to exposure to the stressor. If the perception of the threat persists, however, the body will stay activated. During this stage the body's defense mechanisms are fully at work, gradually using up its energy just to maintain homeostasis. In contrast to the alarm stage, when the adrenal glands secrete their hormones into the bloodstream until these hormones are gone, the adrenals rapidly manufacture new hormones during the resistance stage. Hormone concentrations increase, and this persists until the stressor is reduced or eliminated or until the third stage, exhaustion, begins.

Stage of Exhaustion

Exhaustion sets in when the demands on the body overwhelm its ability to return to homeostasis. The organs (lungs, heart, adrenals, and others) have been working hard to overcome the stressor, and the body's resources become depleted. The body can no longer meet the demands placed upon it and begins to fail or function improperly. Fatigue sets in, and the body becomes vulnerable to a variety of illnesses. Exhaustion can result in damage to the organs, and if severe enough, even death. Intense shock that produces cardiac arrest at the scene of an auto accident is an example of extreme stress resulting in death. In this case, the body cannot meet the extreme demand placed upon it.

The GAS has become the model for stress research, opening the door to understanding the physiological dangers of long exposure to strong, persistent stressors and the relationship between stress and disease. The body's many physiological reactions to stress (the GAS) are the same whether the stressor is physical or psychological, real or imagined, chronic or acute.

Stress and Disease

Among the conditions caused or aggravated by stress are:

Allergies	Kidney disease
Angina	Lupus
Arteriosclerosis	Multiple sclerosis
Cancer	Pancreatitis
Diabetes	Raynaud's disease
Epileptic attacks	Respiratory ailments
Epstein-Barr syndrome	Rheumatoid arthritis
Heart disease	Shingles
Herpes	Stroke
High blood pressure	Tuberculosis
Hives	Ulcers

Stress and Disease

The concept that stress can result in disease is not new. The concept was first formulated by Selye in the 1940s, and extensive research from many allied health fields has provided evidence that chronic stress is correlated with a wide variety of diseases, from the common cold to cancer, in both adults and children. The box above summarizes the major long-term effects of chronic stress. Up to 70 to 80 percent of all health-related illness and the physiological changes that result (such as ulcers) are at least indirectly related to stress wearing down the immune system, which makes people more susceptible to disease.[3] The box above identifies common conditions that are caused by or aggravated by stress. Stress affects each of the five components of health: the physical, the mental, the emotional, the social, and the spiritual.[4]

The relationship between stress and disease is complex, involving the interaction between the nervous, endocrine, and immune systems. What emerges from the research are two categories of stress-related diseases:

1. Diseases related to an over-responsive autonomic nervous system, which produces migraine headaches, ulcers, and coronary heart disease
2. Diseases related to a dysfunctional immune system, which invites colds, influenza, and cancers

Regardless of the disease form, if the stressors are controlled or the stress is managed, the disease might be alleviated.

In children, the more common stress-related diseases are the following:

- **Allergies**. When the body mistakes a harmless substance from the environment as a threat, the immune system triggers the release of hormones that produce an allergic reaction. Allergies to certain foods are common. Frequently, children suffer an asthma attack after experiencing a physically or psychologically stressful event.
- **Influenza, pneumonia, and the common cold**. Although these contagious diseases are directly related to viral or bacterial contamination (see Chapter 5), susceptibility markedly increases, because of a compromised immune system, in children under stress.
- **Cancer**. More and more children are succumbing to lymphomas (e.g., Hodgkin's disease, which is cancer of the lymph glands and lymphocytes) and osteogenic sarcomas (bone cancers and leukemia). These have been linked to increased stressors from the environment.

Sources of Stress in Children

Brian is 8 years old. The older of two children from a middle-class family, he feels loved and has no serious behavior problems. His family just moved to a new city, where his father got another job. Brian had to leave all of his old friends behind and begin the process of making new friends at a new school. This is difficult for Brian because he makes friends slowly, is not good at sports, and is shy and uncomfortable around other children. Arguments between his parents have increased since the move, and he has heard mention that they may separate and possibly divorce. His new teacher thinks Brian is a slow learner and, therefore, placed him in a slow group. Lately, Brian has been listless, sleeping more than usual, making excuses for not going to school, arguing with his new friends and classmates, and being hostile toward adults, including his parents. He is falling behind in his schoolwork, saying it is too hard and he can't do it.

Jean is a bright and precocious 10-year-old. She lives with her parents and younger brother in a close and loving family in a middle-class integrated community. In school she is an excellent student, plays the piano beautifully, and has won several awards in mathematics and spelling. When her friends are socializing and playing, she is studying and practicing. She hopes to win a scholarship to college someday. Her parents are proud of Jean, and she doesn't want to disappoint them.

Brian is experiencing stress, and his behaviors verify that. A person could not say that any particular life event was the cause of his problems. Taken together, though, they add up to a significant set of changes, and therefore stress, in his life. Jean also is experiencing stress, although in her case it might be called eustress. Her drive and need for approval, however, may be internal stressors that could generate symptoms of stress.

These patterns are each typical of a growing number of children as they try to negotiate the complexities of modern society. Childhood is under attack by stressors in contemporary life, and children are not always prepared to cope with them.

The Stress of Growing Up

During development, children face a wide variety of challenges and demands, some generated by the body itself as it grows and matures and others from the external environment as adult demands are placed on them. Most children have concerns about their place and role in society, what Humphrey called "self-concerns that induce stress in children."[5] These stressors include the following:

1. **Meeting personal goals**. These can occur early in life and result in stress if adults set goals or tasks that are too difficult and children strive unsuccessfully to reach them. Sometimes children set unrealistically high goals as they compete with friends or peers. If goals are set too low, though, children become unmotivated and may not realize their potential.
2. **Self-esteem**. These are related to fulfillment of self and ego needs that are readily affected by their surroundings, by parents and friends, and by successes and failures. Self-image develops early in childhood from a variety of family values, attitudes, and personal experiences. Those that are reinforced, whether positive or negative, affect how children view themselves and the extent to which they respond to stressors. Coping skills also can be affected by self-esteem. A positive self-image allows for the development of good skills, and a negative one may not.
3. **Changing values**. Some children do not understand the value system adults impose on them. They may get the message that adults do not value the things children believe are important or that their values are unimportant. This can lead to confusion and strife.
4. **Social standards**. Expectations and standards change with different levels of development and with changes in the peer group and school setting. Children become confused trying to understand social standards that are acceptable at one time and not at another.
5. **Ability and personal competence**. This one seems to especially frustrate children. Lack of confidence in their ability can play havoc with their morale, undermine parental expectations, and create problems in school.
6. **Competition with others**. Children want to be liked, and therefore accepted, by their peers. At the same time, they want to be special. Deviations can induce stress.

Although not all of these are characteristic of all children, the key is to recognize individual differences. What may create serious concern in one child may have no affect on another. In any case, knowing these childhood concerns may make adults and teachers more aware of potential stress in children.

Differences Between Children and Adults

Even though the types of stressors that affect children often stem from the same stressors adults have, the major difference is that children do not have the ability to control the situations that cause them stress, as adults often do. Childhood stressors frequently are created by occurrences in the parent's life. For example, children do not control the break-up of a family or which parent they will live with.

Further, children's physical, intellectual, and psychological stage of development relates to their stressors and how they handle them. Their psychological pain is no less intense than adults, but they have less understanding and less control over it—making them more vulnerable to it. "Emotions are sacred, and unfulfilled needs are profane."[6] They have trouble with notions of causality and timeframes. If they can't understand a cause and a time sequence, they cannot control the associated stress. Hence, telling a child "it will get better later" may fall on deaf ears.

Home and Family Stress

The following factors have been strongly associated with childhood stress:[7]

1. Marital discord
2. Low social status
3. Overcrowding or large family size
4. Paternal criminality
5. Parental psychiatric disorder
6. Admission into the care of local authorities

Other factors, including a parent's well-being, play important roles in a child's adjustments to stress. Parents who are ill, have emotional problems, or experience marital tension tend to be less responsive, less nurturing, less affectionate, and more punitive with their children.[8] The introduction of new parental figures in the home (such as stepparents) is particularly stressful for school-aged children. Other childhood stressors include accidents, injuries, or hospitalizations of a family member; family relocation, separation from parents, and the addition of a sibling.

In political speeches, the subject of the family invariably comes up, and one hears such conclusions as "The family is breaking up. We are losing traditional values. The U. S. divorce rate is the highest in the world. The traditional nuclear family no longer exists. Homeless people too often include children growing up in single-parent families. Many of these are headed by women whose husbands have abandoned them. Where there are two-parent households, both parents have to work, leaving little time and attention for children. Violence and child abuse abound." The litany goes on and on. This presents a dismal picture, suggesting that the American family is undergoing major changes with associated stress in children.

Certainly, morals and values are changing drastically from traditional ones to those that may be confusing to family members. Children are being reared within a greater variety of living styles. Parents, attempting to cope with everyday demands of dual-working families, financial obligations, and more responsibilities, may place undue burdens on their children. Sometimes children are left to carry the overload. These factors and the stress that emerges from them increase a child's risk for physical and mental illness.

The child's response to stress is related to the extent of threat in the life event. Even everyday life stressors—such as daily chores and responsibilities, breaking toys, losing a game, getting to school on time, and poor nutrition—can be stressful. These may result in a variety of behavioral, learning, and emotional problems during the school day.

Coping with Stress

Children are not innately prepared to cope with crises. One of the responsibilities of parents is to help children meet crises by being sensitive to their children, encouraging them to communicate about their feelings, and being good role models. Some children are unable to cry or express anger because they have learned to be afraid to express their emotions and have not learned to use their full range of emotions. Helping them to communicate what is bothering them is a major step in the right direction.

Parents who provide children with clear guidelines and parameters about rights and wrongs create an environment wherein children can test, challenge, accept, or reject parental values and eventually develop a value system of their own.

Stress in School

For several weeks, Mrs. Roth had been preparing her daughter Jane for the big day, the first day of kindergarten. The drive to school was full of excited conversation about who the teacher will be and what the day will be like. As they entered the classroom, Jane's demeanor suddenly changed. She wouldn't speak, did not say "hi" as she normally would, and clung to Mrs. Roth's leg and dress. The teacher picked up Jane in her arms, trying to reassure her, and instructed Mrs. Roth to leave. As she reluctantly left the room, Mrs. Roth heard Jane's plea, "Mommy, Mommy, don't leave me!" Both were experiencing separation anxiety.

This familiar scene has been enacted countless times in day-care centers and kindergartens. It is the first of many school-related stress responses. Jane needs reassurance from her teacher and her parents so her fears of being abandoned in this new environment will dissipate.

A common myth about school is that all children are eager to go. School, however, can be the source of a wide variety of positive and negative stressors and even pain. The fear of school can be real or imagined. In many cases, the teacher, the school itself, the administration, or the organization creates stressors for children. The demands of separation, performance, cooperation and competition, socialization, deadlines, homework, tests as proof of learning, and athletics contribute to a stressful environment. These, coupled with some children's low self-image and beliefs about failure, can produce behavioral problems,

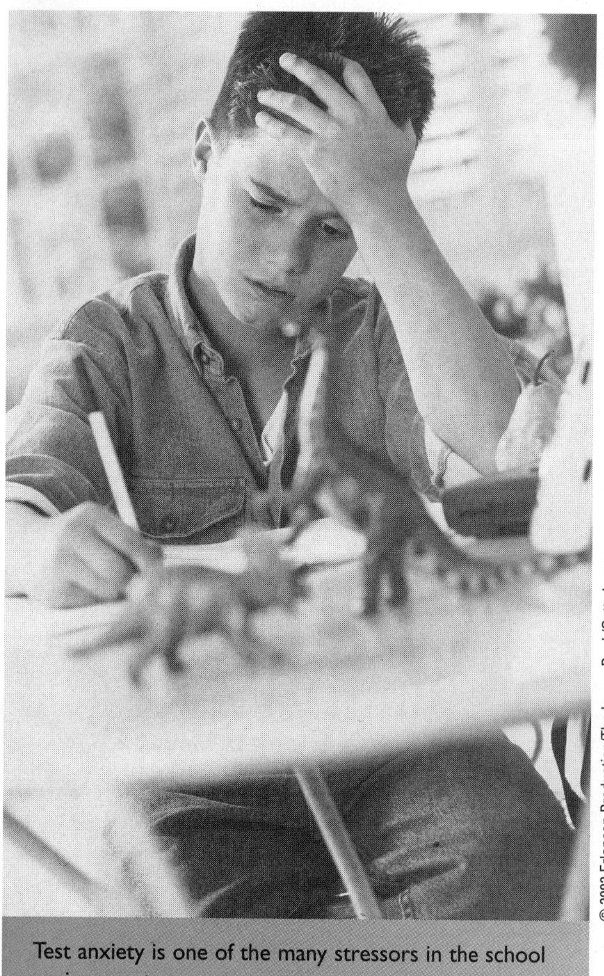

Test anxiety is one of the many stressors in the school environment.

Performance

Stress

Figure 8.3 **The stess/performance curve.**

including social withdrawal or other acting-out behaviors and psychosomatic illness. This may lead to substance abuse and absenteeism later. The major school stressors fall into the following categories:

1. **School adjustment**. The physical environment of the school, the classroom, or even the cafeteria can contribute to a child's stress. Children should perceive the school as a safe place. This translates to well supervised activities, the absence of violence, uncrowded classrooms, display of students' work on walls and bulletin boards, organization and order, and teachers effectively administering the curriculum. If teachers can make the classroom environment a happy place for students, this will reduce stress and facilitate learning.
2. **The learning process**. Because children learn in different ways, they are also motivated to develop learning skills in different ways. Appropriate books, supplies, and resources should be in sufficient supply to meet varying needs. Teachers also have to be concerned not only with studying and learning but also with socializing, security, individual attention, and evidence of self-worth. The teacher can reduce stress in this area by giving positive feedback—a good way to help children relax and feel good about themselves.
3. **Competition**. A child's efforts can be motivated or stifled by too little or too much competition. Competition can produce a sense of success and fulfillment or of anxiety and feelings of failure. Pitting one child against another can cause one of them to feel like a failure and perhaps the other to feel guilty. Having children work together in groups toward an explicit goal can reduce the sense of competition and, thereby, stress.
4. **Subject stress**. If you ask children which subject they like best, the typical response is "recess and lunch." Some subjects cause more anxiety than others: Many people, for example, are familiar with "math anxiety." The anxiety is related to performance demands and the student's perceptions of his or her own ability to meet them. As clearly shown in Figure 8.3, performance declines as stress increases. Reducing stressors can help raise performance. However, some stress is a good motivator for productive activity.

5. **Test anxiety**. Verbal tests produce greater anxiety than written tests.[9] Anxiety is learned from prior conditioning, and its impact is rarely considered when interpreting test results—which are supposed to measure acquired knowledge rather than the ability to perform under stress. The teacher can help reduce text anxiety by repeatedly going over the material, giving practice tests, and reducing the emphasis, where possible, on tests in the learning process.
6. **Parent involvement**. The issuance of report cards is associated with stress. The teacher can alleviate some of this stress by keeping parents informed and involved through parent-teacher conferences and open school nights. This gives parents opportunities to help their children with stressful experiences in school. By the time the report card is sent home, parents and children have been discussing progress, which makes this time less stressful.

Stressors by Grade Level

The most likely sources of stress by grade level (listed in order of intensity) are as follows:

Kindergarten Fear of abandonment, toileting concerns, fear of punishment or reprimand by the teacher.

First grade Fear of riding the bus, toileting mishaps, teacher disapproval, ridicule by other students, first report card, and not going on to second grade.

Second grade Missing a parent or sharing him or her with a sibling; fear of not being able to understand, not being asked to help the teacher, being disciplined, being different in dress or appearance.

Third grade Fear of being chosen last on a team, parent conference, peer or teacher disapproval, tests, not having enough time to complete assignment, staying after school.

Fourth grade Fear of being chosen last, peer disapproval of clothing or appearance, friends not choosing them to share secrets, student ridicule, not being liked by teacher.

Fifth grade Fear of being chosen last, losing a best friend, not being able to complete work, peer disapproval, not being a sixth grader next year.

Sixth grade Fear of being chosen last, sexuality, not going on to junior high, peer disapproval of appearance, being unpopular.[10]

Some of these fears persist through the grades, and new ones appear as children mature. Table 8.1 on page 280 identifies symptoms of stress-induced exhaustion in children—which are often correlated with physical and emotional problems. Teachers can do many things to diminish these sources of stress. Most good teachers are sensitive to these and will respond positively. Comprehensive teacher training, common sense, knowledge of child development, age-dependent changes, and sensitivity to the classroom environment all can help to manage or eliminate these potential sources of stress.

Teaching Children How to Cope with Stress

When children seem troubled, as evidenced by specific symptoms associated with stressors (see Figure 8.1, page 273), some forms of stress-reducing intervention is called for. Children often cannot communicate exactly what is bothering them. Even if they cannot pinpoint the cause, though, they know something is wrong. In cases where stressors cannot be eliminated (illness, death in the family, change in living style, and so on), stress management focuses on activities that alleviate the physical symptoms, thereby regulating the body's adaptive responses to prevent exhaustion.

An initial goal to alleviate stress symptoms (by decreasing or removing the stressors) could begin by helping children recognize their own signs of stress. Children can learn how to pay attention to these signs and the respective warnings their bodies are sending out through symptoms (many such symptoms are listed in Table 8.1 on page 280). For example, fear of doing poorly on an exam can be converted into a physical symptom, such as a stomachache or headache. Sometimes this experience can translate into more chronic test anxiety, even if the original cause is no longer present. The teacher can attempt to get to the problem by eliminating the symptom, control the stressor by altering the child's perception of it, or manage the stress response once it occurs. Ultimately, effective stress management should be directed toward minimizing or altering stressful situations, thus addressing the entire problem.

Perhaps an important step in reducing stress and preventing stress disorders is to help children allocate time for relaxation, thereby lowering stress response thresholds. The following is a brief summary of various techniques that have been used to foster relaxation, followed by a selection of integrated grade-specific Learning Experiences that can be used in the classroom.

Table 8.1
Signs and Symptoms of Stress

Cardiovascular
- Pounding of the heart
- Racing of the heart
- High blood pressure
- Irregular heartbeat
- Chest pain
- Cold, sweaty hands
- Common colds

Mental
- Confusion
- Lack of creativity
- Loss of memory
- Low self-esteem
- Negative thinking
- Lethargy

Respiratory
- Shortness of breath
- Rapid breathing
- Asthma attacks

Sleep disorders
- Accidents
- Insomnia
- Fatigue
- Nightmares

Skin problems
- Acne
- Excessive dryness
- Rashes
- Excessive perspiration

Emotional
- Nervousness
- Unexplained fearfulness
- Martyrdom
- Frustration
- Lack of direction
- Cynicism
- Anxiety
- Emotional instability
- Impulsive behavior
- Depression
- Irritability
- Forgetfulness
- Severe mood swings
- Tearfulness
- Urge to hide
- Difficulty completing tasks
- Changes in eating/smoking/drinking
- Increased dependence on drugs
- Boredom
- Apathy

Musculoskeletal
- Twitching or shakiness
- Neck or back pain
- Headache, including migraine
- Stiffness of muscles
- Tension
- Restlessness
- Accidents

Gastrointestinal
- Dryness of mouth and throat
- Difficulty swallowing
- Grinding of teeth
- Indigestion
- Nausea or queasiness
- Vomiting
- Loss of appetite
- Excessive appetite
- Diarrhea or constipation
- Abdominal pain
- Increased cravings
- Frequent urination
- Weight change

Relational
- Isolation
- Distrust
- Intolerance
- Lack of intimacy
- Loss of friends
- Using people
- Sudden bursts of anger
- Resentment
- Loneliness
- Poor communication
- Nagging

Laughter and Fun

The health benefits of humor are common knowledge. When people are having fun and laughing, they temporarily forget their troubles and often feel better. Humor can reduce stress, ease pain, foster a return to health, and improve a person's outlook on life in general. One widely publicized example is Norman Cousins's recovery from a serious crippling illness, facilitated by watching film clips of Laurel and Hardy, the Marx brothers, and "Candid Camera." Many subsequent research studies have confirmed the stress-reducing benefits of laughter.

Comic books, cartoons, silly toys and games, and funny movies are among effective stress reducers for children. The laughter that emanates from humor can contribute to stress reduction. Thus, encouraging opportunities for laughter during the school day and at home by reading funny stories and telling humorous anecdotes from personal experience can reduce stress in children.

Altering Perceptions

Probably the most pervasive cause of stress is the way a person thinks about the world and perceives situations. A person can perceive a simple comment as a direct attack or as friendly advice. Believing oneself to have only limited choice or to lack control in a given situation can produce stress. Changing the way adults view the world around them can be difficult. The task may be easier with children, because they commonly base their perceptions on limited experience, a brief history, and immediate needs. Each of these factors is accessible to modification. Children are easily distracted by new experiences, and negative perceptions sometimes can be replaced by more positive ones. Children can be helped to expand their alternatives, boosting their sense of control and thereby reducing their stress. Having children share in curriculum development—deciding what to include and what to leave out, openly discussing the relevant issues, and having them come to collective decisions—is a means of broadening their perceptions about the world around them and increasing their feelings of control.

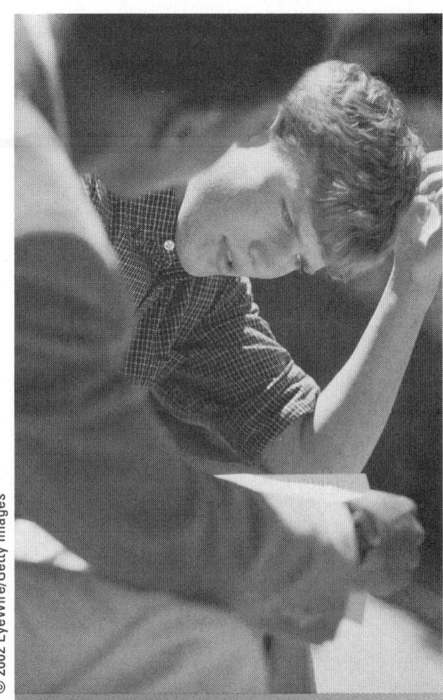

That special attention paid to students by teachers motivates them and promotes positive attitudes about self and school.

Defense Mechanisms for Coping with Stress

People learn to cope with stress in various ways—some of them healthy, some not. The more common defense mechanisms include

- Daydreaming about pleasurable situations.
- Repression—purposely or selectively forgetting unpleasant experiences.
- Denial—flat refusal to believe or recognize that a stressful situation is real.
- Rationalization—coming up with socially acceptable justifications for behavior or situations.
- Reaction formation—adopting behaviors and attitudes that are exactly the opposite of how the person really feels.
- Projection—placing the blame for one's weaknesses or problems on someone else.
- Displacement—redirecting socially unacceptable behavior from the true source to a less threatening substitute.
- Regression—reverting or retreating to childish or childlike behaviors.
- Isolation—detaching oneself from the underlying cause of a stressor.

Revising Attitudes

How children feel about themselves (self-image) and how they interact with others (socialization) have a great influence over their stress reactions. Stress-producing traits include procrastination (putting off work until the last minute, cramming for exams, and the like), lack of assertiveness (being passive, shy, or introverted; avoiding eye contact; fidgeting), and excess of aggression (appearing obnoxious, abrasive, or insensitive; loud and angry). Ways of decreasing stress include building self-image, developing assertive responses that are confident, and expressing needs (as in recognizing more than one "right way" to do so). The teacher, acting as a role model, can effectively demonstrate these characteristics.

Some psychological defense mechanisms can be applied to help reduce stress. Sometimes, these may not produce a positive health state or reactions in others.

Nutrition

A child's nutritional state can be a stressor itself or can be the result of other emotional stressors. Nutrition affects health, and poor nutrition can be the direct cause of a variety of health problems (see Chapter 3). Some food chemicals produce stress by stimulating the autonomic system. For example, caffeine (found in coffee, tea, chocolate, and sodas), if used excessively, can produce hypertension, anxiety, irritability, and an inability to concentrate. Excess sugar (hyperglycemia) intake has similar effects. So, too, does too little sugar (hypoglycemia). Some vitamins received from foods we eat are thought to protect against stress.

Thus, maintaining a well-balanced diet can prolong the state of resistance and maintain homeostasis. Providing a wide variety of foods early in life can prevent a child from becoming a "picky eater." The foods available during snack time or at lunch in schools can be monitored so they do not contribute to stress. Having children construct and implement a lunch or snack menu in the classroom is one learning experience about food (see Learning Experiences at the end of Chapter 3).

The Relaxation Response

> Each of us possess a natural and innate protective mechanism against "overstress" which allows us to turn off harmful bodily effects to counter the effects of the fight-or-flight response. This response against "overstress" brings on bodily changes that decrease heart rate, lower metabolism, decrease the rate of breathing, and bring the body back into what is probably a healthier balance. This is the relaxation response.[11]

Achieving relaxation requires not only preventing stressors from entering the body, but also establishing peace of mind—no easy task. Many people have outlets, things they like to do—not for achieving goals or accomplishments but, instead, for personal satisfaction. This allows them to focus their mental energies on the activity and away from the pressure of everyday life. The diversion can be a physical activity, an artistic or a musical interlude, a class or activity group, or a good book—anything that lowers the level of stress and produces the relaxation response. The main reason for participating in the activity is relaxation.

Helping Children Relax

Many children engage in activities that are nondirective and sometimes unproductive, causing them to become agitated and possibly creating behavior problems. Relaxation techniques can channel their excess energy and help them to focus on one thing for a longer time than they normally would. The techniques that follow have been shown to help resolve stress-related problems, such as tension and migraine headaches, anxiety, peptic ulcers, nail biting, stuttering, and depression.

Physical Activities

Daily exercise or sports is a good release for excess energy. Among the many possibilities are swimming, bicycling, jogging, walking, rollerblading, and team sports such as tennis and handball. These can be excellent stress relievers if the participants feel refreshed and relaxed afterward. Some activities also condition the cardiovascular system and tone the muscles. Helping young people to recognize the stress-reducing qualities of physical activity gives them an important lifelong tool.

Meditation and Yoga

Meditation, thought to be the oldest form of relaxation, is basically a mind-emptying process. Focusing and concentrating increases the awareness of one's inner self and leads to an altered state of consciousness that changes sensory perceptions and reduces heart rate and blood pressure. It produces a state of deep relaxation in a relatively short time, creating an opportunity for people to listen, feel, and connect with what's going on inside their bodies.

Yoga, a form of meditation, attempts to achieve a union of the mind, body, and spirit. **Hatha yoga**, one of the more common forms, consists of a series of movements that combine breathing, stretching, and balance. **Tai chi** is yet another form of movement and balance exercises. Transcendental meditation (TM), a widely used meditative process, is based on the simple technique of repeating a sound, phrase, or word (a mantra) again and again while in a comfortable sitting position. This process reduces distracting thoughts and facilitates peaceful concentration (similar to counting sheep before falling asleep). Regular meditation increases flexibility, improves muscle tone, and creates an inner calmness that seems to contribute to improved self-esteem.

Some teachers use **guided fantasy** to help children relax and meditate. The children assume a relaxed position in chairs or on floor mats with their eyes closed. For about 15 minutes, they visualize something like a country scene, a camp experience, a time on the beach listening to the waves, or other peaceful fantasy. Then they share with the class their experiences and how they felt afterward, introducing a concept of relaxation that some may want to adapt for themselves.

Progressive Muscle Relaxation

Children can achieve deep muscle relaxation by concentrating on relaxing specific muscle groups in an ordered sequence called **progressive muscle relaxation**. This involves systematically tensing then relaxing all the major muscle groups in the arms, head, chest, back, stomach, and legs. In one technique, the child visualizes the body as a huge sack of sand with a small hole at the bottom. Beginning with the head, he or she empties the sack of sand gradually from all body parts and feels each part as it relaxes. After the activity, class members can discuss how they felt.

Using these methods has had positive results in alleviating insomnia, hypertension, headaches, anxiety, and general autonomic system arousal. It can facilitate body awareness, which can be helpful to overactive children, teaching them to have more control over their behavior. The box on the next page lists guidelines for using this technique.

Deep Breathing

Another effective way to relax is through breathing exercises. When the lungs are filled with air, the muscles of the diaphragm expand and contract, and slowly exhaling helps to relax these muscles. This method counteracts the tensions of shallow breathing. Replacing accumulations of carbon dioxide with oxygen slows the cardiovascular system, reduces the pulse rate, and thus decreases anxiety. Breathing exercises are commonly used in conjunction with yoga or meditation.

Autogenic Training

Autogenic training uses aspects of meditation, progressive relaxation, and self-hypnosis. Autogenic means "self-generating." The technique trains children to exercise control over their physiology, thereby alleviating symptoms of anxiety and achieving homeostasis. It involves using mental and bodily functions simultaneously by learning a set of standard exercises. The mind focuses attention on a self-suggestion that produces a variety of controlled sensations and emotional responses. One form takes the child on a guided fantasy trip (as discussed above), perhaps to a quiet place in the mountains or to a

For Your Health

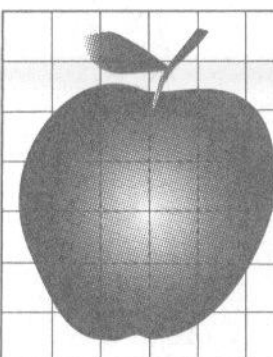

Progressive Muscle Relaxation

Regardless of the routine used for progressive relaxation, follow these guidelines.

- Lie on your back in the most comfortable position possible.
- Take off your shoes and loosen any restrictive clothing.
- Close your eyes, rotate your ankles outward, and place your arms at your sides.
- Make sure you move all major muscle groups in the body. Don't forget your face, including your forehead, eyes, nose, mouth, cheeks, and tongue.
- As you move each muscle group, contract the muscles as tightly as you can and hold the contraction for 30 seconds.
- If you experience pain or cramping during a contraction, release the contraction immediately.
- Concentrate on the dramatic difference in feeling between a tensed muscle and a relaxed one.

beach, and asks him/her to relive a positive experience or to be with a loving person. Studies have shown that these exercises are effective in treating hyperventilation, asthma, constipation, diarrhea, ulcers, irregular heartbeat, irritability, and sleeping disorders. They are known to modify pain responses and increase resistance to stress.

Biofeedback

Biofeedback technique is used to gain voluntary control over certain physiological responses. Looking in the mirror offers a clear analogy. Physical appearance can be modified by simple behaviors—such as combing the hair, putting on makeup, and the like—which are under voluntary control. Until recently, physiological functions that take place inside the body were much more difficult to observe and were considered uncontrollable by conscious effort. However, biofeedback techniques can regulate some internal responses. For example, we cannot see blood pressure; other methods must be used to measure it. Counting the number of times one breathes in a minute, checking pulse or heart rate, and taking body temperature are examples. On a rudimentary level, children can be taught to count the number of breaths a classmate takes in a minute or their own pulse rate per minute. They can identify how these physiological functions change with activities such as running, being frightened, and resting. Chapter 4 includes some appropriate activities.

Clinical biofeedback uses complex instruments, such as an electroencephalograph (EEG) or an electrocardiograph (EKG), to take accurate measurements of body functions. These methods allow children to gain information about the changes in the activity of specific organs (heart, smooth muscle, and so on) and become aware of the parallel change in attitudes or feelings associated with these changes. They learn relaxation strategies to control these physiological changes directly. The concept is closely related to the internal locus of control, in which a child takes responsibility for aspects of physiology or behavior that he or she can control, such as responses to stress.

Summary

A long history of stress research, beginning with the work of Hans Selye, leads us to believe that a person needs stress to live and to motivate action. Stressors are the stimuli that produce stress. They may be generated either externally (from the environment) or internally (from thought processes such as fantasies). Some stressors are positive (eustress), and some are negative (distress). Both cause physiological and mental/emotional changes in the body that Selye called "stress." Stressful lifestyles are not just an adult problem. Children experience significant stressors. They need to learn how to recognize those stressors, what precipitates them, and how to diminish them to avoid compromising health.

Hans Selye defined the term "stress," differentiated good and bad stress, and spawned subsequent research that has identified the stress response, general adaptation syndrome, and specific body conditions resulting from chronic stress. At the same time, the responses to stress are individual and are developmentally related.

Teachers need to recognize students' sources of stress, both in the classroom and in children's living styles, and among parents, family, and friends. It is important to understand how children's stressors differ from those of adults. Teachers can employ meditation, yoga, guided fantasies, and autogenic training that may help to reduce stress in their students. Finally, teachers can teach students how to relax and better cope with stress.

Web Sites

American Institute of Stress
www.stress.org

Biofeedback Information
www.stresscontrol.com

Childhood Disorders
www.emb.org/hll/practical/cdp.htm

Childhood Stress: Has the Clutterbug Got You?
www.clutterbug.net

Childhood Stress: Times of Stress and Anxiety
www.extension.umn.edu

Learn About Children and Stress
www.plainhealth.com

Managing Stress
www.stress.about.com

Promoting Stress Management: The Role of CSHP [in ERIC Digests]
www.ed.gov/databases/ERIC-Digests

Psychological Stress in Infancy, Childhood and Adolescence
www.omni.ac.uk

Relaxation for Children
www.cerebralmessage.com

Stress and Anxiety
www.anxietysupport.org/cciimenu.htm

Stress in Childhood
www.my.webmed.com

Stress Management
www.mtr_i.com

Stress Management and Relaxation Central
www.futurehealth.org

Stress Management in Early Childhood
www.master-quest.com

Stress Management Overview
www.penpages.psu.edu/penpages-reference/28507/2850776.html

Stress Management Training: Helping Kids Cope with Stress
www.bizhotline.com

Stress-Proof Your Children
www.aomc.org

Stress Treatment Center
www.stresstc.com

Resources

American Academy of Experts on Traumatic Stress
368 Veterans Memorial Highway
Commack, NY 11725
631-543-2217

American Institute of Stress
124 Park Avenue
Yonkers, NY 10703
914-963-1200

Notes

1. R. R. Cottrell, *Wellness: Stress Management* (Guilford, CT: Dushkin Publishing Group, 1992).
2. H. Selye, *Stress in Health and Disease* (Reading, MA: Butterworths, 1976).
3. B. L. Seaward, *Managing Stress: Principals and Strategies for Health and Well-Being*, 2nd ed. (Boston: Jones and Bartlett, 1997).
4. M. S. Massey, *Promoting Stress Management: The Role of Comprehensive School Health Programs*, ERIC Digest (Washington, DC Eric Clearinghouse on Teaching and Teacher Education, 1998).
5. J. H. Humphrey, *Children and Stress* (New York: AMS Press, 1988), 8.
6. B. B. Youngs, *Stress in Children* (New York: Arbor House, 1989).
7. See note 5.
8. See note 6.
9. See note 5.
10. See note 6.
11. H. Benson, *The Relaxation Response* (New York: Avon Books, 1975), 25–26.

Learning Experiences

Children undergo continual change in experiences, values, activities, behaviors, and choices. Unfamiliar and novel situations such as a new home, school, or class; new friends, new family members, or a sudden illness are just a few potential sources of tension, anxiety, and stress. Children who develop a positive self-image and effective methods of managing the stressors of everyday life are more likely to be healthier and happier, more energetic and productive. Therefore, children need to develop effective decision-making and problem-solving skills.

Students come to school with a variety of coping skills that change as they grow older. Only experience can demonstrate which ones are most effective. Many of the strategies used to express emotion can also be used when dealing with stress. A few of the ways students cope with stress are denial, sublimation, daydreaming, and humor.

Students can learn the importance of exercising regularly, getting enough rest and sleep, and relaxing. These skills are vital if they are to gain a true and purposeful understanding of the world. Developing these habits early in their education will serve them for the rest of their lives. Coupled with good nutrition, these skills will increase fitness and overall health.

In grades K–6, a wide variety of activities can be used to deliver information about stress. Students in the lower grades can read or be read stories about stress experiences, draw pictures, play stress-reducing games, develop problem-solving skills, and participate in show-and-tell activities and question-and-answer sessions. In the higher grades, dramatizations can be added. Incidents can become teachable moments for discussing stress-related issues. A bulletin board can be used to display items related to stress and ways to reduce stress.

Grades K–2

In these early grades, students can begin to understand basic concepts related to stress: what sensations are, the differences between good and bad feelings, where stressors come from, what the students think about that changes their feelings, activities they enjoy, and methods that help them relax or go to sleep. Having them recall pleasant experiences in games, dance, and other physical activities can help them learn how to reduce stress.

By the end of the second grade, students should be able to

1. Name some body changes that are indicators of stress
2. Identify the primary emotions and express them
3. Describe the differences between good and bad feelings
4. List the five senses and describe what they do
5. Explain the differences between internal and external stressors
6. Explain where stressors come from
7. Describe activities they like and dislike
8. Identify a simple routine for relaxation
9. Identify people they can go to for help when they feel stress

Grades 3–4

In these grades, students build upon their earlier notions of stress and add components of the general adaptation syndrome, what alarms them, components of the nervous system that mediate stress, the kinds of things they fear, the things that make them happy, the difference between eustress and distress, and some of the complex body changes associated with stress. Their learning experience can include finding ways to relax in school through group activities and at home and understanding the values of sports and dance. The students should be able to make the connection between stress and illness and the level of control they have to make things better.

By the end of the fourth grade, students should be able to

1. Develop a list of common stressors and state whether they are external or internal
2. Assess which of the stressors produce eustress and which produce distress
3. Discuss how people respond differently to stressors
4. List the parts of the body affected by stress
5. Explain how stress is related to illness
6. Describe the effects of acute and chronic stress
7. Describe how they can effectively control some of their stress responses
8. Identify support resources for coping with stress in the school and community
9. Identify activities that help them manage their own stress

Grades 5–6

In these grades, students should become fully aware of the general adaptation syndrome and the specific sequence of its first stage (the alarm reaction) and the functioning of associated body systems (nervous, hormonal, immune) during that stage. They should be aware of specific effects of intense, chronic stress. Students should also become aware of the sources of stress from school, home, and community and what support systems are available to help them manage stress. By the end of the sixth grade, students should be able to

1. List the components of the nervous, hormonal, and immune systems and describe how they work
2. Explain the effects of frequency, intensity, and duration of stressors on the body and where they come from
3. Describe ways of controlling the stress response
4. Identify some cultural differences in the way people respond to stress
5. Identify professionals and resources that can help them reduce stress
6. Describe some stress-management techniques
7. Develop an activity for personal stress management
8. Describe some of the diseases associated with stress and how to help prevent them

For suggestions on creating a rubric with which to evaluate student performance of Learning Experiences, see page 13.

Learning Experience 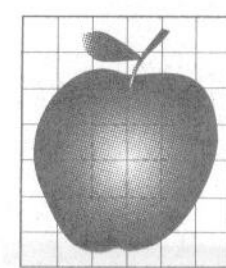 8-1

Soaking Up Stress

Grade Level

K–2

Primary Discipline

Science

Learning Objectives

Following this activity, students will be able to

- Describe some feelings related to stress.
- Identify some causes of stress.
- Describe ways to reduce stress.

Time Required

One session (45 minutes)

Materials

Sponge, pitcher of water, bowl

Description of Activity

Tell students that the sponge represents the body and the water represents stressors from the environment. Ask a volunteer to name a stressor and pour a little water on the sponge. Repeat this until the sponge is saturated, then have another student pick up the sponge and tell how it feels (weight, texture, and so on).

Tell students that the saturated sponge represents tension. Ask students to volunteer healthful reactions to the stressors identified. With each response, squeeze out a little water. Have the students discuss the changes that took place and how it relates to their lives.

Homework

The students ask their parents what stressors they face in life.

Evaluation

Students will be able to

- Describe the characteristics of a sponge when dry and when wet.
- Explain what tension or stress means.
- Describe things that make a person feel "stressed."
- Identify things that make their parents tense or "stressed."

Learning Experience 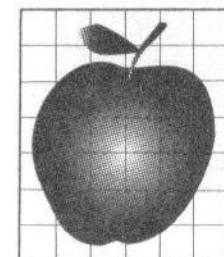 8-2

Getting in Touch with Feelings

Grade Level

K–2

Primary Disciplines

Social Science; Mental Health

Learning Objectives

Following this activity, students will be able to

- Describe feelings.
- Demonstrate individual differences in responses.

Time Required

One session (45 minutes)

Materials

None

Description of Activity

Have students respond verbally to the following:

1. How do you feel when you do something nice for someone?
2. How do you feel when you can't do something you want to do?
3. How do you feel when your parents are angry at you?
4. I feel best when ______________.
5. I feel worst when ______________.
6. How did you feel on the first day of school?
7. Sadness is __________________.
8. Happiness is ________________.

Have the class discuss the variety of feelings people can have and explore ways their bodies responded to happy and unhappy situations.

Homework

Students ask their parents and siblings the same questions.

Evaluation

Students will be able to

- Describe feelings associated with stress.
- Explain the difference between happy feelings and sad feelings.
- Identify situations associated with happy and sad feelings.
- Verbally express themselves about their feelings.

Source: J. H. Humphrey, *Children and Stress: Theoretical Perspectives and Recent Research (Stress in Modern Society, No. 18)*. (New York: AMS Press, 1988). Reprinted with permission.

Learning Experience 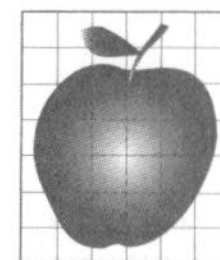 8-3

Body Changes

Grade Level

K–2

Primary Disciplines

Science, Math

Learning Objectives

Following this activity, students will be able to

- Calculate their number of heartbeats in a given time.
- Calculate their number of respirations in a given time.
- Recognize the changes in heartbeat and respiration before and after physical activity.
- Relate the changes to health.

Materials

Stethoscope, paper and pencils to record responses, watch with second hand or display of seconds

Description of Activity

Have students locate the pulse in their wrist (or the carotid artery in their neck). Instructions for finding the right spot:

1. Place the second and third finger of one hand about ½" below the wrist line along the bottom of the thumb of the other hand which is palm up. Press gently until the pulse in discernible.
2. Have the students count and then record the number of pulses while you time 10 seconds, then 1 minute.
3. Have the students repeat the activity using the same fingers to locate the carotid artery in the neck (on either side of the Adam's apple). Remind them to press gently.
4. Then have the students do various calculations, including multiplying the 10-second count by 6 to achieve 1 minute; multiplying by 60 to achieve 1 hour, and so on.
5. Show the children a stethoscope and give them an opportunity to hear their heartbeat through the stethoscope.
6. Have the children repeat the above activities after they have jumped or run in place for 1 minute, then have them repeat after they rest for 1 minute. Explain that these are the contractions of the heart as it sends blood around to the lungs and around the body. Describe how the heart speeds up after activity and how it returns to normal after rest.
7. Discuss the relationship between physical fitness and heartbeat at rest and after exercise and how it could be related to stress. Discuss the part breathing plays in providing the body with oxygen.

Homework

Have the students practice the same activity with a parent and record the calculations. Have them describe the differences between their heart rate and their parent's.

Evaluation

Students will be able to

- Take their own pulse.
- Count their own heartbeat.
- Count their own respiration.
- Perform simple mathematical tasks to calculate heart and respiration changes.
- Describe the changes in pulse and respiration from testing to activity.
- Simply explain the relationship between respiration, heartbeat, and stress.
- Explain why their heartbeat and respiration may be different from their friends' or family members.
- Relate heartbeat and respiration rates to exercise and stress.

Learning Experience 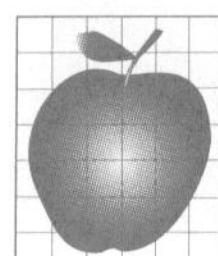 8-4

Ready to Burst

Grade Level

3–4

Primary Discipline

Social Studies; Language Arts

Learning Objectives

Following this activity, students will be able to

- Describe experiences that cause stress.
- Identify ways to manage stress.

Time Required

One session

Materials

Small balloons for each student, paper and pencil

Description of Activity

Have the students brainstorm a list of stressors, then practice reading and spelling the list correctly. As they name each stressor, have them blow once into their balloon. Instruct them to blow harder for strong stressors and easier for weak ones. Continue the exercise until the balloons break.

Have the class discuss how it feels when people are "ready to burst" and also the differences between the things that make some people feel stressed and others not. Ask students what they do to decrease stress. Lead a discussion of why some of the stressors make them feel more tense than others do.

Homework

None

Evaluation

Students will be able to

- Identify common stressors.
- Explain why stressors will affect one person differently from another.
- Explain how stress builds up.
- Describe actions people can take to decrease stress.

Learning Experience 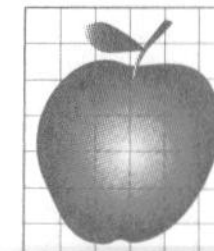 8-5

Showing Anger

Grade Level

3–5

Primary Discipline

Social Studies

Learning Objectives

Following this activity, students will be able to

- Describe the emotion of anger.
- List acceptable ways of expressing anger.
- Identify objects of anger.
- Describe ways they can redirect anger.
- Recognize appropriate from inappropriate responses to anger.

Time Required

One session (45 minutes)

Materials

None

Description of Activity

Using the list below, have the students identify the people toward whom they have been angry and how they express their anger.

WHO	HOW
1. Your best friend	A. Do nothing
2. Your brother	B. Yell
3. Your sister	C. Cry
4. Your parent	D. Slam the door
5. Your pet	E. Walk away
6. Your teacher	F. Refuse to speak to that issue or problem
7. A stranger	G. Throw something at him or her
8. Yourself	H. Hit him or her
9. Other________	I. Other

In small groups, have each student tell a short story about a time they were angry. Present appropriate ways to express anger. Have each group report the story that best describes an appropriate response to anger, then instruct students to write a brief story about an incident involving anger that ended in the angry character expressing his/her anger in appropriate ways.

Homework

The students take the handout home and discuss anger with their parents.

Evaluation

Students will be able to

- Describe situations that make people feel angry.
- Describe different responses to anger.
- Relate anger to stress.
- Explain the difference between appropriate responses to anger and inappropriate responses.
- Effectively relate, in writing, appropriate responses to anger.
- Identify some things that make them angry and their usual responses.
- Describe some alternative responses they can implement in situations that make them angry.

Learning Experience 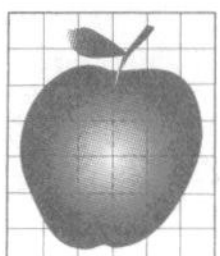 8-6

Progressive Relaxation with Children

Grade Level

K–6

Primary Discipline

Science

Learning Objectives

Following this activity, students will be able to

- Identify the major muscle groups.
- Describe the muscular tension in their own body.
- Explain the principle of progressive muscular relaxation and describe how to relax progressively.

Time Required

30 minutes

Materials

Floor mats for each student and post a chart of muscle groups

Description of Activity

Have the students lie on the mats. For each of the following, have them tense to a count of 5 and relax to a count of 10:

1. Squeeze your eyes shut tightly.
2. Press your lips together tightly.
3. Press your tongue to the roof of your mouth.
4. Pull your shoulders up to your ears.
5. Make a fist as tight as you can with both hands.
6. Make a fist with only one hand. Notice the difference between hands.
7. Pull your stomach way in.
8. Push your knees together hard.
9. Flex your feet: Pull your toes way up toward your knees without moving your legs.
10. Point your toes.
11. Tighten your leg muscles.
12. Now tighten every muscle in your body.

Homework

The students repeat this activity before bed for the next few nights. In class they describe what happened. Were they able to fall asleep faster?

Evaluation

Students are able to

- Point out the major muscle groups using an appropriate chart labeled to fit the grade level.
- Identify muscles in their body and describe how they contract and relax.
- Relate the response of muscles to stress.
- Describe and practice relaxation activities that decrease stress and muscle tension.

Source: J. H. Humphrey, *Children and Stress: Theoretical Perspectives and Recent Research (Stress in Modern Society, No. 18)* (New York: AMS Press, 1988). Reprinted with permission.

Learning Experience 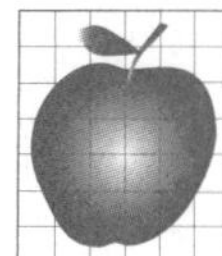 8-7

When It Rains, It Pours

Grade Level

3–4

Primary Disciplines

Social Studies, Creative Arts, Language Arts

Learning Objectives

Following this activity, students will be able to

- Identify the causes of stress.
- Describe the symptoms of stress.
- Identify ways to respond to stressors.

Materials

Oaktag or posterboard, paper, scissors, crayons, paste, handout

Description of Activity

Have students draw and then cut out a number of large raindrop shapes. Organize them into small groups, where they brainstorm stressors and list them (correctly spelled) on the chalkboard. The students label each raindrop with a separate stressor. On the posterboard the students draw a line down the center. On the left side they draw a picture of a person holding a very large open umbrella. On the right side they draw a person without an umbrella. Then they place all of the stressor raindrops on the right side of the picture, above the person.

The group discusses the ways they relieve each stressor. They share their lists with the class while you (the teacher) list the stress reducers on the board. One student at a time reads the stress reducer and moves the related stressor to the other side of the posterboard above the umbrella. When the activity is completed, explain that stress reducers protect against the effects of stress much like an umbrella protects against rain.

Homework

None.

Evaluation

Students will be able to

- Spell the new words correctly.
- Produce a creative product that correctly identifies stressors.
- Identify actions or thoughts that can reduce stress.

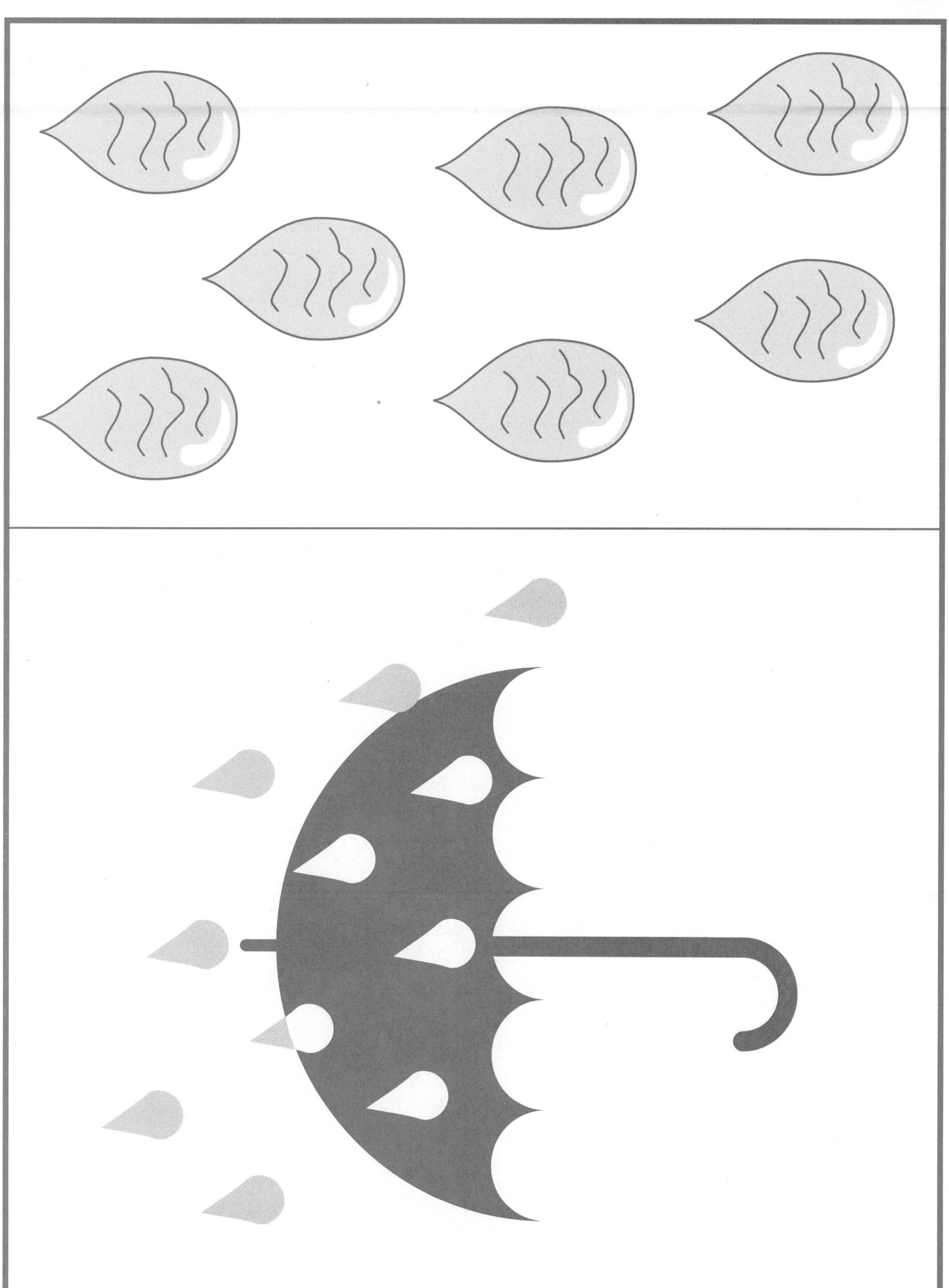

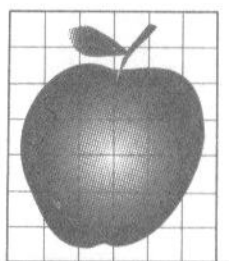

Learning Experience 8-8

The Stress Cycle

Grade Level

5–6

Primary Disciplines

Language Arts, Social Studies

Learning Objectives

Following this activity, students will be able to

- Describe the cycle of stress.
- Identify components of decision-making.
- Identify alternative coping skills.

Time Required

One session

Materials

"The Stress Syndrome" handout

Description of Activity

Have the students read "The Stress Syndrome" aloud and then organize them into small groups.

Ask the students to identify the feeling each incident can cause. Then have them brainstorm common responses to each situation, record each response as negative or positive, and discuss why they thought it was negative or positive.

Have the class as a whole develop a list of positive responses to stressful situations while you write them on the board. Have the students reflect on factors that determine how people respond to stressful situations.

Homework

The students will write their own "Stress Syndrome" incidents and identify one appropriate response for each stressful situation.

Evaluation

Students will be able to

- Relate common responses to stressful situations.
- Identify appropriate alternatives to the common responses.
- Describe common stressful situations they encounter and identify appropriate alternatives to them.
- Express their experiences and feelings in writing.

The STRESS Syndrome

1. Your best friend sits with someone else at lunch and doesn't pay attention to you. You don't like the feeling.
2. You discover you forgot to bring your gym shoes.
3. Your teacher won't allow you to go to the office to call your mother so she can bring your shoes to you.
4. You are so embarrassed you don't want to go to the next gym class.
5. You bump into a desk on the way back to your seat—then you kick it. The student sitting there says, "Watch it, nerd!"
6. You shout back, "You're the nerd!" but the teacher hears only you. You have to go to detention after school for 30 minutes.
7. Because you stayed after school, you can't go to the soccer game with your friends. You had been really looking forward to it.
8. Now that you can't go to the game you were looking forward to all week, you are really mad.
9. Your parents will be upset about your detention. This bothers you because you know you disappointed them.
10. Your brother teases you about having to go to detention, and you respond by hitting him. That makes you feel even worse.

Learning Experience 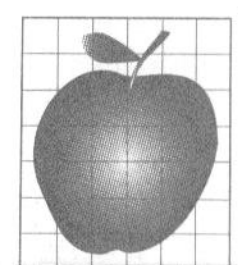 8-9

Get Set . . . Relax

Grade Level

5–6

Primary Discipline

Music

Learning Objectives

Following this activity, students will be able to

- Describe what stress is.
- Identify ways stressors affect them.
- Describe the impact music has on their lives.

Time Required

One session (45 minutes)

Materials

CD or tape player to play recordings of fast and slow music: classical, pop, country, or rock

Description of Activity

Play the different kinds of music played at different speeds and different volume levels. Ask the class what feelings the music elicits. Play the same music again and have the students write their responses to the music on the board. Have the students reflect on individual differences in the way music affects people. Lead a discussion about which music helps them to relax and how they can use music to relax.

Homework

Have the students listen to the tapes or CDs they commonly listen to and label each as either relaxing or stimulating.

Evaluation

Students will be able to

- Relate the effects of music on their responses to stress.
- Identify music that elicits a relaxation response in them.
- Recognize the differences in responses to stress among different people.
- Use music as a stress reducer.

Learning Experience 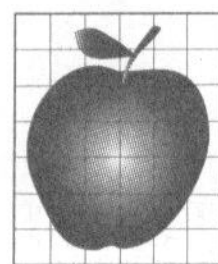 8-10

Stressed Out? How Does It Feel?

Grade Level

5–6

Primary Discipline

Health

Learning Objectives

Following this activity, students will be able to

- Describe the stress response.
- Explain the individual nature of stress responses.
- Identify alternative responses that can mediate stress.

Time Required

One session (45 minutes)

Materials

Pencil and lined paper

Description of Activity

Replay the incident outlined in the vignette that opened this chapter:

Give the following directions slowly and purposefully: "We are going to have a surprise quiz on the work we did during the last session and your homework." Hand each student a sheet of lined paper and ask that they put their name at the top and fold the paper in half vertically, numbering the left side from 1 to 10 and the right side from 11 to 20. Then tell them to fold the paper two more times and throw it in the wastebasket.

Have the students describe their physical reactions to this sequence (tight stomach, lump in the throat, and so on) and their thought processes. Discuss some of the things they might say to themselves or do to mediate the stress, such as: "I know this work, so I don't have to worry"; "What can I do but try my best?" Discuss the idea that students could raise their hands and ask why they are having a surprise test or explain that they are not ready and want to be excused.

Homework

Suggest that, to avoid stress, students study for tests systematically, each week, rather than cram for tests at the last minute.

Evaluation

Students will be able to

- Identify common school stressors.
- Recognize their own responses to stress.
- Relate test anxiety to their own stress responses.
- Describe ways that they can meditate to alleviate test anxiety.

Learning Experience 8-11

How Do You Experience Stress?

Grade Level

5–6

Primary Discipline

Science, Health

Learning Objectives

Following this activity, students will be able to

- Report stressful experiences.
- Identify the places in their body where they experience stress.
- Describe how to manage the stress.

Time Required

45 minutes

Materials

"How Do You Experience Stress?" handout

Description of Activity

Have the students share a story about a recent stressful experience and report how they reacted to that experience. Discuss the different ways they might have reacted or thought about the situation. Have them identify possible physical reactions to stress by referring to the handout. Discuss what happens when the symptoms of stress continue.

Homework

Using a human anatomy outline, the students identify stress sites on or in their body.

Evaluation

Students will be able to

- Identify common physical reactions to stress.
- Identify stress sites in the human body.
- Describe their own common physical reactions to stress.
- Describe ways people react to stress.

How Do You Experience STRESS?

- ☐ Pounding heart
- ☐ Unable to concentrate
- ☐ Shortness of breath
- ☐ Rapid breathing
- ☐ Asthma attack
- ☐ Nervousness
- ☐ Unexplained fearfulness
- ☐ Anxiety
- ☐ Impulsive behavior
- ☐ Depression
- ☐ Urge to hide
- ☐ Difficulty completing tasks
- ☐ Grinding of teeth
- ☐ Loss of appetite
- ☐ Excessive appetite

9

Preventing School Violence

Kathleen Schmalz and Mary Grenz Jalloh

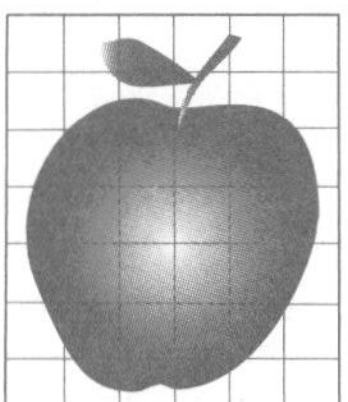

Chapter Outline

Objectives

- Define violence, bullying, sexual harassment, conflict resolution, and social and emotional education
- Explore the types of violence that occur in the school setting and the conditions that enable the occurrence of violence
- Identify the myths and realities of bullying behavior.
- Explain public policy on sexual harassment in the school setting
- Describe current and proposed legislation for reporting violence
- Explore school policy on reporting and following up violence-related incidents
- Explore the classroom teacher's role in violence prevention and resolution
- Explore effective, age-appropriate models for violence prevention and conflict resolution

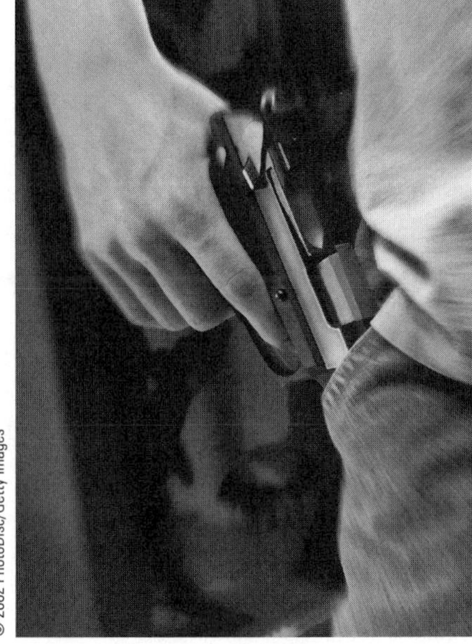

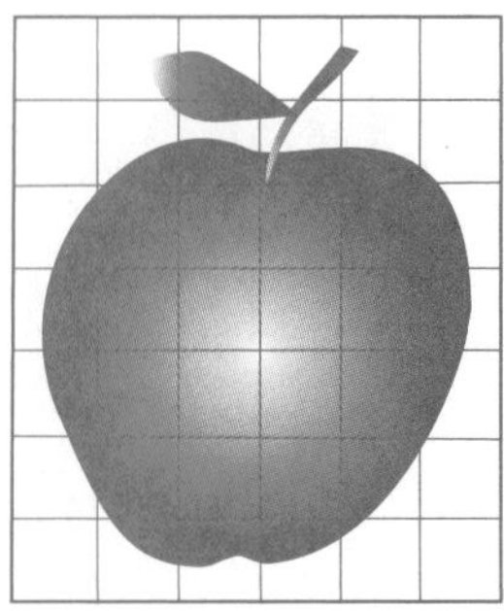

In the wake of the 1999 shooting at Columbine High School, Colorado became one of the first states to pass legislation mandating that every school district implement an anti-bullying policy. The district representative, Don Lee (R), stated categorically that bullying "was one of the factors cited as contributing to what happened at Columbine."[1] New Hampshire and West Virginia have joined Colorado in passing anti-bullying legislation, and similar bills are pending in Illinois, New York, and Washington state.

To many officials, the Columbine tragedy was an unfortunate wake-up call to the reality that, for a growing number of students, schools are not the safe and supportive environment that facilitates learning and social growth. Nearly 30 percent of all students in a nationwide study reported being either the targets or perpetrators of bullying.[2] However, most victims do not come to school with guns for revenge—instead, they often become lonely and withdrawn, and their grades drop. They are more likely to smoke, drink alcohol, and drop out of school. A substantial proportion become bullies themselves: There are always weaker and more vulnerable children.

Most adults remember the bullies from their own school days. There was always a big kid who picked on the smaller kids in the playground. Or maybe the target was the nerd who always got the best grades but had no athletic or social skills. Although the nerd would never act like a bully, one secretly cheered for his/her tormenter or just looked away. Bullying has been going on for so long that many adults have accepted it as normal behavior or just took the approach that, if one were to ignore the problem, it would just go away. In fact, that's the advice that has traditionally been given to victims: "Ignore him and he won't hit you" or "Ignore her and she'll stop teasing you about your clothes." Children who have been bullied know that ignoring the bully does not make him or her stop. It is time for educators to understand that

> Although disagreements are a natural part of growing up, bullying is not. It's a form of violence against the human spirit. It causes students to dread going to school. It wrecks their concentration and destroys their self-confidence. It does untold damage to their academic and personal success. By ignoring it, we're saying to the bully, "You have a right to inflict pain." To the victim we're saying, "You are not worth protecting."[3]

All children must be made to feel that they are worth protecting. Some experts question whether bullying prevention laws will really have teeth at the school level. Respect for others cannot be legislated, but it can be fostered by strategic efforts to defuse violence and make conflict resolution and pro-social behavior an integral part of the school curriculum.

Forms of Violence

A persistent obstacle to confronting violence in the schools has been "lack of a clear and universally accepted definition of violence"[4] Shooting or stabbing a classmate unquestionably qualifies as a violent act, but explosive violence is often the culmination of a series of actions—such as teasing, insulting, or shoving—that are often ignored. Thus, the design and implementation of a successful violence prevention program entails having a clear-cut working definition of the target problems and the strategies for addressing them.

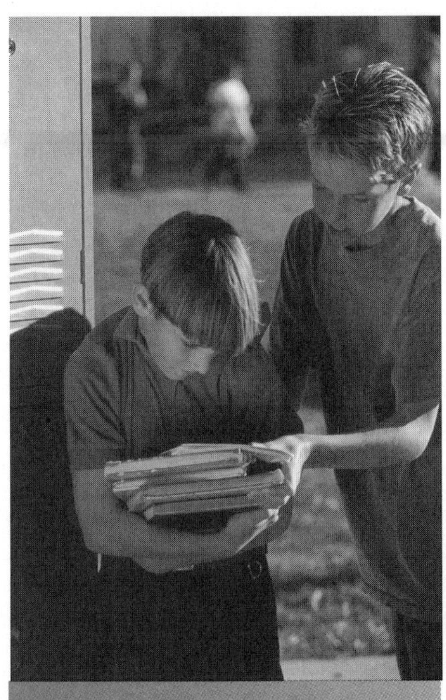
© 2002 PhotoDisc/Getty Images

Bullying can take many different forms, one of which is physical intimidation.

Violence Defined

All violent acts have a single common theme: They all inflict harm, "or threaten harm," to person or property.[5] Although the term "violence" usually invokes the thought of physical harm, non-physical acts, such as teasing, insulting, ignoring, or demeaning gestures or facial expressions, all hold the power to make the recipient feel hurt, disrespected, and devalued. The program Respect and Protect has derived an operational definition that encompasses physical and non-physical violence:

> **Violence** occurs whenever anyone inflicts or threatens to inflict physical or emotional injury or discomfort upon another person's body, feelings, or possessions.[6]

The following definition is simplified for children and adolescents: Violence is any mean word, look, sign, or act that hurts a person's body, feelings, or things.[7]

Working to eradicate school violence begins by understanding that violent acts exist along a continuum. Verbal or gestured abuse does not necessarily escalate to physical violence, but most physical violence begins with the "little things." Physical violence is easy to recognize, although milder forms such as pushing, shoving, or blocking another child's path are often, and misguidedly, ignored. Violence can be divided into two types of physical violence: against person and against property and three types of non-physical violence: social, verbal, and visual.

Physical Violence

A common misconception about bullying is that it usually takes place on the way to or from school, not on the school grounds.[8] While that's a convenient way to make it someone else's problem, a lot of bullying does take place in the school building and playground, particularly in areas that are not monitored by adults.[9] In its definition of violence, Respect and Protect includes incidents on the way to and from school as well as at the school itself. Acts of physical violence commonly perpetrated against students or school staff occupy a range of behaviors from hair-pulling or grabbing to stabbing and shooting. Property violence includes destruction of personal property such as eyeglasses, books, or clothing, as well as destruction or defacement of public property.

Non-Physical Violence: Social, Verbal, Visual

Non-physical violence can be divided into three basic categories, social, verbal, and visual (although there are probably others).

Social violence includes acts that may constitute discrimination or sexual harassment in an adult social context such as unwanted touching or violating another person's civil rights.[10] It also includes acts that may be perpetrated by teachers or other school staff: ignoring a student in class, disregarding requests for help, making fun of a student's cherished beliefs, or betraying a confidence. Among children, spreading rumors is a common form of social violence. Because most children desire peer acceptance, the most devastating form of social violence is ostracism. These actions can also be considered forms of emotional injury.

Verbal violence includes any expression of abuse through spoken or written words. Teasing is the most common form of verbal violence and often goes ignored because it is meant "only in fun." Children (and adults) tease each other in good humor, but attempting to get a laugh at another child's expense is rarely harmless. Name-calling; insults; ethnic, religious, racial, or sexual slurs; lying; constant criticism; taunting; threatening; and making derogatory comments behind a child's back are all forms of verbal abuse.

Visual violence involves the use of visual signals or images to intimidate someone. Visual threats range from glaring, staring, or sneering at someone to threatening them with a fist or a weapon. Among young children, drawing demeaning pictures of peers or imitating mannerisms are common forms of verbal violence that are often downplayed by adults but are hurtful to the targeted child.

Bullying

Like violence, **bullying** has no commonly accepted definition. If one child is seen hurting another, the terms "bullying" and "violence" are often used interchangeably. Bullying has a unique characteristic: Bully/victim conflict takes place within the context of a significant imbalance of power.[11] Specifically,

> Bully/victim violence occurs whenever anyone intentionally, repeatedly, and over time inflicts or threatens to inflict physical or emotional injury or discomfort upon another person's body, feelings, or possessions.[12]

The common stereotype of a bully as a physically big (and often not very bright) child tormenting a smaller one is not always accurate. Some bullies do use physical strength to gain an advantage over other children; others use superior intelligence, street smarts, or emotional manipulation. The idea that bullies lack intelligence is one of many myths that surround bullies and complicate bullying prevention.

One area in which bullies tend to show remarkable intelligence is in hiding their behavior. As with other acts of violence, bullying tends to take place in what has been called "undefined public spaces." Undefined spaces are physical areas that may not be viewed as anyone's responsibility to monitor, and consequently, are where most violent acts take place. In schools, hallways, bathrooms, and playgrounds are "undefined" or "unowned" spaces. As stated by an urban sixth-grade elementary school student, "'Cause there, just everybody beats up on all kinds of little kids all in the bathroom."[13]

In addition to where they know it takes place, students have a lot to say about bullying. A 12-year old boy commented, "I understand why kids kill.... Other kids hit them, tease them, bully them all the time. I would want to hurt them, too."[14] Or this, from a 13-year old boy: "If someone is pushing you around there is no one to tell.... You have to take care of it yourself.... If you run and tell the teachers, they think you're a punk. When they think you're a punk, you know you've got to watch your back."[15]

Sadly, perceptions that nothing can be done about bullying are common among teachers as well as students. Changing the school climate from pessimistic to proactive requires detailed strategic planning and collaboration from all stakeholders: teachers, administrators, students, parents.

A first step for educators and administrators is to understand that, whereas bullying behavior is perpetrated by only a small proportion of students, bullies may be found among children of all ethnic groups, social classes, and intellectual abilities. Bullying exists in similar fashion in rural, suburban, and urban schools. Bullying by girls and boys can take different forms. The behavior of male bullies tends to be more direct and is more frequently labeled "bullying." Boys are more likely to use visible or physical forms of bullying, and usually bully both boys and girls. The behavior of female bullies is often indirect, and therefore, described as "mean" rather than bullying. Girls generally bully other girls, very often through social violence. Boys are more likely to be both perpetrators and victims and more likely to use physical threats or violence, whereas girls often use social manipulation.

According to a U.S. survey of 15,686 students, slightly under 10 percent reported having been bullied, and roughly 6 percent reported having alternately been perpetrators and targets of bullying. Personal features, namely appearance and speech, were much more likely to be targeted than were race or religion.[16]

Bully Busters, a program that addresses the problem, uses the "Double I/R" criteria to distinguish bullying: Bullying behavior is intentional, imbalanced, and repeated. The two basic forms of bullies, aggressive and passive, each has a defining set of characteristics:

Aggressive bullies

- Are the most prevalent type of bully.
- Initiate aggressive acts toward peers.
- Are regarded as fearless, tough, coercive, and impulsive.
- Have a strong inclination toward violence, like to dominate others, and show minimal empathy toward their victims.
- Attack their victims directly (practice "direct bullying").
- Enjoy being in control of others.
- Cognitively misrepresent the meaning of their victim's behavior and tend to overreact in ambiguous situations.
- Have a paranoid view of the world.

Passive bullies

- Are not as common as aggressive bullies.
- Tend to be anxious, insecure, and dependent.
- Generally do not initiate the aggressive acts.
- Intentionally ostracize and exclude others from the group (practice "indirect bullying").
- May lack strong inhibitions against aggression.
- Often follow when they observe an aggressive bully's behavior being rewarded.
- Are eager to be accepted by aggressive bullies.
- May be called "camp followers" or "hangers-on."[17]

Although aggressive bullies are often skilled at shielding their behavior from the eyes of adults, their actions are easy to recognize when observed. In contrast, many teachers have witnessed the actions of passive bullies yet do not regard them as bullying behaviors. The more adept teachers become at identifying the forms violence can take, the more effective they will be at strategically targeting early interventions.

Although the term "bully" is the accepted noun for a person who displays certain behaviors, Title emphasizes that the term should be used to describe a behavior pattern, not label the person. If bullies are labeled, they may internalize the label as an identity: "A bully is who I am." Keeping the focus on the behavior carries the understanding that the behavior is learned, not an innate part of the child. Learned behaviors can be unlearned.[18]

In reality, bullies can always find something to pick on: a wrong answer in class, a mismatched outfit, a bad haircut, or the third strike with the bases loaded. However, certain children can be characterized as passive victims, who are more likely to be singled out and less likely to defend themselves than their peers. Passive victims tend to be insecure and to react anxiously and submissively when attacked. They may seem overly sensitive and often have difficulty asserting themselves.

Male victims, especially, tend to be physically weaker than their peers, although with increasing numbers of girls participating in sports, lack of athletic prowess may predispose both girls and boys to victimization. In contrast to passive victims of bullying are provocative victims. Children with attention deficit disorder (ADD) are common among provocative victims. Like bullies, they are frequently aggressive toward peers, but without the social skills or street smarts that rank bullies among the popular students. The idea that bullies are disliked is a common myth. "More commonly they enjoy average to high popularity."[19] Instead, they seek out weaker students to bully.

According to Remboldt and Zimman, "One thing that can be said of all victims, both passive and provocative, they lack the skills of assertiveness that are necessary for any person to interact comfortably with peers."[20] A well-designed bully prevention program includes a strong component for teaching social skills.

Sexual Harassment

Sexual harassment is defined as unwanted and unwelcomed sexual behavior that interferes with a child's learning or participation in school activities.[21] Sexual harassment spans a range of behaviors included in the categories of physical and non-physical violence. In public schools, sexual harassment is a form of gender discrimination and is consequently prohibited by state and federal law. Whether or not an act constitutes sexual harassment is defined by the targeted student's perception, not by school personnel.

When addressing the topic in class, it is important to emphasize that both girls and boys can be both the perpetrators and targets of sexual harassment. For young children, it may be better to frame certain actions such as pinching, touching or sexual comments simply as bullying behavior rather than attempting to fit children's behaviors into an adult model.

Conflict Resolution

School culture can be either conflict-negative or conflict-positive.[22] Conflict-negative schools assume that all conflict is bad. Conflict is perceived as something to be suppressed, avoided, or denied. As a result, there are no strategies in place for teaching students, teachers, or staff how to manage conflict; after all, paying any attention to conflict just might encourage it.

In the same way that failing to recognize bullying behaviors allows them to escalate, failure to deal with conflict does not stop it from happening; it prevents conflicts from being resolved peacefully. Some philosophers believe that conflict is the essence of change. Conflicts stimulate interest and excitement and, when managed appropriately, lead to new ways of thinking and new ways of doing things. Conflict-positive schools adopt strategies that make schools safe and stimulating learning environments.

School conflict resolution programs are usually designed according to either a cadre or total student body model. In the cadre approach, a small number of students are specially trained to serve as peer mediators. In the total student body approach, all students are trained to manage conflicts constructively. The current emphasis is on having all students take part in activities that facilitate non-violent conflict resolution. Bully prevention strategies include the social skills, problem solving, and teamwork that are integral to conflict resolution.

Social and Emotional Education

In his theory of multiple intelligences, Howard Gardner included interpersonal intelligence, the ability to understand people and relationships, and intrapersonal intelligence, the ability to be deeply aware of one's inner feelings, intentions, and goals.[23] Just like mathematical and linguistic intelligence, these intelligences can be learned and nurtured. Social and emotional education refers to the strategies and techniques used to promote social and emotional competencies. Specifically, social and emotional education is "the process of learning to 'read' ourselves and others and then, using this growing awareness, to solve problems flexibly, to learn, and to be creative."[24] Social and emotional education goes beyond conflict resolution and bully prevention, making the humanistic "personal intelligences" an integral part of the core curriculum.

Reporting Violence

A major reason that violence has been allowed to escalate in schools is that teachers and administrators have been unwitting enablers.[25] Teachers' "most common enabling behaviors are failing to identify and refer students for violent actions. When teachers ignore bullying or disregard students' perceived fears about threats or retaliation, it is not surprising that students should feel that "there is no one to tell. . . . You have to take care of it yourself."[26]

Teachers' Reporting of Violence

Unfortunately, there seems to be more information about teachers' lack of reporting violence than there is on reporting all but the most overt displays of violence or weapons. In order to report acts of violence, teachers must be able to recognize the more subtle forms of violence and the locations in which violence is likely to take place. In fact, reporting initiatives have to be school-wide, because teachers are not the only enablers in the school. Most acts of violence are reported by teachers to administrators and parents who have also been described as unwitting collaborators in a culture of enabling.[27]

Without a formal violence prevention program in place, principals often take disciplinary action independently. Frequently, this involves punitive action without investigating a student's prior actions or the context in which the violence took place. Alternately, principals may choose to ignore violent actions for fear of alienating community members or other school personnel (such as a coach, when the perpetrator is a star athlete).

Comprehensive programs, such as the Comer School Development Program, make parents an integral part of the school governance team. In reality, such programs are few. In most schools, home/school collaboration is minimal, and parents expect correspondence from teachers to be bad news. As a result, they are immediately on the defensive. Reports of violence from teachers are likely to be met with denial.[28]

Denial is especially prevalent in families where children experience physical, sexual, or emotional abuse. Reporting of suspected child abuse is mandated by law. Contrary to popular belief, most bullies are not abused children. However, some definitely are. Teachers who report a child's violent act to a parent and are met with denial or hostility should examine their own feelings about the situation. Has the child shown any signs of abuse? Ignoring the signs of abuse, whether a child has been abused by parents or peers, only allows the problem to continue and intensify.

What to Report

Acts of overt violence in a heavily trafficked school area are easy to identify. Few acts of violence fall into that category, and those that do are likely to be the tragic consequences of actions that went undisclosed or unreported. Actions that should be reported include

- Drug or alcohol use.
- Rumors of planned fights on the school grounds before or after school.
- Hazing rituals.
- Observed or reported weapons-carrying.
- Threats of violence or retaliation against students, teachers, or staff.
- Threatening or violent classroom behavior.
- Sexual harassment.
- Complaints by students who have been victimized.
- Suspected physical or sexual abuse of a child by an adult (i.e., parents or school personnel).
- Property crimes.

School Policy on Reporting Violence

School policy has also been cited as part of an enabling system that allows violence to continue unchecked. Policies are typically unclear and inconsistent. The definition of violence may be too vague or too circumscribed, covering only explicit displays of violence such as physical assault or weapons-carrying. Violence prevention expert Dr. Deborah Prothrow-Smith has denounced anti-bullying legislation, stating:

> I don't think the legal avenue has much promise. I can see this becoming the zero-tolerance fad of today. To the extent that this pursuit of anti-bullying laws takes us further down the punishment track and distracts us from the true preventive activities, it could hurt.[29]

School policies toward violence have traditionally been hampered by focusing only on punishment for offenders rather than providing mechanisms for behavior change. Some zero-tolerance policies are so punitive—and would punish a child who commits a minor infraction as severely as one who waves a switchblade in a classmate's face—that educators, students, and parents are reluctant to support them. As a result, the policy is inconsistently enforced and confusing for students and staff.

New legislative policies unquestionably require the implementation of school-wide interventions. For example, under new Massachusetts guidelines, teachers will be able to physically restrain students who threaten teachers or others after other methods to control them have failed. How teachers will be trained to deal with such situations has been left to the individual school districts, but some form of training is essential. Likewise, teachers need to be formally trained in how to recognize and report violent acts.

Schools need a well–thought-out, well-designed plan that delineates exactly what acts should be reported and to whom. The logical consequences of actions should be embedded in school policy including strategies that support student efforts toward behavior change. Remember that violence takes place along a continuum. Where an act falls along the continuum, school policy should designate who it should be reported to and what actions should take place afterward.

Following a Report of Violence

Reporting a violent act is only the first step. For some students, expulsion may be the only solution. However, this may involve enrollment in an alternative school and the intervention of school support personnel. If the act is reported within the school, collaboration between teachers, principals, and the school counselor, psychologist, or social worker is essential for working with both the perpetrator and the victim. Engaging parents in active collaboration can be complicated, but a clear-cut policy defining the role of each constituent can work to ensure that students receive assistance both at home and at school.

Keeping an up-to-date database can be invaluable for following up on students who have been involved in violence. The important thing is to remember that most students are capable of changing. Tracking a student's behavior is an excellent way to prevent violence from escalating, as well as following up on behavior after violence takes place.

Respect and Protect advocates student support groups for the victims and perpetrators of violence.[30] For victims, the program includes an Empowerment Group. For perpetrators, the levels of support and sanctions increase with the severity of the act.

What Teachers Can Do About Violence

A study on violence in undefined spaces in middle and elementary schools found that in general, elementary school teachers tended to do a better job of monitoring schools, whereas middle school teachers tended to feel that their main responsibility was in their subject specialty classroom. Elementary school teachers felt a sense of personal and professional responsibility for the whole physical plant.[31]

However, certain areas, such as restrooms and playgrounds, were still neglected and, as a result, these were the areas where violence took place. Just as identifying violent behavior is the first step in preventing violence, identifying the contexts where violence takes place is the starting point for taking responsibility for a safe school. Elementary school teachers can employ any of the following strategies to curb violence:

- Collaborate with colleagues, administrators, and parents about monitoring neglected spaces.
- Use the NICE approach. Developed by Bully Busters, NICE stands for

  N = Notice
  I = Increase (Do more of what works.)
  C = Create (Use imagination to create opportunities for bullies and victims to engage in pro-social behavior.)
  E = Encourage (Encourage and celebrate successes, including small ones.)[32]

Also, challenge beliefs and actions that perpetuate bullying, such as ignoring bullying or inconsistently intervening:

- Learn how to identify different types of violence and bullying.
- Learn the skills and techniques necessary to intervene.
- Be accessible to students.
- Serve as a role model for pro-social behavior.
- Integrate violence prevention into the curriculum.
- Serve as a change agent by monitoring your own behavior as well as your students.
- Most important: Believe you have the ability to make a difference![33]

Violence Prevention Programs

Violence prevention programs take a variety of forms. Among the common components are cognitive-behavioral strategies, conflict resolution, teamwork, multimedia, role-play, simulations, role modeling, peer mediation, and pro-social skills development.

Bully Busters

One of the most comprehensive strategies, and one which can be adapted to each individual school, Bully Busters has outlined the "Four Roses" of bully control:

- Recognize that a problem exists.
- Remove yourself or step back from the situation if you do not feel up to the task of effectively intervening.
- Review the situation.
- Respond to the situation: If you feel competent to intervene, do so; if not, help students find other assistance.[34]

The Prepare Curriculum

The Prepare Curriculum is an excellent psycho-educational program designed to teach children and adolescents pro-social competencies. The coordinated courses are specially prepared for students who lack interpersonal skills. Whatever the student is deficient in, the program addresses: Insensitive children are taught empathy, impulsive students receive training in anger management, anxious students learn stress management, and isolated students are involved in group work. This is only a partial list.

Creative Conflict Resolution

Not all curricula encompass all facets of behavior. Some focus on aspects of violence prevention, such as conflict resolution and peer mediation. *Creative Conflict Resolution* is an excellent resource for teachers of all grades. The manual includes "more than 200 activities for keeping peace in the classroom," organized according to the developmental levels of children in grades K–6.[35] By implementing strategies in the early grades, children learn to respect individual differences and develop empathy early on. Most important, they learn problem-solving and teamwork competencies that will help them achieve both academic and social success.

Bully Proof

Bully Proof was developed specifically for fourth and fifth grade students so that each lesson logically follows the next, although the lessons are flexible enough to be adapted to the unique conditions of each classroom.[36] Although not exactly multimedia (although there are cartoons for children to color), the case study format allows for tremendous student input. In short, it allows students to contribute as many perspectives as they can think up.

WIN/WIN

A keynote of successful conflict resolution is achieving a win/win situation. WIN/WIN guidelines can be incorporated into any conflict resolution model:

- Allow for cooling off, if needed; find alternative ways to express anger.
- Using "I messages," each person states the way he/she feels and perceives the problem.
- Each person states the problem as the other person sees it.
- Each person states how he/she is responsible for the problem.
- The conflicting parties brainstorm solutions and arrive at a solution that satisfies both—a WIN/WIN solution.
- Each one affirms her/his partner.[37]

Children can be remarkably creative. Using the WIN/WIN method allows children to envision the solution to the conflict. Through creative, collaborative activities, they learn to explore their own feelings and become aware of the feelings of others. Encouraging the exploration of feelings, thoughts, and experiences enables young children to understand the dynamics of conflict and the obstacles to, and facilitators of, successful resolution.

The HA HA SO Method

Even before Columbine, a number of Colorado school districts were actively engaged in bully prevention. One successful curriculum for teaching children cognitive strategies for identifying bully behaviors and responding effectively employs several imaginative techniques such as the HA HA SO method for responding to aggression: Help, Assert, Humor, Avoid, Self talk, and Own it.

Acronyms seem to be a staple of interventions; another part of the program is CARE, for Creative problem solving, Adult help, Relate and join, and Empathy, which focuses on the problems of students who are victimized.[38]

Second Step: A Violence Prevention Curriculum

This program employs a unique blend of social systems and psychodynamic techniques to help elementary school children deal with the complex dynamics of bullying.[39] The keynote of the approach is that perpetrators, victims, and bystanders are targeted simultaneously. All children take part in all activities, with the healthier children helping those who are more disturbed. Second Step has four components:

1. Zero tolerance for bullying, victimization, and standing by doing nothing.
2. A discipline plan for modeling appropriate behavior.
3. A physical education plan to teach children self-regulation.
4. A mentoring program for adults and children to help children avoid one of the socially undesirable roles.[40]

An evaluation of Second Step demonstrated that a well-planned intervention can successfully achieve the dual goals of academic attainment and social competency. The program elicited significant improvement in academic achievement and fewer school suspensions. In addition, many children who fit the model of the "passive victim" became more verbal and assertive over the course of the program.

Caring, Sharing and Getting Along

Caring, Sharing and Getting Along offers a variety of hands-on activities for young children. Its characters, Kenny and his friends, draws on children's love of animals to illustrate that it is not only humans who have rules for healthy and pro-social behavior.[41] Research has identified a link between animal abuse in childhood and subsequent violent behavior. The use of animals as models not only provides an engaging, age-appropriate way to explore pro-social behavior, but encourages children to have respect for all their fellow creatures.

I Can Problem Solve

Advocates of social emotional learning have a variety of strategies, such as I Can Problem Solve (ICPS), a cognitive strategy for preventing behaviors associated with violence.[42] Like all aspects of social emotional learning, the developmentally appropriate strategy is designed to be incorporated into the school curriculum.

Safe Schools, Safe Students

Safe Schools, Safe Students is based on a comprehensive review that has been adopted by many school districts.[43] The summary list was developed through a detailed review of the literature on prevention of violence, juvenile delinquency, and substance abuse, which generated a synthesis of best practices in prevention. The programs reviewed encompass school, family, and community and have the goals of altering school culture to generate school norms that foster pro-social behavior. Teacher training is an integral part of the programs—as it should be in any program that seeks to replace conditions that enable violence with a culture that prevents violence, promotes peaceful conflict resolution, and rewards pro-social behavior.

Summary

School violence is a pervasive problem that has been perpetuated by an enabling culture. Several states have passed or are in the process of reviewing initiatives that would mandate bully-prevention programs. Educators who take a proactive approach to developing and implementing school programs are effective in bullying prevention. However, legal methods that remain independent of systemic approaches, for combating violence are likely to be ineffective.

First, teachers need to be aware of the continuum of behaviors that constitutes violence—from the most explicit displays to the most subtle cues. Second, schools need to have a clear-cut policy for addressing school violence that is consistently enforced. Third, effective violence prevention entails a collaboration of all constituents, including educators, all school personnel, students, families, and communities.

Many innovative strategies exist to address bullying and violence at all grade and developmental levels. Programs range from specific conflict-resolution interventions to coordinated curricula encompassing all academic and social aspects of the school and home environments. Most are highly flexible and can be adapted to suit the needs of each individual classroom. The most important guideline for both educators and students is the belief that "I can make a difference!"

Resources

Bitney, J. *No Bullying*. Minneapolis: Johnson Institute, 1996.

Center for the Prevention of School Violence, 313 Chapanohe Road, Suite 140, Raleigh, NC 27603, 1-800-299-6054, www.nscu.edu/cpsv.

Delisle, D., and J. Delisle. *Growing Good Kids*. Minneapolis: Free Spirit Publishing, 1996.
28 activities that enhance self-awareness, compassion, and leadership.

Derman-Sparks, L., and A.B.C. Task Force. *Anti-Bias Curriculum: Tools for Empowering Young Children*. Washington, DC: National Association for the Education of Young Children, 1989).
Chapters include why an anti-bias curriculum; creating an anti-bias environment; learning about racial differences and similarities; learning about disabilities; learning about gender identity; learning about cultural differences and similarities; learning to resist stereotyping and discriminatory behavior; and working with parents.

Dunn, L., P. Lewis, L. Hall, I. McAvoy, and C. Pitts. *Conflict Resolution and Peer Mediation*. Chapel Hill, NC: Mediation Network of North Carolina, 1995.
This curriculum teaches negotiation, mediation, and conflict management skills. Uses a "talk it out" strategy to help students negotiate.

Froschl, M., B. Sprung, and N. Mullin-Rindler. *Quit It! A Teacher's Guide on Teasing and Bullying for Use with Students in Grades K–3.* New York: Educational Equity Concepts, 1998.
This book contains nine classroom lessons to help you and your students explore this topic plus problem-solving assignments, literature connections, physical games and exercises, reproducible worksheets, and family activity letters.

Garrity, C., K. Jens, W. Porter, N. Sager, and C. Short-Camilli. *Bully Proofing Your School.* Longmont, CO: Sopris West, 1994. www.sopriswest.com

Gardner, H. *Multiple Intelligences: The Theory in Practice.* New York: Harper Collins, 1993.

Goldstein, A. P. *The Prepare Curriculum.* Champaign, IL: Research Press, 1999.

Hoover, John H., and Ronald Oliver. *The Bullying Prevention Handbook*. Bloomington, IN: National Educational Service, 1996. www.nesonline.com
This handbook provides a comprehensive tool for understanding, preventing, and reducing the day-to-day teasing and harassment referred to as bullying.

Johnson, D. W. and R. T. Johnson. *Reducing School Violence Through Conflict Resolution.* Alexandria, VA: Association for Supervision and Curriculum Development, 1995.

Kane, William M., Magdelena M. Avila, and Hilda Clarice Quiroz. *Step by Step to Safe Schools: The Program Planning Guide*. Santa Cruz, CA: ETR Associates, 2001.

This book explores the roots of violence: bullying, harassment, hazing, and hate-motivated behavior. It offers a blueprint for creating safe schools and safe learning environments, discusses violence prevention education and ways to assist troubled youth, outlines how to develop a Comprehensive Safe Schools Plan.

Kreidler, William J. *Teaching Conflict Resolution Through Children's Literature.* New York: Scholastic, 1994.

The literature and ideas presented are geared for grades K–2. Through the use of language-rich children's literature, the author gives the teacher wonderful ways to teach the concepts of diversity, problem-solving, conflict-solving, caring, respect, and community.

Levin, Diane E. *Teaching Young Children in Violent Times: Building a Peaceable Classroom*. Cambridge, MA: Educators for Social Responsibility, 1994.

This book helps children learn peaceful alternatives to the violent behaviors modeled for them in the media and beyond: a classroom where children resolve their conflicts peacefully; where their critical needs for safety are met; where young children come to respect one another's differences by living and learning in a Peaceable Classroom.

Olweus, Dan. *Bullying at School*. Oxford, UK: Blackwell Publishers, 1993.

Bullying at School is essential reading for all who are involved with children and young people.

Safe Spaces: Creating Safe and Drug-Free Learning Environments. New Paltz, NY: The New York State Center for School Safety, 2000.

Second Step: A Violence Prevention Curriculum

Available through the Committee for Children, 2203 Airport Way South, Suite 500, Seattle, WA 98134, 800-634-4449.

Slaby, Ronald G., Wendy C. Roedell, Diana Arezzo, and Kate Hendrix. *Early Violence Prevention: Tools for Teachers of Young Children*. Washington, DC: National Association for the Education of Young Children, 1995.

Describes practical ways to handle children's aggression, including how to help children become neither aggressors nor victims, but assertive and nonviolent problem solvers.

The Teaching Tolerance Project. *Starting Small: Teaching Tolerance in Preschool and the Early Grades*. Montgomery, AL: Southern Poverty Law Center, 1997. Compiled by Carly J. Reynolds, New York State Center for School Safety.

Videos

Prevent Violence with Groark. Program. Elkind and Sweet Communications. Live Wire Media, San Francisco, 1996. (415) 564-9500.

1: Groark Learns to Control Anger

2: Groark Learns to Work Out Conflicts

4: Groark Learns About Bullying

KidSafety of America. *Managing School Violence In Preschools and Elementary Schools.* 2000. www.kidsafetystore.com

McGruff on Anger, Conflict and Violence

15 minutes; K–6; Aims Multimedia, 800-367-2467

McGruff's Bully Alert

15 minutes; grades K–6; Aims Multimedia, 800-367-2467.

Notes

1. M. A. Zehr, "Legislatures Take on Bullies with New Laws" *Education Week* (2001, May 16): 18, 22.
2. National School Safety Center, *School Safety Update* [Newsletter] (Westlake Village, CA: National School Safety Center, May, 2001).
3. C. Remboldt and R. Zimman, *Respect and Protect.* (Center City, MN: Hazelden, 1996), 78.
4. C. Remboldt, *Violence in Schools: The Enabling Factor* (Minneapolis, MN: Johnson Institute 1994), 5.
5. See note 3, p. 16.
6. See note 4, p. 5.
7. See note 4, p. 6.
8. See note 4, p. 6.
9. R. A. Astor, H. A. Meyer, and R. O. Pittner, "Elementary and Middle School Students' Perceptions of Violence-prone School Subcontexts" *Elementary School Journal* 101 (2001): 511–528.
10. See note 3.
11. B. B. Title, *Bully/Victim Conflict: An Overview for Educators* (Center City, MN: Hazelden, 1996), 4.
12. C. Remboldt, *Solving Violence Problems in Your School: Why a Systematic Approach Is Necessary* (Minneapolis: Johnson Institute, 1994), 20.
13. See note 9, p. 520.
14. D. A. Newman, A. M. Horne, and C. L. Bartolomucci, *Bully Busters: A Teacher's Manual for Helping Bullies, Victims, and Bystanders* (Champaign, IL: Research Press, 2000), 24.
15. See note 14, p. 29.
16. See note 2.
17. See note 14, pp. 58–59.
18. See note 11.
19. See note 3, p. 81.
20. See note 3, pp. 91–92.
21. L. Sjostrum and N. Stein, *Bullyproof: A Teacher's Guide on Teasing and Bullying* (Wellesley College Center for Research on Women, 1996).
22. M. D. Johnson, *Caring, Sharing and Getting Along: Children's Activities in Social Responsibility* (Santa Cruz, CA: ETR Associates, 1993).
23. Gardner, H. *Multiple Intelligences: The Theory in Practice*, N.Y. Basic Books, 1993.
24. J. Cohen, "Social and Emotional Education: Core Concepts and Practices." In *Caring Classrooms/Intelligent Schools: The Social Emotional Education of Young Children*, ed. J. P. Comer and J. Cohen (New York: Teachers College Press, 2001), 3–29.
25. See note 4.
26. See note 14, p. 29.
27. See note 3.
28. See note 3.
29. See note 3.
30. See note 3.
31. See note 9.
32. See note 14, pp. 16–17.
33. See note 14, pp. 29–30.

34. See note 14, pp. 102–103.

35. W. J. Kreidler, *Creative Conflict Resolution* (Glenview, IL: Good Year Books, 1984).

36. See note 19.

37. N. Drew, *Learning the Skills of Peacemaking* (Torrance, CA: Jalmar Press, 1987), 11.

38. L. G. Berkey, B. Keyes, and J. E. Longhurst, "Bully-Proofing: What One District Learned About Improving School Climate," *Reclaiming Children and Youth* 9 (2001): 224–228.

39. S. W. Twemlow, P. Fonagy, F. C. Sacco, M. L. Gies, R. Evans, and R. Ewbank, "Creating a Peaceful School Learning Environment: A Controlled Study of an Elementary School Intervention to Reduce Violence," *American Journal of Psychiatry* 158 (2001): 808–810.

40. See note 14.

41. See note 20.

42. M. B. Shure and A. Glaser, "I Can Problem Solve (ICPS): A Cognitive Approach to the Prevention of Early High-Risk Behaviors. In *Caring Classrooms/Intelligent Schools: The Social Emotional Education of Young Children*, ed. J. P. Comer and J. Cohen (New York: Teachers College Press, 2000), 122–139.

43. Drug Strategies, *Safe Schools, Safe Students: A Guide to Violence Prevention Strategies* (Washington, DC: Drug Strategies, 1998).

44. *Safe Spaces: Creating Safe and Drug-Free Learning Environments* (New Paltz, NY: The New York State Center for School Safety, 2000).

Learning Experiences

Critical to maintaining safe and healthy learning environments is the need to help children understand connections and relationships with others. Developing the awareness of the impact of one's actions on others and awareness of the feelings of others (empathy) is core to the establishment of healthy, non-violent relationships. Essential skills to develop during the elementary years to help children prevent interpersonal violence include communication, self-management, stress management, decision-making, planning and goal setting, and advocacy. With competency in these areas, children can better recognize and appropriately respond to conflicts that could otherwise lead to violence.[44] The following activities, by grade level, are offered as guidelines and a starting point for preventing school violence.

Grades K–2

Demonstrating basic communication skills in everyday classroom activities is the first step in creating a safer school environment. These skills may include listening, following directions, making "I" statements ("I feel ... when you ...."), responding to questions, and respectfully refusing to argue with others. It is important for children to see how these skills are used by adults in their environment so they can model them accordingly. It is helpful to have clear and simple expectations for children at this age and to reinforce those expectations daily in practice and discussion. It is also critical that children understand consequences for violating expectations. This is the beginning of establishing normative behavioral standards, with many practice opportunities for skill development. This establishes the foundation of the skill of self-management.

Grades 3–4

Teachers should continue to reinforce the skills of communication and self-management. Children at this age can begin to express how conflict creates stressful feelings in themselves and learn techniques to reduce and/or manage stress. Discussion circles can help elicit these feelings ("How does it make you feel when you see someone fight?") and develop strategies for response. Classroom activities can emphasize basic decision-making skills at this level by relating real-life situations to the children's experiences. Many classroom situations can demonstrate the skill of decision making as a group, reinforcing what children are practicing independently.

Grades 5–6

Continuously reinforcing and practicing skills internalizes them, ensuring that they will be used daily to avoid conflicts. Children at this age, with the core skills of communication, self-management and decision-making, can practice the skills of planning and goal-setting. This moves children into more abstract thinking and reasoning. If the goal is to avoid conflict with a bully, a plan to achieve success can be developed. Children can identify supports to help ensure success, then practice and review the outcome to refine the plan for greater success.

Once children understand and internalize the skills of communication, self-management, stress management, decision-making, and planning and goal-setting, they can become advocates for a caring community where conflict is minimized and connections and relationships are emphasized. Learning Experience 9-5 ("Is Everyone Here?") sets the stage for children to learn the skill of advocacy through examining, assessing, and changing their everyday environment.

Learning Experience 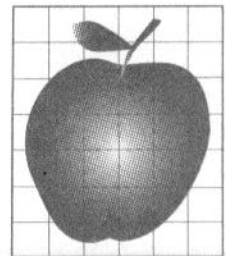 9-1

Discussion Circle—Do We Have to Fight?

Grade Level
3–4

Primary Discipline
Language Arts

Learning Objectives
After this activity, students should be able to

- Describe situations of conflict that can lead to fights.
- Demonstrate strategies for resolving conflicts without fighting.
- Articulate unacceptable ways of dealing with conflict.

Time Required
45 minutes

Materials
Strategy cards, flip chart, and marker

Description of Activity
Before class, prepare strategy cards to introduce as needed. Some of these could include

- Listening to hear another's point of view.
- Using "I" messages instead of "you" messages (that is, express how you feel with an "I" message, such as "I feel bad when you take all the cookies and don't share with me" instead of a "you" message, such as "You always take all the cookies!").
- Take turns.
- Find a compromise (Example: "I'll use this ball while you ride my scooter, and then we'll trade.")
- Ask for help. Although tattling is an unacceptable way to resolve conflict because it is trying to get someone else in trouble, it's OK to ask an adult to help children and their friends to come up with a solution to your conflict.
- Agree on a cooling off time before trying to settle the conflict.
- Violence, through words or actions, is always unacceptable as a means to resolve a conflict.

Ask students to move chairs in a circle, ensuring that the circle is arranged heterogeneously. After everyone is seated, introduce the topic "Do We Have to Fight?" by indicating that conflict is normal and occurs every day in our lives. Sometimes little things can lead to arguments and fights. Ask students for examples of conflicts they have experienced. (Examples may be conflict with a sibling about a TV program to watch or an argument with a friend about whose turn it is to play a game.) Invite students to share how they felt when they experienced conflict. Ask, "Can you think of a time when a conflict happened that almost led to a fight?" Ask, "What can we do to resolve conflicts without fighting?" List strategies students give on the flip chart. Discuss each strategy, indicating whether it is an acceptable or unacceptable way of dealing with conflict. Introduce the strategy cards you prepared.

Invite students to role-play strategies you've discussed using situations they mentioned in the beginning of the discussion circle that have created conflict.

Evaluation

- Students will demonstrate at least two strategies for resolving conflicts.
- Students will identify one adult at school and at home who could help them in a conflict situation.
- Fights with words or hands will be observed with decreased frequency.

Source: For related activities, see Terri Akin et al., *Self-Esteem Activities for the Elementary Grades* (Spring Valley, CA: Innerchoice Publishing, 1990).

Learning Experience 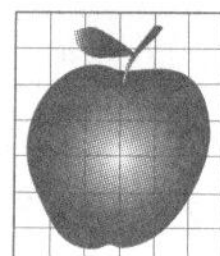 9-2

Bullying Combatants

Grade Level

3–4

Primary Discipline

Language Arts, Art

Learning Objectives

After this activity, students should be able to

- Understand the concept of bullying.
- Increase empathy and activism.
- Use knowledge of ways to intervene on behalf of targets.

Time Required

45 minutes

Materials

Chalkboard, paper, art supplies, five simple bullying scenarios (these should be short, realistic situations where the reader is witnessing someone else being teased), anti-bullying certificates

Description of Activities

Begin by asking the students the following question: "Can anyone tell me what bullying is?"

Allow for many answers to clarify the definition in the students' words, but make sure to highlight the repeated characteristic of power over behavior.

Then ask: "Has anyone ever been bullied or teased before?" Have the students draw a picture of a time that they were bullied, teased, or picked on. If any students have a hard time thinking of an incident, ask them about older siblings' or cousins' behavior. If they still can't think of anything, have them draw an imagined scenario. Ask the students to draw or write how the teasing made them feel. When they've finished, have them share their feelings in a group discussion.

Then ask: "What do you do when someone is teasing you?" Write their responses on the chalkboard. All reasonable responses should fall into one of three categories: "Ignore it," "Get help from an adult," or "Stand up to it." Record the responses in these three groups, then point out the categories by labeling them.

(Allow a discussion of using physical force if the students initiate the idea; however, steer the discussion so that they understand why that would not be productive.)

Then ask: "Because being picked on makes us all feel bad, and we now know lots of ways to handle it, what will you do when you see someone else being teased?" Record these responses under each appropriate category on the chalkboard. Point out which category each response belongs under as you record it. The "Ignore it" category takes on a different meaning when discussing witnessing teasing. If a student suggests doing nothing, remind the class of their drawings and how they all felt. In the course of the discussion, a new category should emerge: "Be a friend." Point out and label this new category. Make a simple drawing or design to represent each of the new categories: "Be a friend," "Get help from an adult," and "Stand up to it."

Next, read the bullying scenario list. After each example, have the students draw the symbol of the category that they would use in that situation. Make the class aware that they can use more than one or all three at any given time. Have a discussion about the various responses after each scenario.

At the end of the lesson, present each student with a certificate indicating that they are qualified to combat bullying for themselves and others.

Submitted by Lorelei Christensen, New York State Center for School Safety.

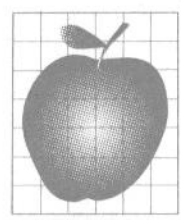

Learning Experience 9-2 continued

Homework

Within a week of the lesson, have the students write an essay about what they learned about bullying and a time when they did, or plan to, combat it using the techniques they learned in class.

Follow Up

Construct a poster with the categories and responses to be hung in a highly visible area of the classroom. Implement a minor reward system for students who use the techniques discussed in class. Create a simple form the students can fill out to nominate a classmate for a reward.

Evaluation

The students' essays can be evaluated on the following basis:

A: Student demonstrates an understanding of bullying, willingness to work actively to combat it, and refers specifically to the categories and various concepts discussed.

B: Student demonstrates understanding of bullying, willingness to combat it, and refers vaguely to categories and concepts discussed.

C: Student demonstrates willingness to combat bullying.

D: Student does not demonstrate willingness to combat bullying.

F: Student does not complete assignment.

Learning Experience 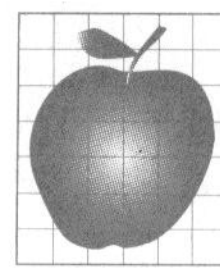 9-3

Using Our Words For Good

Grade Level

K–2

Primary Discipline

Language Arts

Learning Objectives

After this activity, students should be able to

- Understand the impact of words.
- Increase empathy and activism.
- Establish positive alternatives to negative language.

Time Required

45 minutes

Materials

Chalkboard, two puppets, paper, crayons (other art supplies optional), pins that say "I will make others feel good by using my words!"

Description of Activities

Begin by asking the students the following question: "Name some words someone could say that would make you feel bad, sad, or scared."

(Be prepared for vulgar or abusive language students may hear at home, through the media, from other students, or from older siblings. Be aware of any comments that may red-flag an abusive home life. Follow your protocol as a mandatory reporter.)

Write the responses on the chalkboard. Then ask: "Name some words someone could say that would make you feel happy, loved, or safe." Write those responses next to the "bad" ones.

Using puppets, model a scenario using one or more of the "bad" responses. Now refer to one of the puppets and ask the class questions such as: "How do you think [frog] feels right now?" "Why do you think s/he feels that way?"

"What are some different words [skunk] could use that would make [frog] feel good instead of bad?"

Repeat using different scenarios as many times as class interest and time allows. Explain to the students that words are powerful—they can make someone feel good or bad.

Have the students draw a picture of themselves making someone else feel good by using their words. As they work, circulate around the room and ask the students to explain their work, using questions such as: "Who is that you are talking to?" "What are you saying to make them feel good?" Work individually with students that may not have mastered the concept.

When they finish, solemnly make the following announcement:

"Now that you all understand how to use your words to make others feel good, each one of you has a very important job. Are you ready? Raise your right hand. Do you all promise to always use your words to make others feel good?"

Upon agreement, present each of them with their pin confirming individually that they can do it.

Homework

(optional) Send a note home to the parents explaining the exercise, its purpose, and how they can perpetuate the lesson using positive reinforcement.

Follow Up

Display the students' drawings. As often as possible, praise students exhibiting kindness by referring back to the lesson and implementing a minor reward system.

Evaluation

Observing the following behaviors indicate positive outcomes from this lesson. An informal data sheet to track behaviors before and after the lesson will provide more concrete results:

- A decrease in negative language
- An increase in positive language
- Students reminding each other about the need for positive language

Submitted by Lorelei Christensen, New York State Center for School Safety.

Learning Experience 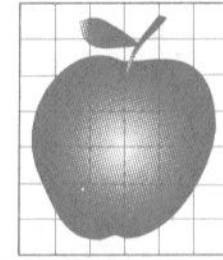 9-4

We're Alike and Different

Grade Level

K–2, 3–4 with added math concepts

Primary Discipline

Math

Learning Objectives

After this activity, students should be able to

- Identify ways members of a group are alike and different.
- Represent similarity and difference in a graph format.
- Explain how they are part of different groups at different times.
- Explain how categories of a group relate to each other.

Time Required

40 minutes

Materials

Post-It notes (1" × 1" or 3" × 3"), sheets of poster-size graph paper

Description of Activity

Children experience non-physical violence when they are excluded, ignored, and made to feel disrespected and devalued. This activity is intended to help children see that they are a part of many different groups at different times. Sometimes they have a unique identity, many times others are linked with them in a group. Give children a series of questions they can answer about themselves, for example:

- Who has a brother or sister at this school?
- How many children have a pet dog? Cat? Fish? Bird?
- How many children are named after a family member?
- Who walked to school?
- Who took the bus?
- Who was dropped off by an adult?
- ...and so on.

For each question, have a graphing poster ready for responses. Children put their name on a Post-It and place it on the bar graph representing their answer. For example, on the graph for "Pet Ownership," one bar is for dogs, one for cats, one for fish, one for birds, one for other, and one for no pets. Children place their Post-It on the bar that represents their pet ownership. Complete graphs in a similar way for other questions posed. For older children, you may introduce the concept of prediction and have them predict how many responses would be in each category, then compare with the actual responses. You can extend the math lesson by asking "How many more (or less) are in one category than another?" or "What percent/fraction of the total class is represented in a category?"

Homework

May be assigned before or after activity. Questions to be used in this activity can be homework.

Evaluation

Following this activity, students will

- Identify how members of their class are alike and different (comparisons and contrasts)
- Explain how they were included as a part of different groups for different questions.
- Read a simple bar graph and tell its meaning

For related activities, see Barbara J. Thomson, *Words Can Hurt You, Beginning a Program of Anti-Bias Education* (Menlo Park, CA: Addison-Wesley Publishing, 1993).

Learning Experience 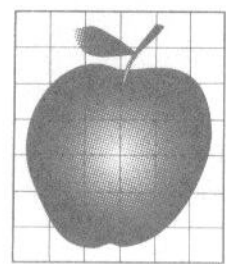 9-5

"Is Everyone Here?"

Grade Level

5–6

Primary Discipline

Social Studies, Art

Learning Objectives

After this activity, students should be able to

- Critically examine their school environment for stereotypes and omissions.
- Identify how their school environment represents various groups.
- Develop recommendations for visually changing the school environment.
- Design images to counter stereotypes.

Time Required

Two 40-minute blocks

Materials

Paper and pencils (Day 1), art supplies (Day 2)

Description of Activity

Introduction

Before doing this activity, be sure to discuss the project with all members of the school community and secure permission from other teachers for your students to examine their rooms in the analysis.

Activity

Being misrepresented or excluded is a form of non-physical violence. In this activity, students will examine their school environment to determine the visual signs of inequality, misrepresentation, and exclusion. Divide students into heterogeneous groups of three to four. Assign each group to a section of the building to assess. Before students venture out (with paper and pencil in hand), have them brainstorm possible findings. Examples include:

- Roles of men and women, boys and girls.
- Activities of boys and girls.
- Numbers and roles of people of color compared with white people.
- Roles of people at different ages.
- Types of families represented.
- Religious and language representations.
- Numbers of people with disabilities.

When students return, have each group report out their findings and summarize the results. On the second day, have students develop recommendations for change and design visual images to counter stereotypes. Involve the art department in this activity. This project can be extended to include an examination of textbooks, literature, television programs, movies, staff in school, and so on. Math concepts can be introduced by graphing and comparing findings. For example, how does the gender/race breakout of students in the building compare with the gender/race breakout of staff? What does this reflect?

Homework

To complete the assignment between days 1 and 2.

Evaluation

Students will accurately identify omissions and misrepresentations. Students will develop new visuals to counter stereotypes in the school environment.

Source: Adapted from Nancy Schniedewind and Ellen Davidson, *Open Minds to Equality* (Boston: Allyn and Bacon, 1998), 213–230.

Learning Experience 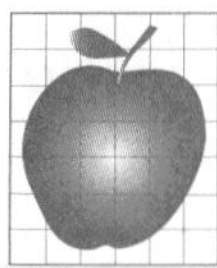 9-6

Contracting Against Bullying

Grade Level

5–6

Primary Discipline

Language Arts

Learning Objectives

After this activity, students should be able to

- Increase empathy and activism.
- Experience cooperative learning and brainstorming.
- Establish, and empower students to use, a classroom reporting system.

Time Required

1 hour

Materials

Chalkboard, paper

Description of Activities

Have the students write a short, in-class essay about a time when they were bullied or witnessed someone else being bullied. Ask them to include what was done about it, as well as what they think should have been done about it.

Make two columns on the chalkboard: "What Was Done" and "What Should Have Been Done." Have as many students as are willing share their stories. Record their responses under the appropriate columns. If the following concepts are not brought up under the "What Should Have Been Done" column, suggest their addition:

- Witnesses should have reported to an adult.
- An adult should have stepped in.
- Someone should have befriended the target.
- Someone should have told the bully to stop.

Once the students feel the "What Should Have Been Done" column is complete, inform them that this will be the basis of classroom bullying contracts. Facilitate a discussion whereby the entire class formulates a contract for each of their behavior expectations in the event that he or she witnesses bullying. Write the final wording on the chalkboard with a space for each to insert his or her name. Have each of the students copy the contract onto a given sheet of paper and sign the contract. Next, discuss a uniform, anonymous system for reporting incidences of bullying to you, the teacher, that you and the class find acceptable. Explain the difference between reporting and tattling:

Tattling is done for personal gain, whereas reporting is done to help someone else.

Finally, commit, by drafting your own contract, to follow up on all reports and do everything in your power to end bullying in the classroom. Read your contract to the class and accept suggestions if possible.

Hang all the contracts in visible places around the room and implement the agreed-upon reporting system.

Submitted by Lorelei Christensen, New York State Center for School Safety.

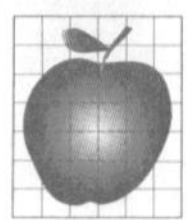

Learning Experience 9-6 continued

Homework

Have each student write an essay outlining an anti-bullying campaign for the entire school.

Follow Up

Uphold your contracted commitments and maintain the reporting system. (Optional: Based on the essays, have the class collectively brainstorm an anti-bullying campaign for the school and submit the idea to the principal.)

Evaluation

The students' essays can be evaluated on the following basis:

A: Student presents a detailed, comprehensive plan including all of the elements the class discussion deemed necessary.

B: Student presents a detailed plan including most of the elements the class discussion deemed necessary.

C: Student presents a plan including some of the elements the class discussion deemed necessary.

D: Student presents a plan including none of the elements the class discussion deemed necessary.

F: Student did not complete the assignment.

Learning Experience 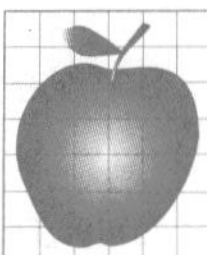 9-7

Express Myself

Grade Level

5–6

Primary Discipline

Health Education

Learning Objectives

After this activity, students should be able to

- Identify their own emotional states.
- Demonstrate stress-management techniques.
- Connect appropriate behavior to situational events.
- Learn to ask for help from others.

Time Required

Two 30-minute periods

Materials

Pieces of paper for role-modeled skits, journals for recording emotions

Description of Activity

Explain to students that emotions can be felt in a range from mild to extreme. Draw a number line on the board and write "mild" at one end, "extreme" at the other, and "happy" in the middle.

Ask students to describe feelings of happiness in a mild form. Responses can include "okay," or "not bad." Ask students to describe the extreme forms of happiness; responses can include "hysterical" and "delirious." Ask for a mid-range description of happy; responses can be "joyful," or "great." Student volunteers will then be handed slips of paper with these different emotional expressions written on each slip.

Students will be asked to role-play typical scenes from everyday life (going to school, going shopping), but others will not know the emotional expression they were given. After a brief role-play, ask the class to guess the emotional state demonstrated. Facilitate a discussion about appropriate emotional expression and ask how this could affect someone if they were sad or unhappy in the extreme sense—how would this behavior look?

During the second session, discuss the ways that students expressed their emotions in the past that may have caused them problems—what did they do when they became upset? Ask students to describe the physical signs of stress: fast breathing, increased heart rate, sweaty palms.

Lead students through deep-breathing exercises (take deep breaths while counting slowly for ten seconds) and ask students to describe how this feels. Suggest that another way students can deal with stress is by discussing feelings with a friend or someone they trust. Have the class discuss the benefits of finding someone to help with problem-solving as a way of relieving stress and seeking validation for their emotional responses.

Homework

Ask the class to record in their journals four noticeable emotional states that caused them stress and to write next to it the event that preceded or caused it. Have students do this same exercise the second week, but have them use the stress management exercise and record its effect. Have students discuss their emotions with a friend and journalize their feelings and ability to problem solve as a result of their conversation.

Submitted by Constance Milland, Hudson Valley Center for Coordinated School Health.

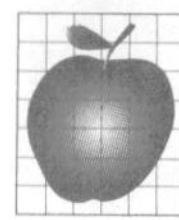

Learning Experience 9-7 continued

Evaluation

A: Students will be able to identify their emotional states and apply stress-management techniques. Students will identify appropriate emotional responses. Students will also identify friends who will assist them in seeking appropriate emotional responses. Students will submit completed journal assignments.

B: Students will identify at least one emotional state and demonstrate the ability to perform the stress-management technique in class. Students will journalize one situation involving emotional stress and record their application of either the stress-management technique or discussing with friends.

C. Students will articulate stress, but not necessarily self-identify. Students will perform stress-management technique in class and will not record events in journal.

D. Students will not participate in class discussion/exercise or complete journal assignment.

Learning Experience 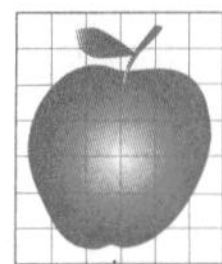 9-8

Communicating with Care

Grade Level

4–6

Primary Discipline

Health Education, mathematical reasoning

Learning Objectives

Following this activity, students should be able to

- Identify the various parts of the communication process.
- Demonstrate sending a message by using different communication methods.
- Correctly interpret the overall meaning of a message conveyed by the sender.
- Correctly identify proportions in a pie chart.

Time Required

Two sessions (30 minutes each)

Materials

Colored art paper, scissors, tape, chalkboard, chalk

Description of Activity

Explain to the class that the act of communicating consists of many parts—the message (or words that you use), the sound or tone of voice, facial expression, and body gestures.

Draw a pie chart on the chalkboard and identify each slice of pie: Message, Tone of Voice, Facial Expression, and Body Gestures. Explain that the pie chart represents the entire communication process and each pie slice is a part of that process. We have to be aware of these different parts of communicating when we send a message, because they help the listener understand our intention.

Ask the class to watch carefully to determine if the messages he/she sends uses equal parts of message, tone of voice, facial expression, or body gestures. Role-model a variety of ways of saying the sentence, "I really care about you." Demonstrate emotions ranging from empathy to boredom, using more or less vivid facial expressions or body gestures for each demonstration. After each role, ask the class to evaluate the performance, re-divide the pie slices to reflect the emphasis placed on facial expression, body language and so on. For example, a message that uses no facial expression will only have a pie with three slices; a message that is mostly gestures will have one large slice and three small slices.

Wait for class response, then re-draw the pie chart after each demonstration to reflect the correct proportion of his/her use of facial expression, body gestures, and so on used in his/her prior demonstration.

Identify the emotional intent of the message (care, distraction, boredom, and so on). Have students role-model their own messages and have class members correctly identify the proportions of their pie chart after each demonstration. Class will also determine the overall emotional content of each message.

Homework

Ask the class to deliver the message "I really care about you" to three people who are important to them (for example, parents, friends, relatives) in three different ways. Have students make up their own pie charts to reflect their message deliveries and discuss this with other students the following week.

Source: Submitted by Constance Milland, Hudson Valley Center for Coordinated School Health. Adapted from New York State Center for School Safety, *Respect* (New York: 2001).

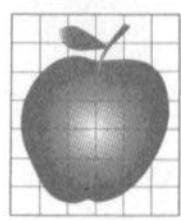

Learning Experience 9-8 continued

Evaluation

For a grade of

A: Students will name and correctly identify the four different parts of the communication process. Students will show an understanding of proportions as demonstrated by the pie chart and through development of their own pie charts with the correct proportions as reflected in the role-modeled demonstrations. Students will identify emotional content of messages.

B: Students will be able to name at least three parts of the communication process. Students will be able to identify the proportions in the pie chart and link these to the role-modeled demonstrations. Students will identify emotional content.

C: Students will name two parts of the communication process. They may or may not correctly match the proportions in their pie charts to the role-modeled demonstrations. Students will not identify emotional content of role-modeled demonstrations.

D: Students will not identify parts of the communication process, nor will they be able to depict the proportions of each role-modeled demonstration to their pie charts.

10

Use of Alcohol, Tobacco, and Other Substances

Michael J. Ludwig

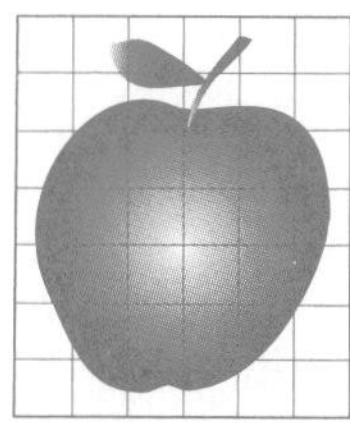

Chapter Outline

Objectives

- Describe the difference between drug education and substance abuse prevention
- Analyze research findings on effective substance abuse prevention programs
- Describe a conceptual framework of substance abuse prevention by naming risk and protective factors in the six life domains.
- Explain the interactive effects of both risk and protective factors as they relate to substance abuse.
- Present a reliable statistical profile of alcohol, tobacco, and other substance use trends, particularly among school-age students
- Define drugs, drug use, drug misuse, drug abuse, dependence, and addiction.
- Classify drugs into appropriate categories
- Explain the routes of drug administration
- Differentiate appropriate and inappropriate alcohol use
- Define alcoholism and describe some effects of long-term misuse/abuse of alcohol.
- Explain the health effects of tobacco use
- Discuss research-based approaches to tobacco prevention as it applies to elementary and middle school students
- Describe the forms of marijuana and their effects on the body
- Describe the forms of cocaine and their effects on health and well-being
- Explain the effects of heroin and the socioeconomic implications of illegal drug use
- Describe the inhalant classification of drugs and their properties
- Explain how anabolic steroids, natural and synthetic, work in the body
- Differentiate prescription and over-the-counter drugs and their appropriate and inappropriate uses
- Give some approaches to drug treatment and some ways in which teachers can promote prevention of drug use in their students

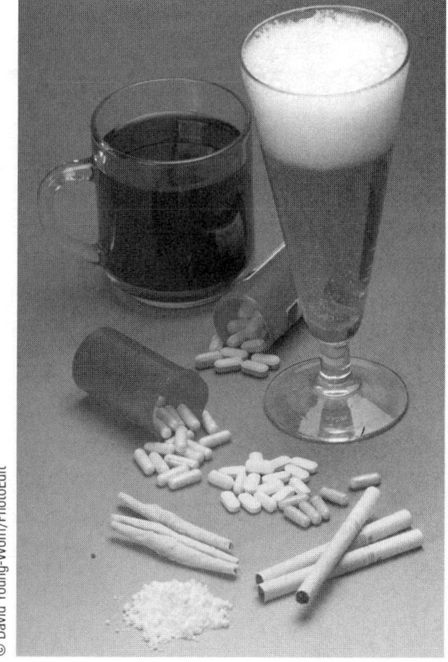

© David Young-Wolff/PhotoEdit

Clarke remembers when he was in third grade and the school counselor came to his class to talk about the problems kids would have if they were to use alcohol and drugs. The counselor described alcoholism and how people who are alcoholics behave. Clarke became alarmed because he realized that his parents were both alcoholics. The teacher said that children of alcoholics often become alcoholics themselves, and that really scared Clarke. He never told anyone about his realization or his fears, but now he is in sixth grade and the kids are all talking about drinking beer and how cool it is to get drunk. Clarke's friend, Whitlin, told him that he knows where to get some marijuana.

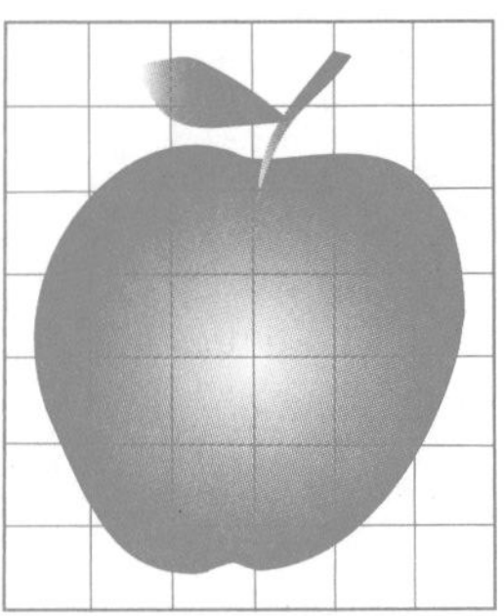

Clarke is clearly confused. What is the difference between a good drug and a bad drug? Will taking a drug from a doctor make him an addict? What messages has he learned at home about drugs and alcohol? Will he be influenced by his peers to drink or take other drugs? What factors contribute to alcoholism or drug abuse? Where can he go for help, and what can he do to help his family with the problems of substance abuse?

Alcohol, tobacco, and other substance use have a long and storied history. They are and have been a part of all cultures' lifestyles, rituals, and values in one way or another. Ancient Greece, for example, accepted and encouraged drinking and drunkenness at festivities. In U. S. society today, drinking is expected at many social functions, and it is included in some religious rituals. Research has identified binge drinking as a common event among many college students.[1]

Drugs other than alcohol and tobacco are also a part of our culture. Aisles at grocery and drug stores are filled with remedies for every conceivable ache and pain. The direct marketing of prescription drugs to the public has exploded since restrictions were lifted a short while ago. We use drugs to keep us healthy, to treat illness, to give pleasure, or to alter our mood.

This chapter will provide classroom teachers with an overview of effective substance abuse programs, practices, and policies as well as a brief description of alcohol, tobacco, and other substances as they affect students' health. Almost everyone uses drugs (aspirin and caffeine are drugs), but a caring and knowledgeable classroom teacher can help students develop skills that may help protect them from the misuse and abuse of drugs. Further, any teacher who better understands both the power and the limits of his/her position can help students become aware of the appropriate use of drugs, alternatives to their use, effects of their use, and means of primary prevention.

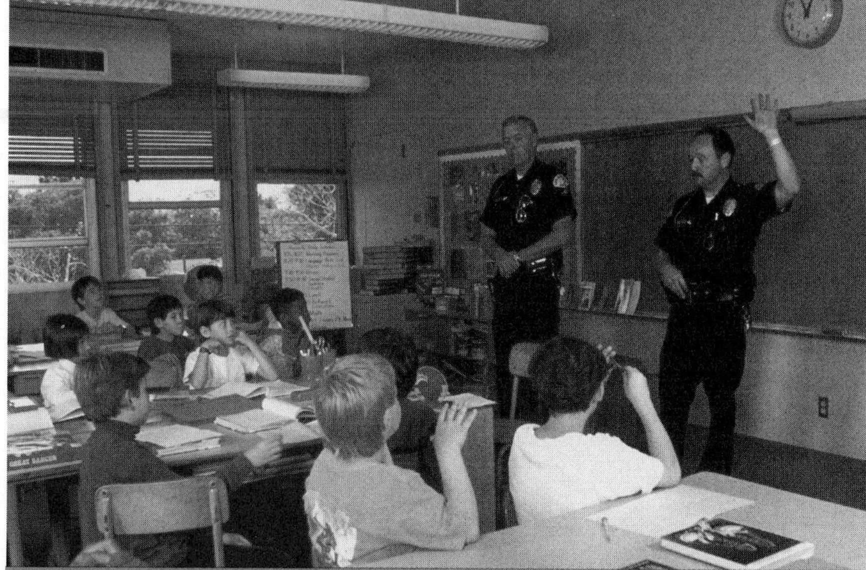
Mary Kate Denny/PhotoEdit

Police officers illustrate community involvement in the schools through their participation in the Drug Abuse Resistance Education (D.A.R.E.) program.

Drug Education and Substance Abuse Prevention: What Do We Know?

Parents, community members, teachers, and students express concern about the use and abuse of alcohol, tobacco, and other substances by young people. The school setting is an excellent place to educate young people about alcohol, tobacco, and other substances. However, although various types and forms of drug education have been going on in the schools for quite some time, a drug problem still exists. Many of the early drug education efforts have been shown to be ineffective.[2]

We have learned a great deal about effective substance abuse prevention programs. Educators, parents, and community leaders often confuse drug education with substance abuse prevention. Drug education is a broad concept that includes substance abuse prevention. For example, drug education should include the proper and safe use of prescription and over-the-counter medications, whereas substance abuse prevention is broadly aimed at influencing people to abstain from illicit drug use.[3]

Prevention work ideally focuses on as many of the factors that influence drug use, misuse, and abuse as possible. Some of those factors can be addressed in the school setting. In the past, prevention work focused on risk factors associated with illicit drug use, misuse, and abuse. This is still the case, but it is also important to recognize the existence of protective factors and that, by focusing on these factors, prevention can be served. The Center for Substance Abuse Prevention's recent publication *Here's Proof Prevention Works: Understanding Substance Abuse Prevention—Toward the 21st Century*[4] provides a conceptual framework for substance abuse prevention (see Table 10.1) that can help teachers (1) better understand the complexity of the issue and (2) formulate the role in substance abuse prevention they can play in the classroom.

As can be seen from Table 10.1, the teacher should not consider him- or herself the first and last line of defense against substance abuse. All members of the family, community, schools, businesses, and media must be involved in order to achieve success. This recognition can be a relief to many teachers who wrongly believe they are the only ones doing anything to reduce the problem of drug abuse. However, that is not to suggest that teachers should stand idly by and expect others to pick up the ball; all involved must participate.

Many teachers may be surprised to realize that effective prevention work does not demand complete and thorough knowledge of all types of drugs. In fact, if teachers are doing the following things, they are doing prevention work:

1. Creating an orderly and safe learning environment for children.
2. Providing children with an appropriate forum for discussing life issues.
3. Teaching social and other skills for coping with peer relations and stress.
4. Helping children gain access to community resources outside of the school.
5. Devising alternative learning strategies for children with reading deficits.
6. Correlating relevant drug-related material with the curriculum.[5]

As is evident, only one of the above listed items deals directly with drug-related material. Each of the items above deals with either ameliorating a risk factor or strengthening a protective factor as described in Table 10.1. For example, Item 3 in the list above deals with social and other skills for dealing with peers. Notice this *does not* say "for dealing with peer pressure." (A wealth of literature portrays peer pressure as a negative force acting only upon children and teens. In fact, peer pressure can be a positive force and everyone, even adults, is susceptible to it.)

Table 10.1
Key Risk and Protective Factors by the Six Domains

Life Area or "Domain"	Protective Factors	Risk Factors
Individual	• Positive personal characteristics, including social skills and social responsiveness, flexibility, problem-solving skills, and low levels of defensiveness. • Bonding to societal institutions and values, including attachment to parents and extended family, commitment to school, regular involvement with religious institutions, and belief in society's values. • Social and emotional competence, including good communication skills, responsiveness; empathy, caring, sense of humor, inclination toward prosocial behavior, problem-solving skills, sense of autonomy, sense of purpose and of the future (e.g., goal-directedness), and self-discipline.	• Inadequate life skills. • Lack of self-control, assertiveness, and peer-refusal skills. • Low self-esteem and self-confidence. • Emotional and psychological problems. • Favorable attitudes toward substance use. • Rejection of commonly held values and religion. • School failure. • Lack of school bonding. • Early antisocial behavior, such as lying, stealing, and aggression, particularly in boys, often combined with shyness or hyperactivity.
Family	• Positive bonding among family members. • Parenting that includes high levels of warmth and avoidance of severe criticism, sense of basic trust, high parental expectations, and clear and consistent expectations, including children's participation in family decisions and responsibilities. • An emotionally supportive parental/family milieu, including parental attention to children's interests, orderly and structured parent-child relationships, and parent involvement in homework and school-related activities.	• Family conflict and domestic violence. • Family disorganization. • Lack of family cohesion. • Social isolation of family. • Heightened family stress. • Family attitudes favorable to drug use. • Ambiguous, lax, or inconsistent rules and sanctions regarding substance use. • Poor child supervision and discipline. • Unrealistic expectations for development.
Peer	• Association with peers who are involved in school, recreation, service, religion, or other organized activities.	• Association with delinquent peers who use or value dangerous substances. • Association with peers who reject mainstream activities or pursuits. • Susceptibility to negative peer pressure. • Strong external locus of control.
School	• Caring and support; sense of "community" in classroom and school. • High expectations from school personnel. • Clear standards and rules for appropriate behavior. • Youth participation, involvement, and responsibility in school tasks and decisions.	• Ambiguous, lax or inconsistent rules and sanctions regarding drug use and student conduct. • Favorable staff and student attitudes toward substance use. • Harsh or arbitrary student management practices. • Availability of dangerous substances on premises. • Lack of school bonding.
Community	• Caring and support. • High expectations of youth. • Opportunities for youth participation in community activities.	• Community disorganization. • Lack of community bonding. • Lack of cultural pride. • Lack of competence in majority culture. • Community attitudes favorable to drugs. • Ready availability of dangerous substances. • Inadequate youth services and opportunities for prosocial involvement.
Society	• Media literacy (resistance to pro-use messages). • Decreased accessibility of substances. • Increased pricing of substances through taxation. • Raised purchasing age and enforcement. • Stricter driving-while-under-the-influence laws.	• Impoverishment. • Unemployment and underemployment. • Discrimination. • Pro-drug use messages in the media.

Source: Data from Center for Substance Abuse Prevention, *Here's Proof Prevention Works: Understanding Substance Abuse Prevention—Toward the 21st Century*, DHHS Publication No. SMA 99-3300. (Atlanta: U. S. Department of Health and Human Services, Substance Abuse and Mental Health Services Administration, 1999).

Facts About Adolescent Drug Use

By the time adolescents reach age 17,

- 62% have friends who use marijuana; 22% indicate that more than half of their friends use it.
- 43% have friends who have a serious drug problem; 28% have more than one friend with a drug problem.
- 79% have friends who are regular drinkers, and 34% know someone with a serious drinking problem.
- 40% have observed the sale of drugs in their neighborhood.
- Only 1 in 3 is willing to report a drug user or seller to school officials.

Source: National Center on Addiction and Substance Abuse (CASA), *Cigarettes, Alcohol, Marijuana: Gateways to Illicit Drug Use* (New York: Columbia University, 1996).

Instead, Item 3 identifies the set of skills needed to develop positive and health-enhancing peer relationships, including

- Being able to make friends and to recognize when someone is not a friend;
- Being able to distinguish between health-enhancing actions and health-threatening actions;
- Being able to resist and refuse health-threatening actions in a way that reflects one's own and one's family's values; and
- Being able to recognize stress and having effective and healthful ways of dealing with it.

Some Statistics

Many reliable sources of statistics can help describe the parameters of who is using and abusing drugs. One of the most important reasons to have access to reliable sources of data is that children and teens (as well as many teachers) have wildly exaggerated notions of the levels of drug use and abuse. The common belief is that everyone is using illicit drugs. The judicious use of reliable statistics can help counter that belief—an approach known as "social norm reinforcement"—and provide reassurance that most teens are not abusing alcohol, tobacco, or other drugs. The Web sites listed at the end of this chapter offer a wealth of statistics relating to children's and teens' use and abuse of drugs:

However, many children and teens have used drugs. For example, by the 8th grade, 52 percent of youth have tried alcohol, 41 percent have smoked cigarettes, and 20 percent have tried marijuana. Furthermore, by the 12th grade, about 80 percent have used alcohol, 63 percent have smoked cigarettes, and 49 percent have used marijuana.[6]

As startling as these statistics are, a closer examination reveals that many of those who have tried one or more of the above substances have done so on a one-time only basis or are periodic experimenters. Clearly, those who try or experiment with drugs are more likely to develop problems than those who do not. However, most experimenters are just that—experimenters. It is important to distinguish among experimenters, social users, and abusers. Although each of the categories present a potentially dangerous health risk and teachers are not in the business of condoning any level of use, there are distinct differences between someone who is experimenting and someone who is addicted. These distinctions are often lost on many who read and interpret statistics.

A closer look at the Monitoring the Future (MTF) data can offer a further example of how statistics may be misleading. Lifetime prevalence of illicit drug use for the year 2000 is as follows: 26.8 percent of 8th graders, 45.6 percent of 10th graders, and 54.0 percent of 12th graders have used an illicit drug.[7] An illicit drug is defined (by MTF) as including marijuana, LSD, other hallucinogens, crack, other cocaine, heroin or other narcotics, amphetamines, barbiturates, methaqualone, or tranquilizers not under a doctor's orders.[8] These statistics therefore reveal a level of illicit drug use that is of concern to parents, educators, and our society.

However, if one looks at these same categories for illicit drug use just during the year 2000, the data are 19.5 percent for 8th graders, 36.4 percent for 10th graders, and 40.9 percent for 12th graders. Further, in the same categories for use of any illicit substance in the last 30 days, the data are 11.9 percent for 8th graders, 22.5 percent for 10th graders, and 24.9 percent for 12th graders. Of course, these data still are much higher than they should be and are rightfully a cause for concern.

However, the truly startling data regarding drug use concerns the use of the legal drugs—alcohol and tobacco. Lifetime prevalence for alcohol use in the year 2000 is as follows: 51.7 percent of 8th graders, 71.4 percent of 10th graders, and 80.3 percent of 12th graders. Lifetime prevalence for cigarette use in the year 2000 is as follows: 40.5 percent of 8th graders, 55.1 percent of 10th graders, and 62.5 percent of 12th graders.[9] (See Table 10.2.)

"Legal" drugs are obviously the most prevalent subjects of abuse. The ability to critically examine statistics is a skill teachers need to understand and, as developmentally appropriate, that elementary students can begin to learn about.

Table 10.2
Drug Use Statistics

	Used During Lifetime			Used During Year 2000		Used in Last 30 Days		
	Any Illegal Drug	Alcohol	Tobacco	Any Illegal Drug	Alcohol	Any Illegal Drug	Alcohol	Tobacco
8th graders	26.8	51.7	40.5	19.5	43.1	11.9	22.4	14.6
10th graders	45.6	71.4	55.1	36.4	65.3	22.5	41.0	23.9
12th graders	54.0	80.3	62.5	40.9	73.2	24.9	50.0	31.4

Source: Data from L. D. Johnston, P. M. O'Malley, and J. G. Bachman, *Monitoring the Future National Survey Results on Drug Use, 1975–2000. Volume I: Secondary School Students,* NIH Publication No. 01-4924 (Bethesda, MD: National Institute on Drug Abuse, 2001).

Definitions

A commonly used definition of the term "**drug**" is any chemical or biological substance that has no food value and, when taken into the body, causes changes in the structure or function of the body. Drugs can affect cell functions by stimulating, depressing, or blocking a reaction or response, or by replacing normal chemicals in a reaction (for example, cocaine replaces a neurotransmitter substance in the brain).

Drugs can destroy or deactivate a cell. They can irritate cells to achieve abnormal or exaggerated levels of activity. Drugs can cause the body to slow down or to speed up, sleep, mask pain, swell up, shrivel, or even grow abnormally. If processes in the body slow down enough, the person dies. Drugs can be life-saving, like antibiotics, or life-threatening, like poisons.

How drugs are used determines whether they are good or bad for an individual. "Good" uses include relieving pain and curing illness and disease. These include both prescription and over-the-counter (OTC) drugs. When a drug causes more trouble than it prevents or cures, such as **psychoactive/** psychotropic "street" drugs, it is considered "bad." The notion of good and bad is also related to the dosage. That is, good drugs can be bad if too much is taken. Drug use, whether good or bad, is complex and specific to the individual. Therefore, good drugs should be used with caution; bad drugs should not be used at all.

Drug misuse is the inappropriate or improper use of a drug that results in impairment of the user's physical, mental, social, or emotional well-being. The misuse can be accidental or purposeful. Examples include taking an outdated prescription or one not intended for the user; taking an incorrect dose; using a drug for a purpose other than the one for which it was intended; taking one or more medicines simultaneously, without a doctor's recommendation, or against a doctor's advice; self-medicating over an extended time; or combining any two drugs from the same class (for example, combining alcohol with sleeping pills or tranquilizers—all CNS depressants) to increase their effect.

Drug abuse is the chronic, deliberate, and excessive use of any drug, prescription or over-the-counter medicine, legal or illegal, that results in impairment of the user's physical, mental, emotional, or social functioning. Using a drug can result in dependence. Overdosing is always possible. Drug abuse can result in suicide ideations, destroyed relationships, lack of control, fetal alcohol syndrome, inability to function in school, criminal behavior, and other problems.

The reasons for drug misuse and abuse are as numerous as the number of people using drugs. Whatever the reasons, abuse of drugs is a high-risk activity.

A **risk** can be defined as any behavior that people perceive as having some danger or thrill associated with it. Perception is a key word here, because each of us sees things differently. Though we appreciate that willingness to take risks can be an asset and act as a motivator for progress, risks have to be weighed against benefits. In the case of drug abuse or misuse, what factors make young people willing to take the risks associated with it?

Drugs can make people feel good, bad, or totally indifferent. They can help children feel happy, "up," talented, energetic, accepted, and even loved. Drugs can make them feel confident, competent, and able to do anything. We all desire these feelings. The desirable feelings that drugs can create, however, can be attained by other, safer, acceptable, and enjoyable means. The problem is that many students do not know how to get these feelings in safer ways. The less access people have to good feelings, the more vulnerable they are. When young people use drugs to attain good feelings early in their lives, they do not develop the skills to achieve these feelings in other, healthier ways.

Drug dependence is the physical or psychological need to use a drug despite adverse consequences. In physical dependency, and the stronger term, **addiction**, the user's body comes to rely on the drug to maintain homeostasis or a balanced functioning. Physical dependency can result in increasing tolerance for the drug, requiring the user to increase the dosage or frequency of use to produce the same effect. Because the person's body has adapted to use of the drug, withdrawal is difficult or, in the case of addiction, has serious side effects.

Psychological dependency, also called **habituation**, occurs when people feel they cannot maintain themselves without the drug. They have a craving for the drug they cannot overcome. People who are psychologically dependent may or may not be physically dependent. Both physical and psychological dependency are serious conditions that leave the user feeling out of control.

The focus of public concern about drug use revolves almost exclusively around the psychoactive effects on the brain or psychotropic, mind-altering properties. These chemicals may be classified according to how they affect thinking, feeling, perception, mood, or behavior. Following are the commonly used classifications of these drugs:

1. **Narcotics/Opiates** are powerful painkillers, including analgesics, that also induce sleep. Examples include opium, heroin, and morphine.
2. **Depressants and sedatives** slow down the central nervous system (CNS) or affect other body systems to produce lethargy and sleep. Alcohol is a major CNS depressant; this category also includes many types of prescription medications that have the potential for misuse and abuse.
3. **Stimulants** speed up CNS reactions, increasing alertness and excitability. Caffeine is the most common stimulant in this category. Cocaine and crack are two other examples.
4. **Psychedelics** or hallucinogens can produce false perceptions of reality called **hallucinations** and misinterpretations of either real or imagined events, called **delusions**. Included in this category are LSD, psilocybin mushrooms, MDMA (ecstasy), and others.
5. **Inhalants** are volatile chemical drugs (such as nitrous oxide) or nondrugs (such as paint thinners or model airplane glue) that are breathed in and affect the brain in ways similar to CNS depressants.
6. **Steroids and human growth hormones** are chemicals found in the body or produced synthetically that induce the build-up of proteins in tissue.
7. **Marijuana and hashish** are both derived from the *cannabis sativa* plant family; both contain the active ingredient delta-9-tetrahyrdrocannabinol (**THC**). The effects of either substance are varied: It can be excitatory in nature, it can have a sedative effect, in high doses it can cause hallucinations. It is the most widely used illicit drug.

Routes of Drug Administration

For a drug to work, it must enter the body's circulatory system, which enables it to reach all parts of the body. The route of administration determines how quickly a drug works, how long its effects will last, and how intense the reactions will be. Several common methods of administration are as follows:

1. Orally ingested doses pass through the digestive system. This method is convenient, permits easy self-use, and avoids injection. It results in slower absorption and, therefore, a slower effect (approximately one-half hour from administration to observable effects) than the other methods.
2. Sniffing/snorting and other forms of absorption get drugs into the body through one of the interior membranes. This method is convenient for self-medicating and has a much faster effect than ingestion. Examples include intranasal administration (as is used with cocaine or snuff tobacco), sublingual administration (where the drug is placed beneath the tongue), rectal administration (in the form of a suppository), and transdermal administration (a new technology that transmits the drug through the skin, as in the nicotine patch).
3. Inhalation and/or smoking through the mouth and/or nose and into the lungs is the most efficient and quickest way of getting a drug into the bloodstream.
4. Various forms of injection includes **intramuscular** administration, which introduces the drug directly into the muscle tissue and takes effect within a few minutes; **intravenous** administration, which places the drug directly into the bloodstream through a vein and takes effect almost immediately; and **subcutaneous** administration, which places the drug immediately beneath the skin (sometimes called "skin popping") and takes effect in about 10 minutes. Injection allows for an accurate dose and a rapid response that bypasses the digestive process. It reduces the unpredictability of the response and the possibility of dose-error, which could lead to overdose. In legal uses, this administration is performed only with sterile equipment.

After administration, the chemical is circulated, metabolized, and eventually eliminated. Some substances remain in the bloodstream for long periods; some are distributed uniformly throughout the body; and most are distributed unevenly depending on their ability to be absorbed into different tissues. Few actually become concentrated in tissues or organs. Metabolism is the process that eventually leads to elimination. The drug is prepared for elimination, primarily by a liver enzyme. The kidneys are responsible for excretion in urine, although some excretion is carried out by saliva, gastric juices, feces, breast milk, and the lungs.

Many factors determine what, when, and where a drug works. The dose of the chemical is a primary factor. It can range from the **threshold dose** (the lowest dose at which the drug will work) to an overdose that will kill the user. Age is another factor affecting a response: The very old, the very young, and the middle-aged respond differently to a given dose of drug, probably because of differences in metabolism. Body weight and the amount of fat present also affect responses. Heavier people require a larger dose than lighter people.

The **dose-response time** (the time from administration to initial response) varies with the method of induction. Illness, pregnancy, menstruation, and other factors affect a drug's behavior. Some drugs that are taken simultaneously can compound the body's reaction, known as a synergistic effect. Other influencing factors include mindset or the user's expectations (referred to as "set"), the user's previous experiences with the drug, and emotions that lead to gastric and hormonal changes. Some drugs—particularly the psychedelic and hallucinogenic drugs—are affected by the setting, the people the user is with, where they are, and the time of use.

Commonly Abused Drugs

Commonly abused drugs include alcohol, tobacco, marijuana, cocaine, heroin, inhalants, anabolic steroids, and a variety of "club drugs" that have rapidly become popular among young people. Prescription and over-the-counter drugs can be misused as well.

Alcohol

Although alcohol is often thought of as a stimulant because, in small doses, it relaxes people enough to make them feel "up" and have a good time. In reality, it depresses and slows the central nervous system (CNS). Alcohol can affect brain function, adversely affecting speech and motor skills, slowing reactions, and inducing drowsiness. An overdose can lead to death if the vital centers of the brain shut down.

The effects of alcohol vary from person to person and even within the same individual from time to time. These effects depend on factors such as size and weight (larger, heavier people usually take longer to feel the effects than smaller people); the size of the drink and the amount of alcohol in it (called "proof"); the amount of food in the stomach at the time of drinking (food slows absorption of alcohol into the bloodstream); and how long and how rapidly the person drinks. People who have consumed drinks in the past know better what to expect, but this does not mean they will escape the effects.

Appropriate and Inappropriate Drinking

Because drinking is a legal form of drug use, proper and safe use of alcohol is a major concern. Deterrents to drinking include family and peer attitudes, religious beliefs and influences, and a dislike for the taste. Where, when, and how much drinking may be appropriate are functions of an individual's values but may be heavily influenced by others. Responsible drinkers are in control of when and how much they drink and how they behave when they are drinking. People can learn how to drink responsibly. On the other hand, problem drinking occurs when people are not in control of their drinking or the behaviors associated with it, although they often think they are. They abuse alcohol to cope with life's problems, to socialize more easily, or to feel good about themselves.

Alcoholism is a treatable condition that requires considerable help for the drinker and all of the people important in his or her life. There seems to be a genetic predisposition toward alcoholism. In families with a history of alcoholism, the problems may be more difficult to treat. The millions of adult children of alcoholics can attest to the lifelong ramifications of growing up in an alcoholic family. How can we measure the cost to society of a broken family, of abused children, of lost school time or work time by members of an alcoholic's family? The monetary costs include lost time on the job or loss of the job itself, medical costs associated with chronic alcohol abuse; damage to vehicles and personal property, and the resulting increase in insurance costs to everyone.

Sources of Help for Problem Drinkers

Most communities have agencies in place to help problem drinkers and their families. These include medical and psychological resources, places of worship, schools, and various 12-step programs such as Alcoholics Anonymous and Alanon. Both the drinkers and their families need help. Most large corporations and municipal services, such as police and firefighters, offer specialized services for people who are willing to admit to a problem.

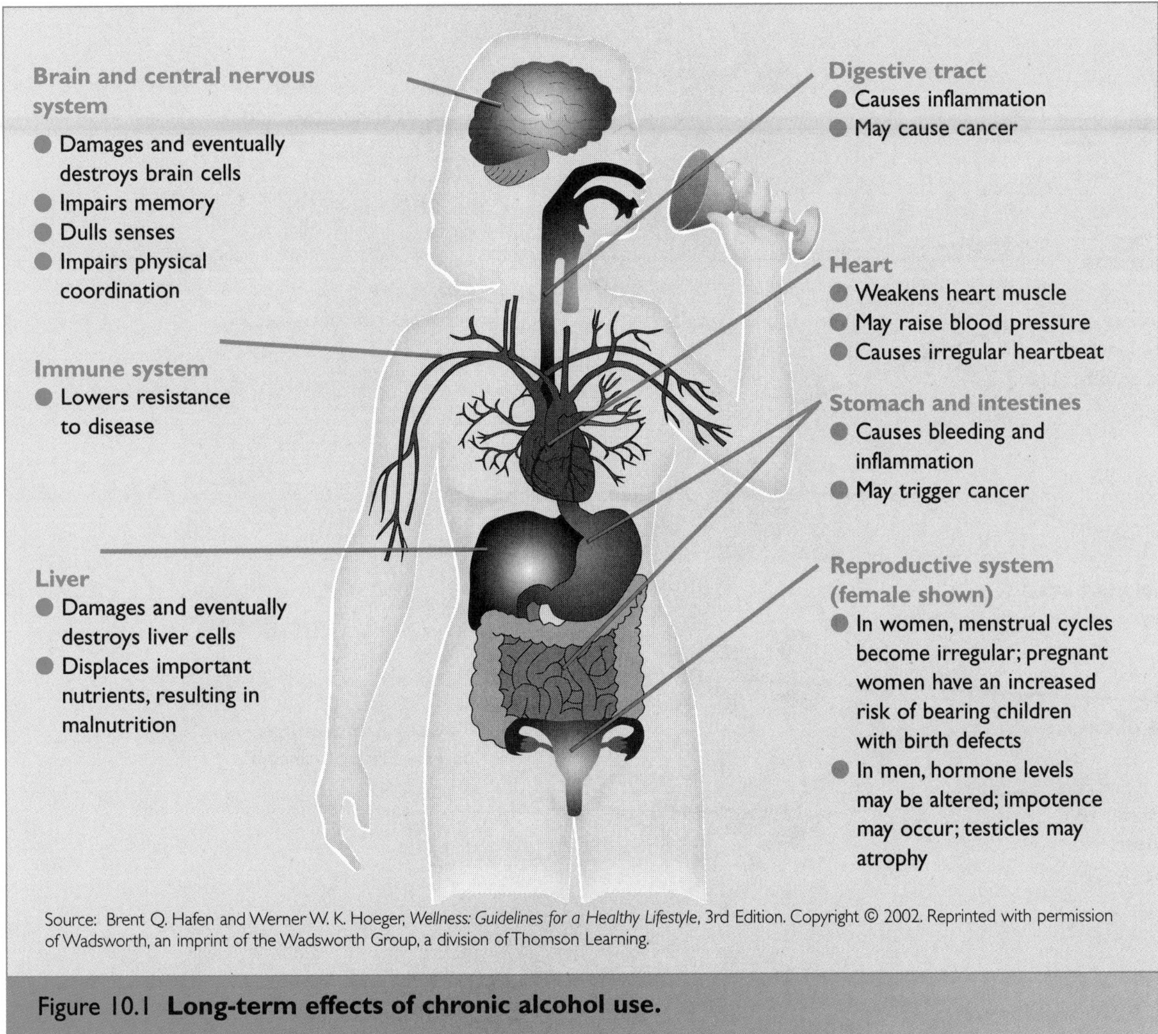
Brain and central nervous system
Damages and eventually destroys brain cells
Impairs memory
Dulls senses
Impairs physical coordination
Immune system
Lowers resistance to disease
Liver
Damages and eventually destroys liver cells
Displaces important nutrients, resulting in malnutrition
Digestive tract
Causes inflammation
May cause cancer
Heart
Weakens heart muscle
May raise blood pressure
Causes irregular heartbeat
Stomach and intestines
Causes bleeding and inflammation
May trigger cancer
Reproductive system (female shown)
In women, menstrual cycles become irregular; pregnant women have an increased risk of bearing children with birth defects
In men, hormone levels may be altered; impotence may occur; testicles may atrophy

Source: Brent Q. Hafen and Werner W. K. Hoeger, *Wellness: Guidelines for a Healthy Lifestyle*, 3rd Edition. Copyright © 2002. Reprinted with permission of Wadsworth, an imprint of the Wadsworth Group, a division of Thomson Learning.

Figure 10.1 **Long-term effects of chronic alcohol use.**

Guest speakers from helping facilities welcome the opportunity to talk to school classes. Alert teachers can reach out to the school's mental health resources to help students who show signs of inappropriate use or exhibit behaviors that suggest parental alcoholism.

Early education about alcohol use, misuse, and abuse can result in students seeing responsible drinking as both a personal and a group decision. It should be stressed that these behaviors are both illegal and dangerous and that the consequences can be long-term and unpleasant. A sensitive curriculum can also provide students with hope and places to go for help when they are experiencing alcoholism in their family or among their friends. The curriculum might include effects of alcohol on the body (see Figure 10.1), drinking and driving, withstanding peer pressure, and safety issues (such as drinking while participating in sports and other physical activities).

Tobacco

Illnesses associated with tobacco use make up the largest group of preventable illnesses in the United States. Nicotine, the addictive substance in tobacco, is rated one of the most difficult addictions to break—therefore, the emphasis must be on not starting. If a person smokes already, quitting as soon as possible will improve the smoker's health and reduce the probability of developing a smoking-related illness.

The ways in which people are exposed to tobacco include cigarettes, pipes, cigars, chewing tobacco, and snuff. The dangers involved in tobacco are attributed to the products of burning tobacco, chemicals in the tobacco itself, and the impact of secondhand smoke. One of these toxins is the carbon monoxide produced during smoking. This gas replaces oxygen in the blood, so the person tires quickly. At high enough levels, carbon monoxide can cause death by asphyxiation. Although this will not occur from smoking tobacco, it may become inconvenient: Many homes now have carbon monoxide sensors to

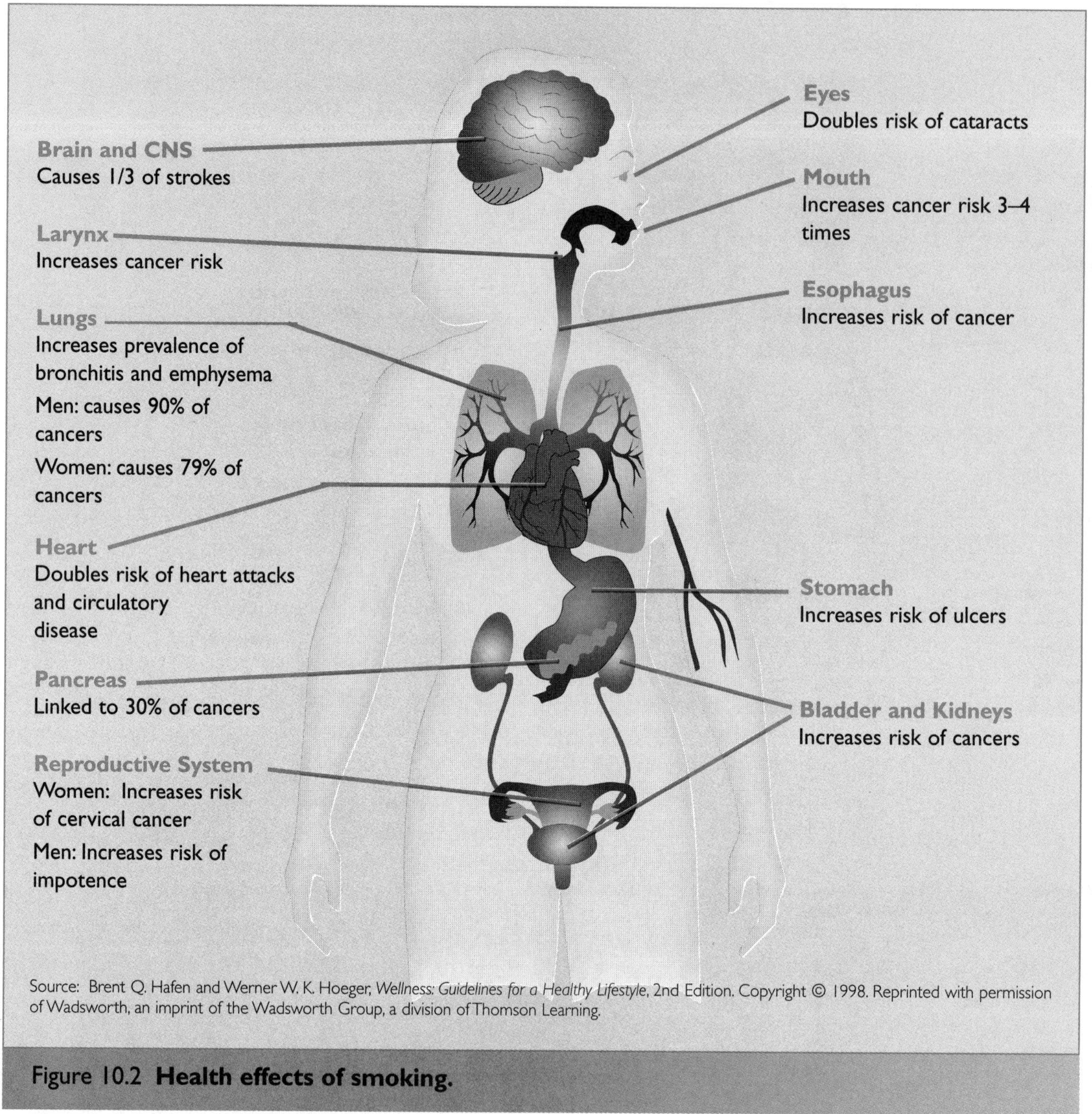
Brain and CNS
Causes 1/3 of strokes
Larynx
Increases cancer risk
Lungs
Increases prevalence of bronchitis and emphysema
Men: causes 90% of cancers
Women: causes 79% of cancers
Heart
Doubles risk of heart attacks and circulatory disease
Pancreas
Linked to 30% of cancers
Reproductive System
Women: Increases risk of cervical cancer
Men: Increases risk of impotence
Eyes
Doubles risk of cataracts
Mouth
Increases cancer risk 3–4 times
Esophagus
Increases risk of cancer
Stomach
Increases risk of ulcers
Bladder and Kidneys
Increases risk of cancers

Source: Brent Q. Hafen and Werner W. K. Hoeger, *Wellness: Guidelines for a Healthy Lifestyle*, 2nd Edition. Copyright © 1998. Reprinted with permission of Wadsworth, an imprint of the Wadsworth Group, a division of Thomson Learning.

Figure 10.2 **Health effects of smoking.**

avoid deaths from carbon monoxide poisoning.

The irritant effects of tars and other chemicals in tobacco smoke and the heat with which it burns can damage the lining of the mouth, nose, throat, and lungs. This includes damage to the **cilia** (small hairlike projections lining the membranes of the bronchioles) and interference with the alveoli (which enable the exchange of gases in the breathing process). These changes may be permanent. Chronic tobacco use puts the user at risk for developing common colds, bronchitis, emphysema, and other diseases of the respiratory system. Tobacco also damages the teeth and gums, leading to decay and loss of teeth, as well as periodontal disease.

The chemicals in tobacco are known to temporarily increase heart rate, blood pressure, and constriction of the peripheral blood vessels. Quitting after chronic use does not allow the body to recover fully between uses and eventually leads to serious, if not fatal, diseases. In any case, cardiovascular disease is two to three times more common in chronic smokers than in nonsmokers.

The rate of strokes, often a result of weakened blood vessels and heightened blood pressure, is much higher in tobacco users. Strokes can result in motor and speech loss, and long-term or permanent disability. Also more common in tobacco users are cancers of the kidney and bladder, peptic ulcers, and cirrhosis of the liver. In pregnancy, tobacco use is a factor in low birth weight babies, a condition that puts the health and well-being of the newborn at considerable risk. Women who smoke during pregnancy also have a higher risk for spontaneous abortion (miscarriage), premature birth, and a higher fetal death rate. These health effects are depicted in Figure 10.2.

Some of the reasons young people smoke include

- **Peer pressure**. Their friends smoke and urge them to join in.
- **Curiosity**. Their friends, parents, or sports or music idols smoke.
- **It looks "grown up."** Young people want to look older to impress a prospective date; to get into "forbidden" places such as social clubs, concerts, or bars; or to look as "grown up" as their friends.
- **Advertising**: Young people want to emulate the beautiful models shown enjoying tobacco in idyllic settings and the macho men appearing in fantasy-like advertisements. (This area can be a fruitful avenue to use in the development of lessons in media literacy. Young people need to develop the critical skills to break down tobacco advertisements and expose the lies behind them. They also can produce more accurate advertisements as a form of counter advertising, as suggested in Learning Experience 10-9.)

Smoking Prevention Programs

A body of research on smoking prevention has demonstrated effectiveness in reducing tobacco use. Its findings include the following:

School-based smoking-prevention programs that identify social influences to smoke and teach skills to resist those influences have demonstrated consistent and significant reductions in adolescent smoking prevalence, and program effects have lasted one to three years. Programs to prevent smokeless tobacco use that are based on the same model have also demonstrated modest reductions in the initiation of smokeless tobacco use. The effectiveness of school-based smoking-prevention programs appears to be enhanced and sustained by comprehensive school health education and by community-wide programs that involve parents, mass media, community organizations, or other elements of an adolescent's social environment.[10]

These research-based programs are listed on the Centers for Disease Control and Prevention's Web site (listed at the end of this chapter). Societal pressures are converging to fight tobacco use by young people. The schools can take the lead in antismoking campaigns, and many school districts maintain smoke-free (and drug-free) environments.

Marijuana

Marijuana is one of the most controversial drugs in the United States today. The cannabis plant is the source of marijuana, one of the oldest known drugs. Also called the Indian hemp plant, *Cannabis sativa* flourishes in many parts of the world. The psychoactive ingredient—one of more than 400 chemicals isolated from the plant—is tetra-hydro-cannabinol, or THC. The leaves of the marijuana plant are dried and then, most often, smoked in either a pipe or as a hand-rolled cigarette, commonly known as a joint.

Shredded leaves also may be sprinkled on salads, baked into cookies or brownies, or added to cooked foods. The most potent product of the *Cannabis* plant is hash (a shortened form of "hashish"), the dried resin of the plant, which may be up to 50 times more potent than the dried leaves.

The marijuana user experiences an altered state of consciousness often described as "wasted" or "high," though descriptions of this state vary considerably. Typical descriptors range from "relaxed" to "energized." Some users say they are totally alert, and others say they are "spaced out" or dazed. The drug is a mood enhancer, meaning that it does not create one single mood; rather, it exaggerates the existing mood. The more a user expects, the greater the effect will be.

Cannabis is considered to be addictive. The user develops a psychological dependency and there is evidence of some experiencing physical withdrawal symptoms. **Reverse tolerance**, in which the user actually requires less of the substance to achieve the desired results, is common.

Because THC is fat-soluble, it is stored in fatty tissues in the body and can be found in the bloodstream for up to 30 days after ingestion. The following three factors make marijuana smoking at least as dangerous to the cardiorespiratory system as cigarettes and maybe even more toxic:

1. The marijuana joint generates greater heat.
2. The smoker inhales deeply and holds it as long as possible.
3. The smoker smokes the joint down to the butt (where chemicals are most concentrated), using a roach clip to prevent burning the fingers.

These factors are thought to increase the carcinogenic potential of marijuana smoke and are known to cause chronic respiratory irritation and distress. Some other possible adverse effects of marijuana include all of the problems cigarette smokers have with coughs and odors, plus distortion of time and vision and a lack of initiative.

Some positive medical uses have been identified. The drug has properties that act as an appetite stimulant, an anti-asthmatic broncho-dilator, and a muscle relaxant. THC-synthetics are now available to help reduce intra-ocular pressure in people with glaucoma, to help reduce nausea associated with chemotherapy, and to improve appetite. As a result, there is a growing movement to legalize marijuana for distribution by medical people to relieve the pain and suffering of several different types of illnesses. Many young people do not see it as a dangerous drug, so they are less fearful of using it. However, it is the most commonly used illicit drug. It should be stressed that smoking of any kind is dangerous and that marijuana is an illegal drug whose possession or sale both carry severe penalties in most of the United States.

Cocaine

Many temperature climates are hospitable to the growth of the coca leaf. For thousands of years, its potent chemicals enabled native populations of the high Andes mountains to cope with hard work in a low-oxygen atmosphere. Today these leaves are processed and sold as cocaine hydrochloride. This white crystalline powder and its more addictive offshoot, crack, are two of the most dangerous street drugs. Figure 10.3 shows the forms of **cocaine**. Crack can be made in any kitchen at a low cost. Cocaine is one of the most addictive of the known drugs. "Coke," as it is familiarly called, is a stimulant to the central nervous system (CNS). Doctors use it as a local anesthetic. When smoked or injected, it also temporarily numbs subjective or emotional pain. Dentists and others commonly use legitimate synthetic derivatives during surgery.

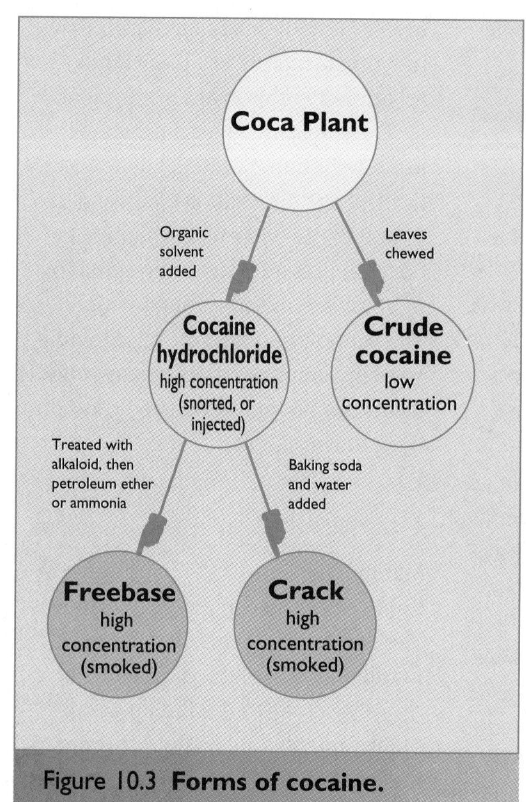

Figure 10.3 **Forms of cocaine.**

When misused, cocaine is most often snorted into the nostrils. It may also be injected, skin-popped, or smoked. Crack is most commonly smoked in a pipe. Cocaine-snorting leads to many physical and psychological problems. The physical ones include erosion of the mucous membranes in the nasal cavity (chronic running nose), numbing of the upper respiratory area, and frequent nasal bleeding. Cocaine abusers often display chronic agitated behavior, delusions, and severe weight loss. The psychological problems include depression (from deprivation), intense anxiety, and mental aberrations such as "snow lights," in which victims see flashing starlike lights, or "snow bugs," wherein they believe they are being attacked by bugs.

Crack may be the most volatile abusive drug of all. Its effects are of short duration (a high may last only a few minutes), thus requiring frequent exposure. Users often become violent and exhibit irrational behavior. Because it creates quick feelings of euphoria, the user feels compelled to use it constantly, to the eventual exclusion of all other interests. Sometimes people use a CNS depressant (frequently alcohol) to come down from the excitable, exhilarated state, which accounts for the high incidence of dual addictions. The drug is especially addictive to persons who do not have significant positive outlets in their everyday lives. Accidental deaths from cocaine use have been attributed to rapid increases in high blood pressure and heart rate. Because most people lack knowledge of hidden coronary conditions, this characteristic of the drug means that every exposure is like playing a game of Russian roulette. We have read of athletes, the best known of whom is Len Bias, and entertainers who died suddenly after cocaine use.

Heroin

Heroin is a semi-synthetic drug made from **morphine**, which comes from the opium poppy. It is called by common street names—such as junk, skag, and hard stuff—or by a trade name such as China white or China brown (the latter two describe the origin and color). Heroin is a white crystalline powder, usually packaged in small glassine bags and sold as "nickel" or "dime" bags (the former costs $5; the latter, $10). The cost varies with the drug's availability and purity (heroin is usually cut or diluted with a powder that looks like it, such as milk sugar or quinine) as well as with the current demand.

The risk of overdose is related to variations of heroin in any bag sold on the street. A bag may contain anywhere from 0 to 60 percent heroin, the rest being any of the cutting powders. One of the most highly addictive substances known, heroin produces a brief euphoria followed by a somnolent state, manifested by the user being "on the nod," or practically asleep. The more common methods of administration are by mainlining (injecting directly into a vein), skin-popping, snorting, and smoking.

Heroin and the related drugs opium, morphine, codeine, and Percodan are CNS depressants. Pharmacologically they are intended to be painkillers. Addiction is characterized by increased tolerance requiring larger or more frequent doses over time to achieve the desired results and by withdrawal symptoms ranging from a flu-like runny nose, body aches, lassitude, severe cramps, vomiting, profuse perspiration, yawning, and exaggerated anxiety. These usually begin 4 to 6 hours after the last dose wears off and, if monitored, can terminate in 3 or 4 days. Psychological dependence is more difficult to overcome, because the user often returns to the environment that engendered its use. Thus, aftercare is essential if the addict is to have a chance at rehabilitation.

Heroin is expensive because it is illegal, and the addict needs as many as six doses daily. The cost may reach hundreds of dollars per day. Crime and prostitution often are the only ways to get this much money. The risks of this lifestyle are the obvious: entanglement with the law, contracting sexually transmitted diseases (AIDS is prevalent in intravenous drug users), loss of family, job, and so on. Other risks associated with IV heroin use include the possibility of hepatitis, bacterial infection, abscesses and sores, blood disorders, and collapse of the veins being used.

The socioeconomic implications of illegal drug use are embodied in heroin, which currently is undergoing a resurgence of popularity. Addicts most often steal portable, marketable property to support their habits. Because they cannot get full value for the stolen items, this translates into $50,000 to $75,000 of stolen goods per year per addict. The costs to society for crime prevention, courts and lawyers, incarceration, insurance, and rehabilitative services are in the billions of dollars annually. The cost to society in terms of lost resources, broken families, and emotional distress cannot be measured.

Inhalants

The inhalant category of drugs includes gasoline and other petroleum derivatives, airplane glue, and certain aerosol sprays. Government intervention has almost eliminated aerosol sprays through legislation, and manufacturers are required to replace some dangerous chemicals with more benign ones. Abuse of inhalants warrants more attention because many of these products are legal, easy to obtain, and therefore more accessible to youngsters. Too often glue-sniffing and similar activities represent a child's first experience with drugs. The abusers are predominantly preteens who have been turned on by older children. Use is enhanced by ready availability. The abuse of these chemicals appears to be widespread, although tracking this problem is difficult because the immediate symptoms of abuse can be short-lived and therefore may go undetected. Also, parents are reluctant to have their children prosecuted and may not be willing to risk police reports.

The physical risks involved in using inhalants should not be taken lightly. They include suffocation or asphyxia from inhaling the substance from a plastic or paper bag—one of the more popular ways to inhale. A user can lose consciousness and possibly die. Long-term use can lead to kidney, bone marrow, liver, and brain damage, low blood pressure, and chronic weight loss. Fire is an additional risk inherent in the misuse of petroleum-product inhalants such as gasoline, kerosene, lighter fluids and paint removers. All inhalants are highly flammable.

Suggestions for reducing inhalant use include the following:

1. Laws requiring the addition of nausea-inducing substances to model airplane glue.
2. Regulation of the sale of chemicals in retail outlets.
3. Education of adults regarding proper storage of volatile home products.
4. Requirement of childproof containers for dangerous chemicals.
5. Education of the public in general about the inhalant category of substance abuse.

Anabolic Steroids

Anabolic steroids are compounds found naturally in the human body as hormones or produced synthetically. They induce the buildup of protein and other body tissue. Some steroids are oil- or fat-soluble and are stored in the body, where they can remain for up to a year. However, most steroids are not fat-soluble and leave the body within a few hours after ingestion. Steroids are most commonly taken by mouth and less commonly by injection. In cases where a physician believes the person must have steroids to help with an abnormal growth pattern, they are available by prescription.

People who are interested in a large-muscle appearance also use steroids. The recent increased interest in physical fitness has led many to seek "quick fixes." Young athletes sometimes use steroids because of their reputed ability to increase strength, size, speed, and endurance. All major league sports have rules against the use of steroids, and most have testing programs to enforce these rules.

Sellers of steroids may frequent places where young athletes, weight lifters, and body builders work out. No reputable health club or training facility condones the use of steroids.

Much of what we know about the abuse of steroids comes from the testimony of people who have used them and suffered from their use. Probable effects include alteration of liver chemistry, changes in blood vessels, shrinking of testicles and lowered sperm count, breast enlargement in men, slowing or halting of bone growth, increase in cholesterol count, severe acne, hair loss, behavioral disorders, and severe aggression and hostility. These risks seem to be present only during and immediately after use and usually disappear when the use stops. Because anabolic steroids have been in use only 25 years or so, the long-term effects are not well documented. Yet, there is some suspicion that the results of use over time may include prostate cancer, atherosclerosis, rapid aging, and adverse effects to the immune, endocrine, and nervous systems.

Club Drugs

The mission of the National Institute for Drug Administration (NIDA) is to bring the power of science to bear on drug abuse and addiction. This charge has two critical components: The first is the strategic support and conduct of research across a broad range of disciplines. The second is the rapid and effective dissemination and use of the results of that research to significantly improve drug abuse and addiction prevention, treatment, and policy. Further information on the drugs addressed in this section can be found on NIDA's Web site (listed at the end of this chapter).

Concern about the use of the following substances has been growing: MDMA (ecstasy), Rohypnol, GHB (gamma hydroxybutyrate), and ketamine. Each of these substances are associated with young people and teens who attend nightclubs and raves (an all-night dance party that takes place in large warehouse-like settings). Although most nightclub and rave attendees do not take these drugs, a growing number are attracted to their relatively low cost, their ability to increase stamina (the most popular drug, ecstasy, is a form of speed), and the high that allegedly magnifies the rave experience.

Ecstasy (3-4 methylenedioxymethamphetamine or MDMA) is a synthetic psychoactive substance with both stimulant and hallucinogenic properties. Street names for MDMA include ecstasy, Adam, XTC, hug, beans, and love drug. MDMA has been used by some psychiatrists who believed that it had the ability to enhance empathy. However, a "NIDA-supported study has provided the first direct evidence that chronic use of MDMA, popularly known as 'ecstasy,' causes brain damage in people and that heavy MDMA users have memory problems that persist for at least two weeks."[11] Ecstasy causes both psychological and physical difficulties, including confusion, depression, sleep problems, severe anxiety, paranoia, muscle tension, involuntary teeth clenching, nausea, blurred vision, faintness, and chills or sweating. The stimulant effects of MDMA, which enable users to dance for extended periods, may also lead to dehydration, hypertension, and heart or kidney failure.

Gamma-hydroxybutyrate (GHB) is predominantly a central nervous system (CNS) depressant. It is colorless, odorless, and tasteless. It can be produced in clear liquid, white powder, tablet, and capsule forms and is often used with alcohol. Given that alcohol is also a CNS depressant, the combination is particularly dangerous. Street names for GHB include grievous bodily harm, G, liquid ecstasy, and Georgia home boy. GHB has been implicated in poisonings, overdoses, date rapes, and fatalities. It was available over-the-counter in health food stores until 1992 and was used mainly by body builders to aid in fat reduction and muscle building. GHB's intoxicating effects begin 10 to 20 minutes after the drug is taken. The effects typically last up to 4 hours, depending on the dosage. At lower doses, GHB can relieve anxiety and produce relaxation; however, as the dose increases, the sedative effects may result in sleep and eventual coma or death.[12]

Rohypnol (flunitrazepam) is a benzodiazepine. It is not approved for use in the United States, but it is approved in Europe and in more than 60 countries as a treatment for insomnia, as a sedative, and as a presurgery anesthetic. Street names include roofies, rophies, roche, and forget-me pill. It is colorless and tasteless and dissolves easily. When mixed with alcohol, it can incapacitate victims. It has been implicated in an increasing number of sexual assault and rape cases. Rohypnol can also produce a short-term amnesia, wherein individuals may not remember what happens to them while under the effects of the drug.[13]

Ketamine is an anesthetic that has been approved for both human and animal use in medical settings since 1970. Almost 90 percent of ketamine is legally sold for veterinary use. Street names include Special K, K, vitamin K, and cat valiums. Lower doses of ketamine can cause dream-like states and produce hallucination. At higher doses, it can cause delirium, amnesia, impaired motor function, high blood pressure, depression, and potentially fatal respiratory problems.

Drugs Used Medicinally

Medicines are used to relieve pain, cure illness, prevent the spread of disease, and prolong life. They may be **prescription drugs** (those that only a licensed professional practitioner can order), or they may be **over-the-counter (OTC) drugs**, which an adult can buy in a store (see Chapter 15). In either case, education must emphasize proper use

For Your Health

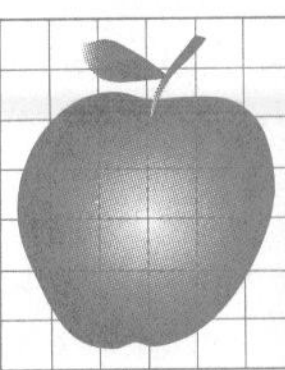

Safe Use of OTC Drugs

- *Do not* take more than is recommended.
- *Do not* take the medicine longer than is recommended.
- *Do not* use medications that have expired.
- *Do not* give medications to children under age 12 unless the label lists a recommended dose for children.
- *Do not* continue taking the medication if the symptoms persist or get worse.
- *Do not* combine medications.

of these drugs, only with the supervision of a medical professional (for prescription drugs) or parent in the case of OTC drugs.

Procedures for proper use of medicines should be stressed beginning in the earliest grades. Following are some precautions adults can take:

1. Always take medicines as directed by the prescribing physician or the label.
2. Never take another person's medicine, especially a prescription drug.
3. Carefully store medicines to avoid accidental use (accidental poisoning is a leading cause of death in children).
4. Properly dispose of drugs when they are outdated or no longer needed.
5. Buy medicines in childproof containers.
6. Be sure labels are clear and readable.
7. Avoid candy-flavored medicines, because children may be unable to distinguish them from candy, with possibly dangerous results.

Young children are curious and inventive about getting to and opening bottles and jars and putting these products into their mouths. Drugs and common household chemicals (such as bleach or cleansers) are potentially lethal. Some precautions that adults can take include

1. Keep all of these products (including alcohol) out of reach (chairs, stools, and countertops can add to their reach).
2. Lock up all chemicals, even if they are out of reach.
3. Place refrigerated drugs, especially those stored in common food containers, in childproof containers.

The effects of misuse of medicines are often difficult to predict because many factors are operating. Size, age, sex, nutritional status, other chemicals present, and recent consumption of food or beverage can affect what a drug does to the body. People must be aware of drug interactions if they are using more than one drug. Possible side effects of prescribed drugs should be discussed with the physician or pharmacist. Children should learn to identify side effects of medicine, including stomach distress, fever, headache, pain in another area, and loss of a normal sensation such as touch or taste. The box above lists common-sense rules to follow when using OTC drugs.

Proper use of medicines, including vaccines, is a shared personal and community responsibility. Developing a list of medicines commonly found in the home, along with information pertinent to their use, will help educate citizens about drug categories, uses, hazards, and sources. Parents and teachers working together can help children understand that medicines are helpful when they are properly used and dangerous when improperly used. Education in this area can mean life or death.

Approaches to Drug Treatment

Many treatment approaches have been tried to help addicts overcome their addiction. One plan consists of a short inpatient stay (21–30 days), followed by outpatient or day treatment programs in which addicts are medically withdrawn from their drug and then supported through the psychological hard times. Outpatient centers are staffed by professionals and sometimes ex-addicts, supported by medical personnel, and work with the user's family to encourage continuation in the program. A major drawback to some of these programs is their policy of voluntary entry and withdrawal, which makes it difficult to estimate or measure their success. Addicts may be terminated and then select another center after they use again. Also, some addicts take advantage of programs simply to decrease the amount of drugs they need.

Another avenue through which an addict may be helped is psychiatric treatment. It may be accomplished by pharmacological drugs that counteract or decrease the need for a drug. For example, **methadone**, a synthetic opiate, is used in place of heroin because it does not get the user high but does satisfy the craving for the drug. Maintenance on methadone is relatively inexpensive compared to illegal heroin, and the user is able to function normally. Most big-city hospitals have methadone maintenance programs, and most also have long waiting lists.

One of the more popular types of treatment is the 12-step program. Groups such as Alcoholics Anonymous and Narcotics Anonymous are organized brotherhood/sisterhood, peer-supported programs with a strong spiritual component. Many have found 12-step programs helpful in overcoming addiction, but success rates are unavailable because of the confidential nature of the programs.

Staying Drug-Free

Almost everyone who has children, or is responsible for them, has contemplated the problem of drug use. Today, more people are abusing drugs at earlier ages, more often, and in greater quantities than anyone would say is an acceptable level. People like what drugs do to them. That's why they take drugs. There are drugs for every feeling a person could ever have, imagine having, or be afraid of not having. The cost is immeasurable: loss of life, loss of function in the family and community, breakdown of the family, increased crime, and the enormous economic costs related to each of these factors.

The many theories about how to stay drug-free indicate that there is no one solid path to that goal—and that a solitary focus on being drug-free does not empower people to become critical thinkers. Maybe that should not be the goal. Rather, we should be looking at how to use drugs in effective and health-supporting ways; how to make personal, mature decisions about their use; and how to avoid drug misuse and abuse even as we set expectations for students to abstain and be drug-free.

A great deal of emphasis has been placed on education, and certainly it has its place. In his book *Seduction*, the author presented a concept he called "DAPS and PADS": Drugs Are People Substitutes and People Are Drug Substitutes. According to the author, people who relate well to others have a better chance of avoiding drug abuse than people who do not have good interpersonal relationships. Hence, if children can be helped to relate better to their peers, communicate more effectively, and be aware of how their relationships affect their behavior, they may have a better chance of staying drug-free.[14]

Another of his concepts is that a person who is internally motivated is more likely to be protected against the possibility of drug abuse than one who is externally motivated. Another way of saying this is that people who are more secure and self-confident within themselves and who do not have to rely excessively on others for approval or drugs for their feelings will have a better chance of avoiding the things that lead to drug abuse. We are all aware of peer pressure as a factor in drug abuse. The pressure to be accepted, liked, and similar to one's chosen peer group is strong. Social pressure, such as that experienced by a teenager at a party where alcohol is being consumed illegally or in a car where illegal substances are being used, comes from risky situations involving peer pressure. Low self-confidence and self-esteem increase the allure of peer pressure, compounded by the lack of ability to initiate resistance or refusal skills (the "how to say no" strategies) when an individual wants to feel accepted.

Children of parents who abuse or misuse drugs are also at greater risk. Regardless of whether we believe that the propensity for alcohol and other drug abuse is genetically or behaviorally passed from one generation to another, children in abusing families need to know that, just because family members abuse drugs, they do not have to follow that path. They need to learn how to counteract the negative behaviors modeled in their abusing families. These behaviors commonly include poor communication styles, self-destructive behaviors, critical parenting, unhealthy ways of relating to others, confused values and attitudes, and unclear or inconsistent boundaries and limitations.

Children must learn that substance use and misuse is not acceptable, even in a society where the media constantly bombard us with messages suggesting that some forms of drug use are acceptable. Children must be taught to differentiate socially approved behavior from that which may lead them into trouble. When, where, and how to use drugs and medicines are vital parts of this education, as is the ability to make independent decisions that support their well-being.

Awareness and Staying in the "Now"

In his book *Awareness*, J. O. Stevens identified three levels of awareness that continue to be pertinent today.[15]

1. We are aware of immediate external stimuli through our senses: touch, taste, sight, hearing, and smell.
2. We are aware of immediate physiological sensations of our body, including things such as pain, itching, bowel sounds, and a host of others. These, Stevens claims, are the only true reality of life; everything else is fantasy.
3. Fantasy is all of our memories (which Stevens claims are, for the most part, vague and inaccurate), all of our projections of what will be in the future, and all of our imaginings of what we think is "now," without the input of our own senses.

Most of us, especially children, are encouraged to spend an inordinate amount of time worrying about what the future will hold, anguishing about the past, trying to be someone or something we think others want us to be. Too much time spent in fantasy prevents us from dealing with reality. Staying in the "now," dealing with perceptions of what is, holds promise for many. It rejuvenates the "one day at a time" phenomenon that has been a successful message in 12-step programs. Being aware of what we are and how we behave is a step toward improving our daily existence.

How are our behaviors formed? Where do our attitudes come from? Why do we behave as we do? These questions may arise as our awareness level of the present increases.

To help students increase their awareness of the "now" concept and connect with it, the teacher might have them close their eyes and follow these instructions:

With your eyes closed, listen carefully and try to identify all the sounds you can hear, including those that may be coming from your own body (breathing, heartbeat, restless movement in your seat). Once you have identified the sounds and located them, with your eyes still closed, what else are you aware of in your "now"? Are any other living things present—for example, humans, pets, plants? How do you know? These are your senses at work in the present, the only real time we have. Now, open your eyes.

Many of us spend a great deal of time and effort living in the past or the future. We often act or make decisions based on what we believe happened in the past or will happen in the future. What we know of the past is based on memory—ours if it's our past, someone else's if it is not ours. Examples of the latter are books and artifacts describing the past by someone who may have lived during that time. To see how this may be of questionable accuracy, ask anyone if he or she can describe an event in the recent past (a week or a month ago). What did he or she eat? Where did he or she go? Who was the person with? What was said? You will soon see that actions based on what we believe happened in our past may be based on faulty thinking.

The bottom line is that drug misuse and abuse usually exist because drugs make people feel better, less unhappy, less alone, less alienated, less different and less concerned about things they have done in the past or what will happen in the distant future. It makes them feel good. It fulfills needs that all people want but that abusers don't know how to fulfill in other, healthier, more constructive ways.

Look for these signs of abuse in students or peers, and get help.

- Major changes in behavior
- Sudden changes in mood
- New friends who are suspected of abusing drugs
- Drop in school performance
- Changes in appearance
- Irresponsible decision-making/poor judgment
- Aggressiveness
- Lying, cheating
- Forgetfulness, withdrawn attitude
- Loss of memory
- Poor coordination
- Slurred speech
- Attention-getting behaviors
- Denial of any problems

Summary

Drug use by school-age students in the United States is the highest among industrialized countries in the world. The highest usage rates are for alcohol, tobacco, and marijuana and, to a lesser degree, drugs such as cocaine, ecstasy, and heroin. Glue-sniffing and other inhalant use is most prevalent in upper elementary school children. Anabolic steroids are used by athletes and others who want to improve their physical appearance and performance. All of these drugs have deleterious effects on the human body, especially if they are used to excess and over time.

Drugs are classified as narcotics/opiates, depressants/sedatives, stimulants, psychedelics/hallucinogens, inhalants, marijuana, and steroids. They enter the body orally, by sniffing or snorting, by inhalation or smoking, by absorption, or through injection. Prescription and over-the-counter drugs also have the potential for misuse and abuse.

Among the many conditions drugs can cause or exacerbate over time are cardiorespiratory and cardiovascular ailments, certain types of cancer (notably lung cancer in smokers), liver deterioration (from excessive alcohol), and defects in the newborn babies of drug-using mothers.

Early education is a means of helping children develop the confidence and security to withstand the need to escape into drugs or succumb to peer pressure. It is important to remember that information about specific drugs is often *not* developmentally appropriate for elementary age students. Rather, drug education must be a diverse strategy that includes classroom activities focused on developing personal and social skills as well as other developmentally appropriate activities and learning experiences. In addition, drug education and prevention must involve the family, the community, and the cultural environment, particularly the media. One form of effective drug education by teachers is being a responsible and caring role model. Treatment approaches include psychiatric treatment coupled with prescribed medications, 12-step programs such as Alcoholics Anonymous and Narcotics Anonymous, and other support systems within the community.

Drugs are likely here to stay. They are part of cultural, religious, and social rituals and activities. The medical profession prescribes drugs as part of its treatment for various diseases. The challenge for educators is to pave the way for students to know when not to use drugs and, when they do, to use them in ways that will complement their lives and health.

Web Sites

American Council for Drug Education
http://www.acde.org

Center for Alcohol and Addiction Studies
http://center.butler.brown.edu/
Located at Brown University, the center's mission is to promote the identification, prevention, and effective treatment of alcohol and other drug use problems in our society through research, publications, education and training.

Centers for Disease Control and Prevention
http://www.cdc.gov/tobacco/edumat.htm
The CDC maintains a list of research and educational material for tobacco prevention.

Monitoring the Future Study, University of Michigan
www.isr.umich.edu/src/mtf

Centers for Disease Control and Prevention (CDC)
http://www.cdc.gov

ClubDrugs.Org
http://www.clubdrugs.org
This site, set up by NIDA, provides the latest information on these substances.

National Clearinghouse for Alcohol and Drug Information
http://www.health.org/
This is the information service of the Center for Substance Abuse Prevention of the U.S. Department of Health and Human Services. NCADI is the world's largest resource for current information and materials concerning substance abuse prevention.

Substance Abuse and Mental Health Services Administration
http://www.samhsa.gov

Tobacco Facts Website
http://www.tobaccofacts.org/
An excellent site related to many facts and resources regarding tobacco use.

Tobacco Research Center
http://www.hsc.wvu.edu/mbrcc/trc/trc_home.htm
The TRC brings together all the resources—scientific, medical, social, psychological, and administrative—for a coordinated approach to problems arising from tobacco use.

The Nicotine and Tobacco Network
http://www.nicnet.org/
From the University of Arizona, this excellent resource contains links and information on research, news, programs, resources, and other items relating to nicotine and tobacco.

National Institute on Drug Abuse
http://www.drugabuse.gov
This site contains information on the NIDA, including its organizations, calander of events, communications, grants and links to other related Web sites.

National Inhalant Prevention Coalition
http://www.inhalants.com/
This is a very comprehensive page devoted to disseminating accurate information about inhalants.

SteroidAbuse.Org
http://www.steroidabuse.org
This site is maintained by the National Institute on Drug Abuse.

Notes

1. H. Wechsler, J. Lee, M. Kuo, and H. Lee, "College Binge Drinking in the 1990s: A Continuing Problem: Results of the Harvard School of Public Health 1999 College Alcohol Survey." *The Journal of American College Health* 48 (2000): 199–210.
2. G. Botvin, "Principles of Prevention," in *Handbook on Drug Abuse Prevention,* ed. R. Combs and D. Ziedonis (Needham Heights, MA: Allyn & Bacon, 1999), 19–44.
3. S. Weinstein, *The Educator's Guide to Substance Abuse Prevention* (Mahwah, NJ: Lawrence Erlbaum Associates, 1999).
4. Center for Substance Abuse Prevention, *Here's Proof Prevention Works: Understanding Substance Abuse Prevention—Toward the 21st Century,* DHHS Publication No. SMA 99-3300 (Washington, DC: U. S. Department of Health and Human Services, Substance Abuse and Mental Health Services Administration, 1999).
5. See note 3, p. 22.
6. U. S. Substance Abuse and Mental Health Services Administration, Office of Applied Studies, *Summary Findings from the 1998 National Household Survey on Drug Abuse* (Rockville, MD: U. S. Substance Abuse and Mental Health Services Administration, Office of Applied Studies, 1999).
7. L. D. Johnston, P. M. O'Malley, and J. G. Bachman, *Monitoring the Future National Survey Results on Drug Use, 1975–2000. Volume I: Secondary School Students,* NIH Publication No. 01-4924 (Bethesda, MD: National Institute on Drug Abuse, 2001).
8. See note 7.
9. See note 7.
10. U. S. Department of Health and Human Services, *Preventing Tobacco Use Among Young People: A Report of the Surgeon General* (Atlanta: U. S. Department of Health and Human Services, Public Health Service, Centers for Disease Control and Prevention, National Center for Chronic Disease Prevention and Health Promotion, Office on Smoking and Health, 1994).
11. National Institute on Drug Abuse, "Ecstasy Damages the Brain and Impairs Memory in Humans," *NIDA Notes* 14, no. 4 (November) (Washington, DC: U. S. Department of Health and Human Services, National Institutes of Health, 1999).
12. National Institute on Drug Abuse, *Club Drugs: Community Drug Alert Bulletin,* in U. S. Department of Health and Human Services: National Institutes of Health (January, 2001) available at http://www.drugabuse.gov/ClubAlert/Clubdrugalert.html
13. NIDA, 2001
14. P. H. Blachly, *Seduction* (Springfield, IL: Charles C. Thomas, 1970).
15. J. O. Stevens, *Awareness: Exploring, Experimenting, Experiencing* (Moab, UT: Real People's Press, 1971).

Learning Experiences

Several learning objectives should be considered when developing curricula and activities for preventing alcohol and other drug abuse. The intent is that students will understand why people abuse drugs, how to prevent them from becoming abusers, and how to find alternatives to drugs for attaining the feelings they want.

Grades K–2

In the early grades, learning about the use and abuse of substances is necessarily limited. At this age students should be taught skills related to the development of self-image and decision making about appropriate and inappropriate behaviors. They can begin to develop their refusal skills, which can later be applied to refusing peer pressure for drug use. They could become aware of different forms of substances (pills, capsules, liquid, powder) and their common names. They also should learn the content of the medicine cabinet or where medicines are housed, what they are, and what they can do. They need to know that people are available to reach out to in case members of their family are abusing drugs. By the end of discussions of alcohol and other drugs, students should be able to

1. Differentiate harmless substances and potentially dangerous drugs.
2. Explain when medicines should and should not be taken.
3. Identify the difference between alcoholic and nonalcoholic drinks.
4. Present some reasons why people drink alcoholic beverages or use drugs inappropriately.
5. Describe some physical effects of alcohol and other drugs.
6. Identify responsible adults to talk to about problems with drug abuse in their family.
7. Identify healthy ways to make themselves feel good.
8. Identify ways to refuse activities they don't want to do.

Grades 3–4

As the students continue to develop, they need to know which beverages contribute to their growth and health (for example, milk, juices) and which they should avoid (for example, alcoholic beverages). They should understand the difference between prescription and OTC medicines and precautions about using them. At the same time, they should be informed about the beneficial use of some drugs. By the end of their exposure to this information and in addition to what they learned in K–2, students should be able to

1. Describe how medicines are used safely.
2. Relate how peer pressure can force children to abuse drugs.
3. Demonstrate refusal skills.
4. Describe how the media influence drug-taking behaviors.
5. Relate the differences between legal and illegal use of drugs.
6. Describe the difference between OTC and prescription drugs.
7. Identify and access programs and resources that assist people and their families with substance abuse problems.
8. Identify alternative behaviors and activities to drug use.

Grades 5–6

Helping children to be aware of themselves and their attitudes and behaviors is vital to their avoiding substance abuse. By these grades, they should understand the social and physical effects of smoking and secondhand smoke and how smoking affects their performance. They should be able to associate the need for drugs and medicines with human problems—emotional, social, economic, and political—and know how difficult it is to stop after starting. In addition to further developing the outcomes from grades K–4, students in grades 5–6 should be able to

1. Describe how peer pressure promotes the use of drugs.
2. Describe how to use refusal skills when feeling pressured.
3. Identify the commonly abused drugs (including OTC, prescriptive, illicit).
4. Explain some problems in social, physical, and emotional health engendered by drugs.
5. Develop appropriate alternatives for getting the feelings that drugs produce.
6. Identify drug-free peers that can support their well-being.
7. Describe the effects of anabolic steroids.
8. Describe how drugs affect decision-making, performance, achievement of goals, and the like.
9. Compare their own attitudes and values surrounding the use of drugs with those of society.

Presenting Information by Discipline

Science

Examine the derivation of various opiates from the poppy, how coca leaves become cocaine, the various kinds of alcohol and how they are made, including fermentation and distillation. Demonstrate the effects of alcohol and tobacco on body tissue. Discuss diseases and the risks of drug use, including HIV/AIDS.

Math

The amount of alcohol differs with the beverage. Beer is about 3–6 percent alcohol; wine about 10–12 percent; spirits such as rye and gin, about 40–50 percent. A standard-size drink of each contains the same amount of alcohol (12 ounces of beer, 5 ounces of wine, and 1½ ounces of spirits all contain 1 ounce of alcohol). Proof and percent of alcohol can be discussed with a comparison of various beverages.

English

The school library and the Internet are good sources for books, periodicals, and other information relating to drug use. These could inspire book reports, summaries, and oral presentations.

Social Studies

Countries of origin of many problem drugs, such as heroin and cocaine, can be explored, along with reasons these countries allow or encourage the drug trade and how the United States tries to deal with this. Some of the relevant places are Mexico, Asia, and Central and South America. Another good topic is ethnic drug use (wine as a religious symbol, use of peyote by the Native American Church, and others). A discussion of drug use laws is appropriate, including their history in the United States and other countries, notably the legal heroin experiment in Britain.

Art

Posters, dioramas, cartoons, and bulletin boards can feature substance abuse issues.

Physical Education

Students can discuss the "high" possible through various strenuous exercises and how this is a viable alternative to drug highs.

For suggestions on creating a rubric with which to evaluate student performance of Learning Experiences, see page 13.

Learning Experience 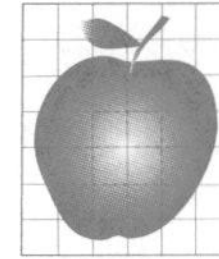 10-1

The Medicine Story

Grade Level

K–2

Primary Discipline

English

Learning Objectives

Following this activity, students will be able to

- Recognize safe from unsafe medicine use.
- Describe circumstances in which medicines are used to keep us healthy.

Time Required

One session

Material

The story below, paper, and pencil. Read the following story:

The kids in the neighborhood belong to a little league softball team. One Sunday morning Tommy and Chuckie decide to get up early to get ready for their game that afternoon. They call their friend Phil and ask his mom to wake him up so they can practice. Phil is the team pitcher. During the practice Tommy falls and bangs his head and badly bruises his arm. He says his arm hurts and he has a headache. Phil tells Tommy that his own mother gave him an aspirin to put in his backpack, to take at lunchtime, and that Tommy could have it instead. Chuckie says he has some "red medicine" in his bag to take for his cold and that Tommy could have that.

Tommy says he thinks children shouldn't take medicine unless it is given by a grown-up or if the doctor says so. Besides, Tommy says, medicine should not be shared. Medicines are not like candy or food even if they sometimes taste and look the same. Chuckie says that maybe Tommy should go home and ask his mom to take him to the doctor. Perhaps the doctor can help him.

The boys go home with Tommy, and Tommy's mom takes them all with her to the medical center down the street from the park. The doctor who examines Tommy cleans up the arm and puts a small bandage on the bad scrape. He gives Tommy's mom a prescription for a special medicine and directions for taking it. The doctor says it will make Tommy's headache feel better. The doctor also gives Tommy an injection to make sure he does not get an infection.

Tommy's mom stops at the drugstore, fills the prescription, and gives the medicine to Tommy as the doctor ordered. Soon Tommy is feeling much better and is playing softball again with his friends.

Description of Activity

Ask the following questions:

- Did you like the story?
- Why didn't Tommy want to take the aspirin?
- Why didn't Tommy want to take the medicine Chuckie offered?
- Why did Tommy take the special medicine the doctor prescribed?
- Why did the doctor give Tommy an injection?
- If your friend offers you his or her medicine, will you take it?

Homework

The students ask their parents if they are allowed to take medicine from someone.

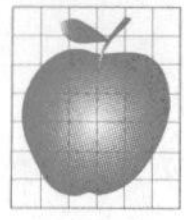

Learning Experience 10-1 continued

Evaluation

The students are able to define the two new vocabulary words introduced (injection and prescription). Each student identifies two reasons why they would not take medicine from their friends.

As additional criteria, students will be able to

- Identify adults they would go to if they or a friend were to feel ill.
- Explain the difference between a medicine and a food or candy.
- Explain the circumstances under which they would take medicine from someone.
- Identify what medicines are supposed to do.

Learning Experience 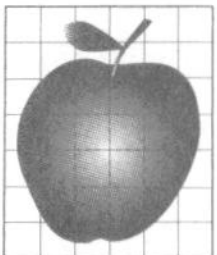 10-2

Defining Substance Abuse and Misuse

Grade Level

4–6

Primary Discipline

Health/Substance abuse prevention

Description

Substance use is often addressed in the upper elementary grades. This topic can be extremely difficult to present. To help students understand the difference between substance use, abuse, and misuse, this lesson provides students with an opportunity to role play a variety of situations.

Goal

The students will understand the difference between substance use, misuse, and abuse.

Objectives

The student will list, on the chalkboard, two reasons why people use, misuse, and abuse drugs. The student will, in a group of four, role play a situation that relates to drug abuse or misuse. The students will list, on a sheet of white roll paper, the characteristics that differentiate drug abuse from misuse.

Background

This activity can be used at the beginning or at the end of a substance abuse unit. The type of role play situations used during this lesson may depend on the maturity of the students. An important reminder is the audience commentary. The student audience may respond only with personal reactions or positive comments.

Concepts

Students will be able to:

1. Differentiate between substance abuse and misuse.
2. Identify the factors that influence substance use, misuse, and abuse.

Material

- Overhead: definitions of substance use, misuse, and abuse
- Role play situations, one per group of four students
- 1 large sheet of white roll paper

Anticipatory Set

A. Ask the the students what soda pop, aspirin, antiperspirant, coffee, and wine have in common.

B. Write these responses on the board.

Input

A. Discuss with the students why they chose to answer the introductory question the way they did.

B. Using the overhead of definitions, define and discuss drug abuse. After presenting this definition, ask the student to provide some examples.

c. Define and discuss misuse. Ask the student to provide some examples. If no one wants to participate, initiate the discussion with an example.

D. Using letters, divide the students into groups of four. Each group is responsible for one role play situation. Randomly pass out one role play situation to each group. Give the students 5–7 minutes to prepare an informal presentation.

Modeling

The teacher will demonstrate a variety of role play ideas. This demonstration will include vocabulary review and presentation expectations.

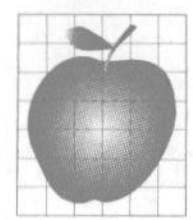

Learning Experience 10-2 continued

Guided Practice

The student will briefly rehearse the role play situations. Offer assistance as needed. If a group member cannot decide on a presentation approach, designate roles or offer suggestions.

Independent Practice

A. Each group will role play the provided situation. This role play will include a brief summary on the presentation choice.

B. The students will comment on the presentation choice or offer personal situations.

Closure

A. Ask the students to describe the difference between drug abuse and misuse. Write these differences on a sheet of white role paper.

B. Ask the students to write their own definition of the word "drugs."

c. Ask the students to compare this definition to the definition before the unit was presented "Why did the definition change?"

Useful Internet Sources

CLN Substance Abuse Theme Page
http://www.cln.org/themes/substance_abuse.html

Drug Related Street Terms and Slang Words
http://www.addictions.org/slang.htm

ERIC Clearinghouse on Teaching and Teacher Education—Health, Physical Education, Recreation and Dance Division
http://www.ericsp.org/pages/healthpe/index.html

Learning Experience 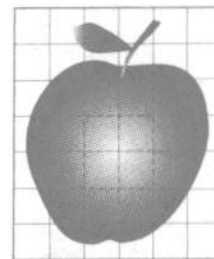 10-3

How Much Alcohol in the Drink?

Grade Level

5–6

Primary Discipline

Math

Learning Objectives

Following this activity, students will be able to

- Describe the relationship between proof and percent of content.
- Use math skills to find out how much alcohol a certain beverage may contain.
- Explain how any beverage containing alcohol is potentially dangerous to health.

Time Required

One lesson (45 minutes)

Materials

Labels and ads brought in for homework

Description of Activity

Have students refer to ads or labels to identify alcohol content by proof or percent. They convert the information to ounces or other liquid measurement. (How much alcohol does a person actually consume in a glass of wine, whiskey, beer?)

Homework

Students bring in labels and ads of alcoholic beverages.

Evaluation

Students are able to

- Calculate the ratio of alcohol to other fluids in a beverage.
- Calculate the amount of alcohol in a glass of wine, beer, or other alcoholic beverage.
- Explain the concept of "proof" in a given beverage.
- Describe the effects on drinkers of higher and lower proof.
- Describe the relationship between alcohol and health.
- Identify this information embedded in advertisements.

Learning Experience 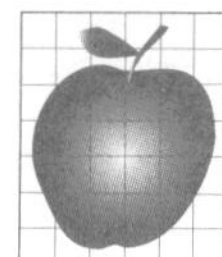 10-4

Who Uses Drugs?

Grade Level

5–6

Primary Discipline

Health

Learning Objectives

Following this activity, students will be able to

- Find out who uses drugs, including alcohol, by age, gender, occupation, or other demographic feature.
- State appropriate uses for drugs.
- Suggest alternatives to drug use.

Time Required

Three 1-hour sessions

Materials

Labels and ads brought in for homework

Description of Activity

The students research drug use nationwide by contacting the agencies that collect the data delineated in the learning objectives. Each group of 4–5 students could be assigned a different source to contact. Some of these sources are 1993 National Household Survey on Drug Abuse (U.S. Department of Health and Human Sources); Public Health Service; National Institute on Drug Abuse. A general number is National Clearinghouse for Alcohol and Drug Information, 800-729-6686. Students generate some appropriate uses for drugs, with specific examples.

Homework

Students write sample interview questions on these topics.

Evaluation

Students are able to

- Prepare questions relevant to an interviewing assignment.
- Collect reliable information about an assigned topic.
- Describe the characteristics of a person who uses alcohol and other drugs.
- Differentiate appropriate uses and inappropriate uses of alcohol and other drugs.
- Identify alternative behaviors to the use of alcohol and other drugs (particularly by peers and teenagers).

Learning Experience 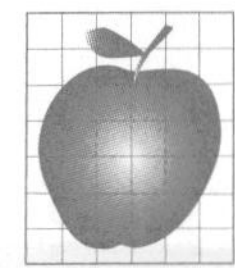 10-5

Risk Taking

Grade Level

5–6

Primary Discipline

Social Science

Learning Objectives

Following this activity, students will be able to

- Define risk taking.
- Describe levels of risk and characteristics of risk-takers.
- Report which level of risk-taker they tend to be.

Time Required

One session

Materials

Pencil and paper

Description of Activity

Have students develop a list of 10 behaviors they perceive as risky (examples: smoking in school, lying to a parent or the teacher, trying out for a team or a play). Write these on the board and ask students to rank them from 1 to 10 on a sheet of paper.

Divide the class into groups of five or six to discuss the following concepts:

- People perceive risk levels differently. What may be risky to you may be just fun for a friend.
- You don't always know the consequences, but you should try to identify them before you assume the risk.
- You should seek alternatives, especially if the risk is high.
- A person should not take risks solely to impress someone or respond to peer pressure.
- When should someone take a risk?

Homework

None

Evaluation

Students are able to

- Define risk taking and give examples of risks.
- Differentiate great-risk and low-risk behaviors and give examples of each.
- Identify the high-risk behaviors for students their age.
- Describe the steps one could take when deciding whether to take a given risk.
- Describe their own risk taking style.

Learning Experience 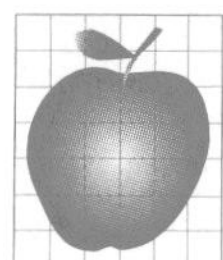 10-6

Tripping Without Drugs

Grade Level

5–6

Primary Discipline

Social Science

Learning Objectives

Following this activity, students will be able to

- Discuss the many ways to "trip" without drugs.
- Describe the good feelings they can get from things they do without drugs.

Time Required

One session

Description of Activity

1. Have the students relax by using a relaxation exercise (deep breathing or progressive muscle relaxation—see Chapter 8, page 282) wherein they visualize a trip to their favorite place.
2. Have students concentrate on things they like to do that excite them (painting, reading a book, singing, playing a musical instrument, playing sports, going for a bike ride, sewing, surfing, writing, joining a group, and so on).

Homework

Have students make a list of all of the things they enjoy doing and bring it to class to share.

Evaluation

Students are able to

- Identify the reasons why people use alcohol and other drugs.
- Identify things people do, other than taking alcohol and other drugs, to feel good or competent.
- Describe the strategies they can use to relax and feel good.
- Identify new things they have learned from their friends or classmates that they have not yet done that would make them feel excited.

Learning Experience 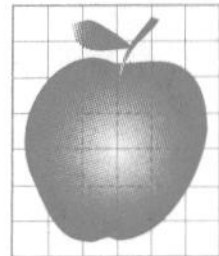 10-7

Tobacco Use

Grade Level

5–6

Primary Discipline

Social Studies, Science, Language Arts, Creative Arts

Learning Objectives

Following this activity, students will

- Have accurate information about the effects of tobacco on the body.
- Be able to describe the dangers of smoking and secondhand smoke.
- Be able to work with others to develop a smoking prevention plan.
- Be able to describe the local laws associated with tobacco use among young people.
- Know how to contact their congressperson and advocate for a health cause.
- Be able to create a poster and a public service announcement.

Time Required

Four sessions

Materials

Magazines, scissors, paper, pencils, envelopes, colored pen, brief written description of smoking laws in their community or town

Description of Activity

In groups of no more than four students, have the groups identify one person as the recorder who will take notes about the group's work; one person as the group spokesperson who will report the work to the larger group; one person who will be responsible for collecting the materials and other products of the group's work and keeping them in a folder; one person who is in charge of keeping the group on task.

Sessions 1 and 2

Task One: Give each group three or four commonly read adult magazines. Have the students cut out pictures of the different types of smoking ads (cigars, cigarettes, pipes, chewing, and so on) they find in the magazines. Discuss the pictures in the ad and the people used to advertise. Make a list of important things they notice about the product and the people in the ads.

Task Two: Take the students to the library or use the resources available in the classroom. In their group, have the students develop a fact sheet about the use of tobacco and the effects of tobacco on people.

Reconvene all students, and have each group spokesperson summarize some of the discussion. Put the information on the board, and have each groups' recorder add things missing in their lists.

Task Three: Have each group produce a poster that represents the information they have gathered.

Session 3

Task One: Provide each group with information about smoking laws in their community. Have the students discuss the laws and render a group opinion that they will report to the larger class.

Task Two: Have the students develop a program that includes rules for their own school that will prevent tobacco use by students their age and in middle school. Tell the students that the program must be easy to follow and able to be carried out.

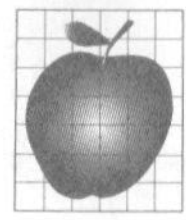

Learning Experience 10-7 continued

Session 4

Identify the names of state congresspeople who represent the school district. Discuss with the students what makes a good public service announcement. You might want to bring in some taped examples. In groups have the students develop a public service announcement that would help prevent the use of tobacco.

Homework

Have students each bring in a letter they have written to their congressperson describing the dangers of smoking for young people. They should include a description of the public service announcement and the prevention plan they have developed. Have the students ask their congressperson to support antismoking programs and laws.

Evaluation

The following rubrics will help assess the poster and the public service announcement. Additional criteria can be added to address the content of the primary discipline.

Evaluation of Poster

Criteria	4	3	2	1
Content	Content is accurate and complete.	Content is accurate, but incomplete.	Content is accurate, but the message of poster is unclear.	Content is vague or inaccurate.
Design	Placement of graphics and information is logical; poster includes at least one graphic.	Placement of graphics and information is logical; poster includes at least one graphic.	Placement of graphics and information is logical; poster includes at least one graphic.	Placement of graphics and content is poor.
Effectiveness	Spelling, grammar, and punctuation are correct; poster communicates information clearly and attractively.	Spelling, grammar, and punctuation are correct; poster communicates information clearly and attractively; project is submitted late.	Spelling, grammar, and punctuation are correct; poster communicates information clearly and attractively; project is submitted late.	Spelling, grammar; and punctuation are incorrect; design is poor; poster does not communicate information effectively.

Evaluation of Public Service Announcement

Criteria	4	3	2	1
Content	Content is accurate; PSA includes clear message about dangers of drug use.	Content is accurate; PSA includes clear message about dangers of drug use.	Content is accurate, but message of PSA is unclear.	Content is vague or inaccurate.
Design	Graphics and information are logical; PSA includes at least three important facts about drug use.	Placement of graphics and information is logical; PSA includes at least two important facts about drug use.	Placement of graphics and information is logical; PSA includes at least one important fact about drug use.	Placement of the graphics and content is poor; PSA includes at least one important fact about drug use.
Effectiveness	Grammar is correct; PSA communicates information clearly and attractively.	Grammar is correct; PSA communicates information clearly and attractively; project is submitted late.	Grammar is correct; PSA communicates information clearly and attractively; project is submitted late.	Grammar is incorrect; PSA does not communicate information effectively.

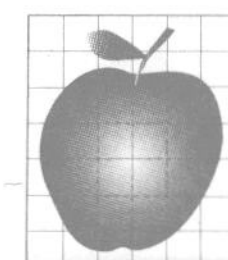

Learning Experience 10-8

Antismoking Song

Grade Level

5–6

Primary Discipline

Creative Arts, Language Arts, Science

Learning Objectives

Following this activity, students will

- Know important facts about smoking and health.
- Differentiate myths and facts about smoking.
- Be able to explain why it is important not to start smoking.
- Know where to go for help to stop smoking.

Time Required

Three sessions

Materials

Antismoking Song handout

Description of Activity

Introduction

Relate the following information:

Some people might think smoking tobacco can't be all that bad—there are so many people who do it! Many people continue to smoke because nicotine, one of the harmful substances in tobacco, causes smokers to become addicted. Nicotine, tar, carbon monoxide, and other chemicals in tobacco are responsible for many diseases, including cancer, high blood pressure, heart disease, and lung disease. Although there are many reasons not to smoke, teenagers and adults often begin smoking because of peer pressure or advertising from tobacco companies. There are ways to stop smoking, and organizations as well as medications that can help people quit.

Activity

Divide the class into groups of 3–4 and give the following instructions and provide a handout with a list of tasks to be accomplished by the group.

In your group, you will write an original rap or song. Pretend that each of you is a member of an influential music group that wants to write a song with a clear antismoking message. The lyrics to your song, or the words of your rap, will include facts about how smoking tobacco and secondhand smoke can affect people's health and about the harmful substances in tobacco that cause diseases. They will also tell how to avoid pressure to smoke from peers or from advertisements. This will require several days of gathering information.

Most songs include several stanzas and a chorus or refrain. The one- or two-line chorus is repeated between the verses. Your chorus should be an antismoking slogan that people will remember. For example: "Your lungs can't work when they're coated with tar. And when you try to run, you won't get far."

You will present your rap or song lyrics with other students in the class, as well as other students in your school. Think about the kind of songs that appeal to your audience. Think, too, of songs you know that have a positive message.

Homework

None

Evaluation

For the grades listed below, the song or rap meets the associated criteria:

A: The song includes four to six factual pieces of information about tobacco and the health dangers associated with tobacco use. The song strongly conveys originality in dealing with the relationship between smoking and poor health (heart disease, cancer, emphysema) and the choices students have about starting to smoke. The song's message suggests other positive ways to handle stress and peer pressure. The whole song works

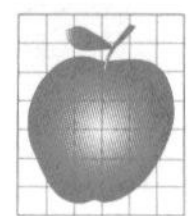

Learning Experience 10-8 continued

extremely well for an antismoking message for the intended audience.

B: The song includes two or three pieces of information about tobacco and the health dangers associated with tobacco. The group has composed an original antismoking song that shows limited choices in dealing with smoking and poor health. The song mentions that students have an alternative way to deal with tobacco use and peer pressure. The lyrics and the music work together to achieve the desired effect on the audience.

C: The song lacks factual information about tobacco and the health dangers associated with smoking. The song only mentions the act of smoking without clarifying its relationship to poor health. The organized structure lacks ways of dealing with peer pressure and other ways of handling stress. The group does not make use of an appropriate antismoking message. The words and music do not convey important facts about tobacco to achieve the desired effect on the audience.

D: The song is disorganized, unoriginal, and lacks factual information about tobacco. The song mentions only the act of smoking without additional information on poor health. The lyrics do not convey the necessary messages about the dangers of tobacco or alternative ways to handle pressures to use tobacco. The words and music lack clarity for the audience.

Antismoking Song

Check the following boxes to indicate your group progress.

- ☐ 1. Select your audience.
- ☐ 2. With your group, research and review the main health problems associated with smoking tobacco, breathing secondhand smoke, and using smokeless tobacco. Which are the most important facts for teenagers to know?
- ☐ 3. Discuss and record how peer pressure affects teens in our school. Exchange ideas about ways to avoid the pressure.
- ☐ 4. Talk about ways to present your lyrics to your audience. You could make a tape of your rap or song at home and bring it to school. You could say or sing the lyrics aloud. You could perform your lyrics with music if someone in your group can play a musical instrument.
- ☐ 5. List the main facts you want to present about how smoking damages the body. Include some facts about the diseases caused by smoking and the parts of the body harmed by smoking.
- ☐ 6. As a group, investigate how song lyrics are constructed. Find printed lyrics included in tape cassettes, CDs, and music magazines. The chorus should have a clear, easy-to-remember antismoking message.
- ☐ 7. Write the first draft of your research and lyrics. Will your song rhyme? To get started with the lyrics, list words that rhyme with a key word (for example, cancer, answer; disease, ease; smoke, joke; cool, fool, rule, drool).
- ☐ 8. Read over your research and song drafts. Make sure they include the facts listed in Step 5. Continue to revise your song so it is both informative and entertaining.
- ☐ 9. Prepare a final written version of your research paper and your lyrics.
- ☐ 10. Present your lyrics to your audience and your research paper to your health teacher.

Learning Experience 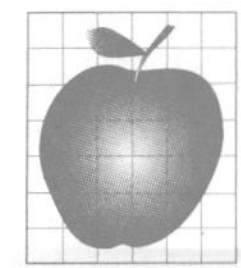 10-9

Fruit Juice Drink

Grade Level

5–6

Primary Discipline

Creative Arts, Language Arts, Science

Learning Objectives

Following this activity, students will

- Know important facts about alcohol and its effect on the body.
- Differentiate myths and facts about alcohol use.
- Be able to explain why a person should not use alcohol.
- Be familiar with support groups pertaining to alcohol use.

Time Required

Three sessions

Material

Posterboard, computer (optional), magazines, handout

Description of Activity

Introduction

Provide the following background and a handout with a list of tasks to be accomplished by the group:

When people think of alcohol, they may think of the many advertisements that show happy, healthy people enjoying a party or a game of volleyball on the beach. But alcohol is a drug that can prevent you from enjoying good social, mental, and physical health. Alcohol can also cause diseases of the liver, heart, and stomach. Alcoholism, a physical and an emotional dependence on alcohol, afflicts many Americans. Traffic accidents—the leading cause of death among teenagers—are often related to alcohol use.

Your best chance to avoid having problems with alcohol is not to use it. Many organizations and support groups are available to people whose lives have been affected by alcoholism. Teens and adults alike, can learn how to refuse alcohol.

Activity

Give the following instructions:

In your groups, you will write a magazine advertisement for a carbonated fruit-juice beverage that does not contain alcohol. You will create a name for the beverage. Your advertisement will be aimed at teenagers who do not use alcohol. The company that makes the fruit-juice drink wants the ad to contribute to teenagers' awareness of the dangers of alcohol.

Your ad will include some facts about alcohol use and alcohol-related problems, such as driving after drinking. It will also suggest that drinking the fruit-juice beverage is much "cooler" than drinking alcohol.

In an advertising agency, writers and graphic designers often team up to make a presentation of the ad they think will sell the product to the targeted audience. You will work as a team to make your presentation on a posterboard. Your presentation should include a picture or some other graphics (made on the computer if possible).

Your audience will be teenagers and other members of your health class. Think about which magazines and other printed material teenagers like to

Source: Darlene Kurth, Health Educator, Bellmore-Merrick, C.H.S.D., Merrick, NY. Reprinted with permission.

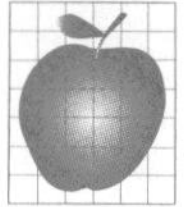

Learning Experience 10-9 continued

read. In your group, look at and discuss the advertisements in those magazines to see how they appeal to teenagers.

Advertisements often use a celebrity spokesperson to help get a message across. The group might want to use a celebrity spokesperson who does not use alcohol, and whom teenagers admire, as a spokesperson for the ad. You could also use unknown teens as spokes people, or a cartoon figure that you invent, or a teacher.

Homework

The students collect magazine ads relevant to this activity.

Evaluation

For the grades listed below, the display meets the associated criteria:

A: The display is eye-catching and conveys a strong message for drinking a nonalcoholic beverage. The graphics, statistics, and informational displays are done with great artistic and technical skill. Organization of facts is creative and thoughtful. The display shows a factual balance between nonalcoholic drinks and alcoholic beverages. The whole display communicates the health risks of alcoholic beverages (illnesses, unsafe driving, violence) versus the health benefits of the nonalcoholic beverage. The idea of choice is conveyed to the audience.

B: The display is convincing for the use of a nonalcoholic beverage versus an alcoholic beverage. The group has selected and arranged the physical objects so the theme is carried out clearly. Graphics, statistics, information, and places to get valid information are included. Organization of facts is creative and thoughtful. The advertisement is eye-catching. The display is neat and presentable. It accomplishes its intended purpose with the target audience.

C: The theme selected is not appropriate for the concepts to be conveyed. It does not clearly show alternatives, the health risks of alcohol abuse, or the safety issues dealing with alcohol. The selection and organization for a nonalcoholic beverage advertisement show little thought or effort. The graphics are incomplete or inaccurate and do little to carry out the theme. The display is not neat and presentable. The display does not accomplish its purpose with the intended audience.

D: The display is disorganized and conveys little or no information. It fails to offer alternatives to alcohol and lacks important facts about the health risks of alcohol abuse. The selection and organization for a nonalcoholic advertisement are totally inaccurate and lacking a theme. The display has little effect on the audience.

Fruit Juice Ad

Check the following boxes to record your progress.

☐ 1. With your group, brainstorm ideas about how to reach your audience. Think about how you can get teenagers to pay attention to your ad's message.

☐ 2. Work with your group to review important information on alcoholism and alcohol's effect on the body. Write an informational report. Include facts from this report in the advertisement.

☐ 3. Research additional information. You may want to contact SADD, Alateen, or AA for further information and statistics. Doctors and clinics may also have pamphlets about teens and drinking. Your ad could include telephone numbers of organizations that give help and support.

☐ 4. To get your group thinking of ideas for your advertisement, look in magazines and newspapers to see how ads are organized and presented.

☐ 5. Write a draft of the text of the ad. As you do, keep your purpose in mind. Find ways to make the fruit-juice drink sound appealing and alcohol just the opposite.

☐ 6. Read the advertisement. Will teens be convinced that drinking the fruit-juice drink is "cool?" Check to make sure you have included the information you listed in Step 2 and any information gathered in Step 3.

☐ 7. Cut out pictures or make drawings for the ad.

☐ 8. Copy the ad onto posterboard. Add the pictures or drawings. You may want to use the computer for graphic designs.

☐ 9. Present the ad to your class. After the class has reviewed all the ads, class members should discuss which ones they liked the best and why. Which is the best name for your fruit-juice beverage?

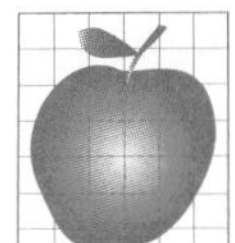

Learning Experience 10-10

Drug Information Boards

Grade Level

5–6

Primary Discipline

Creative Arts, Language Arts, Science

Learning Objectives

Following this activity, students will

- Know the classifications of drugs.
- Understand the effects of the various drugs on the body.
- Be able to explain why a person should not use drugs.
- Be familiar with support groups pertaining to alcohol use.

Time Required

Three sessions

Material

Posterboard, handout

Description of Activity

Introduction

Provide the following background:

There are several categories of drugs. Medicines cure or prevent disease, but if they are used incorrectly, they can cause health problems. Prescription medicines can be purchased legally only with a written order from a doctor. Some of these medicines—such as stimulants, depressants, and narcotics—can be addictive if they are abused. Over-the-counter medicines, such as cough suppressants, can be bought without a prescription.

Crack, hallucinogens, inhalants, and other street drugs are bought and used illegally. Using street drugs is dangerous for many reasons: They can harm the body and the brain; cause addiction; lead to diseases such as AIDS through the sharing of needles; and get you arrested. Drug addiction can be cured, but withdrawal is a long and painful process. Support organizations can help people overcome addiction, and many treatment programs are available to help teens and adults remain drug-free.

Activity

Give the following instructions and provide a handout with a list of tasks to be accomplished by the group.

Working as a group, make several information boards for your school. Organize newspaper and magazine articles according to categories, write titles for the categories in your displays, and include group research about the drug discussed in the article. Use of the computer is suggested.

Each person in the group will collect two articles about drug abuse. For each article, write a short paragraph explaining the nature of the drug and the health problems it causes. For example, if your article is about children who are born addicted to crack cocaine, your paragraph should explain that crack cocaine is a stimulant and that it is addictive.

Homework

Students collect newspaper and magazine articles about drug use.

Evaluation

For the grades listed below, the board display meets the associated criteria:

A: The board display with appropriate articles dealing with consequences of drug abuse. It is attractive, creative, interesting, and informative. The message comes across strongly that drug abuse can destroy people, lead to jail, and cause serious health consequences. The information and research for the drug mentioned in the articles is factual and well-presented. The display is neatly done and clearly organized for the intended audience.

Source: Darlene Kurth, Health Educator, Bellmore-Merrick, C.H.S.D., Merrick, NY. Reprinted with permission.

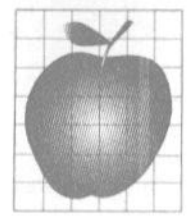

Learning Experience 10-10 continued

B: The board conveys the importance of not abusing drugs. The message is clear, and the information presented is appropriate and accurate regarding the concepts of drug abuse. The information is correct and effective in dealing with the importance of staying drug-free. The organization of graphics and statements helps clarify points of drug abuse. The board is informative and presentable to the intended audience.

C: The board is not interesting and lacks clarity of information on the drugs researched. The intended message about the importance of staying drug-free is not clear. Information is missing or incorrect. The design is cluttered or disorganized. The mix of words, statements, and other graphics does not help much to accomplish the purpose of the board. The board is not neat and presentable.

D: The board is disorganized, with little mention about the importance of staying drug-free. Articles and the required research are missing. Some information is given, but it lacks a connection between the drug mentioned in article and the research.

Drug Information Boards

Check the following boxes to indicate your progress:

☐ 1. As a group, review your information about medicines and drugs. Discuss drug misuse and abuse, recalling any recent articles that members of the group had read about drug abuse.

☐ 2. Talk about where you are likely to find articles about drug abuse. Your local library is a good source for magazines, newspapers, and other periodicals. You can make copies of articles in the library to use in the board displays.

☐ 3. As members of the group collect articles, make a list of the drugs mentioned in them. Organize and assemble articles according to the drug classifications.

☐ 4. Prepare a short informational report for each drug. You can look in the library and find pamphlets in clinics, treatment centers and doctors' offices.

☐ 5. Write an explanatory paragraph for each article, stating the following:

   a. The drug mentioned in the article.

   b. How the drug is classified (depressant, stimulant, narcotic, hallucinogen).

   c. How the drug affects the body.

   d. Whether the drug is addictive and how long it takes to become addicted to the drug.

☐ 6. Write a first draft of each paragraph. Reread the paragraphs to make sure you have included all the points in Step 5. Then write a final draft.

☐ 7. Cut out the articles and use a paper clip to attach the paragraph that goes with each one.

☐ 8. With your group, sort through the articles. Decide how to categorize the articles for your boards. You could choose to organize them by the type of drug (for example, inhalants) or by some other classifications.

☐ 9. Choose the articles you will use for the boards. Write attention-getting titles for each board and category. Use the computer. Organizing the boards by making categories will make them easier for the audience to read.

☐ 10. Make the informational boards. Save all the articles not on the board. After a couple of weeks, you can remake the boards with those articles.

Learning Experience 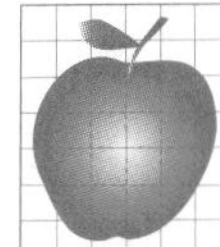 10-11

Natural Highs

Grade Level

5–6

Primary Discipline

Social Science

Learning Objectives

Following this activity, students will be able to

- Discuss the many ways to get a "high" without drugs.
- Describe the good feelings they can get with the things they do and the people they are with, without drugs.

Time Required

One session

Materials

Paper and pencil for interviews

Description of Activity

Give the following instructions:

1. Sit comfortably in your seat.
2. Close your eyes and breathe deeply in and out several times.
3. Count backward from 10 silently while I speak the count slowly (10, 9, 8 . . .).

Talk the students through the muscle relaxation sequence given in Chapter 8 (page 283). Ask the students to imagine taking a fantasy trip with you to their favorite place—someplace they go when they have a wonderful time. Maybe it is the beach, maybe it is the mountains, maybe it is to camp. They silently imagine themselves in that place and see who they are with and what they are doing. They see themselves in that place. What are they feeling? How do they look? After a minute of silence, the students follow the count back from 1–10 and then slowly open their eyes.

Have students write a little story about what they did, whom they were with, and what they were feeling. After they have written their story, they list the kinds of things they did and the people they were with generically (best friend, sibling, grandparent, or parent, and so on). Then they discuss what made it such a good time.

Homework

The students interview two of their best friends and their parents, asking them to identify two activities that make them feel like that they are having a great time. The activities must be limited to things they can share with others openly and are healthy.

Evaluation

Students will be able to orally identify three ways to feel good that do not involve drugs.

11

Child Abuse Prevention

Alane S. Fagin

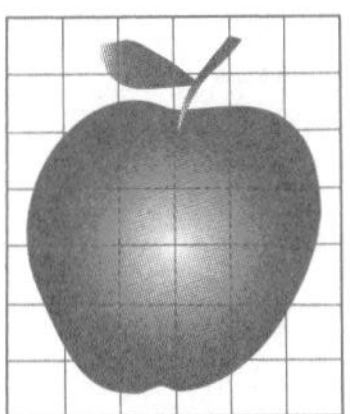

Chapter Outline

Objectives

- Define child neglect, physical abuse, sexual abuse, and emotional abuse
- Identify typical indicators of neglect
- Discuss signs of physical abuse
- Discuss indicators of sexual abuse
- Explain emotional abuse and why it is difficult to pinpoint
- Describe laws for reporting child abuse and neglect and the role of mandatory reporters
- Explore school policy on reporting and following up child abuse
- Delineate the basic concepts of instruction in personal safety
- Discuss developmentally appropriate activities and materials for use in preventing abuse

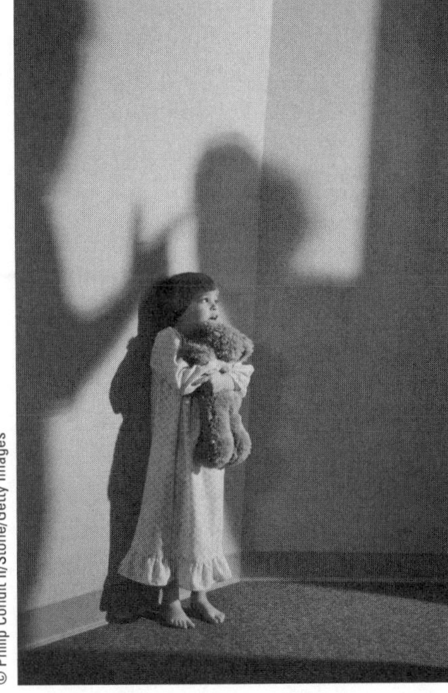

Sara has always been a wide-eyed, bubbly child in school. Lately, though, she's been falling asleep during class and has lost interest in her schoolwork. Her grades have fallen significantly.

The bus driver has started to notice that, for the past two weeks, Jon has gotten anxious as the bus approaches his stop. Some days he balks at getting off, even though his babysitter is waiting for him at the stop.

Tyrone usually comes to school hungry. He rarely brings his own lunch, and his mom often "forgets" to give him lunch money despite the many "reminder" notes sent home to her. Tyrone's teachers often find him asking his classmates for food or taking food from their trays in the cafeteria. Some of the teachers have started giving him money so he can buy lunch.

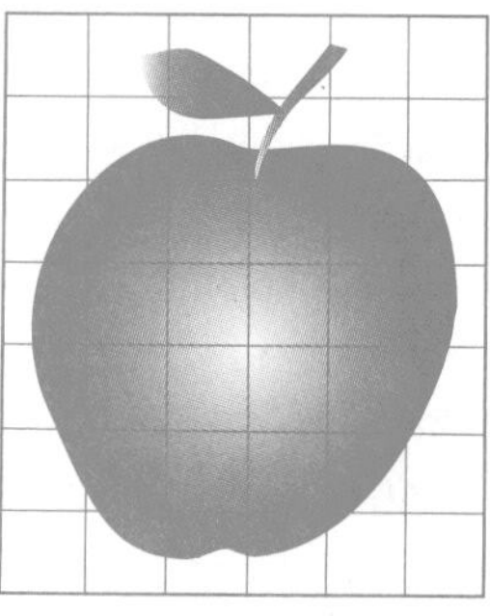

Sleeping in class and chronic fatigue can be indications of child abuse or neglect. Nurturing adults can help develop a child's sense of trust in self and others. Might these behaviors signal abuse or neglect? Who is responsible for recognizing these signals, and where should people who suspect a problem go?

Child abuse and neglect has many faces—from the young girl who is sexually abused nightly by her mother's live-in boyfriend to the 9-year-old boy who is afraid to go home because of an abusive babysitter to the student who comes to school dirty and hungry. Sometimes the abuse is as blatant as a black eye or a strap mark across the back, and other times no physical signs are evident. Some cases of abuse are clearly identified; others are more subtle.

Some Definitions

Although the legal definitions of child abuse and neglect or maltreatment vary from state to state, they are based on some fundamental premises. An abused or neglected child is generally defined as one whose physical or mental health or welfare is harmed or threatened with harm by the acts or omissions of his/her parent(s) or other person(s) responsible for his/her welfare.[1] Abuse and neglect are separated into four broad categories: child neglect, physical abuse, sexual abuse, and emotional abuse.

Child Neglect

Child neglect is characterized by a parent's or caregiver's failure to provide for a child's physical, educational, or emotional needs. Some of the more common indicators of neglect are the following:

Physical neglect: lack of food, shelter, and clothing; failure to provide adequate and appropriate nutrition and safe, sanitary shelter; inadequate clothing that is appropriate for the weather, poor hygiene; lack of appropriate and adequate supervision (such as leaving a child alone for an extended time); failure to provide appropriate medical, dental, optometrical, or surgical care.

Educational neglect: failure to ensure that the child attends school regularly and/or inattention to special education needs.

Emotional neglect: refusal or failure to provide psychological care (such as failure to help the child develop a positive self-image or to give positive feedback and reassurance); chronic/harmful exposure of the child to spouse abuse (either implicit or explicit); permission for the child to use drugs or alcohol.

Whereas physical abuse is often episodic, neglect tends to be chronic. When one form of neglect is observed, usually other forms of neglect are present as well. Neglect constitutes the greatest number of reports made to child-abuse hotlines. Its effects on a child can have long-lasting consequences. Neglected children can exhibit serious social problems in the school setting. Children who come to school unbathed, dirty, and unkempt are often ostracized by the other children and may be excluded from play. This sets them apart from their classmates and makes it difficult to maintain positive relationships. If neglected over time, many of these children do not develop the social and verbal skills necessary for interacting with their peers, and they might exhibit behavioral and conduct disorders as well.

Lags in emotional development and behavioral extremes can be manifested by over-compliance and passive or aggressive behavior. These children might appear listless and fatigued and even fall asleep at their desk. Some children might have responsibilities at home that are not developmentally appropriate or suitable for their age, such as having to care for younger children, prepare meals, or do the family laundry.

Many of these children go home to an empty house at the end of the school day ("latchkey kids"). Others might have to stay outside in the cold and dark until a parent returns. Responsible parents, when they are required to be away from the home, seek out alternatives such as after-school programs and other forms of supervision.

Some children have unmet medical needs or untreated physical problems. Letters sent home to parents may be to no avail, and the medical problem remains unattended.

Children are required by law to attend school regularly. Unexcused and frequent absences should be reported to appropriate school administrators. They should be addressed early, before the problem becomes chronic.

Neglected children tend to be more self-destructive, inattentive, nervous, and withdrawn than typical children, and in many circumstances demonstrate more problems than physically abused children.[2] Teachers must be sensitive to and aware of the indicators of neglect. The teacher is in a position to identify problems early before they become chronic and report the neglect, which can lead to the provision of needed services.

Physical Abuse

Physical abuse is non-accidental injury or threat of injury caused by the child's caregiver. Some of the more common indicators are unexplained bruises, welts, and bite marks; unexplained burns (from cigarettes or cigars) or lesions (caused by instruments such as irons, forks, rope, or immersion in hot water); unexplained fractures; head and face injuries (hair pulled, black eyes); cuts and bruises; lacerations or abrasions (to mouth, lips, gums, eyes, and body).

The abuse may be a one-time violent reaction to a child's behavior, or it can be episodic or repeated. In many cases the child is unaware that he or she has done something wrong. Children who are physically abused might appear to be wary of contact with parents or other adults. They might become apprehensive when other children cry. In the school setting, they might exhibit behavioral extremes, from withdrawal or depression to aggressive or acting-out behaviors. Children who have been physically abused might come to school early, remain on school grounds after hours because they are afraid to go home, or appear reluctant to get off the bus at the end of the school day (as in the vignette at the beginning of this chapter). To hide their bruises, their caregivers might dress them inappropriately, as for example, in long-sleeved shirts or long pants in warm weather or the child might refuse to dress for gym.

Children who have been physically abused often deny the abuse and fabricate stories that are inconsistent with the injury they have received. These children might be embarrassed or frightened by the abuse and seem to protect their parents from possible allegations. They keep the abuse a secret because they may be hurt more if the abuser finds out about the disclosure.

Parents or caregivers of these children may offer explanations that are inconsistent with the type of injury or developmental stage of the child. At one level, some may view the abuse as normal disciplining of a disruptive child. At another level, parents know that others would not condone their behavior. Thus, many abusive families live in isolation with few social contacts. The children, therefore, may have limited opportunities to socialize with other children and to learn appropriate social skills. This reinforces their lack of self-esteem, which further contributes to their feelings of inadequacy.

In the classroom, children who have been abused usually show a lack of self-esteem. They have little confidence in their abilities, which may be exhibited in poor school performance or poor peer relationships. Studies indicate that these students lack motivation, demonstrate less readiness to learn, and consequently are often underachievers.[3]

Sexual Abuse

Sexual abuse is characterized as any contact or interaction between a child and an adult in which the child is used for the sexual gratification or stimulation of the adult. All states' laws acknowledge that minors are not capable of consent to sexual interactions with adults. Therefore, these forms of behavior are considered abusive. Sexual abuse encompasses a wide range of behaviors or activities such as inappropriately touching a child's genitals, buttocks, breast, or other intimate parts; engaging or attempting to engage in sexual intercourse; forcing a child to engage in sexual activity with other adults or children; exposing a child to sexual activity; permitting a child to engage in sexual activity that is not appropriate to a child's age or development; and using a child in a sexual performance for child pornography or prostitution.

In 80–90 percent of sexual abuse cases, the offender is known to the child. In half of these cases, the offender is a family member or resides in the home.[4] These statistics underscore the need for prevention education, particularly programs that focus on "appropriate and inappropriate touch" rather than "stranger danger."

Certain behavioral indicators exhibited by school-age children might lead school personnel to suspect sexual abuse. Foremost of these are overly sexualized behavior or developmentally inappropriate knowledge of sex; avoidance of touch; avoidance of certain adults, certain places, or being left in certain situations; unwillingness to dress for gym or dressing inappropriately for the weather; regression (thumb sucking or bed wetting); or running away. These behaviors usually are accompanied by changes in academic performance, behavioral changes, inability to concentrate, disruptive behaviors such as regression or withdrawal.

Sometimes a child makes indirect hints that he or she is being abused.

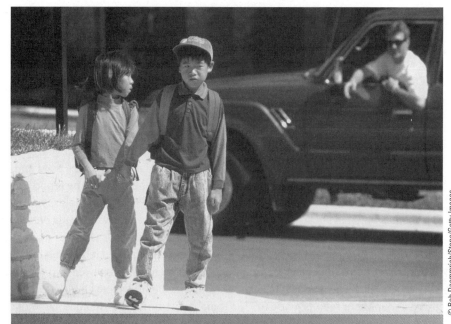

"Stranger danger" education is a preventative measure against child abuse.

© Bob Daemmrich/Stone/Getty Images

These indirect disclosures, along with behavioral indicators, should be taken seriously.

In most cases, there is no physical evidence of sexual abuse. These indicators, therefore, can serve as "red flags." Observance of any of these indicators in and of itself might not be enough to report abuse. Observance of several of these indicators, however, might be reasonable cause to suspect abuse and follow up.

Emotional Abuse

Emotional abuse or psychological maltreatment is defined as any act that results in impairing a child's psychological growth and development. Many believe that it is the most insidious, damaging form of abuse, yet it is the most difficult form to prove. Emotional abuse underlies all forms of abuse and neglect. Some physical indicators of emotional abuse are speech disorders, lags in physical development, failure to thrive, and eating disorders.

Emotional abuse takes many forms, including verbal assaults, constant belittling, shaming, condemning, and insulting. It is often characterized by a lack of parental concern for the child. Five forms of psychological maltreatment have been conceptualized: terrorizing, rejecting, isolating, ignoring, and corrupting.[5]

Emotional abuse erodes a child's self-esteem and confidence and undermines a child's sense of well-being. It can make a child constantly anxious, depressed, withdrawn, or fearful for his or her safety. These toxic forms of abuse leave scars that can last a lifetime.

Effects of emotional abuse can be observed in the school setting. Some children develop learning disabilities because of developmental delays. Some behavioral indicators of emotional abuse or psychological maltreatment are speech and language disorders; habit disorders (such as biting, rocking, and sucking); conduct disorders (antisocial, destructive, delinquent behavior, and the like); behavioral extremes; compliant, shy, aggressive, demanding, overly adaptive behavior (inappropriately adult or infantile); and suicide attempts.

Indicators of all forms of abuse and neglect are clues, pieces of a puzzle that help create a better picture or understanding of what is going on with a child and a family. The set of indicators is neither all-inclusive nor definitive. The repeated presence of an indicator or several indicators in combination, however, should alert school personnel to the possibility of abuse or maltreatment. Educators should keep in mind that some of these indicators can be present in families where there is no abuse or neglect (as in the case of learning disabilities), but where there might be other problems that require attention.

Children with disabilities are often at greater risk for being maltreated and neglected by their caregivers. The teacher has to be particularly sensitive to the special needs of these children.

A student's physical and behavioral indicators in the school setting is often the basis for a teacher's suspicion of abuse or neglect. Some characteristics and behaviors of abusive and neglectful parents also can contribute to the educator's assessment of a potentially abusive or neglectful situation. Adults with a greater potential for abuse are often immature, have a history of maltreatment or neglect, are alcohol or substance abusers, are unskilled as parents, and have few coping skills. A parent's lack of knowledge of child development can result in inappropriate expectations, impulsiveness, inadequate care, and excessive punishment. If teachers are sensitive to and aware of these clues, they will be better equipped to identify abused children.

Reporting Child Abuse and Neglect

Data from the National Committee for the Prevention of Child Abuse indicate more than 3.1 million reports of child abuse and **neglect** in the United States annually.[6] A Carnegie Foundation survey of 22,000 teachers found that almost 90 percent recognized the problem of child abuse in their students. In a survey conducted by the National Center on Child Abuse Prevention Research, 74 percent of a sample of teachers indicated that they had suspected a child of being abused or neglected at one time or another.[7] Therefore, teachers should be sensitive to the statistical likelihood of having at least one abused or neglected child in their classroom.

Teachers' Reporting of Child Abuse

Since the early 1970s, all 50 states have enacted legislation that requires certain professionals to report suspected child abuse and neglect to their state hotlines. Although the legislation differs from state to state, as do mandated reporters (individuals required by law to report abuse), all states require teachers and school officials to report abuse and neglect. Most professionals who come into regular contact with children are considered mandated reporters. In about 20 states, under the law, everyone is considered a mandated reporter.[8]

Educators account for the greatest percentage of abuse reports from mandated sources. This is not surprising, given that teachers come in contact with children regularly, 5 days a week. Teachers are keen observers of children's physical state, behavior, and academic performance. They need to be educated in child development and aware of the range of developmentally appropriate behaviors. Teachers are often the first to notice both the imperceptible and the dramatic changes in a child's demeanor. Particularly in the elementary school setting, the child perceives the teacher as a confidant, a trusted adult, a person who cares, and therefore is receptive to both direct and indirect disclosures of abuse.

Perhaps more powerful than the legal requirement or mandate to report suspected child abuse is a teacher's strong commitment to the well-being of his or her students. This moral, ethical, and personal sense of obligation to report is often the underlying reason for a teacher's persistence and tenacity in seeking help for a child.

The state mandate to report is so strong that failure to report suspected child abuse and neglect, in violation of state law, can result in a misdemeanor, a jail sentence, or a civil suit. Furthermore, it is assumed that mandated reporters are reporting in good faith and, therefore, are immune from liability.[9]

What to Report

State legislation requires that when a mandated reporter has reasonable cause to suspect child abuse or neglect, it should be reported to the state's central register or child abuse hotline. Reasonable cause to suspect is based on suspicion of abuse and can be the result of a direct disclosure, physical evidence, or a cluster of indicators that suggest the possibility that abuse has occurred. The role of the mandated reporter is not to prove the abuse but, rather, to identify and report suspicion of abuse. Proving that abuse or neglect has occurred is the responsibility of child protective services and professionals whose role it is to investigate the reports.

The child abuse hotline receives reports of abuse 24 hours a day, 7 days a week. Some states (for example, New York) have a "mandated reporter's hotline" specifically established to facilitate calls from mandated reporters. In some jurisdictions, submission of a written report by the mandated reporter is required following an oral report of suspected abuse.

School Policy on Reporting Child Abuse

Enactment of policies and guidelines pertaining to the identification and reporting of child abuse within the school setting has become much more widespread in recent years. Policies usually support state laws and regulations.[10] These policies define the protocol for reporting and identify key support personnel within the district. They establish guidelines and inform the staff about legal requirements and procedures. In some states the law permits schools and other institutions to notify a primary administrator, or his or her designated agent, who then assumes the responsibility for making reports to a hotline. The designated reporter facilitates the reporting of suspected cases and also expedites the handling of these cases. Some schools have established teams to review these reports and provide follow-up or assistance to the classroom teacher.

Some jurisdictions require annual in-service programs on school policy and the identification and reporting of child abuse. The annual review of school policy by the faculty can be quite helpful in reminding educators of the legal responsibility for reporting, the role of the school in preventing child abuse, and the support that community resources can provide by working with the school district. A comprehensive school policy that is updated periodically and reflects current child abuse legislation and community resources is an important tool for educators in carrying out their mandate to report suspected child abuse and neglect.

Following a Report of Child Abuse

Although the school's legal obligation might be fulfilled by merely filing the necessary reports, the teacher can be of invaluable assistance to professionals responsible for the investigation. Providing information on academic and behavioral observations of the child, interactions between parent and child, and other relevant information can be of critical importance in assessing the allegation of abuse or neglect. After the report is made, the classroom teacher can be an advocate for the child, ensuring that the child receives support and concern, providing input in remedial services, and helping the child through this potentially difficult period.

What Teachers Can Do About Child Abuse

Elementary school personnel can take a leading role in identifying, reporting, and preventing child abuse. Some states require child abuse prevention programs; others require sexual-abuse prevention, child abduction prevention, or child safety programs.

Who are appropriate teachers of this type of material? What should the content be? In what format should programs be administered, and for how long? Many curricula are available. Prior to implementation of either a curriculum or lessons addressing child abuse and neglect, the teacher should understand the scope of the problem, how it may appear in a classroom setting, reporting procedures, and handling disclosure. The teacher also should be aware of the guiding principles or concepts behind programs that address child abuse or personal safety (see also Chapter 14).

The first step is to understand what constitutes abuse and neglect. By learning to recognize and identify abuse, the teacher is able to initiate a process that can protect a child from further harm. The teacher can become an advocate for the child, providing support and guidance to the child as well as his or her family.

Once abuse or neglect has been identified, the next step for the teacher is to understand his or her role and the role of other school personnel. What state laws pertain to reporting abuse? What are the most effective and appropriate means for intervention in suspected cases of abuse and neglect? Does the school have a specific policy on reporting suspected cases? Does the school have a child abuse or child study team that assumes responsibility for handling these cases and adopting a plan for intervention? What programs are in place within the district (special education or parent education, for example) that address the needs of at-risk families or families in which abuse has been identified? The classroom teacher should attempt to get the answers to these questions.

The key to prevention is education. Research indicates that prevention programs do work, that children can be taught important safety skills to prevent abuse, and they can become empowered to protect themselves. After having been exposed to a comprehensive victimization prevention program, victimized and threatened children were more likely to use recommended self-protection strategies, perceived themselves to be safer, and were more likely to disclose the incident to someone.[11]

Child abuse and neglect cuts across all socioeconomic, ethnic, racial, and religious lines, and parenting styles differ from culture to culture. Any program, audiovisual aid, or classroom exercise should be culturally sensitive and respect inherent differences among students.

Finally, teachers need to develop a degree of comfort with the materials they use so children will feel comfortable to disclose abuse. Attitudes about abuse, preconceived notions about parenting and sexuality, and their own past histories shape teachers' response or ability to respond to a child's direct or indirect disclosure of abuse. A sensitive, appropriate response to a child's disclosure can have a positive effect on a child and reinforce the feeling that he or she did the right thing by telling. In contrast, a response of disbelief or panic might make children feel ashamed, that they are to blame for the abuse, or might even encourage them to recant the disclosure.

Child Abuse Prevention Programs

Recognizing and reporting child abuse is the first step in ensuring that children are protected and safe. Elementary-school teachers are in a unique position to help prevent child abuse by offering child abuse prevention programs in their classrooms. These should include some basic personal safety concepts that underlie most abuse prevention programs in grades K–6. The following are ten basic concepts of personal safety instruction:

1. Touch is a part of children's daily life. Everyone needs to be touched. It makes people feel good about themselves. It makes them feel loved and wanted. Touch is a part of good health, along with good nutrition, exercising, and taking care of themselves.
2. There are different kinds of touch. Most touch makes us feel good and safe. Some touch makes us feel bad. It might hurt and make us feel unsafe. Some touch can be confusing. If a child is touched in a way that he or she does not like or does not understand or makes him or her uncomfortable, the child should speak to a trusted adult.
3. Some parts of the body are private. Children need to know that they have a right to privacy and a right to say "no" to anyone who wants to touch the private parts of their body unless it is for health reasons.
4. Children should trust their feelings. If something doesn't feel right, if they feel that they are being tricked, forced, or manipulated into a situation that feels wrong or dangerous, they can say "no" and speak to a trusted adult about it.
5. Children have the right to say "no" to touch they do not like. They can say "no" in many ways, both verbally and with body language. Children need to practice saying "no."
6. Sometimes children are in situations where they can't say "no." Children are never to blame for abuse, however, nor should they ever feel responsible if they are unable to stop or prevent the abuse from occurring.
7. Sometimes children need to tell several people before something is done. Adults may not respond to their pleas for help, or they may not want to believe the abuse is occurring. Children need to keep telling until someone believes them.
8. Children can go to many trusted adults for help. Children need to be able to identify the family members, friends, and professionals who could be of assistance to them.
9. Children need not feel they are alone. Child abuse and neglect is a widespread problem. Children need to know they are not the only ones who have been abused.
10. Help is available for abusive families and abused children. Many professionals, agencies, and organizations work with abused children and their families. Many community resources are able to intervene in the cycle of abuse and treat families.

Although the concepts are universal for all elementary schoolchildren, the depth and manner in which they are taught differ according to grade and developmental level.

Over the past 15 years, materials addressing the issue of child abuse have proliferated from coloring books and pamphlets to videos and curricula. Some of the materials are of a general nature and cover a broad range of safety topics; others are more specific and cover one facet of personal safety, such as child abuse prevention.

These materials vary widely in quality. Some have not been developed using currently accepted research. Some of the materials might not be suitable for certain age groups. Therefore, all material should be previewed prior to use in the classroom, with particular attention to developmental appropriateness for a given grade and age level.

Prevention messages should be simple but concrete and suitable for that age. The curricula selected for implementation should offer ample opportunity for students to role-play and participate in class discussion. Children need to learn skills they can practice to keep themselves safe and prevent abuse. Rehearsal, repetition, and reinforcement are important to the success of any program.

A comprehensive curriculum can be developed by the health teacher, nurse, school counselor, social worker, and any trained specialist in prevention education, in association with classroom teachers. The latter are in a unique position to go beyond a fixed curriculum. They can integrate lessons throughout the year in all components of a child's education, reinforcing basic concepts and giving students the tools to protect themselves. The Learning Experiences at the end of this chapter indicate how safety concepts can be incorporated into language arts, social studies, and science lessons.

Summary

Child abuse and neglect are problems that children bring to the classroom. As mandated reporters in all states, teachers need to be alert to the signs and indicators of the various forms of abuse, as well as the laws and school policy on reporting suspected abuse. Neglect is the most common of these forms and may be easiest to observe, as it often is manifested in children's appearance, hygiene, and signs of hunger. Physical abuse also leaves the child with behavioral and physical indicators, often covered by clothing inappropriate for the season. Sexual abuse is more difficult to identify, as it leaves no obvious physical damage and the child usually tries to keep it a secret. Nevertheless, a constellation of indicators, including shrinking from adult touch and fear of certain situations and places, are clues for closer observation.

Emotional maltreatment is the most damaging aspect of all forms of abuse. It erodes the child's sense of worth and esteem and can make a child constantly anxious, depressed, withdrawn, or fearful. The teacher can institute a variety of activities, using available resources, to be an advocate for the child.

Education focusing on prevention is an important component of the school curriculum. A wider support system in the community is a valuable resource of which teachers and students alike should be aware. Many printed and video products are available. These should be reviewed carefully for developmental appropriateness and in the specific context of the child's culture and community.

Web Sites

American Humane Association
www.americanhumane.org
National organization involved in identifying and preventing the causes of child abuse and animal abuse and neglect.

Childhelp USA
www.childhelpusa.org
National child abuse hotline, dedicated to prevention and treatment of child abuse and neglect.

National Center for Child Abuse and Neglect
www.calib.com/nccanch
National resource for professionals seeking information on child abuse and neglect and child welfare.

National Center for Missing and Exploited Children (NCMEC)
www.missingkids.com
National resource center for child protection, child safety, and missing children.

National Clearinghouse on Child Abuse and Neglect Information
330 C Street SW
Washington, DC 20447
800-384-3366
www.calib.com/cbexpress

Prevent Child Abuse America
www.preventchildabuse.org
National organization dedicated to the prevention of child abuse.

Resources

Examples of Comprehensive Child Safety Curricula

Kids and Company: Together for Safety

A personal safety curriculum for grades K–6, providing children with skills, information, self-confidence, and support that will enhance their self-esteem and help prevent abduction and abuse. This multimedia curriculum provides engaging activities, puzzles, songs, and games, as well as video-based role-playing. Available through the Adam Walsh Children's Fund, 407-775-7191.

No-Go-Tell: Child Protection Curriculum for Very Young Disabled Children

A personal safety curriculum designed to facilitate the understanding of concepts of sexual abuse as concretely as possible for very young children.

Safe and Okay: A No-Go-Tell Curriculum for Disabled Children (grades 3–6).

Available from James Standifeld & Co., 800-421-6534.

The Safe Child Program

A child abuse prevention curriculum for grades K–3 that teaches prevention of sexual, emotional, and physical abuse, prevention of child abduction, and safety. This multimedia curriculum introduces concepts and demonstrates skills through videotaped modeling and role-play in age-appropriate segments. Available from Coalition for Children, PO Box 6304, Denver, CO 80206, 800-320-1717.

Second Step: A Violence Prevention Curriculum

A multimedia violence prevention curriculum that includes large photographs with discussion questions in the areas of empathy training, impulse control, and anger management. Video accompanies lessons. Lessons and concepts are individualized for grades 1–3, 4–5, 6–8. Available through The Committee for Children, 2203 Airport Way South, Suite 500, Seattle, WA 98134, 800-634-4449.

Talking About Touching: A Personal Safety Curriculum

A child sexual abuse prevention program with physical abuse and neglect supplement. Photographs and stories serve as the basis for classroom discussion about decision making and personal safety. Individualized for grades 1–3, 4–5, 6–8. Available through The Committee for Children, 2203 Airport Way South, Suite 500, Seattle, WA 98134, 800-634-4449.

Videos for Children, K–6

The following videotapes are a sampling of materials in child abuse prevention, child assault prevention, child abduction prevention, anger management, and violence prevention. All videotapes should be previewed prior to showing to determine suitability for the audience.

All About Anger

Teaches basic, easily comprehensible concepts about anger, along with some simple techniques to help youngsters deal with their anger in an appropriate manner. 15 minutes; elementary; available through Sunburst Communications, 800-831-1934.

Anger: Handle with Care

Uses dramatic vignettes to show children how to handle their anger. 12 minutes; upper elementary; available from Barr Films, 818-338-7878.

Being Safe

A series of videotapes designed to support a developmental elementary school curriculum in child-abuse prevention. Aims to create a sense of self-worth in children. Three videos; 20 minutes each; K–6; available from Altschul Group Corp., 800-421-2363.

Believe Me

Teaches the difference between good and bad touch. 21 minutes; elementary; Coronet/MTI, 800-255-0208.

Better Safe Than Sorry

Deals with stranger awareness, stressing good judgment as different situations are presented and viewers are challenged to handle the problems. 15 minutes; elementary; Altschul Group Corp., 800-421-2363.

Better Safe Than Sorry II

Three simple rules that can help children prevent or deal with potential sexual abuse: Say No, Get Away, Tell Someone. 14½ minutes; primary; available from Altschul Group Corp., 800-421-2363.

Better Safe Than Sorry (second edition)

Sexual abuse prevention in situations where the offender is known to the child. 16 minutes; upper elementary, available from Altschul Group Corp., 800-421-2363.

Break the Silence: Kids Against Child Abuse

Profiles four courageous children who have survived child abuse. Unique combination of live interviews and animation; 30 minutes; grades 3–6; available from Aims Multimedia, 800-367-2467.

Bully No More: Stopping the Abuse

Strategies for dealing with bullying. 20 minutes, grades 4–6, Aims Multimedia, 800-367-2467.

Child Sexual Abuse: A Solution

Offers a solution to sexual abuse by giving the message that your body belongs to you and you can control who touches it, using concrete examples of sexual molestation and abuse. Six segments, 10–15 minutes each; grades K–1, 2–4, 5–6, Parents/Teachers; available from James Standifeld & Co., 800-421-6534.

Emotional Abuse: How to Cope

Three stories portray different types of emotional abuse and the ways in which each child learned how to handle the situation. 26 minutes; upper elementary; available from Altschul Group Corp., 800-421-2363.

It Happened to Me

Developed for boys 6–9 years old, designed to educate them about sexual abuse prevention. 15 minutes; available from Boy Scouts of America, 972-580-2295.

John Walsh: Talk It Out With Adults You Trust

Talking and listening to an adult when a child needs advice, as part of a safety plan for children. 20 minutes; elementary; available from Coronet/MTI, 800-255-0208.

Nobody's Home

The story of a young mother intent only on her needs and a young boy who feels responsible for what happens to his family; one of the few videos that focuses on neglect. 20 minutes; upper elementary; available from Altschul Group Corp., 800-421-2363.

Solving Conflicts

Using role-play and real situations in the video, 11-year-old students search for better ways to handle conflict. 18 minutes; upper elementary; available from Churchill Films, 213-657-5110.

Spider-Man: Don't Hide Abuse

Spider-Man helps a young girl solve her problem of how to disclose her father's physical abuse. 11 minutes; elementary; available from Coronet/MTI, 800-777-2400.

Two Kinds of Touch

Young children learn the difference between "good touching" and "bad touching" and about their right to say "no." 14 minutes; primary; available from Altschul Group Corp., 800-421-2363.

What Hurts: Emotional Abuse

Two classmates, victims of emotional abuse, come to the attention of their teacher. The children's response provides a model for discussion. 15 minutes; elementary; available from Altschul Group Corp., 800-421-2363.

What Tadoo

A combination of original music, live action, and clever puppetry teach fundamental rules to protect young children from hurt and danger. 18 minutes; primary; available from MTITeleprograms, 800-777-2400.

Who Do You Tell?

Young children are encouraged to bring their problems and concerns out into the open and to identify and make use of support systems available to them. 11 minutes, primary; available from Coronet/MTI, 800-777-2400.

Yes You Can Say No

One boy's success in stopping his sexual victimization. Demonstrates assertiveness skills for personal safety. 20 minutes; grades 2–6; available from AIMS Media, 800-367-2467.

Notes

1. D. Koralek, *Caregivers of Young Children: Preventing and Responding to Child Maltreatment* (McLean, VA: The Circle, 1995).
2. E. Goldson, "The Affective and Cognitive Sequelae of Child Maltreatment," *Pediatric Clinics of North America* 38 (1991): 1481–1496.
3. See note 2.
4. D. Finkelhor, N. Asdigian, and J. Dziuba-Leatherman, "The Effectiveness of Victimization Prevention Instruction: An Evaluation of Children's Responses to Actual Threats and Assault," *Child Abuse and Neglect* 19 (1995): 141–153.
5. J. Gabarino and A. C. Gabarino, *Emotional Maltreatment of Children* (Chicago: National Committee for the Prevention of Child Abuse, 1987).
6. C. T. Wang and D. Daro, *Current Trends in Child Abuse Reporting and Fatalities: The Results of the 1997 Annual Fifty State Survey* (Chicago: National Center on Child Abuse Prevention Research, 1998).
7. N. Abrahams, K. Casey, and D. Daro, "Teacher's Knowledge, Attitudes, and Beliefs about Child Abuse and Its Prevention," *Child Abuse and Neglect* 16 (1990): 229–238.
8. C. Tower, *Understanding Child Abuse and Neglect*, 4th ed. (Needham, MA: Allyn and Bacon, 1999).
9. D. Besharov, *Recognizing Child Abuse* (New York: Free Press, 1990).
10. C. Tower, *The Role of Educators in the Prevention and Treatment of Child Abuse and Neglect* (McLean, VA: The Circle, 1992).
11. See note 4.

Learning Experiences

The following, by grade level, outlines child abuse and neglect concepts for furthering children's safety:

Grades K–2

As children in grades K–2 progress from their limited view of the world through their family to learning more about the neighborhood and community, this is an ideal time to introduce the concept of personal safety to them. Children at this age are moving from fantasy thinking to more concrete thinking. Therefore, they need concrete examples that leave little to their imaginations.

Many excellent videos can be used with this age group. Also at this age, personal safety can be introduced as one form of the broader area of safety that includes fire and bike safety (see also Chapter 14). Activities that incorporate art, music, dance, and creative expression will help to reinforce the concepts. Encouraging young children to express themselves verbally, practice "telling," and to identify and label their emotions will enhance learning.

Lessons should not be too long, and information should be simple and basic. Imagination should not be allowed to run wild, and the lessons should not incite unnecessary fear of strangers. After being exposed to lessons on child abuse and safety, the students should be able to

1. Say how their bodies belong to them.
2. Name the different kinds of touch (good, bad, confusing).
3. Use the strategy Say no! Get away! Tell someone!
4. Identify adults they can ask for help with an abuse problem.

Grades 3–4

At this level, children can handle more freedom and independence. They are often involved with many activities beyond school. Their sense of neighborhood is expanding, and their exposure to adults has increased. Children at this age spend as much time as possible in the company of peers. They are concerned with rules, what is fair and just. Their verbal and written skills are becoming more sophisticated. Activities should include ample opportunity for students to work cooperatively with their peers. Role-play and rehearsal of assertive strategies will enhance learning and empower students to feel that they are in control. Prevention content should include some discussion of bullies. Cooperative and collaborative activities will enrich learning of concepts at this age. After exploring their world further, they should be able to

1. Identify adults who are part of their personal support system.
2. List people within the school setting who are available to assist them with problems.
3. Practice telling someone when they have a problem.
4. Identify safe and unsafe touch.
5. Practice "Say no, Get away, Tell someone" responses.
6. Discuss rules for personal safety with their family.

Grades 5–6

Children at this level are becoming more and more independent. Their neighborhood continues to expand, and they venture farther and farther away from home. Their contacts with adults expand as well, with parents reluctantly relinquishing control and supervision.

At this age, children may be left home alone for longer periods. They are much more aware of current events and are influenced greatly by peers and the media. As these children are gaining control over their lives, they need to have skills that can keep them safe and secure. They often feel conflicting impulses—wanting to affect bravado and independence but simultaneously feeling inner fearfulness of certain situations. Because of the reluctance on the part of boys, particularly, to disclose when they are being abused, children should understand clearly that abuse happens to both girls and boys. Boys, too, should be encouraged to speak to an adult about abuse problems. After lessons about abuse, the students should be able to

1. Describe potentially dangerous situations and know how to respond to them.
2. Trust their instincts and report danger signals.
3. Identify professionals who know how to handle specific types of problems.
4. Describe the basic needs of all individuals (versus neglect).
5. Say "no" to touch and situations that do not feel right, get away from dangerous situations or situations that feel uncomfortable, and tell someone.
6. Keep on telling until they are believed.
7. Help a friend tell an adult if he or she is being abused.

For suggestions on creating a rubric with which to evaluate student performance of Learning Experiences, see page 13.

Learning Experience 11-1

People I Can Tell

Grade Level

K–2

Primary Discipline

Social Studies

Learning Objectives

Following this activity, students will be able to

- Define what a support person is.
- Identify important adults in their support system.
- Describe situations when they should tell one of these adults about a problem.
- Tell an adult when they have a problem.

Time Required

30 minutes

Materials

Construction paper, paste, scissors, magazine pictures of adults

Description of Activity

Have students create a book of pictures of important people in their life. They will include family members, relatives, and people in their school community and neighborhood. They will point out adults who can help them if they are afraid of someone.

Homework

Children look through magazines and bring pictures to class of adults including doctors, nurses, police officers, and so on.

Evaluation

Students can identify adults who will form their support system. You might develop a rubric with the following criteria to assess students' performance:

A: The student will define a support system and will identify at least one adult each in the family, the school, and the community (total of three adults) and will be able to articulate what a problem is and who to go to. They will create the book.

B: The student will identify at least two adults (one in the home, one in the school/ community) and will create the book.

C: The students will identify one adult and will hand in a paper with cutouts.

D: The student did not complete the assignment.

Learning Experience 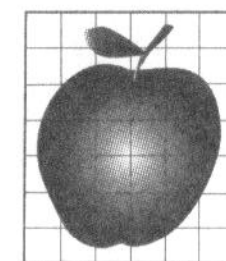 11-2

Important People Puppet Show

Grade Level

1–2

Primary Discipline

Social Studies, Creative Arts

Learning Objectives

Following this activity, students will be able to

- Define a support system
- Identify important adults in their support system.
- Describe situations in which an adult should be told about a problem.
- Tell an adult when they have a problem.

Time Required

Two lessons, 30 minutes each

Materials

Sticks, cardboard, pictures from magazines of adults who can help (parents, grandparents, neighbors, doctors, nurses, teachers, firefighters, police, crossing guards, child-care workers, and so on)

Description of Activity

Introduction

Define a support system. Have students identify adults in helping professions who can be a part of their support system.

Activity

Have students make puppets of these important adults using magazine pictures mounted on cardboard and attached to sticks to hold them up. Once each student has his/her own puppet, ask each student to either (a) explain who the person is and how he/she can help children, or (b) participate in a play in which different members of the support system help a child. Give students the opportunity to practice telling the puppet about a problem.

Homework

Students cut pictures from magazines in preparation for this activity.

Evaluation

Students can identify adults in helping professions who are a part of their support system. The teacher might develop a rubric with the following criteria to assess students' performance:

A: The student will define a support system, identify a minimum of four adults in the support system, create stick puppets, and actively participate in the explanation and/or play.

B: The students will define a support system, identify a minimum of three adults in the support system, create stick puppets, and actively participate in the explanation and/or play.

C: The students will not be able to define a support system, will identify only one adult who can help with a problem, will create stick puppets, but will not participate in the explanation and/or play.

D: The student did not complete the assignment.

Learning Experience 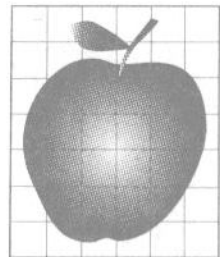 11-3

My VIP Phone Book

Grade Level

3–4

Primary Discipline

Social Studies

Learning Objectives

Following this activity, students will be able to

- Define a support system.
- Identify important adults in their support system.
- Describe situations in which an adult should be told about a problem.
- Tell an adult when they have a problem.

Time Required

30 minutes

Materials

Lined paper, construction paper, stapler, scissors

Description of Activity

Introduction

Define a support system.

Activity

Students will make a list of important adults in their life (parents, grandparents, doctor, teacher, relatives, and so on). Then, introduce different professions and have students define their roles. Have students alphabetize the list (either by name or by profession) and include their phone number. Have students create a small book to write the names in.

Homework

Once students have a complete list of names, they will have to get phone numbers (and addresses) at home. This project will involve parents.

Evaluation

The teacher might develop a rubric with the following criteria to assess students' performance:

A: The student will define a support system and define roles, identify four adults to be included in their phone list, alphabetize list correctly, and complete assignment accurately and neatly.

B: The student will define a support system and identify two adults to be included in their phone list, but have difficulty alphabetizing list. Student will complete assignment.

C: The students will be able to identify helping adults, but will not be able to define their roles. Student will have difficulty alphabetizing list but will complete assignment.

D: The student did not complete the assignment.

Learning Experience 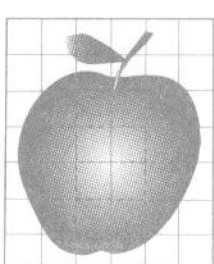 11-4

My Handy Phone Card

Grade Level

3–4

Primary Discipline

Social Studies

Learning Objectives

Following this activity, students will be able to

- Develop a list of helping professionals.
- Identify their own personal safety support system.
- Describe the importance of telling an adult about a problem.
- List school personnel who work with children (guidance counselor, social worker, psychologist, school nurse).

Time Required

30 minutes

Materials

Colored cardstock, string (or hook-and-loop fasteners), lamination supplies (if possible)

Description of Activity

Have students brainstorm a list of adults who can help children in all aspects of their lives. Each type of professional and service will be defined. Have students create their own safety support card to hang on their door, bulletin board, or other handy place. Names and phone numbers will include parent's office, doctor's office, school, police, fire department. A hole is punched at the top, and the string affixed. If possible, the card is laminated.

This project would be enhanced by inviting relevant school personnel into the classroom to introduce themselves and explain to the class their function in the school.

Homework

Students will identify adults who would be important sources of help and get their phone numbers. This is an ideal opportunity to engage parents in this activity.

Evaluation

The teacher might develop a rubric with the following criteria to assess students' performance:

A: The student will develop a list of a minimum of six professionals, define their specific roles, and complete assignment accurately and neatly.

B: The student will develop a list of four professionals, define their specific roles, and complete the assignment.

C: The student will develop a list of three professionals and define their roles, but finished product will be incomplete and inaccurate.

D: The student did not complete the assignment.

Learning Experience 11-5

Helpful Community People

Grade Level

5–6

Primary Disciplines

Language Arts, Social Studies

Learning Objectives

Following this activity, students will be able to

- Develop a list of support services in the community that help children.
- Define the roles that individuals play in protecting children.
- Report to classmates about a selected profession.
- Identify potential problems and professionals who would be appropriate to handle them.

Time Required

30 minutes

Materials

None

Description of Activity

Have students develop a list of helping professions and agencies in their community. Assign each student to write a letter to an agency or professional requesting information on the services provided. After the information arrives, have students report to the class. If time does not permit oral presentations, a class book or folder can be created.

Homework

Letters can be written in class or as a homework assignment.

Evaluation

Letter could be used as evaluation, or students could be asked to define or describe each of the professionals/support services listed by the class. You might develop a rubric with the following criteria to assess students' performance:

A: The student will develop a list of a minimum of five support services in the community that work with children, define their roles, and write a grammatically correct business letter to one organization or individual.

B: The student will develop a list of a minimum of three support services in the community that work with children, define their roles, and write a letter with few grammar/spelling errors.

C: The student will develop a list of a minimum of three support services in the community that work with children and define their roles, but will be unable to write an appropriate letter to an organization.

D: The student did not complete the assignment.

Resource: Child Abuse Prevention Services, PO Box 176, Roslyn, NY 11576.

Learning Experience 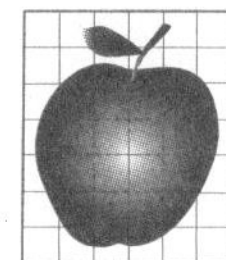 11-6

Class Book About Feeling Good

Grade Level

K–2

Primary Discipline

Language Arts

Learning Objectives

Following this activity, students will be able to

- Identify different types of safe touch.
- Identify the feeling and emotion associated with good touch.
- List words that make them feel good and label emotions associated with safe, unsafe, and confusing touch.
- Talk about their feelings.

Time Required

30 minutes

Materials

Magazines, glue, scissors

Description of Activity

Introduce concept of good/safe touch and emotions and words associated with safe/good touch. Have students cut out pictures of good touch, things that make them feel good, and words that make them feel good (happy, love, like, kiss, hug, and similar words). In class, have each student make a collage of his/her cutouts. Pages will be put together to create a book for the class or a large collage for the bulletin board. Continue the class discussion of unsafe/bad touch—touch that does not feel good. Help students identify and label actions and emotions.

Homework

Pictures can be cut out at home. (Parents can become involved in this activity.)

Evaluation

The teacher might develop a rubric with the following criteria to assess students' performance:

A: The student will be able to identify four different types of safe touch (such as handshake, holding hands, and hugs or kisses from appropriate people) and words that make them feel good. Student will cut out at least four pictures.

B: The student will be able to identify three different types of safe touch and words that make him/her feel good. Student will cut out at least three pictures.

C: The students will be able to identify two different types of safe touch and words that make him/her feel good. Student will bring in two pictures.

D: The student did not complete the assignment.

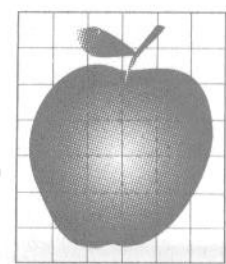

Learning Experience 11-7

Rewriting Fairy Tales

Grade Level

3–4

Primary Discipline

Language Arts

Learning Objectives

Following this activity, students will be able to

- Identify abusive and unsafe situations.
- Formulate plans to make them safe.
- Describe how to help a friend when he or she is in an unsafe or abusive situation.
- Say no! Get away! Tell someone!

Time Required

30 minutes

Materials

Grimm's fairy tales (specifically *Hansel and Gretel*, *Red Riding Hood*, and *Rapunzel*)

Description of Activity

Define the four forms of abuse: physical, sexual, emotional, and neglect. Have each student read one fairy tale that depicts abuse.

Afterward, have the class discuss the fairy tales and the types of abuse depicted. Ask students what they would do in similar situations, whom they would tell, and what measures could have been taken to protect the children from abuse.

Have students rewrite each fairy tale, eliminating the abuse and making the children safe.

Homework

Children read the fairy tale at home. They also could review old nursery rhymes to assess the different forms of abuse.

Evaluation

The teacher might develop a rubric with the following criteria to assess students' performance:

A: Student will define the four forms of abuse, read one fairy tale, and rewrite one fairy tale with an appropriate new ending. Fairy tale will be grammatically correct.

B: Student will define the four forms of abuse, read one fairy tale, and rewrite one fairy tale with a new ending. The assignment will have some grammatical/spelling errors.

C: Students will identify two forms of abuse and read one fairy tale, but will be unable to rewrite the story.

D: Student did not complete the assignment.

Learning Experience 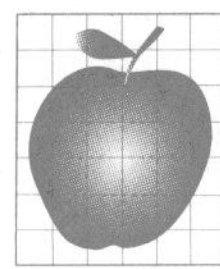 11-8

Writing an Advice Column

Grade Level

5–6

Primary Discipline

Language Arts

Learning Objectives

Following this activity, students will be able to

- Identify situations that might be unsafe.
- Describe the situation and problem-solve what to do.
- Say no! Get away! Tell someone!
- Help a friend.

Time Required

20 minutes

Materials

Paper, pens, index cards

Description of Activity

Introduction

Present several safety issues for discussion either by showing a video (such as *Better Safe Than Sorry*) or by initiating a class discussion. Suggested topics include bullies, talking to strangers, accepting a ride from strangers, and not following family safety rules.

Activity

Have students cut out applicable copies of Ann Landers or Dear Abby columns from the newspaper, then have students write a letter to Dear Abby on an index card, using one of the safety issues. Each student then will get an index card from another student to write a response to the question. The letters can be "published" in a class newspaper or be used for class discussion of the responses.

Homework

Students can cut out copies of advice columns to bring to class and to use as a sample. Letters can be written at home or in class.

Evaluation

The teacher might develop a rubric with the following criteria to assess students' performance:

A: Student will identify a minimum of four situations that might be unsafe, write a "Dear Abby" letter, and write a grammatically correct, appropriate response.

B: Student will identify a minimum of three situations that might be unsafe, write a "Dear Abby" letter, and write an appropriate response. There will be few grammatical/spelling errors.

C: Student will identify two situations that might be unsafe and write a short "Dear Abby" letter and response. Writing will include many errors.

D: Student did not complete the assignment.

Resource: *Better Safe Than Sorry* video is available from Altschul Group Corp., 800-421-2363.

Learning Experience 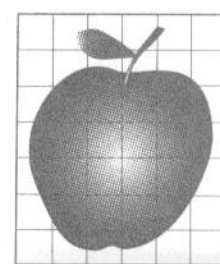 11-9

Children's Bill of Rights

Grade Level

5–6

Primary Discipline

Social Studies

Learning Objectives

Following this activity, students will be able to

- Define basic needs of all individuals and the specific needs of children.
- Describe the responsibilities of parents.
- Describe what happens when needs are not met.
- List children's rights and responsibilities.

Time Required

30 minutes

Materials

Copies of the Bill of Rights to U.S. Constitution, butcher paper (or other parchment-like paper) and pencils (or chalkboard)

Description of Activity

This activity can be a cooperative effort with "Children's Bill of Rights" written on the chalkboard, compiled by the students, or an independent writing assignment. First, have students read the Bill of Rights and discuss it in class. Ask them to brainstorm the specific needs of children. Discussion should include issues of cultural differences and special needs. If you have each child write his/her own "Children's Bill of Rights," it can be done on parchment paper.

Homework

Before the activity, students can read the Bill of Rights at home.

Evaluation

The teacher might develop a rubric with the following criteria to assess students' performance:

A: Student will read Bill of Rights, actively participate in classroom discussion, and prepare a thoughtful, well-written Children's Bill of Rights with a minimum of eight items.

B: Student will read Bill of Rights, participate in classroom discussion, and prepare a Children's Bill of Rights with a minimum of six items.

C: Students will read Bill of Rights and prepare a Children's Bill of Rights with a minimum of four items.

D: Student did not complete the assignment.

12

Children's Experience with Loss, Dying, and Death

Carole Smitten and Jane Colgan

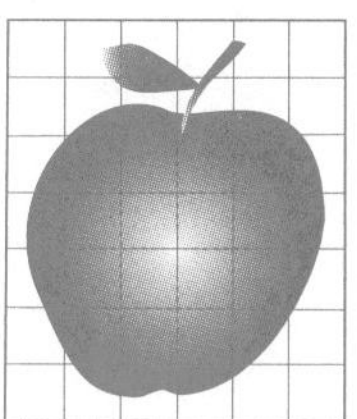

Chapter Outline

Losses in Childhood
Dying
Those Left Behind
Special Cases
The Aftermath of Death
Classroom Responses to Death
Spiritual Aspects
Understanding Children's Grief

Objectives

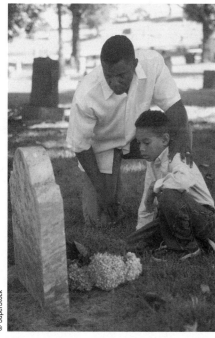

- Explain the types of losses and define grief, bereavement, and mourning
- List some typical losses during childhood: divorce of parents, loss of a grandparent, and death of a pet
- Identify the five stages of dying
- Describe how children perceive death by developmental level
- Identify some grieving behaviors in children
- Explain what magical thinking is and what the teacher's response should be
- Discuss the particular aspects of suicide and signs of suicidal ideation
- Define and explain near-death experience
- Discuss how to deal with a death in the school
- Describe the spiritual aspect of dying and death
- Discuss the aftermath of death: wakes, funerals, and other rituals that have developed to cope with death
- Present some ideas for dealing sensitively with a child who returns to school after the death of an important person in his or her life.

Danny's mom had been sick for a long time. Once last year when she was in the hospital, Danny had to leave school and go to live with his grandmother in another state. Danny has been sad since he came home. He and his mom recently moved in with his Aunt Alice. Back in school, he told the class that different nurses have been living with them. Last week, when Danny didn't come to school at all, the children in the class asked the teacher if he went to his grandmother's place again. She told them that Danny's mom had died. The children in Danny's class wrote special sympathy cards to Danny and told him how much they missed him and hoped he would come back to school soon. All of the children felt sad and didn't know what they would say to Danny when he came back.

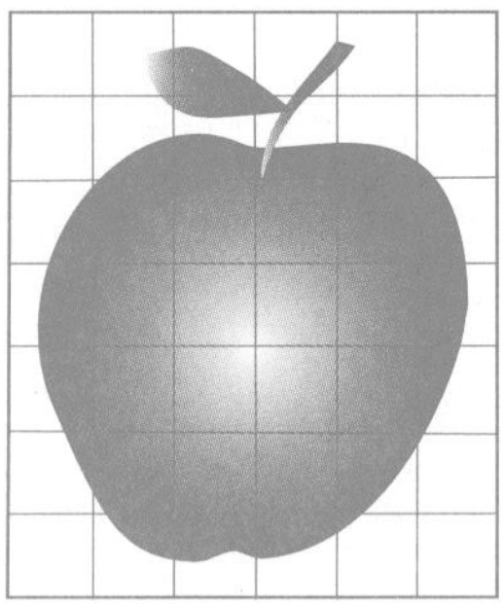

Should you shield the canyons from the windstorms, you would never see the beauty of their carvings.[1]

What are the concerns of children who have experienced a death of a friend's parent such as the one in the vignette above? How vulnerable and fearful might they be feeling about their own or their parents' potential death? What kinds of cultural, religious, or ethnic experiences have they had with death? How can they approach their friends with kindness and appropriate sympathy? These are among the many concerns and questions children might bring to the classroom when death has entered their immediate environment. They require the teachers' responses to questions dealing with issues related to illness, dying, and death.

The United States has changed from a society that once embraced the concept of dying and having funerals at home to one in which deaths occur in hospitals and funeral directors orchestrate the family's mourning. Death is a topic that is "out of sight, out of mind." It is rarely discussed in the home.

A child, by age 14, will witness an estimated 18,000 deaths on TV, usually in the form of violent murders. According to Goldman, 12 percent of all childhood deaths are caused by guns in accidents, suicides, and murders. Auto accidents are the leading cause of accidental deaths of children. Drownings are second. In a school system of 6,000 students, an average of 4 students die each year, and 20 percent of today's children will have experienced the death of a parent by the end of high school.[2]

The media perpetuate myths about death by showing cartoons in which characters fall from cliffs or dive off buildings and are miraculously unharmed, even bouncing back to resume the activity. Characters in soap operas and films die only to reappear as other characters in other TV series and films. Actual deaths from war and violence are often reported in the news without mention of the associated emotional pain and grief. Those who travel the information highway, too, receive stimulating but not necessarily helpful or accurate messages about death.

Recent violent events in our nation —the Columbine massacres and the terrorist attacks on the World Trade

Center and Pentagon—brought death and bloodshed into our children's minds and into our homes. Thousands of families were thrown into unfathomable grief. Our sense of safety and security was breached in a moment. Domestic tranquility was torn from our suburban communities. Our children were witness to the horror itself *and* to our responses and reactions to these horrific events. Children learn what they experience.

Many adults, parents and teachers alike, hesitate to speak about these events for fear of scaring, scarring, or further upsetting the children. But, how often do parents or teachers take the time to discuss with children the reality or unreality of these media messages? How often do parents or teachers talk about the little deaths—the death of a leaf from a falling tree as it loses its green color and falls to the ground, or the ant rendered motionless by a simple spray from a can. These are healthy and appropriate ways to discuss death. We have allowed death to become an unreality or an enemy instead of the natural passage or the culminating life stage that it is.

All children experience losses in one form or another. Teachers can acknowledge these experiences and give their students permission to feel, to cry, to grieve. They can help to demystify loss and death so children do not feel so isolated and alone. Frequently, children believe they are going crazy and no one will understand them. Sometimes the classroom teacher is the only adult they can turn to. This is a major responsibility, and the teacher may feel inadequate to approach the task. This chapter may offer help and alleviate the anxiety of classroom teachers surrounding discussions of dying and death.

Teaching about dying and death in the schools is particularly challenging. Probably no other word strikes terror in the heart than the word "death." What exactly is it? At what moment does life end and death begin? If people believe in an afterlife, do they truly die? The more we search for an answer, the more we realize that dying and death have different meanings for each person.

Does life end when our brain or our heart stops, or when the soul leaves the body? When we think of dying and death, beliefs, values, and fears come to the fore. Teachers and their students alike will feel many emotions as they discuss loss, dying, and death as part of the life process.

Losses in Childhood

Losses fall along a continuum ranging from relatively minor to catastrophic. When experiencing loss of any kind, the person enters a state of **bereavement**. **Grief** is the emotional suffering the loss causes. Grief or **mourning** is an emotional process that progresses through stages until the bereaved become involved with life once again.

Common losses in childhood include the following:

- Parents' separation or divorce
- Loss of a grandparent
- Death of a sibling
- Death of a pet
- Unavailability of a parent emotionally
- Loss of a favorite toy or object (blanket, teddy bear, and so on)
- Loss from environmental hazard (fire, flood, hurricane, tornado)
- Moving and changing schools
- Loss of self-esteem from physical, sexual, emotional, or deprivational abuse
- Loss related to skills and abilities (being held back in school, not chosen for team sports, overweight, or injured; having illness, physical disability, dyslexia, ADHD, or developmental differences)
- Loss related to habits (cessation of thumb sucking, biting fingernails, or twirling hair; experiencing a change in eating patterns or daily routines, such as beginning or ending the school year)

The first four items are the most common of the major losses a child will experience.

Divorce of Parents

To children, a divorce is the death of their family. They mourn the loss as they would mourn a death. What makes this loss even more difficult is that they often are triangulated by two angry or bitter parents. Children may fear losing the love of one or both parents. They often blame themselves for the events leading to the divorce and feel sad. They typically engage in magical thinking about getting their parents together again.

Loss of a Grandparent

Children are often attached to their grandparents in a very special way. Grandparents frequently give unconditional love, and children respond to that. The loss or death of a grandparent may therefore be especially traumatic for children. Grandparents may move away to a warmer climate. They may become ill and possibly hospitalized or go into a nursing home. Ultimately they die. This is frequently the first significant loss for children.

When a classmate's grandparent dies, other children in the classroom sometimes fear it will happen to their grandparents. Allowing students to share their experiences of loss and death with each other will lessen the pain and, at the same time, prepare other children for the experience.

Death of a Sibling

Frequently, parents and other caring adults try to protect the surviving siblings from knowing the truth about death. Mommy's miscarriage is not discussed. Some children are never told they had a twin. If a brother or sister dies, they may not know the circumstances of the death. Yet they are aware that the family is going through something traumatic. In a way, these children suffer a double loss: the loss of the sibling and the temporary loss of their parents, who are in deep grief. Often, the children are left to suffer alone. They see Mommy and Daddy crying so hard and for so long that they may become afraid.

Frequently, children blame themselves for the death. They may have wished, during a sibling's illness, that he or she would die so the family would stop suffering or would pay more attention to the well child.

An excellent question for the teacher to ask is "What are you afraid of?" Teachers can seek out the parents to learn how they explained the death to the child and offer support to the parents as well. They can encourage the parents to plan outings with the siblings so they know they are still important and loved.

Death of a Pet

The death of a pet may be the child's first experience with death. The child should be encouraged to mourn the loss and take part in whatever rituals are appropriate to help with that process, including a funeral and burial. Some veterinarians allow family members to be present when a pet is euthanized. Children could be included in this. The family is saying goodbye to one of its members. Too often parents replace the dead pet before the children have been given the chance to mourn the loss.

Dying

Elisabeth Kübler-Ross, whose monumental work with dying patients changed how American society views dying and death, identified five stages of dying that the person goes through.[3]

Stages of Grief

1. *Denial.* When a person learns that he or she is terminally ill, the person doesn't believe it. This helps to cushion the reality of impending death.
2. *Rage and Anger.* In the next stage the person asks, "Why me?" and becomes angry at the thought of dying while others are alive and healthy. Often the person rants at God. Kübler-Ross encourages people to do this. "God can take it," she says.
3. *Bargaining.* This is the stage when the dying person says, "Yes, me, but . . ." and attempts to strike a bargain with God for more time.
4. *Depression.* In the fourth stage, the person begins to mourn past losses, things not done, wrongs committed. Often he or she engages in "preparatory grief," getting ready for the arrival of death. In this stage, the dying person may become quiet and not want to see family members. They are ready to let go.
5. *Acceptance* is not a happy stage, nor is it unhappy. The patients are simply ready to die.

Not everyone passes easily from one stage to the next, and not everyone will reach acceptance.

The Dying Child

Children who have terminal diseases have special needs. Most of the time their parents try to give them some "normalcy," and the teacher may be called upon to help with that task. Educationally, the teacher supports the child by giving him or her work to do at home or in the hospital.

Children often bravely try to make this time easier for their parents by not talking about their fear of dying. They sometimes turn to other trusted adults, including the classroom teacher. This teacher will have to know exactly what the parents have told the child about his or her disease. School personnel should help parents understand that open communication is critical. All members of the family should be involved in helping each other through this difficult time. As Kübler-Ross wrote:

> If people doubt that their children are aware of a terminal illness, they should look at the poems or drawings these children create, often during their illness but sometimes months before a diagnosis is made. . . . It needs to be understood that this is often a preconscious awareness and not a conscious, intellectual knowledge.[4]

Bluebond-Lagner, a researcher, worked with a group of terminally ill children between ages 3 and 9 who, she believed, understood the seriousness of their illnesses. As a result of her study, she described the experience of dying children. First, they become aware that the illness is "serious." They learn the name of the drugs they take and their side effects. They learn the purposes of treatments and procedures. They experience the disease as a series of relapses and remissions that eventually will cease with death.[5]

Kübler-Ross would concur that dying children are aware of the seriousness of their illness. Through the use of spontaneous drawings, children have illustrated clearly that they are aware of their condition. Even though children are aware, they quickly assess the feelings of the adults in their life to determine if it is safe to discuss it with them. If they determine that it makes Mommy cry, they will not bring it up. Instead, they may turn to the classroom teacher to answer their questions. Teachers can prepare themselves to help the dying child. Without mentioning the disease itself or the word "dying," they might first ask the child, "What is it that you are afraid of?" The answer to that question may open many doors.

The adult hospice movement has shown the need for children's hospices. Children and their families are supported through the final stages of dying. The philosophy is the same: to give comfort, to control pain, and to help the families cope with their caregiving role. The family is encouraged to bring the child home so that the child can be among familiar surroundings.

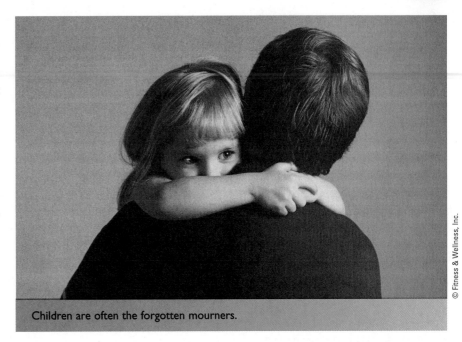

Children are often the forgotten mourners.

© Fitness & Wellness, Inc.

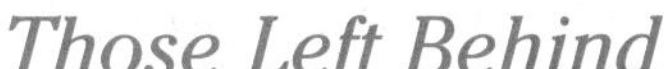

Those Left Behind

After a person has died, we turn to the needs of those who are left to mourn. The feelings created by loss can be disorienting and confusing. People suffer through the grieving process until they emerge on the other side. Adults often reach out to friends and loved ones for support. They may join a counseling group. Grief has no timetable, and the process often takes years. Yet, when children grieve, an adult's reaction may be "She doesn't really understand" or "He'll get over it" or "They won't remember it." These assertions could not be farther from the truth. Children suffer as much as adults do, perhaps more. If children are old enough to love, they are old enough to mourn.[6]

Children's Grieving

Other reasons for overlooking children's grief may be that the adults in their lives are grieving also or because adults try to protect children from pain. So children frequently are left to mourn alone, to find their own way out of what they believe is a bottomless abyss. They become the forgotten mourners who suffer silently for years and who often suffer severe and long lasting emotional damage.

Also, children grieve differently than adults do. Because they can tolerate less grief at one time, they take longer to grieve. When they are numb, they may appear to lack feelings and be unaffected by the loss—adults must not be deceived by this appearance. Because children may not be able to verbalize their feelings, adults in their lives have to respond to their nonverbal messages. If parents are deeply immersed in their own grief, they may misread these stages and think children are insensitive or unaware. Adults may distance themselves, leaving the children to mourn alone.

Wolfelt wrote about the dimensions of childhood grief and ways children express themselves. Children may exhibit, at various times, any of the behaviors below as they move toward acceptance or reconciliation.[7]

1. Initial shock/denial/disbelief/numbness: "Daddy isn't dead. He'll come back." Slowly, reality re-enters the child's life. This may take 6 to 8 weeks.
2. Overt lack of feelings: Often misinterpreted by adults to mean the child doesn't care; children's natural reaction to intolerable pain is to wall themselves off.
3. Physiological changes: These include sleeplessness, fatigue, headaches, skin rashes, stomach aches, and others. Like adults, children may develop the symptoms of the person who died (such as chest pains resembling a heart attack).
4. Regression: Children may regress any time during the grieving process. These behaviors include sleeping with a parent, returning to infantile behavior and baby talk, or refusal to go to school.
5. "Big man or big woman" syndrome: Children take on adult roles as a symbolic way of keeping the person alive and to protect themselves from the sense of hopelessness or helplessness. This reaction may be reinforced by an overwhelmed parent. A comment such as, "Now you have to be the man [woman] of the house" can have serious negative implications for the youngster.

6. Disorganization and panic: This stage often occurs suddenly and unpredictably from 1 to 6 months after the death. It may be manifested through dreams, restlessness, irritability, crying, and not making sense.
7. Intense emotions: The primary feelings are pain, helplessness, and frustration. Also, the child may be angry at the person who died, at God, at self, or those whose loved one didn't die.
8. Acting-out behavior: The child may act out emotions, primarily anger directed toward others to keep them from getting close.
9. Fear: Children fear abandonment (emotional and physical), fear loving again, fear the death of other loved ones, or fear their own death.
10. Relief: Children may be relieved after a loved one dies following a lengthy illness. Children are confused by this feeling and need to know that it is natural.
11. Emptiness/sadness: An empty feeling sets in slowly, usually between 6 and 10 months after a loss, leading to depression. Children should be encouraged to express these feelings through play, artwork, or writing.
12. Guilt and self-blame: Children sometimes feel responsible for the loss. This is particularly true in divorce.
13. Eventual reconciliation: This final state is achieved when a whole and healthy person emerges from grief with the recognition and acceptance that life will be different without the loved one.

In addition, most children, including adolescents, engage in magical thinking. Youngsters may believe their bad thoughts or anger caused the death. Or a child might get angry at a parent and wish the parent were dead; then, if the parent does die, the child believes he or she caused the death.

Developmental Stages

Children react to death according to their developmental stage. Kübler-Ross explained:

> Very young children have no fear of death. Later on, children are naturally afraid of separation, because the fear of abandonment and the absence of a loving caretaker is very basic and meaningful.[8]

According to Hungarian psychologist Maria Nagy, the following developmental stages occur in children's attempts to cope with death:[9]

Stage One: Before age 5, children view death as reversible, like a sleep from which the deceased will awaken. They recognize that the deceased is gone and view the death more as separation or abandonment. Children at this age are literal. Thus, adults should not use terminology such as, "Grandpa is sleeping" or "Daddy is on a long trip."

> When his grandfather died, a three-year-old was told that Grandpa was in heaven playing with other children. The child became very agitated. He told his mother that he wanted his grandpa to come back and play with him. He thought his grandpa left him to play with other children, and he cried.[10]

Stage Two: From ages 5 or 6 to age 9, death becomes personalized. Death is the bogeyman or a skeleton that comes down to take people away. This is a terrifying time for children.

Stage Three: After age 9, children are more aware that death is irreversible and will happen to everyone.

Most follow-up studies indicate that exposure to the computer, the Internet and other mass media have caused children to move more quickly through the stages. There is less of a tendency to personify death and more of a tendency to describe death in terms of a computer shut down and other references to technology. Children who are intellectually superior with advanced verbal skills have a more mature understanding of death.

Grief is complex and varies from child to child. It has no specific timetable. Children can be encouraged to express their grief and not be ashamed of it or try to hide it. Often, the intensity of their feelings frightens them. They need to be constantly reassured that what they are feeling is normal, and that it will eventually subside.

> Once a student had an argument with her grandfather. They had always had a loving relationship, with no disagreements. That night he died of a heart attack. [The student] was ten years old. For years afterward she blamed herself for his death. She suffered in silence because no one took the time to explore the experience with her. Finally, when magical thinking was explained to her five years later, she was able to release the guilt.[11]

Special Cases

Three forms of death warrant special attention. These are suicide, near-death experiences, and death in school.

Suicide

Suicide in families is the most tragic death of all. It is one that usually has no answers. Also, this form of death is the most taboo. Yet, it is the death that is the most important to discuss. Often the family feels guilty. Family members may look back over the life of the deceased and believe they could have intervened to save that life.

The classroom teacher has to know the circumstances and how the family is handling the death. Although the school has counselors and psychologists, the teacher may be the first school person the family contacts. He or she needs to be prepared.

Even very young children commit suicide. It is important to recognize that suicidal ideations may develop early in childhood, and their fatal outcomes may be manifested later in life. Nonetheless, most attention has been directed at adolescent and elderly suicides. Even the American Association of Suicidology, a clearinghouse for the latest research on the topic, has little information about childhood suicide. Pfeffer wrote one of the few books on the topic.[12]

The suicide death of a family member or friend is devastating to a child. They feel an incredible amount of shame; often the children feel responsible. Perhaps they discovered the body. It is important that the child be told quickly and honestly by someone the child trusts.

One of the best books written on this topic is *How Do We Tell the Children?* wherein Dan Schaefer and Christine Lyons recommend being honest and speaking about the death in simple terms.[13] Some people's bodies get sick and just don't work right; and sometimes a person's mind doesn't work right. These people can't see things clearly and they feel the only way to solve their problems is to take their lives, to kill themselves. This is never a solution to problems, though. The only reason they thought of it is that they weren't thinking clearly.

Although suicide is not inherited, it is often repeated in families. The act may be viewed as a way to solve problems. This book is an enlightening guide. It emphasizes that not discussing a suicide and not mourning it can lead to severe emotional problems.

Even though young children may be unaware of the finality of death, they can still engage in self-destructive acts. Children who come from abusive or alcoholic homes or homes in which parents are severely depressed are more likely to be self-destructive. Children who engage in these behaviors are violent toward others, or have frequent accidents, are at risk for suicide. The very quiet child, too, may present cause for concern; this child may be hiding his or her pain and may be extremely depressed. Depression, whether acted out or repressed, is a breeding ground for an attempted suicide.

Young children have attempted suicide by jumping from buildings or ingesting poisons. Sometimes they wish to join a loved one who has died, particularly a grandparent. Adults and children alike should know the signs of potential suicide and report these children to appropriate authorities. Children may know about their friends' troubles long before a trusted adult becomes aware. Teachers can encourage classmates to help each other and to tell a trusted adult.

Another important sign to look for is a recent loss that may be catastrophic to the child. Some children express their pain in their drawings or in their writings. Sometimes they are able to relate how they feel. The teacher may be the only one who recognizes the signs. Helping a suicidal child can be emotionally exhausting. Classroom teachers should seek help from other school professionals. Together, they can plan an appropriate intervention.

Near-Death Experiences

In his text *Life After Life,* Dr. Raymond A. Moody, Jr. explained the **near-death experience** through descriptions of his patients who had cardiac arrest or other life-threatening trauma and then were revived.[14] Some gave accounts of feeling unconditional love and seeing a beam of light. Some saw a life review or loved ones who had died. Others had a sense of leaving their bodies and seeing the activity at the scene. At some point in their journey, they were told they had to return, that it was not their time.

The International Association of Near-Death Studies was formed at the University of Connecticut by Dr. Kenneth Ring and Dr. Bruce Greyson, whose research paralleled that of Dr. Moody. Near-death experience has had a profound effect on these people, often altering their view of living and dying. Many had difficulty coming back and living in a materialistic world. Most dedicated their lives to the service of humankind. All had difficulty talking about their experience with their families and medical professionals.

Dr. Melvin Morse has been studying near-death experiences of children who have been declared clinically dead and then revived.[15] He recounts story after story of children who "died" and entered the tunnel of light. Professionals should be aware that children in the classroom may have had these experiences or heard about them. They may not have told anyone because of their fear of being told they are crazy or of being ridiculed. Introducing the topic of the near-death experience in school may create an environment wherein children feel safe enough to discuss their experiences, understandings, and fears surrounding death.

Death in School

Incidents of violence and death in school have increased. Children have been killed on field trips and in bus accidents. Perhaps a beloved custodian or administrator died of a heart attack during the school day. In some cases, children and teachers have been held hostage, and some have been murdered. Administrators and teachers need to introduce activities that allow the students to express themselves and to grieve. Often, social service agencies and counselors are called in for support. Parents, too, should be involved and encouraged to talk with their children and express their own grief.

Experiencing a sudden death is like having the rug pulled out from under one. Suddenly the person is gone. When this happens, families react with much emotion and may remain in shock for a long time. It is the same with children. Sometimes they believe that the person went away or disappeared and will search for them. Often they will worry that others of importance in their lives could also leave suddenly. They look to the adults in their lives to help them externalize their feelings. If the death is violent, much anger accompanies the loss. Children listen to the way adults react to police and medical personnel. Teachers can help children to resolve and externalize their **unfinished business** by talking about what they would have said if they were able to say goodbye.

A phenomenon called **survivor guilt** often arises when someone has survived a traumatic event. He or she may think, "Why did it have to be her? Why couldn't it have been me? I could have saved her!" This guilt complicates recovery. School personnel can help to mediate the grief. Meanwhile, teachers may require support themselves.

In the aftermath of a violent or traumatic death, some children develop post-traumatic stress disorder (PTSD). The child will experience flashbacks and behave in irrational and bizarre ways. They develop fears and have nightmares. Immediate referral is crucial to these children. Children look to adults in their lives to see how they are coping with loss. Healthy modeling will help children recognize appropriate expressions of sadness and grief. Specific activities can be planned, such as planting a tree or writing a poem.

The Aftermath of Death

When someone is known to be dying, loved ones enter **anticipatory grief**. They prepare for the eventual death. It is a time of intense activity, in which the family and loved ones begin to set things in order. Plans are made, words are said, people are forgiven. Children need to be a part of this. Unlike sudden death, the survivors have a chance to plan the rituals for the aftermath of death. In catastrophic losses such as earthquakes, floods, terrorism, and plane crashes, grief resolution takes many years.

Wakes and Funerals

According to Schaefer and Lyons,[16]

> Children, like adults, need a vehicle to mourn their loss, to say goodbye and get on with living again. Families deprived of this catharsis because their loved ones were missing in action or lost at sea often have a hard time coming to terms with the loss. Unless they are able to face death squarely, acknowledge the loss in some kind of ritual, and bury the one they loved, the grief doesn't go away.

Children need to be part of the rituals surrounding death. Sheltering them from the pain and not allowing them to say goodbye can have long-term and sometimes permanent implications. Wolfelt urges parents to describe, in a non-frightening way, what the children will see and then ask them if they want to attend.[17] Goldman believes children should be part of the commemorating ritual.[18]

Saying goodbye is as important to a child as it is to an adult. According to Kübler-Ross:[19]

> Siblings should have their own private time, preferably accompanied by a person of their own choice with whom they are comfortable and unashamed to ask questions. Children do not want to be sheltered from the truth.

In one instance the parents did not tell their child that, while she was away at camp, her cousin had died. The child wrote letters to him and wondered why he didn't answer her. When she returned home, she learned of the death and funeral. She was outraged, felt betrayed, and wondered what other secrets her parents would keep from her. She grieved her cousin's loss as well as the loss of trust.[20]

Children are naturally curious. They may want to view the body, touch it, look inside the hearse. The choice should be theirs. They should not be forced to participate. Part of the commemorating ritual may be for the children to place mementos in the coffin. All of this should be encouraged and supported. The book *How Do We Tell the Children?* may answer many of their questions.[21]

According to Wolfelt, children are capable of reconciling grief if the following conditions are present:

- The relationship with the deceased was secure.
- Children are given prompt and accurate information about the death (especially suicide).
- Questions are allowed and encouraged, and adults respond honestly.
- Children participate in the family mourning and ritual.
- Children have the supporting presence of a trusted adult.[22]

Returning to School After a Loss

Children are naturally self-conscious and do not want to be singled out as being different. When they return to school after a loss, they may feel embarrassed. Peers and adults, too, may feel uncomfortable in their presence. They don't know what to say. Students have reported that they feel like everyone is avoiding them.

School personnel should reach out to them. Ideally, the classroom teacher has prepared the class by having the students send condolence cards, go to the funeral, and offer other signs of support. The students should have the opportunity to talk about what they can say or do to make the returning child feel welcome and comfortable.

When teachers discuss with the child the circumstances of a death, how the person died and what kind of relationship he or she had with the deceased, one question they can ask is, "Do you feel responsible for the death?" Teachers might even consider exploring magical thinking with students as a class exercise. This can help students realize that being angry at someone and wishing for his or her death does not cause death.

Classroom Responses to Death

More and more, teachers are being called upon to help families with their problems. Taking in-service courses and continuing education courses related to death and dying will prepare teachers to meet these needs. These courses also can help teachers work through their own unfinished business. Moreover, knowing when to encourage the family to get professional help and where resources are available are important services.

The topic of death and dying taps into many emotions. Many of the concerns of children and their families are beyond a teacher's ability to help. Part of the study of death and dying for classroom teachers is to develop an understanding of their boundaries and the differences between education, supportive behaviors, and psychotherapy.

The school psychologist, counselor, and principal should be sought when in-depth interventions are needed; they can be encouraged to develop a school plan and a list of mental health professionals in the area for referral. This plan should include establishing a crisis intervention team specifically trained to help in sensitive and emergency situations. The school plan then must be made known to all teachers. The best gift teachers can give their students is a caring heart and a place for children to go. Children know when the teacher is their friend.

Teachers who hesitate to deal with death in the classroom can rest assured that their students already do so. Young children often are observed playing imaginary games involving killing and death themes in which one or more of the participants die for the fun of it all. When asked during a recent puberty lesson what they feared most about growing up, almost one-third of a sample of fifth-graders filled in the blank with one of the following words: death, dying, AIDS, getting killed, violence. For some kids, growing up is synonymous with getting closer to death.

At a recent visit to a local cemetery, a child of approximately 5 years of age was overheard directing the following questions to his mother and grandmother: "So which one is his?" (referring to the tombstones). "Oh, here he is.... I see the name! ... How'd they get him under there?" (He was looking at the thick sod, which had successfully hidden any indications of digging.) "How'd they get him in that little slot?" (referring to the space occupied by the narrow headstone). "Why don't we just dig him back up again?" The adults were involved in their own thoughts and in quiet conversation, so the child's questions went unanswered, ignored, and unaddressed—at least at that moment.

Perhaps these questions will come up again in a classroom somewhere. Perhaps the child will be heard by a teacher who has the courage to answer the questions honestly and directly and with a large dose of compassion.

A fifth-grader, Anthony B., who had the unhappy experience of discovering the dead body of his beloved grandfather, reported to his teacher and to the class at large:

"We were all at a birthday party except my grandpa hadn't gotten there yet. So my mom asked me to walk across the street to find out when he was coming. She would always ask me to go because we had this special relationship, my grandpa and me. So I went across the street, and as soon as I walked into his house, I knew something was different. The air felt different . . . it's hard to explain. I wasn't scared, but it just felt . . . different. When I got to the bedroom, I saw that he was just lying there. I knew right away that he was dead. You could just tell. I wasn't scared. It was all fine. I felt so peaceful and comfortable with him in his bedroom . . . so calm. He had such a peaceful look on his face.

"But then, after a while the adults came. They all started screaming and crying. It was scary then. They started taking his pulse and pushing on him I don't know why. It was so obvious that he was dead. I'm just glad I had some quiet time alone with him before they all got there. I guess I kind of understand why they were all yelling. After all, it was a surprise. But they kind of ruined the peace that was in the room . . . and then they just ignored me. It was as if I was not even there. They weren't trying to be mean. It's just that they were all upset that he had died. But we're all going to die someday anyway, right? I just think it was his time."

The wisdom of youth.

The 9-year-old niece of one of the authors died after a sudden, tragic 3-week illness. Her teachers, who came to share our grief, expressed fear that they would not be able to deal effectively with her classmates. When children die, the event seems so unnatural. Childhood death defies our expectations about the normal chronological progression of life. We are left bereft, confused, broken-hearted, and often numb with pain. But the truth is that death comes to the classroom the same way it comes to our homes—as an often unwelcome and unexpected visitor. And we must learn to deal with death effectively because, like it or not, death is very much a part of our lives.

A large part of dealing effectively with death as a teacher has to do with the three modes of learning: cognitive, affective, and behavioral. Therefore, presenting accurate information, demonstrating an open and honest attitude, and modeling a set of behaviors consistent with the values taught are the three essential components of any curriculum on death and loss. In some ways these may seem simple; in other ways they require a type of preparation and an inward journey not involved in other classroom themes.

Cultural norms, religious customs, family values, ingrained belief systems, and media messages enter the classroom as well. Teachers should not minimize the effects of these factors on their own and their students' personal development—all of which, obviously, may be quite different.

When Jimmy, a fifth-grader, was asked how he enjoyed learning about puberty, he replied, "I really didn't like it so much because it reminded me that I'd be dying soon." Jimmy had no reason to assume that his death was imminent. This presented his teacher an ideal opportunity to address his fears about death, to validate the certainty of the event at some point in the future, and to put his mind at ease for the present moment.

Open-ended questions are often the key: What is it that scares you most about death and dying? Why do you think many people are afraid of dying? How can you handle the fears you have? Most often, other children in the class will offer suggestions. The teacher should create a safe environment by allowing students to express their fears without suffering the embarrassment of putdowns by classmates.

Parents are often surprised when they realize just how much their own children have been affected by the deaths of grandparents and other relatives, friends, or neighbors with whom the children have had minimal contact. One boy, who wrote an essay about his dead grandfather, shocked his mother by describing the closeness he felt to the man who lived thousands of miles away for most of the young boy's life.

Spiritual Aspects

Many children are very spiritually aware. Children often feel the presence of or have dreams about the departed one. Other times they smell a familiar perfume or have similar sensory experience that brings up a vivid memory. This seems to be a kind of knowing that they are not alone. Validating their experiences helps them externalize their grief. They want to be assured that they are not crazy.

Some students have told of having a **premonition** that someone was going to die. Within the classroom, this topic may arise spontaneously when discussing funeral and other rituals that help people grieve. Asking the question, "Did you feel your loved one's presence at any time after his [her] death?" can introduce the topic for class discussion or through drawings or writings. Whatever a teacher's beliefs, he or she needs to provide an environment wherein children can express their thoughts and feelings about death.

We as teachers are honored to have an opportunity to enter into this sacred part of a child's being. Humility is a quality that will benefit all. When listening to profound stories from students, we may have to suspend our own belief so we can find a truth deeper than the one from our own life experience.

Understanding Children's Grief

Teachers can reach out to these silent sufferers if they know and understand how and why children react to loss, especially as it affects their school performance. Before teachers can help others, however, they need to look at their own experiences with loss and death and recognize their own issues and unfinished business.

Some questions teachers can ask themselves in search of understanding are: How was death treated in my family when I was a child? What were my family's messages about death? Have I mourned the losses in my life? Can I talk about death? Am I comfortable allowing children to cry and externalize their grief? Only when teachers are aware of and work through their own issues can they teach about death and help others. Otherwise children can immediately sense their teacher's discomfort and may censor their responses accordingly. Understanding how children mourn will help teachers to be more responsive to their needs. When children see adults being sad, it can empower them to acknowledge their own feelings.

Children's literature is filled with themes about death and dying. Many of

For Your Health

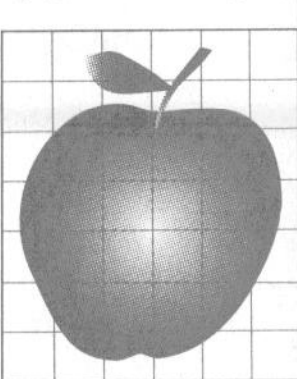

Constructive Grieving

Children often express many of their deeper insights in various art forms. To help students grieve constructively:

- Encourage students to draw, sculpt, and write.
- Have students tape-record stories about their experiences with loss, dying, and death.
- Tell students stories involving death. Storytelling is particularly helpful.
- Play appropriate music for students while they draw or write leisurely in the classroom.
- Encourage students to jointly write a play about their experiences and enact the drama for the class.

the Learning Experiences (at the end of this chapter) can be adapted easily in a literature- or other creative arts–based curriculum or where thematic units are employed. Other activities are listed in the box above.

Cultural Expectations

When discussing death in the classroom, the teacher needs to be aware of the cultural context within which a family experiences death. In some cultures the children are included in the mourning ritual; in others they are excluded. Teachers should educate themselves about ethnic diversity, attitudes about death and mourning, the rituals that surround it, and beliefs about afterlife. Which adult caregivers are responsible for the child, and what are the family's religious beliefs?

Family Conference

When dealing with grieving children, teachers might invite parents in for a conference. When teachers reach out to grieving families on behalf of their children, they can suggest that they share their grief. Involving parents can be most worthwhile.

Schaefer and Lyons advise caregivers and parents to communicate clearly: "We are sad because Grandpa died. That means his body has stopped working."[23] Most children at any level can understand this. They may ask if they or their parents will die. One way to answer such questions is to acknowledge that every living thing dies.

Embrace the totality of the students' lives by embracing the totality of your own. The gift of inspired teaching may be one they hold dear long after their schooling is over. May the teacher's gifts endure.

Summary

Children are often the forgotten mourners after a loss. Adults may believe that children are not old enough to understand losses or that they do not have the depth of feeling that adults do. In actuality, children mourn intensely, though their concepts of loss differ from those of adults according to their developmental level.

The most common losses during childhood are the separation or divorce of their parents (in which they often feel they are to blame), the loss of a grandparent (either because of a move away or death), the death of a sibling, or the death of a pet. Children should be encouraged to work through their loss, whether it is a "small death" or one that is catastrophic.

Elisabeth Kübler-Ross, pioneer researcher on death and dying, stated that dying people go through five stages:

denial, rage and anger, bargaining, depression, and acceptance. Surrounding people should recognize what stage the person is in so they can provide optimum support.

In school, the teacher can do much to support the student and family by providing a trusting environment in which the child feels free to express himself or herself and by educating the class about issues surrounding dying and death. Listening is an important facet of the teacher's role. Classmates might help by sending school-made cards and, if the circumstances warrants, attending the funeral. The teacher should be aware of cultural, ethic, and religious differences in beliefs and rituals surrounding death.

Suicide is a special case that requires special attention by school personnel because of the stigma that often surrounds taking one's own life. A situation that requires a special response is death within the school.

Resources and Web Sites

American Association of Suicidology
2459 S. Ash
Denver, CO 80222
303-692-0985
www.suicidology.org

Center for Loss and Life Transition
3735 Broken Bow Rd.
Fort Collins, CO 80526
970-226-6050

Centering Corporation
Catalog of Grief Resources
www.centering.org

Children's Hospice International
1101 King Street,
Suite 131
Alexandria, VA 22314
703-684-0330

The Delta Society
(resource for pet death)
321 Burnett Ave. South, Third Floor
Renton, WA 98055-2569
206-226-7357
www.petsforum.com

Griefnet
www.griefnet.org

Hospicenet: Death and Dying, Caregiving and Grief
www.hospicenet.org

Parents of Murdered Children
www.pomc.survivorships.com

Notes

1. E. Kübler-Ross, *On Children and Death* (New York: Macmillan, 1983), 19.
2. L. Goldman, *Life and Loss: A Guide to Help Grieving* (Indianapolis: Accelerated Development, 1994).
3. *Death: The Final Stage of Growth* (Newark, NJ: Prentice Hall, 1975).
4. See note 3, p. 134.
5. R. A. Kalish, *Death, Grief and Caring Relationships* (Monterey, CA: Brooks/Cole, 1981).
6. A. Wolfelt, *Helping Children Cope with Grief* (Indianapolis: Accelerated Development, 1983).
7. See note 6.
8. See note 1, p. 64
9. Robert J. Kastenbaum, *Death, Society & Human Experience*, 11th ed. (Needham Heights, MA: Allyn and Bacon, 2001).
10. See note 1, p. 226.
11. R. J. Kastenbaum, *Death, Society and the Human Experience*, 10th ed. (Needham Heights, MA: Allyn and Bacon, 1995), 232.
12. C. Pfeffer, *The Suicidal Child* (New York: Guilford Press, 1986).
13. D. Schaefer and C. Lyons, *How Do We Tell the Children?* (New York: Newmarket Press, 1990), 105–106.
14. R. A. Moody, Jr., *Life After Life* (New York: Bantam Books, 1988).
15. M. Morse, *Closer to the Light* (New York: Random House, 1990).
16. See note 14.
17. See note 6
18. See note 2.
19. See note 1, p. 198
20. See note 14.
21. See note 6.
22. See note 14, p. 28.

Learning Experiences

Experiences with loss and death are not age-defined. Children are touched by them in different ways throughout their elementary education. In a society that has trouble speaking about death as a part of the life experience, children grow up with fears and feelings that they often do not express. Activities that develop skills that enhance children's ability to talk about death; cope with their own experiences with loss and death; empathize with others' pain, grief and fear; recognize the symptoms, seriousness, and permanency of death (especially as it relates to suicide); and appreciate life have an important place in the school curriculum. Both developmental stage and common life experiences that are happening in the particular community can have considerable influence on curricula in death and dying education. If there are terminally ill children in the school, if there has been a suicide or accident that resulted in a death among the students, if the parent of a child or a teacher in the school has died, one might expect more attention to be paid by children to activities that address these issues. The following competencies can be expected at various grade levels K–6 after effectively planned sessions on death and dying. The students will be able to

1. Identify feelings associated with loss and dying including sadness, grief, fear, guilt, relief, and so on.
2. Identify common human reactions to death including anger, rage, silence, hysteria, and so on.
3. Differentiate between what can be controlled and what cannot be controlled with regard to death and dying.
4. Describe some rituals that are followed as a part of the closing process, particularly those that are followed by their own family, religious, or cultural group.
5. Explain the physical changes that occur as a result of death.
6. Express an elementary understanding and personal definition of life and death.
7. Identify ways to help sick or dying people and those who love and care for them.

8. Prepare and express personal memorials for people and things lost or dead.
9. Identify warning signs of suicide.
10. Identify sources of help in the school, community, and family.
11. Recognize when they need help with grief, loss, or feelings of hopelessness and helplessness.

For suggestions on creating a rubric with which to evaluate student performance of Learning Experiences, see page 13.

Learning Experience 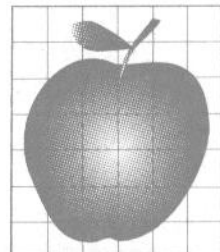 12-1

Magical Thinking: "If Only I . . ."

Grade Level

K-6

Primary Discipline

Language Arts

Learning Objectives

Following this activity, students will be able to

- Describe their belief systems about death.
- Discuss the relationship between cause and effect.
- Name the limits to their personal power.
- Identify sources of help in and out of school.

Time Required

One session

Materials

Easel, markers, bulletin board or display wall

Description of Activity

Introduction

Magical thinking and egocentrism are normal developmental processes for growing children. They can bring problems with grieving, however, because children often blame themselves for the events causing death. They may feel guilty and believe they could have stopped the event "if only. . . ." These beliefs are often shrouded in silence or tears as well as rage and anger, and it takes some artful open-ended questioning on the part of the adult to help children get beyond the unnecessary guilt, self-blame, and shame that result from magical thinking.

Activity

1. Divide easel paper into two columns and add the headings "Accidents/Sickness" and "We Feel." Using the easel to record responses, explain that people often get sick, have accidents, get hurt, and so on. Ask the question, "What are some things that cause accidents?" (Answers may include drunk drivers, carelessness, confusion, lack of order, mistakes.) Q: "What are some things that cause sickness?" (A: germs, smoking, drug abuse, allergies, genes, contaminated food, poor habits).
2. After developing the lists, ask the students how they feel when someone they love is hurt or gets sick. Record their responses on the easel under the "We Feel" column (responses may include sad, scared, angry, guilty, ashamed).

   Define guilt and offer a personal experience so students will identify the feeling in themselves. (Example: "When my dog died five years ago, I felt guilty because I thought for a while that I should have been home to take care of him, but I was at the movies with my friend.")
3. Ask the students to draw a picture that represents one or more of these life events or feelings. Display the pictures on a bulletin board with an appropriate title (for example, "Sometimes Life Is Difficult").
4. Explain that we cannot control many things about life. No matter how much we wish or hope or pray, and no matter what we do, no human being can control life and death. List on another sheet of easel paper "Things We Cannot Control" (for example, the weather, sickness, the past, death). Ask students for suggestions, making sure to include other people's behavior (what other kids and adults do), death, and tragedy. List on easel paper "Things We Can Control," which will include our behavior, our thoughts, our habits, our tone of voice, and the way we react to our feelings, among others. Explain that sometimes people feel sad or guilty or angry because they are not so powerful. (We cannot stop Mom or Dad from abusing substances; we cannot change our

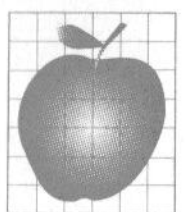

Learning Experience 12-1 continued

families; we cannot stop divorce or fighting, or disease process, or death). We *can* get help from others when we feel sad. We can't change what has already happened, but we can ask for help.

5. Ask "Who can help?" Develop a list of helpers available to students, including in-school and out-of-school resources. Bear in mind that grieving parents may be unavailable for their children; therefore other adults are important alternatives for help. Younger students could draw pictures of the resource personnel for the bulletin board.

Follow Up

The easel paper or a bulletin board could be displayed during the year as a reminder of the sources of help for difficult situations.

Homework

Grades K–1
Students draw two pictures, one entitled "Things I Cannot Change" and another called "Things I Can Change."

Grades 2–3
Students list three things they cannot change, three things they can change, and three things they wish they could change.

Grades 4–6
Students write a story entitled, "Sometimes Life's Not So Much Fun" or "If Only I . . ."

Evaluation

Students will be able to

- Identify situations that result in accidents or illness.
- Differentiate events that we can control from events that we cannot control.
- Define and explain emotions including anger, sadness, and so forth.
- Identify people and other resources in and out of school where they can go to when they feel sad, afraid, or need help.
- Describe what they and their family believe or know about death.
- Identify belief systems other than theirs about death.
- Identify things they wish to change in their lives and describe which can be changed and which cannot.
- Produce creative products including poster and bulletin boards.

The serenity prayer:

"Grant me the serenity to accept the things I cannot change, the courage to change the things I can, and the wisdom to know the difference."

Learning Experience 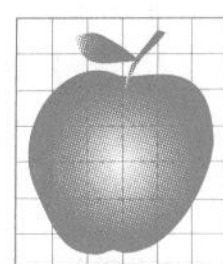 12-2

Photographs

Grade Level

K–6

Primary Discipline

Language Arts

Learning Objectives

Following this activity, students will be able to

- Demonstrate writing skills.
- Transform inner experience into written or oral form.
- Relate human relations to loss.
- Name resources available for help.

Time Required

Three teaching periods

Materials

Several magazine photos of people whose facial expressions and body posture might indicate sadness, depression, or anger (trim away all print); mounting paper (or laminate); pencils, paper, crayons

Description of Activity

Introduction

This activity provides a safe, nonjudgmental environment in which the students will feel free to express themselves. This activity could follow the reading of a relevant literature selection, or it could be used in a unit on feelings or friendship. The aim is to encourage students to speak about their losses and their feelings in general and to identify sources for help and healing. Talking about loss often elicits responses about death.

Activity

Grades K–1

Gather students around. Hold up one photo of a sad person. Tell the children that something is causing the person to feel very sad. She has lost something precious to her. Ask, "What do you think she lost?" "How does she feel?" "Do you think she felt differently before the loss?" "What will she do now?" "Do you think anyone can help this person?" "Have you ever lost anything?" "How did you feel?" "Who do you talk to when you're feeling sad?" "Where in school could you go for help?" (Here, identify psychologist, social worker, counselor, by name.) "Outside of school, where could we find help when someone dies?" (Suggest relatives, counselors, clergy). Ask students to draw a picture of two people who could help them if they ever become very sad. Ask how they could contact this person.

Grades 2–6

Copy a photo for use by the entire class or direct students to choose one from a selection you provide. Students work independently during this writing exercise. Explain that different people experience different emotions when faced with similar events in life. Getting lost, a pet's dying, getting sick, losing a game, or failing a test will cause different responses in different people. Explain that the person in the picture has just experienced a major loss. Following is one way to organize the three sessions:

Class Session 1: Have students write a story about the person in their photograph. Ask them "Who is this person? How does he/she spend the days? What kind of family does he/she come from? What kind of friends does he/she have? What happened to cause the feelings the person is showing in the photograph? What will happen now? Who can help? What will he/she do to feel better?"

Class Session 2: Create an experience chart entitled, "Death Makes Us Feel . . ." Using their writings from Session 1, the students will highlight various emotional reactions to loss or death. Sadness, sorrow, depression, anger, rage, emptiness, relief, fear, terror, confusion, numbness, and even joy can be expected in a grieving person. List the

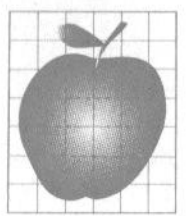

Learning Experience 12-2 continued

emotions on the chart and say: "These feelings can be very powerful. I realize that they were taken from fictional stories that you wrote about someone you've never met, but the feelings themselves are very human. When death occurs, it is natural to have strong feelings. How do people handle such strong feelings?"

Create a second experience chart entitled, "Emotions/Feelings Can Cause. . ." and have students fill in the blank. (Responses may include crying, hitting, yelling, sickness, accidents, hugs, laughter, giggles, isolation, deeper friendships). Avoid judging reactions, but point out that violence doesn't make the grief disappear; that grief is a process and people need time to heal inner wounds. Those of us who are friends will be most helpful if we learn patience, tolerance, kindness, understanding, and compassion for the grieving person.

Class Session 3: Introduce the stages of grief described by Elisabeth Kübler-Ross (*On Death and Dying*). Break the class into dyads or triads. Using the photos from Session 1, distribute one or more to each group. Ask the students to try to determine which stage of grief is being expressed in each photo: denial, anger, bargaining, depression, acceptance. What clues helped them to determine their answers? Is it always easy to determine a person's inner feelings? Is it helpful to know the truth about a person's inner feelings? Why or why not?

Note: Kübler-Ross' Stages are not meant to be applied as a "ladder of progression" to demonstrate dominance over grieving. These stages are experienced in various depths and degrees by each grieving person and will vary with each loss. They will follow no set sequence, and individuals may move in and out of each stage several times as grief is healed.

Homework

None

Evaluation

Students will be able to

- Describe emotions and other needs from a visual experience (a photo, a person) and effectively and accurately describe the situation they see, in writing or orally.
- Describe the need for, and then make written or oral suggestions about, support persons or organizations if a person feels badly or needs help.
- Describe the meaning of "loss" and give some examples of their own or other people's experiences with it.
- Explain their feelings and attitudes about death and describe other peoples feelings and attitudes.
- Describe stages of grief that people may experience after a loss.

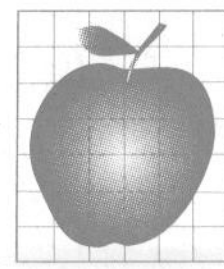

Learning Experience 12-3

Seed to Flower; Cocoon to Butterfly; Egg to Chick; Life to Death

Grade Level
K–6

Primary Discipline
Science

Learning Objectives
Following this activity, students will be able to

- Describe properties of living things.
- List the physical changes of death.
- Explore spiritual aspects of death.

Time Required
Several weeks

Materials
Seeds for perennials, soil, containers; or chrysalis and container; or eggs and incubator.

Description of Activity
Introduction
Teaching about death is teaching about the process of life. Many children have been exposed to media messages about death in which violence and bloodshed abound. In the face of this high exposure, they have been insulated from the natural cycle by our high-tech environment, by institutionalization of the weak and the dying, and by the need of many adults to "protect" them from the "sad facts of life." Classroom teachers have a marvelous opportunity to openly explore death as a natural process.

Choose the activity that suits the teacher's needs or those of the age group.

Activity
Prepare a corner of the room by decorating a bulletin board entitled " The Cycle of Life" or "Living Things" or "Life Is Beautiful." Select appropriate children's books for a literature table or shelf. Explain to the children that they will be examining life cycles. Discuss the conditions necessary to support various or specific forms of life. Ask, "What conditions will destroy life?"

Plant seeds (or prepare incubator, or set up chrysalis container according to the needs of the organism). Over time observe changes, prepare experience charts, collect data, and make predictions. (The degree of difficulty will depend on the level of the students.)

Questions for Discussion
- What do you hope will happen with our experiment?
- What do you think will happen?
- What is the difference between hoping and thinking?
- Why do we hope for life?
- How will you feel if the seeds never bloom (the eggs never hatch, the butterfly never emerges)?

Alternative
If some seeds do not bloom, or if eggs don't hatch, or butterflies do not emerge, use the event to talk about the feelings associated with death and loss. Do not deny the event by hiding the truth from the students. This is the teachable moment. Here, as in the unhappy event of the death of a classroom pet, many opportunities abound for teaching about the sanctity of life in all its forms, about the tender responses of the human heart, and about the compassion we can offer each other.

Homework
Extend discussions into creative expression by assigning a writing activity: If classroom example did not live, have students write a letter to the unbloomed flower (or unhatched egg or unformed butterfly). If/While the classroom example lives, have students write a poem about hope and life or draw a picture titled "What's happening under the soil?" (within the egg? inside the cocoon? within your hopeful heart?).

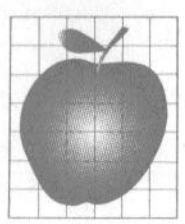

Learning Experience 12-3 continued

Evaluation

Students will be able to

- Describe the properties of living things and give examples.
- Describe some of the conditions that support life and some that destroy life, and provide examples of each.
- Describe the physical changes that occur after death.
- Give some examples of what people can do to be supportive to someone who is grieving.

Resources

4-H groups, Cornell Cooperative Extension, local nurseries, farms, hospices.

Learning Experience 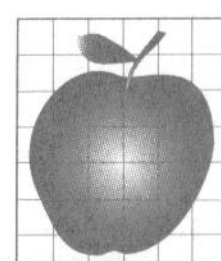 12-4

Timelines

Grade Level
2–6

Primary Disciplines
Math, Social Studies

Learning Objectives
Following this activity, students will be able to

- Identify units of time measurement: second, minute, hour, day, week, month, year, decade, century.
- Practice measuring and measurement skills.
- Discriminate between time well spent and time poorly used.
- Evaluate the quality of human life.
- Predict outcomes of behavior.

Time Required
Open-ended

Materials
Rulers or meter sticks, pencils, colored markers, erasers, paper; (optional: magazines for pictures, scissors)

Description of Activity

Introduction

Early elementary students are beginning to understand the relationship between the passage of time and its measurement. Using a timeline is an excellent way to help them understand these concepts. Older students often need help with time management and will benefit from looking toward the future when making behavioral decisions. It is helpful to orient oneself with regard to time when studying history. Timelines are easily adapted to the study of life and death.

Using a timeline is an excellent way to concretize the finite nature of life. These activities will facilitate discussion on a variety of topics related to life and death, including

a. importance of good decision-making
b. time well-spent and wasted
c. value of human life (including effects of violence)
d. human development/learning
e. habit formation/addictions
f. aging

Demonstrate timelines using examples from references (history texts, encyclopedias) and explain to the students that they will be creating their own timelines—perhaps a reflection of their own lives or that of family members. Demonstrate the importance of accurate measurements between intervals on the line (especially if this is a math lesson!).

Activity

With students, establish the limits: When will the line begin? When will it end? (This will depend on your goals for the lesson.) A line is drawn across the middle of the page with appropriately spaced intervals. The following significant dates/timeframes might be noted:

a. birth
b. death
c serious illness
d. accident
e. hospitalization/interventions/treatments
f. education
g. jobs
h. travel/trips/vacations
i. marriages/divorce
j. birth of children
k. deaths of significant people and other significant losses
l. retirement
m. birth of grandchildren
n. creative times/times of sadness or depression

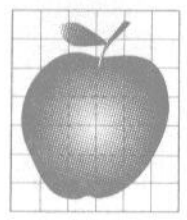

Learning Experience 12-4 continued

Questions for Discussion

What is a high point? What is a low point? Who determines the meaning of the events in an individual's life? How do people recover from major illnesses? From deep sadness? From painful losses? What criteria are used to determine the success of an individual's life? Is it money earned, position, or power? What are the greatest gifts life has to offer? Can death teach us anything?

Homework

Have students write an essay entitled, "Life Is Pleasure . . . Life Is Pain" or write a biography using their own timeline.

Other Activities (depending on content area)

Social Studies

The students create a timeline for a historical figure they have studied in class.

Math

Students find the midpoint and quarter points of an individual's life. Students measure life in decades and in fractions. What is a full life? Is life a whole? Does death cut life in half?

Related Activities

We're All Connected: Students create a timeline for an older relative (plot death if applicable), including significant life events, (awards, accidents, births of grandchildren, graduations, historical events, highs and lows, and so on). They draw a parallel timeline several inches below the first to represent the birth and life of the student.

Students plot significant moments of shared time between the student and the chosen relative and connect the dots. They draw pictures in the space between the lines to represent the shared events and connect the lines in the appropriate places. Have students note the length of the older person's line and that much of life occurred before the birth of the student. Ask what the student has learned from the older person. Will the student continue to learn from that person? Can the student imagine being important in the life of another person? To whom is the student important today? What does "quality time" mean? How can we have more quality time in relationships? After death, does our life have meaning?

Superstars: Have students draw a timeline for a famous figure indicating highs and lows by plotting points above and below the line (birth of first child, loss of job, sickness/suffering). This finished line will indicate the hills and valleys common to all human life. Often we idealize the life of celebrities and concentrate only on their successes. We forget that all people experience sadness during life. Stress that all must learn to deal with loss and gain, life and death.

Evaluation

Students will be able to

- Calculate units of time (day, month, year, decade, and so on).
- Identify and then calculate the average time needed to complete various common tasks or activities (for example, baseball game, homework, vacation, bout with a cold, life span)
- Identify the components of time management.
- Develop a daily or weekly time management plan.
- Describe the factors that determine quality time and quantity of time.
- Explain and give examples of limited time.

Learning Experience 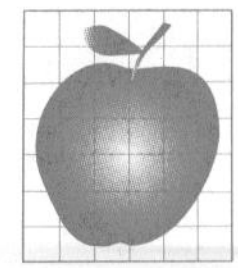 12-5

Rubbings

Grade Level

4–6

Primary Disciplines

Language Arts, Social Studies

Learning Objectives

Following this activity, students will be able to

- Discuss the meaning of death and life.
- Practice related writing skills.
- Report on human history.

Time Required

Two or three sessions

Materials

Visit to a local cemetery, a large sheet of newsprint for each student, masking tape, chalk, crayons, charcoal for each student

Description of Activity

Introduction

This activity helps to dissipate the mystique of cemeteries that has long been a source of children's nightmares and fears and that has had a resurgence with modern horror movies. It provides an opportunity for students to ask questions about burial, cremation, and cultural customs regarding death.

Make arrangements with personnel at a local cemetery. A small, private cemetery, where older grave markers are in abundance, is best. The activity is an appropriate extension of lessons about American history, immigration, genealogy, and related topics.

Remind students about the need for respect and reverence for the dead.

Before the day of the trip, have the class participate in discussions about burial customs and experiences, ancestors, human potential, legacies of our national heritage, and the legacy of our ancestors. Stress the notion here that one human life can make a difference.

Activity

Upon arriving at the cemetery, have students pair off to examine the headstones that mark each grave. They may find one with a familiar family name, or one with a date of historical significance, or they may simply be intrigued with the stone carving itself. Direct each student to select one monument, tape a sheet of newsprint to the stone, and rub over the surface of the paper with the side of the crayon or charcoal. The resulting impression is used to complete the lesson. Have students note all information on the headstone.

Other Activities (depending on content area)

Language Arts

Using the rubbings, have students create an imaginary biography about the individual buried at the gravesite. Ask "Why was this person's life important? What special gift did this person offer those who knew him/her? What struggles did the individual face and overcome? What talents and traits did this person have? What did people miss most when the loved one died?"

Social Studies

Have students use the rubbings to construct the larger history surrounding the life of the individual buried at the gravesite, including details of political struggles; social change; and major regional, national, and world events that shaped this person's life. (The age of the individual is critical for correct inferences.) Math skills are also needed here.

Follow Up

1. A member of a veterans' association could be asked to speak to the class about the need to honor the dead.
2. The class could examine the burial/funeral rites of other cultures.
3. Visit memorials in parks, U.S. veterans' memorials and monuments, and so on.

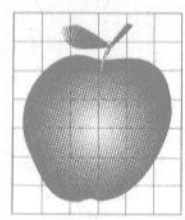

Learning Experience 12-5 continued

Homework

Students ask their parents to visit the graves of relatives buried in the local area or they visit a local war memorial or monument erected in honor of someone and report to the class in written or oral form.

Evaluation

Students will be able to

- Describe the rituals that families follow just after a person dies, their meanings, their origins, and the part they play in the grieving process.
- Describe the rituals their family follows and explain where their rituals originate.
- Identify some of the writings on tombstones and discuss their relationship to the person's life.
- Verbalize their own death or loss experiences.

Learning Experience 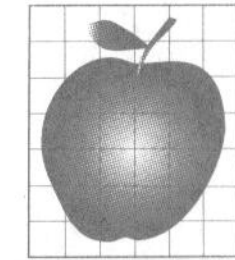 12-6

Grief Rocks

Grade Level

4–6

Primary Discipline

Language Arts

Learning Objectives

Following this activity, students should be able to

- Identify common emotions experienced in grief.
- Use storytelling as a means of oral expression.
- Translate images into language.

Time Required

One class session

Materials

Selection of rock or stones (enough to provide one for each student), container to hold the stones

Description of Activity

Introduction

Referring to a piece of literature with which the group is familiar (for example, *Bridge to Terabithia, Diary of Anne Frank, The Giving Tree*), say, "When someone or something dies, those who are living must adjust to life with a loss. They must learn how to live without the person (or animal, or plant). They often have strong feelings about this loss. Today, we are going to have a chance to examine some of those feelings—an opportunity to talk with each other about them."

Activity

Ask the students to sit in a circle. Show them the container of stones. Remind them that each stone is different: Some are smooth, some rough, some large, some small, some pink, gray, or brown. The stones represent the different feelings people experience following a death. Feelings change through time. One moment we may feel one way, and a few hours later a new emotion may replace it. Also we can feel more than one feeling at a time, which can cause emotional confusion. And the same event can give rise to different emotions in different people. Use the literature to illustrate these points.

Have students choose one rock to represent or remind them of an emotional response to the reading or to a loss in their own life. Model the activity by selecting one stone and sharing with your students whatever feeling this stone represents to you and why. (Examples: "Today I'm choosing this pink stone because pink makes me feel hot and angry. When my grandma died, I was very angry. I wasn't ready for her to leave me." or "Today I'm choosing this cold black rock. When my dog died, I felt black inside, like my insides were a dark cave" or "When I realized that Anne Frank had died so young and so innocently, I realized that death doesn't happen to just bad people. I'm choosing the white stone to represent innocence.")

Allow enough time for each student to share. Draw parallels in the experiences of the students and allow for the various emotional responses. Each is indeed unique.

Homework

Students write a cinquain, a poem, or a letter reflecting the lesson of grief rocks.

Evaluation

Students will be able to

- Recognize the emotions people experience when they have had a personal loss or death.
- Describe the emotions they felt after a personal experience with loss or death.
- Communicate through a creative product (poem or letter) their understandings, learning, attitudes, and emotions about death.
- Explain the permanency of death and the vulnerability of all living things (including young ones).

Learning Experience 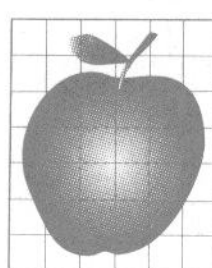 12-7

The Cry Guy

Grade Level

2–6

Primary Discipline

Language Arts

Learning Objectives

Following this activity, students should be able to

- Identify the emotional responses to death and loss.
- Share feelings about personal loss.
- Identify the processes of grief.

Time Required

One session

Materials

Poem in box on page 423

Description of Activity

Introduction

Reading a poem aloud adds a beautiful dimension to language arts classes. The poem in this activity, and many others, can be used as a starting point for discussion and examination of the grieving process, to stimulate awareness of the needs for compassion, to address the topics of death and dying as universal challenges in life. Remind the students that grief can last a long time and that the stages are not proscribed. As unique individuals, we experience and express our grief in a variety of ways.

Activity

Read the poem aloud to the class, then follow this procedure:

Grades 2–3

Ask the children to draw pictures of the main character both before and after the death of his dog. Ask children to write about a time when they felt similar to the "Cry Guy." Ask students to write a letter to the "Cry Guy," helping him understand that it is okay to feel sad.

Grades 4–6

Have a class discussion about compassion in the face of grief. Define the stages of grief as described by Elisabeth Kübler-Ross (see page 400). Ask the students to write a story or a poem describing a loss they have experienced in their own lives. Remind the students that loss is not felt only in the presence of death, but that people grieve in the face of divorce, loss of friendship, and so on.

Homework (grade level 4–6 only)

The students talk to an adult at home and ask him/her about losses he/she has experienced.

Evaluation

Students list and describe the stages of grief. Students will also be able to

- Describe the characteristics of poems.
- Describe some of the ways people react to death or loss.
- Define and give examples of compassion for people who are sad or ill.
- Speak with their parents about death.
- In class, share personal experiences with death or loss.
- Recognize and be able to describe the stages of death described by Kübler-Ross.

Resource

Elisabeth Kübler-Ross, *On Children and Death* (New York: Collier Books, 1993).

The Cry Guy

Like falling rain
The tears streamed down
Upon his face.

The cry guy
Didn't hide
A single tear.

Mary called,
"Crybaby! Crybaby!"

He said,
"Not crybaby
But the cry guy,

I'm strong and brave
Enough to cry,
To touch my tears,
To breathe a sign,
To feel the storm
That's passing by,
Like the tall oak
In a rainy sky."

The children laughed,
"Sissy! Sissy!"
He said,
"Not sissy, sissy,
But the cry guy."

The teacher said,
"The tears must fall
For all;
Even the mighty oak
Bends and quivers
In the rain."

The cry guy
Held a picture
Tightly in his hands
Of a boy
And a speckled
Black-and-white
Puppy,
And said,
"It's so hard
To say good-bye.
I remember him

When I cry."
The rain fell gently
On his cheeks
Until he felt
Better.

Source: Kalli Kakos, *If You're Not Here, Please Raise your Hand.* Reprinted with permission of Simon & Schuster Books for Young Readers, an imprint of Simon & Schuster Children's Publishing Division.

Learning Experience 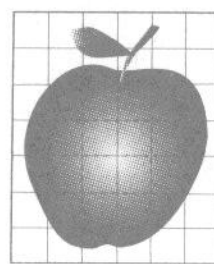 12-8

Important Events

Grade Level

4–6

Primary Discipline

Language Arts

Learning Objectives

Following this activity, students will be able to

- Identify significant life events.
- Practice critical thinking skills.
- Practice writing techniques.

Time Required

Two class periods

Materials

Essays (pages 425 and 426), Important Events Worksheet (page 427 and 428), paper and pencils

Description of Activity

Read the essays. Have the students complete the Important Events Worksheet. Discuss volunteered responses to the questions. (Children often access deeper feelings and share their life experiences more readily when others model these experiences and behaviors.)

Homework

Students each write a brief essay about an important event in their life that involved loss or death.

Evaluation

Students respond to the questions on the Important Events Worksheet. Assessments include students' ability to describe their feelings verbally and explain the reactions of the characters in the stories.

A rubric can be developed to evaluate students' ability to complete the homework assignment. Some of the criteria that could be measured include the students' ability to

- Differentiate important events and less important events.
- Describe events and explain the emotions associated with them in an organized and creative way.
- Write comprehensively and clearly, using correct grammar, without spelling errors and with appropriate terminology.

Resources

Losing Uncle Tim, Sedako, Diary of Anne Frank

An Important Event

Tara Donohue, Age 10

The most important event that went on in my life was my grandfather's death. This event was important to me because my grandfather suffered a whole lot. It was as if he was trapped, nowhere to go. Then God made a special place for him in heaven.

I also feel that it was a way for me, my sisters and brothers to actually feel the love of everyone around us, the concern of other people coming toward us.

The best part about this event was that my grandfather and I were close to each other. So close that we watched "Murder, She Wrote" together. We tried figuring out the mystery during commercials.

Another important part was he felt peaceful.

I wasn't actually there when he died, but I've heard the story many times. He was in a coma for a couple of weeks. Then on St. Patrick's Day he opened his eyes, looked at my grandmother, took a deep breath, and that was it.

I always think of his death as a fairy tale because he was so strong. He lasted the two years that the doctors thought he was going to die within. My mother thinks he lasted this long because of us kids.

At the funeral parlor I slipped a best-friend heart into his pocket. I have the other half and wear it almost every day, close to my heart, and close to his heart.

I'll never forget this important event. My grandfather will always be in my heart.

Source: Reprinted by permission of N. Donohue.

My Important Event

Michael Stengel, Age 10

Many events happen in my life, but only one of them I will never forget. The important event was when my poppy died. I pretty much knew my poppy when he died. I was only about 7 or 8. Even though he died, I still remember him deep down. The reason he died was because he had cancer and the doctors had cut off his legs. It was so sad seeing that. He used to put on prosthetic legs to walk, but now he can't. When I went down to Florida, I usually went down to see him and nanny. Now when I go down, I go to see him at the cemetery.

This event was important to me because I love him a lot and miss having him around. I also loved when he used to pull my teeth out so I could get more money from the tooth fairy. He also gave me $20 when I found the Afikoman on Passover. Now I still get $20, but it's just not the same when my nanny gives it to me instead of my poppy. He used to have catches with me and he even taught me how to take a slap shot.

Out of all the events that happened in my life, this was the most important. I will never forget all of the things he taught me, and I will never forget him.

Source: Reprinted by permission of R. Stengel.

Important Events Worksheet

1. What event was of greatest importance in each of the two essays?

2. In Tara's essay, she writes that this is a sad way to learn about love. How has sadness taught you about love?

3. How do you know that you are close to another human being? Does "close" always mean that you can actually reach out and touch that person with your hand?

4. When have you felt close to a person who is not with you? How did it feel?

5. Tara's grandfather lived for years even though he was very sick. What could be some reasons for this unexpected happening? Why do some people live long lives?

6. When Michael writes that he can "still remember him deep down," what does he mean? Is there someone or some event you will always remember "deep down?"

7. Michael says that now when he goes to Florida, "I go to see him at the cemetery." What does Michael mean when he writes about "seeing" his grandfather?

8. What kinds of things do you want your grandchildren to remember about you?

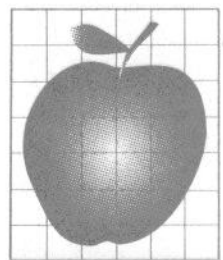

Learning Experience 12-9

Of All the Things I Ever Lost . . .

Grade Level

3–6

Primary Discipline

Language Arts

Learning Objectives

Following this activity, students will be able to

- Describe the worth of material possessions.
- Practice writing skills.
- Predict consequences of personal habits.

Time Required

One session

Materials

Paper, tape player (or CD player), pencils, calming instrumental music on tape or CD, handout (page 431)

Description of Activity

Introduction

Children lose much during the course of their young lives. Strong emotional reactions to loss are common and natural, though often unexpected and powerful. Equally common in children is an almost baffling facade of seeming apathy in the face of the death of loved ones. Adults often confuse this apparent lack of interest with a lack of emotion. This activity enables students to access, through creative visualization, many hidden memories associated with loss. The writing exercise provides a vehicle for expression of associated feelings and may help students deal more compassionately with one another.

Activity

Part 1

Explain to the students that they will be experiencing a two-part activity that will be done in silence with music in the background. Ask the students to relax, close their eyes, and remain still while you play the tape and read the following visualization in slow, modulated tones:

Imagine that you are walking alone along a path in the country. Perhaps it's a trail through the woods or a country road that's safe to walk on. Pick your favorite place. You are dressed comfortably for a walk outside. Smell the air; feel the warm sunshine on your face and the earth beneath your feet. If there is water nearby, notice it. Listen for the sounds of birds. As you walk along, you begin to think about your life, and you remember all the things you have lost during your lifetime. You've lost teeth; you've probably lost a toy or two; or books, maybe from the library; a pair of favorite sneakers, or maybe just one of the pair; a piece of jewelry. Everyone loses things. Some things that we lose are more valuable than others. Sometimes we find the things we have lost, but sometimes the things we lose stay lost forever. Sometimes we lose people, like when a friend moves away, or when a loved one dies. Life is filled with losses, and on your journey through the woods today, you are remembering the losses *you* have experienced.

As you're thinking and walking, you spot a picnic blanket along the side of the road. Near the blanket is a basket. The basket is for you. Your name is on it, written very clearly. Open up the basket! Look inside! In it is a reminder of something or someone you lost some time ago; something you valued; or someone you wish you hadn't lost. What a surprise! Here in your basket is a little reminder that makes you feel connected to something you lost. Examine it! Notice all the details, and then put it back into your basket. It will be safe there. You can come back and get it whenever you wish.

As you replace the object in your basket, you notice something else inside. It is a letter addressed to you. The letter is a very loving message from someone you have not seen in a long time. The person might not be alive today, but the letter was written to *you*. Open it! Read what it says. It is a very special note telling you some very wonderful things about you. Give

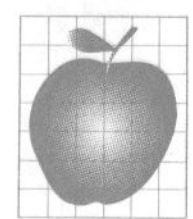

Learning Experience 12-9 continued

yourself plenty of time to read the message. When you are finished reading, put your letter back in the basket. Remember, you can come back and visit any time you want.

Now close your basket. Get up off the picnic blanket and begin walking on the road back to this room. As you walk, notice the plants and flowers if any are growing near your path. Notice the temperature of the air. Put your face up to the sun and breathe in the fresh air as you return. And when you feel comfortable, open your eyes slowly and return to this room.

Part 2

Distribute the handout. Ask students to respond by writing in silence or ask students to draw pictures that represent the treasures in their basket.

Questions for Discussion

After students have completed the written work, many will want to share their experiences orally. Lead the discussion by asking open-ended questions. Avoid judgments and critiques at all costs. Ask

- What did you enjoy about the activity?
- Were you surprised at the contents of your basket?
- What feelings did you experience during your walk?
- How do you feel about being able to return to your place whenever you wish?
- What makes a possession valuable?
- Must something of value be expensive?
- How do we learn to care for our possessions?
- How can we show respect for the possessions of others?
- What makes a person valuable to us?
- How can we show loved ones that they are valued?

Homework

None

Evaluation

Students will be able to

- Identify the objects they consider important.
- Recognize the values of other people.
- Describe what makes objects valuable.
- Explain how strong emotions equate with experiences.
- Describe what makes people valuable to one another.

Resources

Suggested music for this activity: George Winston's "Winter," "Spring," "Summer," "Fall"; Windham Hill's "Guitar Sampler"; Nature Company's "Last Great Places on Earth."

My Lost Friend

Make a copy of the letter you found in your basket.

Dear ____,
(Your Name)

As you create the letter, think about these things:

What is the treasure you found in your basket?

What makes it so special to you?

Why is it so hard to lose things we love?

Write about the person whose letter you found.

Why is he/she so special?

Why did you enjoy being with the person?

How did you spend time together?

How did this person act toward other people?

How did this person treat you?

Why is it sometimes painful to say goodbye?

Learning Experience 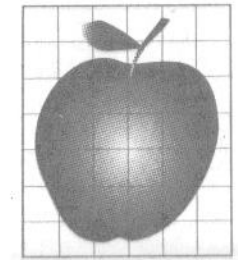 12-10

Memory Quilts

Grade Level

5–6

Primary Disciplines

Social Studies, Math, Creative Arts

Learning Objectives

Following this activity, students will be able to

- Practice measuring skills.
- Describe properties of various geometric shapes (squares, rectangles, and so on).
- Write memorials for deceased relatives/friends.

Time Required

Two or three sessions

Materials

Scissors, colored construction paper, plain drawing paper, pencils/markers/crayons/colored pencils, 1"-grid graph paper, rulers, yard/meter sticks, brown craft paper, fabric, needles and thread, fabric glue, fabric markers

Description of Activity

Introduction

This activity can be done as a memorial after the death of a person well known to the students, as a way to help students express feelings about a death that occurred some time ago, or as a response to a literary theme.

The quilt is poignant because, when complete, it represents the total expression of grief of a community, yet maintains each person's personal expression. Class members may choose a common theme (hope, giftedness, feelings) to unify their individual experiences. Associated decisions might include color schemes and an examination of cultural differences.

Some teachers have successfully created quilts out of fabric with young students. Colored felt is easiest to work with, because hemming is not necessary and glue can be used instead of needles and thread.

Note: This lesson requires accurate measurements and perpendicular placement of each square. The whole will be equal to the sum of its parts, both in mathematical accuracy and in emotional expression. This is an ideal opportunity for cooperative learning.

Each student will complete at least one square; some students may contribute more than one. You may choose to have students draw significant pictures and write names, dates of birth and death, or quotes and phrases in each individual square. The background squares will be used as "mats" for the students' work. The colors of the mats will determine the pattern of the quilt as well as the contents of the square.

Activity

1. Count the students who will participate in this activity. Determine the size, shape, colors, and pattern of the finished quilt by using the graph paper and student input. When assembled, the quilt will consist of a collection of equal-sized squares or rectangles set in a defined pattern. The pattern can be as simple as a two-colored checkerboard, or it may be something more elaborate.
2. Begin the lesson by reminding students that death is a part of life. Death causes varied responses in the people who remain alive. As time passes, we tend to forget some of the funny or important parts of the person's life. Because we don't want to forget, we often make something that will last perhaps even longer than our memories.

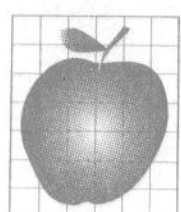

Learning Experience 12-10 continued

3. Have students measure a perfect square, or give each child a perfect square of drawing paper or fabric. Ask them to draw a picture or print words that reflect the theme chosen for the class quilt (examples are a special day they shared with the person, or the most important gift they received from the person, or unforgettable words the person spoke, or one reason they are glad the person lived). Students will then mount their contributions on the appropriate color "mat." (If the pictures are 4 × 4, the mats should be perfect squares somewhat larger to provide contrast for patterning.)
4. Glue individual paper quilt squares to brown craft paper, or sew or glue fabrics in the pattern chosen.
5. After the quilt is complete, give each child an opportunity to verbalize the meaning of his/her individual square.

Homework

Before the activity in class, students could research quilt patterns by finding books or magazines in the library.

Evaluation

Students will be able to

- Work cooperatively to complete a task.
- Identify items, life events, and the like that can describe the meaningfulness of a person's life.
- Select a theme and develop a product that describes the theme.
- Produce a creative and aesthetic product.

Resource

AIDS Quilt Project

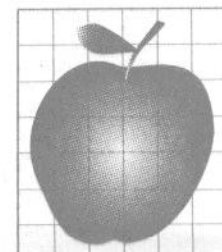

Learning Experience 12-11

Suicide and Children

Grade Level

3–6

Primary Discipline

Social Studies

Learning Objectives

Following this activity, students should be able to

- Describe warning signs of suicide.
- Identify depression, sadness, hopelessness, fear.
- Recognize hope as a healthy alternative.
- Identify sources of help in their community.

Time Required

One session

Materials

Poem (page 436)

Description of Activity

Introduction

Children are exposed continually to violence. Stories in the media and, sadly, stories from their own lives may even include tales of suicide. Suicide is a sad subject that can be even more difficult for families and friends to bear if it is laden with judgments and harsh criticism or shrouded in denial, guilt, and shame. If suicide comes to the classroom, teachers can help by encouraging students to learn healthier attitudes by suspending judgments and criticism. No religion teaches that any of its followers is the ultimate judge of another person.

Activity

Teachers prepare the students by explaining that the poem they are about to read was found among the possessions of a young man who had recently committed suicide. It is not known if the poem was actually the boy's work, but it was given to his teacher.

Questions for Discussion

- What is suicide?
- What types of feelings could cause a person to want to end his/her own life?
- Why is suicide so sad?
- How is the human community diminished by the loss of one life?
- Who can help us when we become extraordinarily sad? (Develop list of professionals.)
- How would we help a friend who had such deep sadness? (Never keep secrets where life is endangered!)
- How do we deal with sadness, failure, loss, grief, and so on, in healthy ways? (Develop responses.)
- Have the class develop a list of community and in-school resources that will point students toward interventions and necessary help.

Homework

None.

Evaluation

Students will be able to

- Define and explain suicide, including its permanency.
- Discuss the signs of a potential suicide.
- Identify symptoms of depression, hopelessness, sadness.
- Describe alternative thinking to feelings of hopelessness and thoughts of suicide.
- Identify actions to take when a person has feelings of hopelessness and thoughts of suicide.
- Identify resources in the family, school, and community that they can call upon for themselves or if they suspect a suicide.

If You're Not Here, Please Raise Your Hand

He always wanted to explain things
But no one cared.
So he drew.
Sometimes he would draw,
and it wasn't anything.
He wanted to carve it in stone
or write it in the sky,
and it would be only him and the sky and
the things inside him that needed saying.
It was after that he drew the picture.
It was a beautiful picture.
He kept it under his pillow
and would let no one see it.
He would look at it every night
and think about it.
When it was dark and his eyes were closed,
he could still see it.
When he started school,
he brought it with him,
not to show anyone,
just to have along like a friend.
It was funny about school.
He sat at a square, brown desk,
like all the other square, brown desks.
He thought it would be red
and his room was a square, brown room,
like all the other rooms.
It was tight and close and stiff.
He hated to hold the pencil and chalk,
his arms stiff, his feet flat on the floor, stiff,
the teacher watching and watching.
The teacher came and spoke to him.
She told him to wear a tie
like all the other boys.
He said he didn't like them.
She said it didn't matter!
After that, they drew.
He drew all yellow.
It was the way he felt about morning.
and it was beautiful.
The teacher came and smiled at him.
"What's this?" she said, "Why don't you
draw something like Ken's drawing?
Isn't that beautiful?"
After that his mother bought him a tie.
and he always drew airplanes
and rocket ships
like everyone else.
And he threw the old pictures away.
And when he lay alone looking at the sky,
it was big and blue and all of
everything,
but he wasn't anymore.
He was square inside and brown,
and his hands were stiff.
He was like everyone else.
The things inside that needed saying
didn't need it anymore.
It had stopped pushing.
It was crushed.
Stiff.
Like everything else.

(From the *Long Island Press*, Feb. 17, 1970)

Learning Experience 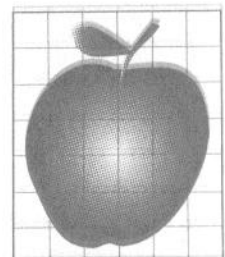 12-12

Eulogy

Grade Level

5–6

Primary Discipline

Language Arts

Learning Objectives

Following this activity, students will be able to

- Examine the lasting gifts of human life.
- Name positive character traits and human virtues.
- Continue practicing writing skills.

Time Required

One or two sessions

Materials

Attached eulogy (page 438) or obituaries from daily newspapers, chart paper, pens, paper, highlighting pens.

Description of Activity

Introduction

Eulogies address the finest of human qualities. They present human accomplishments. This lesson provides an opportunity for students to identify, examine, and recognize fine human traits in their friends and relatives, as well as people they do not know.

Activity

1. Provide copies of a eulogy (use the example on page 438 or obituaries from newspapers) for each student. Ask the students to identify desirable human qualities and character traits by highlighting the applicable words or phrases in the eulogies or obituaries.
2. Using student input, develop a comprehensive list of traits on chart paper.
3. Ask students to compose a eulogy for themselves and one for someone who is a youth role model.

Homework

Students can prepare for the lesson ahead of time by selecting obituaries from local or national publications.

Evaluation

Students will be able to

- Explain the purposes of a eulogy.
- Explain the relationship between the eulogy and the person's life.
- Discuss how families choose the person who eulogizes.
- Discuss the kinds of things they would like said about them after their death.
- Produce a creative writing sample of their own eulogy, indicating their ability to express themselves in writing.
- Name some of the things other people think are important to them.

A Eulogy

It was first grade, and I was on a mission: Find someone you love, and ask them about their first job. Armed with a marble notebook and a pencil, I took my customary seat on the floor, at the Cat's feet. At the Lion's feet . . . he was already a lion by then. He was larger than life to me even then—that much never changed. Grandpa always had a mystical quality about him I think it stemmed from his phenomenally strong faith, coupled with his utterly selfless and boundless love—a man who gave to all he touched in such an enormous way that it was apparent that God flowed directly through him.

So when he told me he was a police officer, it made sense to me. But I knew that he wasn't the intimidating kind. Although he was larger than life, he was much more protective than scary. To protect and serve, that's what lions do, too. True, they are cats with many lives: Husband, Father, Grandfather, Uncle, Friend, Role Model, Golfer, Volunteer, Head Custodian (he straightened up every mess he came across), but in each of his lives, the Cat, the Lion protected and served. All in the line of duty.

My grandfather was the best at what he did. I have never seen a man more wise, more intelligent, and still so simple. Never arrogant about what he knew, he gave perfect advice without making you seem like a lesser person. He commanded and gave respect like no other. He loved like no other.

As all of us in one way or another are his children, so was he a child of God. His faith was astounding—unshaken, inspiring, complete. He always knew that no matter what the circumstances were, no matter how far he was thrown, the Lion would always land on his feet. When I had my own crisis of faith this year, I asked him if he was frightened of dying. "To tell you the truth, Jonathan," he responded, "I never really gave it much thought."

He didn't worry about the things we spend our time worrying about every day—money, death, sickness, the future. He convinced me to let go of the uncontrollable. He embraced today like he embraced all of us—without fear, with complete confidence, with his Lion's heart. When we lacked strength, he provided. When we lacked courage, he gave us support—the Lion's share.

Even his own death did not shake him. He accepted it long before any of us began to, like the joke he always told: A Lufthansa plane was flying over the Atlantic, and the stewardess came up to the cabin to announce, "The left wing has fallen off, and we will have to make an emergency landing. All those on the right side of the plane will exit through their windows. And as for those on the left side of the plane—thank you for flying Lufthansa." This time he was stuck on the left side of the plane. But there were never any complaints, never any bitterness. I asked Grandpa what he believed heaven to be. His answer: "70 degrees, a Spring day, on a golf course, with the people I love around me."

And if any man deserved a heaven on earth, Grandpa did. The Lion's beauty, grace, integrity, and strength live beyond his body. His love lives in all of us.

Jonathan Mastro
July, 1994

Source: Reprinted by permission of J. Mastro.

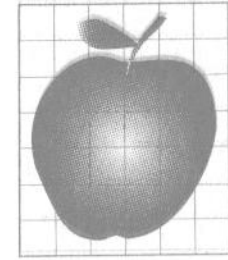

Learning Experience 12-13

Yarn Party

Grade Level

3–6

Primary Discipline

Social Studies

Learning Objectives

Following this activity, students will be able to

- Name several communicable and non-communicable diseases.
- Identify several ways in which infectious diseases are spread.
- Examine emotional reactions to disease.
- Report on the values of the community.
- List several ways to help sick or dying people.

Time Required

One or two sessions

Materials

Lengths of yarn in five or six different colors, scissors for each student

Description of Activity

Introduction

This activity may elicit strong emotional reactions from the students. The teacher might refer to Chapter 5 and its activities on communicable diseases and be prepared to deal with human reactions of shock, horror, fear, dread, and relief.

Activity

1. Ask students what they usually share with one another at parties. (Answers may include food, drink, games, fun, gifts, laughter, time, pizza, and so on.) Tell the students that today they will be attending a "make-believe party." They will be visiting each other the way people visit each other at a party.
2. Tap a student on the shoulder, which will signal "a party visit." This student will carry scissors and yarn to any other student in the room. (Review safety rules for walking with scissors.) The "visiting" student will share his/her yarn with the other student by cutting each strand in half. Both students will now have two strands of yarn. On a subsequent visit, each student must share both colors with the new visitor.
3. Continue to tap students until they have made many "visits" and exchanged many colors.
4. Stop the activity when some students have five strands of different colors. Some may have only the original strand or fewer than five.
5. Remind the students that many things are shared at parties—lots of good times, fun, and sometimes germs. Each of the colors they have just shared represents a disease with which they may have come into contact during the party. Disclose the meaning of the colors (see below) and allow time for emotional reactions and discussion.

Blue — Chicken Pox
White — Pneumonia
Yellow — Flu
Green — Measles
Red — Common Cold
Orange — AIDS

Each disclosure opens up opportunities for discussion on a variety of topics, for example:

- communicable versus non-communicable diseases
- modes of transmission
- physical and emotional needs of sick people
- prevention behaviors
- reactions of sick and dying people

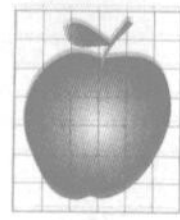

Learning Experience 12-13 continued

- reactions to sick and dying people
- the effects of inclusion and exclusion
- sickness and health and the value of living with the best possible health

Homework

Students compose a letter to a sick friend or relative, or write an essay titled, "Disease and Fear" or "Anger and Illness," or compose a story, "I Am Me—I Am *not* My Disease."

Evaluation

Students will be able to

- Describe behaviors that people who are seriously ill or dying typically show.
- Describe behaviors that people in contact with the seriously ill or dying typically show.
- Recognize the difference between myths and facts about serious illness that make people afraid.
- Identify acceptable behaviors that can comfort or help sick or dying people.
- State ways they would like to be treated if they were sick or dying.

13

Environmental Health

Efrem Rosen and Kathleen Zammett Walter

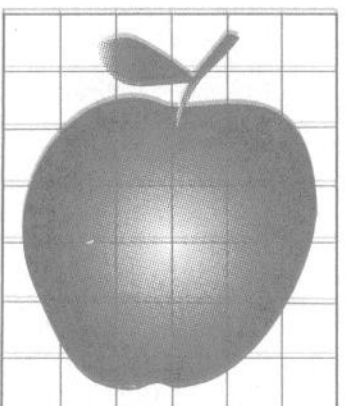

Chapter Outline

Objectives

- Define and describe ecology, the ecosystem, the biosphere, and the sustainable ethic
- Explain the relationship between the environment and people's physical and emotional health
- Identify outdoor and indoor air pollutants and their effects
- Explain how water becomes polluted and identify some water pollutants
- Discuss other forms of pollution, including thermal pollution and oil pollution
- Explain noise pollution and decibel levels; identify their sources that can produce negative health effects
- Explore the concepts of greenhouse effect and deforestation
- Discuss waste accumulation and identify some hazardous wastes, including pesticides and other health-harming chemicals
- Discuss laws to protect endangered species
- Identify some things a person can do to contribute to healthier people and a healthier environment

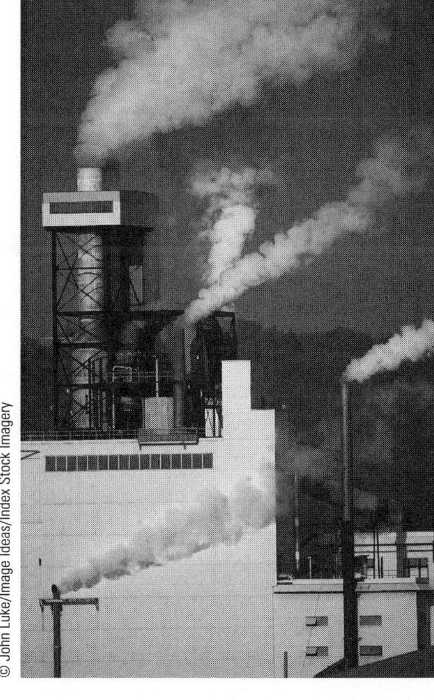

Tiffany and Joey are 10 years old. They and their classmates went on a class trip to the zoo. The children brought lunch from home, and the teacher provided paper cups for drinks and small bags of pretzels for snacks. They ate lunch under the trees. After lunch, the teacher insisted that all of the children gather their garbage and dispose of it in the trash can. Some of the kids left crumbs, cups, and wrappings from their snacks on the ground when they left. The teacher was angry.

• • •

After school Tiffany's parents took them to the lake to swim. When they got there, they saw several dead fish near the shore and a big sign that said "No Swimming Today." Lots of motor boats were on the small lake. Tiffany heard her mom telling her dad about how clear the water used to be when she was a young girl. "You could actually see your toes in it," said Tiffany's mom. Their swimming day was ruined.

• • •

The children in the small country town that Tiffany and Joey live in used to pick the berries from the bushes near the park and eat them. They were sweet blueberries. Over the past few years, they have been told that the blueberries are no longer healthy to eat. They have a white film on them that the children were told is poisonous and will make them sick. The white film comes from the spray the town is using to keep the mosquitoes away.

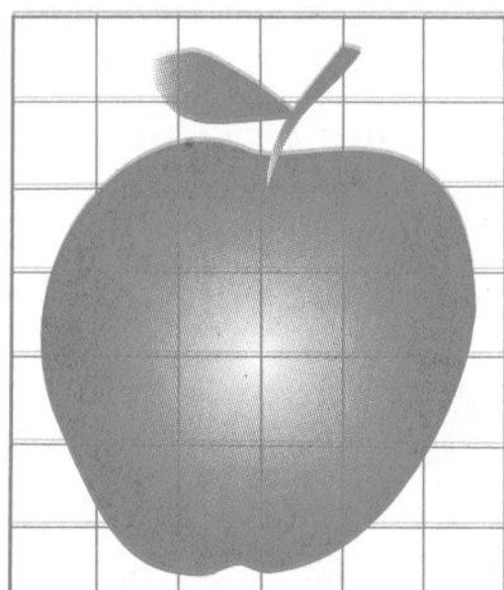

What do Tiffany and Joey need to know about their environment that will help them understand how their own lives have been changed by a lack of environmental concern? How can they come to recognize the consequences of their behavior on human health? How can they become concerned citizens who will acknowledge the importance of protecting their environment? They will need to gain a lot of information about their environment and how it affects their health. Because all environments interact, directly or indirectly, Tiffany and Joey would then have to learn how their own environment interacts with their friends' environment, their neighborhood's, their city's, their country's, and ultimately, their planet's.

Have you ever driven through a large city on a sunny day and couldn't see the tops of the taller buildings through the haze? Have you seen gulls flying above a low hill alongside a highway that, as you got closer, turned out to be a garbage dump? Have you ever walked along the shore at a sandy beach, looked down at the bottoms of your feet, and found they were black from stepping into an oil slick? Have you ever turned on your water faucet to find that the water looked brown? If you have experienced any of these situations, you already are aware of several changes in the environment. Each of these changes has implications for maintaining health.

A diminishing supply of pure water, increasing pollution of the air, the accumulation of hazardous wastes, or the loss of farmlands or wetlands, affects most communities. The biosphere is facing many threats that affect our health. Preparing children to make intelligent decisions about their environment and their health is the challenge of a curriculum about environmental health. Providing the facts and skills needed to make wise decisions can reap social and psychological benefits for society and will help ensure the welfare of the planet.

Ecology

We do not inherit the Earth from our ancestors; we borrow it from our children.

— Ralph Waldo Emerson

Ecology is the study of living things in their natural environment. Ecologists study interactions within and among ecosystems, investigating, for example, the food webs of plants and animals and how they affect each other. Understanding ecology requires recognizing and appreciating the following four basic ecological principles:

1. Interactions occur between producers (plants), consumers (animals), decomposers (such as bacteria and fungi), and the physical environment.
2. A cyclic flow of matter (nutrients and water) takes place within the planet's biosphere.
3. Once created, nutrients are never destroyed but are recycled (that is, they continue to flow within the ecosystem) in one way or another.
4. Sunlight, as a form of energy, powers the cycles of nutrients and water, but it flows in only one direction. It enters the planet's atmosphere as light energy and is converted into plant energy (which is then used for food by consumers). It then leaves the planet as heat (entropy). These processes, therefore, convert nutrients into energy that is used by the system.

Thus, the amount of food in an ecosystem, generated by the process of photosynthesis, is finite. What people do affects the flow of energy and the cycling of nutrients. Any change, disturbance, or destructive action within these processes can have a serious impact on living things. The choices people make—including the decisions made in industry, agriculture, and government—affect the ecosystem. If sustainable solutions (procedures that support the environment rather than exploit it) for ecological problems are found and if we learn to use our resources well to meet our needs, other species will be able to meet their needs and have adequate resources; the survival of future generations will be assured.

The principle of a **sustainable ethic** encourages people to reduce the exploitation of environmental resources. This principle holds that humans are part of nature and subject to its laws. Thus, people have to cooperate with the forces of nature. To put this ethic into practice, people need to follow the ecological principles of conservation, recycling, use of renewable resources, restoration, population control, and adaptability.[1] Residents of a sustainable community work to improve public health and a better quality of life for all the inhabitants by limiting waste, preventing pollution, maximizing conservation, promoting ecological efficiency, and developing local resources to sustain the local economy. A sustainable community resembles a living system in which all resources—human, natural and economic—are interdependent and draw strength from each other.[2]

The Ecosystem

The word "**ecosystem**" has two components, "eco" or "oicos" (which in Greek means house or home) and "system"—which means that it has input (in this case, sunlight), an internal structure (the set of living things), and an output (including unusable energy and waste material). Another example of a system is a car: a man-made system that also has input (gasoline), an internal structure (the engine, frame, and electrical parts), and output (1. the energy to move the car and 2. carbon dioxide, a waste product).

All living things are a part of ecosystems that are composed of plants, animals, and decomposers. These dynamically interact with the nonliving components such as air, water, sunlight, and minerals. Also, living things within an ecosystem interact reciprocally, forming a self-contained ecological unit—that is, altering the biotic environment will affect the physical environment, and changing the physical environment will transform the biotic environment. Some ecosystems are natural (for example, a grassland); some are man-made (for example, a city). Examples of ecosystems are a woodland, an ocean, a desert, or even a farm.

Like a beehive hanging from a tree, many smaller ecosystems are found within larger ones. The bees collect nectar from plants for food. In doing so, they help the plants reproduce by fertilizing the flowers. Other animals, bears for example, use the product of the hive, honey, for food. Bears, in turn, will be food for other organisms, and on and on. Size varies greatly: The size of an ecosystem can be as small as the branch of a tree or as large as the Atlantic Ocean. This is just one example of a complex set of interactions called a **food chain** or food web that is the basis for all ecosystems. Upsetting this finely tuned balance of nature can destroy the ecosystem.

Ecosystems are in continuous interaction with one another and are united by the actions of the various physical and biotic environments. These form biomes, which are large geographical areas with similar plants, animals and decomposers. You may be familiar with the more common biomes such as tropical rain forests in South America, the tundra near the cold Arctic, evergreen forests of the Northwest, or deserts like the Mojave. Each of these large communities contain a set of species that are adapted to its varying concentrations of water, nutrients, and soil.

Finally, these biomes combine to form a global ecosystem called the **biosphere**. All living things depend on this biosphere, which is also a self-contained life-support system with complex global relationships. The relationships within our biosphere have a direct impact on our personal health and well-being. Almost everything people do affects the environment in some way, and the environment, in turn, affects people, their diet, the air they breathe, and thus, their health. Drinking contaminated water, breathing polluted air, or living in overcrowded conditions jeopardize health and well-being.

Environmental Health

One cannot consider the fundamental connection between the environment and health without thinking about the tragic events of September 11, 2001, when the World Trade Center in New York City was so viciously destroyed by international terrorists. The smoke that emanated from its ashes for the next several weeks created a long list of health problems, such as respiratory ailments, skin irritations or even cancer, each affecting the health of the environment, the survivors, and the many hundreds of rescuers. So far, extensive tests of air, dust and water in and around Ground Zero have not uncovered major risks to people's health, but higher levels of air contaminants (asbestos, airplane fuel, dioxin) are present. What the long-term effects will be remain to be seen.

Environmental health focuses on issues that relate health status to ecology, such as indoor and outdoor air pollution, temperature changes, water pollution, acid precipitation, noise, solid waste disposal, pesticides, and radiation damage. Each of these problems can affect the health of individuals and populations who are exposed to them. Thus, in considering environmental health, it is also important to learn about dynamics of the global environment as a basis for implementing environmentally sound practices.

The following key concepts are presented:

1. We depend on the environment for the necessities of living: air, water, and food.
2. Environmental pollution is a worldwide concern that affects the health of populations.
3. Environmental pollution is caused by a combination of factors.
4. The solution to environmental problems will be found through both people's behaviors and through science and technology.
5. Environmental pollution comes from air, water, and noise, solid waste accumulation, and excessive use of potentially toxic pesticides—each of which has implications for health.
6. Individuals can affect their environment in positive and healthful ways.

All living things are involved in the cycling of energy and nutrients from the sun, water, air, and soil. Our influence over the environment is reciprocal. We can plant an apple tree, and its beauty and bounty will nourish the body and heart; or we can throw garbage into the sea, and the death and destruction of aquatic life will sicken the body and heart. People can do both. In order to protect the environments of the future, children need to become aware of the links between all things in nature, from the smallest microbes to the largest whales in the ocean, from the plants in a rain forest to the Eskimos of Alaska. They can be taught to understand how they fit into this biosphere. When children feel a deep-rooted connectedness with the natural world, they will more readily appreciate the need to protect the earth's life-support system.

Studying Environmental Health

How do researchers study the connections between the environment and health? The first and most important technique is epidemiology, which links an environmental contaminant to personal and community health. This is the type of research that, after many years, linked smoking cigarettes to lung cancer. Another tool is using laboratory animals for screening tests. By exposing these animals to contaminants, at various concentrations, researchers can determine causal links between the contaminant and a health problem. A third technique is testing the effects of potentially harmful chemicals on cell cultures and/or suspensions of microorganisms in the laboratory. From these studies, the genetic or cellular effects of specific contaminants can be determined.[3]

Environmental Education

The impetus for environmental health education was first driven by the publicity surrounding several key events that focused our attention on the critical problems facing us. Publications such as Rachel Carson's *Silent Spring* in 1962 and Paul Ehrlich's *The Population Bomb* in 1968 raised our awareness of the need to take action to preserve our resources. Catastrophic events—such as the nuclear power plant accident at Three Mile Island, Pennsylvania, in 1979; the death of nearly 3,700 people caused by the leakage of 40 tons of methyl isocyanate gas at a Union Carbide plant in Bhopal, India, in 1984; the contamination of large areas of northern Europe caused by the breakdown of the Soviet nuclear power plant at Chernobyl in 1986; the death of thousands of animals caused by the 11-million gallon oil spill from the *Exxon Valdez*, the oil tanker that ran aground in Prince William Sound, Alaska, in 1989; and the air pollution and other environmental damage caused by the war in Kuwait in 1991—all brought worldwide attention to environmental issues.

In 1970, the International Union for the Conservation of Nature and Natural Resources (IUCN) defined "Environmental Education in the School Curriculum":

> Environmental education is the process of recognizing values and clarifying concepts in order to develop skills and attitudes necessary to understand and appreciate the interrelatedness among man, his culture, and his biophysical surroundings. Environmental education also entails practice in decision-making and self-formulation of a code of behavior about issues concerning environmental quality.[4]

In addition, the aim of environmental health education is to teach students that their actions can benefit the environment and preserve their health. This goal can be achieved by providing experiences that foster an interest in the environment and by developing attitudes and increasing levels of awareness that lead to a personal environmental ethic.

In 1977, UNESCO set out three goals of environmental education:

1. To foster clear awareness of, and concern about, economic, social, political, and ecological interdependence in urban and rural areas.
2. To provide every person with opportunities to acquire knowledge, values, attitudes, commitment, and skills needed to protect and improve the environment.
3. To create new patterns of behavior of individuals, groups, and society as a whole toward the environment.

Elementary schoolchildren can begin to learn the importance of caring for nature and the environment. Schools can play a vital role in nurturing students' appreciation and respect for the environment. Students who learn that their well-being and that of the earth are intertwined will come to understand that they are part of the overall ecosystem and that they have responsibilities concerning the environment. Encouraging students to develop environmentally sound habits, measures that create a way of life that coexist in harmony with the environment, will increase the possibility that our future will be led by adults who establish policies and practices that nurture the earth, discourage the exploitation of its resources and then, by definition, support and respect human existence. Students can begin by caring for their immediate environment—their home, yard, school, and community.

The National Institute of Environmental Health Sciences, a division of the National Institutes of Health, describes 20 easy steps that will extend life, improve fitness and enhance the environment:[5]

1. Learn to read the labels on house and garden chemicals, food products, and prescription and nonprescription drugs. See if the directions for use or warnings have changed. Even before you buy a chemical product, compare the labels to be sure that you are buying the safest product. Note any protections required (such as gloves), restrictions of use (such as inside or outside the house), or side effects.
2. Teach children how to minimize exposure to loud sounds and noises. Exposure to very loud noises can cause damage to hearing. Many musicians wear ear plugs to extend the life of their ears (and perhaps their professional lives). Loud music, firecrackers, small arms fire, and even low-flying jet planes can damage hearing.
3. Minimize exposure to carbon monoxide from cars or home heating appliances. Installing a carbon monoxide alarm in the home can reduce accidental death from this poison.
4. Grow plants in the home—not only because they are nice to look at, but also because there is evidence that they clean pollutants from the air.
5. Keep vitamins and all drugs (such as aspirin or other pain relievers) out of the hands of children. They can kill; lock them up. The same is true for paint thinners, detergents, and other home and yard chemicals. (See Chapter 14 on injury prevention and safety.)

6. Teach children what physical activities are potentially dangerous. Climbing up a ladder or lifting heavy objects can produce painful back or leg injuries that can be permanent.
7. Install air filters or air conditioning; vacuum carpets often. What you thought were colds actually may be allergies. Children may be allergic to dust mites, mold, the cat's dander, pollen from trees or plants, or the dust in carpeting or curtains.
8. Teach children to drink only safe water. Clear streams or lakes may be nice places to swim, but they may contain bacteria that may cause stomach or skin problems. When away from home, bottled water may be more suitable.
9. Inspect your home for old lead-based paint. Although lead has been eliminated from the home environment and from gasoline, there may still be flaking paint from pre-1950 buildings that can cause damage. Even low doses of lead can cause developmental problems with learning, remembering, and concentrating in children.
10. Have your home tested for radon, a gas that you can't smell, see, or feel. It comes from uranium in the soil and is radioactive. It increases the risk of lung cancer and is especially dangerous if people in the home smoke.
11. Teach children to exercise sensibly. Children can keep fit by exercising, but excess heat is dangerous. Children need to exercise during cooler hours and to drink plenty of water to keep from dehydrating.
12. Show children how to watch for ozone alerts in newspapers, TV, and radio weathercasts. Ozone is a form of oxygen that can irritate and damage tissues in the nose, throat, and lungs. It can make breathing hard, especially when exercising outdoors or if sensitive to respiratory illnesses.
13. Stress handwashing. Children, especially those who have frequent colds, should wash their hands on a regular basis, especially after handling raw meats or going to the bathroom—as should anyone who handles food.
14. When spraying plants with pesticides, make sure that children are not in the way of the spray. Also, washing raw fruits and vegetables can reduce the exposure from unwanted or even toxic chemicals.
15. Teaching children to eat a good diet, especially with plenty of fresh fruits and vegetables, is essential to health. (See Chapter 3 on nutrition.)
16. Some nutritionists recommend a regular intake of vitamin supplements to maintain good health.
17. Be sure that children wear seat belts, helmets, and other recommended protective gear. Good safety habits can save the lives of children from accidents. (See Chapter 14.)
18. Teach children, at an early age, when appropriate, about their sexuality to help an prevent an illness or an unwanted pregnancy. More and more children are becoming exposed to sexually transmitted diseases, including HIV/AIDS. These infections can lead to cancer, infertility, or even death.
19. Teach young children about the dangers of smoking and remove tobacco smoke from their environment. Smoking cigarettes, cigars, and pipe tobacco kills more people than HIV/AIDS, drug abuse, accidents, murders, and fires combined. The negative effects of smoking are well documented and advertised, yet many young people get addicted at an early age.
20. Help children avoid sunburn. Getting a sun tan is an attractive leisure sport, because it helps people feel good and look good. But the temporary pain of sunburn may result in not only wrinkling of the skin, but the possibility of skin cancer years later. Ultraviolet light from the sun or sun lamps are linked to cataracts that dim vision.

Pollution

Pollution occurs when waste products are deposited in the air, on the water, or land. All ecosystems produce waste products, but normally they do not accumulate; they break down and are recycled within the system. Pollution is also caused by manufactured, nonbiodegradable products that do not decompose and, therefore, do not return to natural cycles. Instead they accumulate, causing dirty, unhealthy, or hazardous conditions. Pollution also is caused by producing too much or too little of natural substances, thus disturbing the natural cycles of nutrients. We are faced with numerous potential health hazards from air, water, and noise pollution, solid-waste accumulation, and dangerous pesticides.

Air Pollution

The air is precious. It shares its spirit with all the life it supports. The wind that gave me my first breath also received my last sigh. You must keep the land and air apart and sacred, as a place where one can go to taste the wind that is sweetened by the meadows flowers.

— Chief Seattle[6]

Air is needed to sustain life. We obtain oxygen from the air we breathe. The Earth's atmosphere consists of about 78 percent nitrogen, 21 percent oxygen, less than 1 percent argon, about 0.04 percent carbon dioxide, and some traces of inert gases. Air also contains varying amounts of water vapor and natural contaminants emitted by volcanic eruptions, forest fires, and decaying vegetation. The quantity of air is limited and must be recycled and reused. The air we breathe is cleansed by natural processes such as rain, which removes many pollutants by carrying them to the ground or into the oceans. The oxygen in the air that is removed by the respiration of all living things is replenished by photosynthesis.

Air pollutants are contaminants in the atmosphere in such large quantities and of such persistence that they pose hazards to all living things, negatively affect human health, and can cause the destruction of the environment. Manmade air pollutants come largely from three sources: automobiles, power generators, and industrial plants. Natural sources, such as volcanic eruptions, also contribute large amounts of air pollutants. They can be carried hundreds of miles from their source, contaminating forests and farms far away.

By creating pollutants, many of the technological processes and products we depend on can actually threaten our health and shorten our lives. Regularly breathing pollutants increases the likelihood of our developing a variety of diseases such as lung cancer and emphysema. Polluted air can also increase the severity of respiratory ailments such as allergies, asthma, colds, and pneumonia. Major air pollutants that are harmful to health include carbon monoxide, sulfur oxides, nitrogen oxides, hydrocarbons, carbon dioxide, chlorofluorocarbons, PCBs, lead, radiation, and toxic chemicals such as mercury. Sulfur dioxide, nitrogen oxide, hydrocarbons, and carbon monoxide often react with moisture and with one another to form secondary pollutants such as sulfuric and nitric acids, which fall to the earth as acid precipitation, ground-level ozone, and photochemical oxidants.[7]

The U. S. government has passed a number of laws to regulate pollutants, and the Environmental Protection Agency (EPA) is responsible for enforcing them. One of the first was the Clean Air Act, passed in 1963 which empowers the government to set limits on the amount of air pollutants that factories and automobiles can release into the air. In 1967, the Air Quality Act divided the nation into regions for monitoring air pollution and set new air quality standards. In 1970, the first Earth Day was celebrated and air pollution became a major political issue. In 1977, amendments to the Clean Air Act aimed at maintaining clean air and restricting automobile emissions were enacted. The Clean Air Act of 1990 added restrictions on acid rain, ozone depletion, smog, and airborne toxic chemicals, and increased funding for additional scientific research into all aspects of air pollution. These tighter restrictions included more stringent automobile emission standards. The Clean Air Act of 1990 added 182 items to the list of airborne toxic substances regulated by the EPA.

Air pollutants occur in two categories: particulates (such as ashes, smoke, and dust) and gases or vapors (such as fumes and mists). When fossil fuels such as coal, oil, and natural gas are burned, many substances are released into the air, including sulfur dioxide, nitrogen compounds, and particulates. These primary pollutants travel through the air and react with each other in the presence of sunlight to form secondary pollutants, such as sulfuric and nitric acids.

Carbon Monoxide

Carbon monoxide is an odorless, colorless, poisonous gas produced by the incomplete burning of carbon in any product. The automobile is the chief source of carbon monoxide in the environment. Keeping the car running in a closed garage can emit enough fumes to permeate the house or kill someone sitting in the car. Poorly vented appliances and tobacco smoking can also produce carbon monoxide indoors. The health effects of carbon monoxide poisoning, caused by the molecules entering the blood and blocking the blood's ability to carry oxygen, include fatigue, headaches, dizziness, rapid heart rate, and in high concentrations, loss of consciousness and sometimes death.

Sulfur Oxides

Sulfur oxides are gases created from burning coal, fuel oil, and transportation fuels. These gases form sulfur dioxide, a poison that causes itching eyes and skin and damage to the respiratory passages. Sulfur dioxide is a colorless gas produced by combustion at power plants and certain industrial sources. A mixture of sulfur oxides and water is the liquid byproduct of burning coal in power plants and industrial processing, which send the molecules into the atmosphere. When this mixture falls to earth, it is called acid precipitation ("acid rain"), which often falls far from its origin (that is, industrial pollutants in XX are likely killing trees in YY)—secondary pollutants are often carried by winds in this way. Acid precipitation kills trees, plants, and fish, destroys stone and metal, and damages lungs. Children with asthma are particularly sensitive when playing outdoors; overexposure can cause reduced lung function.

Nitrogen Oxides

Nitrogen oxides are gases resulting from the high-temperature combustion of energy sources, such as coal and oil, by power plants and motor vehicles. They can also be produced by inadequately vented gas ranges, gas pilot lights, and gas or kerosene heaters. They damage plants and severely irritate the lungs, resulting in respiratory distress and other lung diseases. They also produce nitric acid, a component of acid precipitation.

Hydrocarbons

Hydrocarbons are gases that produce smog from the burning of fuel oil and transportation fuels. Exposure to hydrocarbons such as propane, benzene, and ethylene can lead to respiratory distress and lung cancer.

Dioxins

Dioxin is the common name for a complex organic chemical, also called TCDD. Other compounds, such as PCDD, PCDF, and polychlorinated biphenyls (PCBs), have similar structure and activity as dioxin. Collectively, they are referred to as dioxins. They are formed during the combustion of waste products, in forest fires, the burning of trash, and in the manufacture of herbicides and paper. Dioxins are present in low levels in food and can accumulate in the body in fat tissue, resulting in several forms of cancer and altered reproductive, developmental, and immune system functions. More research by the EPA is needed to establish the health effects of low levels of dioxin contaminants.

Ozone

Ozone is a form of oxygen created when the rays of the sun change the chemical state of the molecules into photochemical oxidants. When it combines with sulfur dioxide that has been mixed with rain to make sulfuric acid near the ground, it becomes toxic. This ozone-acid mix can cause rubber to crack and can damage plants and other living things. Humans exposed to this form of ozone can develop headaches, coughing, and shortness of breath.

Ozone high in the atmosphere is helpful, providing a barrier to the harmful radiation from the sun. The ozone layer is about 15 to 35 miles above the earth in the stratosphere and acts as a filter, protecting us from the cancer-causing ultraviolet rays of the sun. Acute exposure to ultraviolet rays is thought to cause damage to the eyes and skin. Industrial chemicals (for example, chlorofluorocarbons [CFCs], methyl chloroform, carbon tetrachloride, halons, and methyl bromide), when sprayed into the air, destroy the protective ozone layer. This thinning of the ozone layer permits the ultraviolet rays to infiltrate the lower atmosphere and damage forests, crops, and other living things.[8] **CFCs** are odorless nontoxic chemicals formerly used as aerosol propellants and in refrigerators. In 1988, an international agreement was reached, restricting and eventually eliminating the production and use of CFCs.

Indoor Air Pollution

Toxic substances, combined with inadequate building ventilation, cause health problems such as eye, nose, and throat irritation; sinus discomfort; headache; sneezing and coughing; respiratory infections; and fatigue. Office equipment, classroom supplies, and construction materials are frequent sources of indoor air pollution. Electrical equipment may emit ozone. Common office supplies such as glue, rubber cement, and inks release vapors and dust in poorly ventilated areas that can cause a variety of skin and respiratory problems. Solvents used in roofing, painting, and renovation work can cause respiratory irritation, dizziness, and nausea. Chemicals such as ammonia, solvents, paint strippers, and cleansers can cause respiratory irritation, chronic lung disease, and eye irritation.

Lead Poisoning

Lead, a heavy metal found naturally in soil, groundwater, and surface waters, can be highly toxic. Poisoning can occur by the ingestion of particulates containing lead, such as from lead paint, or by inhalation of fumes containing lead (from burning leaded gasoline and other fuels) and of lead-filled dust. Old water pipes and lead-soldered pipe joints in buildings can release lead into the water supply. The use of lead in many products has been banned by the United States government.

Each year, humans release 450,000 tons of lead into the air, mostly through vehicle exhaust. Lead poisoning can damage the brain and nervous system. Signs of lead poisoning include behavioral problems, anemia, decreased mental functioning, vomiting, and cramps. Children may ingest lead by eating paint chips containing lead. They absorb lead more easily and therefore are more vulnerable to its destructive properties. Lead requires time to build up in a pipe before it reaches hazardous levels. Running the water in a tap for a short time can significantly reduce the water-borne lead that may have accumulated overnight.

Asbestos

Asbestos, a mineral widely used in construction and manufacturing, is found in fireproofing materials, shingles, floor tiles, and insulation. Exposure to friable (flaking) asbestos increases the risk of lung cancer and cancer of the digestive tract. If the asbestos becomes airborne, the fibers can be trapped inside the lungs, causing lung and other cancers. The development of these cancers may not be evident until many years after exposure.

Radon

Radon is a naturally occurring radioactive gas that is odorless, colorless, and tasteless. It is emitted from uranium. When radon is released into the air, it is harmless; however, it poses a health hazard when it is released from soil through the cracks in the foundation of a house and becomes trapped in an enclosed space such as the basement. Particles become trapped in the lungs, increasing the risk of lung cancer. This risk is greater for smokers than for non-smokers.

Water Pollution

The shining water that moves
in the streams and rivers
is not simply water, but the
blood of your grandfather's
grandfather.

Each ghostly reflection in the
clear waters of the lakes
tells the memories in the
life of our people.

The water's murmur is the
voice of your great-great-
grandmother.

The rivers are our brothers.
They quench our thirst.

They carry our canoes and
feed our children.

You must give to the rivers
the kindness you would
give any brother.

— Chief Seattle[9]

Water is the earth's most abundant resource. More than 75 percent of the earth's surface is covered with water, which stores vast quantities of heat, thus playing a major role in climate control. About 97 percent of all water is salt water, the major component of oceans. Only 3 percent of the earth's water is fresh and found in lakes. Two percent of the fresh water is locked in ice sheets. Less than 1 percent is suitable for human consumption,[10] as illustrated in Figure 13.1.

Like air, water is essential to life. Our bodies consist of two-thirds water. The average person in the United States uses 125 gallons of water each day. Water cannot be used up. It evaporates into the atmosphere and returns to the earth's surface in the form of rain, snow, sleet, or hail.

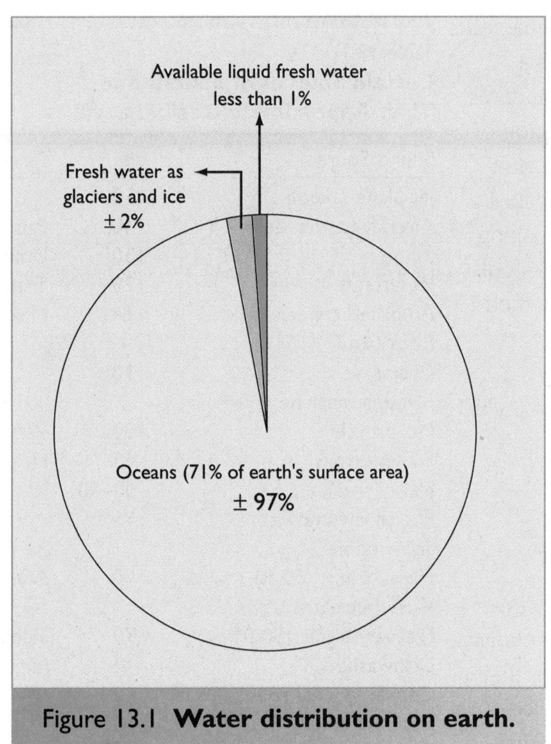

Figure 13.1 **Water distribution on earth.**

We threaten the quality of our water supply by dumping everything from fertilizers and detergents to industrial wastes and sewage into this precious resource. The main sources of water pollution are industrial wastes, animal fertilizers, human sewage, and thermal pollution.

When pollutants are channeled into non-flowing bodies of water such as lakes, eutrophication can occur. **Eutrophication** is the accelerated growth of algae that thrive on the inorganic pollutants, especially nitrogen and phosphorus. When the algae die and decompose, oxygen is consumed, thereby depriving fish and other living things of this life-sustaining element.

People who drink polluted water are in danger of getting serious diseases such as typhoid fever, cholera, parasitic worms, and dysentery. These are not a serious problem in the United States, but polluted water kills at least 25 million people in developing nations each year.[11] Dysentery, which is spread by disease-causing microbes that are frequently found in polluted water, causes severe diarrhea.

Viruses found in human wastes can contaminate water, causing hepatitis. Bacteria carried in polluted water can cause intestinal disorders. Swimming in polluted lakes and rivers also threatens one's health, because these harmful microbes can enter the body through the mouth and nose. Pollution can cause an increase in sodium concentrations in the water, presenting additional health risks to people with high blood pressure. Sewage, animal wastes, and agricultural chemicals increase the amount of nitrates in the water and can kill fish and animals. Infants who drink water contaminated with nitrates are at risk of contracting blood diseases.

Sediment consists of bits of solid matter from loose soil, dead plant and animal matter, and human wastes. Sediment clouds the water and carries bacteria that can cause disease.

In 1973, the U. S. government enacted the federal Water Pollution Act as a means of developing national standards for water quality. Under the direction of the EPA, each state sets pollution standards for drinking water and for lakes and other bodies of water, thus making fresh water safe to drink, to use for cooking, or to swim in. To think that bottled water from "natural springs" is any less polluted than water from the tap is a misconception. Tap water is tested daily; spring water used for bottled water is tested from time to time.

Thermal Pollution

Thermal (or heat) **pollution** occurs when water is warmed by power plants that use the water as a coolant for their equipment. Before being channeled back to its source, the water absorbs heat from the equipment and is then released back into the environment. The higher-than-normal temperatures reduce the amount of oxygen in the water, thus killing fish, aquatic animals, and water plants such as algae that produce the needed oxygen.

Oil Pollution

Oil spills from tankers and offshore drilling operations and waste oil from cars and other machines prevent sunlight from penetrating the water, thereby killing birds and fish and harming sea life. Oil can enter the tissue of shellfish, causing a health hazard to humans who eat them. Birds with oil-soaked feathers cannot fly and will drown or die.

Noise Pollution

Like other forms of pollution, noise is not just a nuisance; it can have an adverse affect on health. Noise pollution is created by transportation, industry, and loud music. Noise levels are calculated in decibels (db). One **decibel** represents the minimum level of hearing for humans. A sound that is 10 times louder is 10 db; another sound 100 times louder is 20 db; one 1,000 times louder is 30 db. Noise 80 to 85 db and above is considered loud. Table 13.1 shows sound levels from selected sources.

Table 13.1
Certain Sources of Sounds and Their Approximate Decibel Level

Sound Source	db	Response Criteria
Jet plane takeoff	150	
Aircraft carrier deck	140	Painfully loud
	130	Limited amplified speech
Jet aircraft flyover	120	Threshold of pain
Amplified guitar	114	Maximum vocal effort
Rock band		
Chainsaw	110	
Riveting machine		
Motorcycle	100	Very annoying
Subway train	95	Hearing damage (after 8 hours)
Heavy truck	50–90	Threshold of annoyance
Power lawnmower	90	
Snowmobile		
Heavy traffic (50 ft)	80	Annoying
Vacuum cleaner		
Freeway traffic (50 ft)	70	Telephone use difficult
Dishwasher		Intrusive
Conversational speech (3 ft)	60	
Business office	50	Quiet
Average residence	40	
Library	30	Very quiet
Broadcast studio	20	
	10	Just audible
	0	Threshold of audibility

Our ears function well as receivers of sound vibrations. When sound waves produce vibrations so strong that they are distorted, they can cause discomfort and possible damage to the ears. Even limited exposure to a loud noise can cause temporary hearing loss. Noise increases stress levels, resulting in headaches, tension, sleep disturbances, and increased anxiety.

An estimated 20 million people are regularly exposed to noise levels that can cause hearing loss. In addition to causing hearing damage, exposure to loud noise can cause an increase in blood pressure, constriction of blood vessels, and increases in blood cholesterol levels.

The Greenhouse Effect

Also called **global warming**, the **greenhouse effect** is a natural process that occurs when certain gases present in the atmosphere (such as carbon dioxide, water vapor, methane, chlorofluorocarbons [CFCs], ozone, and nitrous oxide) allow much of the sun's visible radiation to pass through the atmosphere to the earth's surface but trap the infrared heat reflected from the sun-warmed earth and redirect much of this heat back to the surface. These heat-trapping gases act like the glass panels of a greenhouse and provide the heat needed for our existence on Earth.

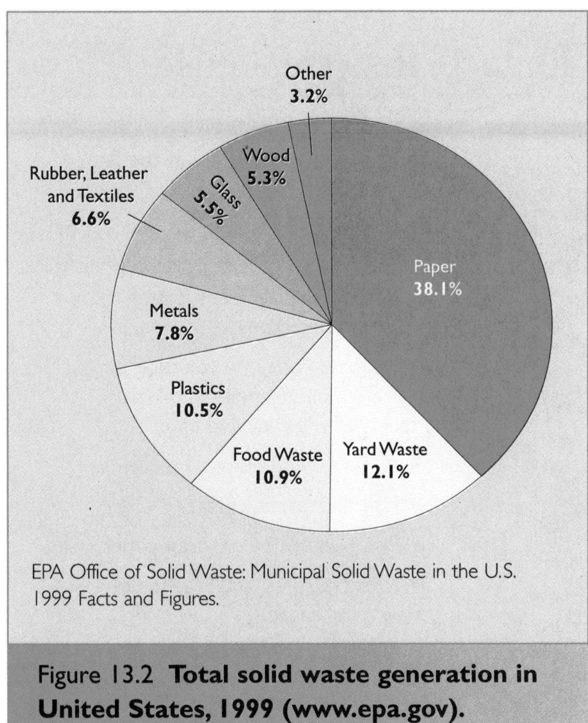

EPA Office of Solid Waste: Municipal Solid Waste in the U.S. 1999 Facts and Figures.

Figure 13.2 Total solid waste generation in United States, 1999 (www.epa.gov).

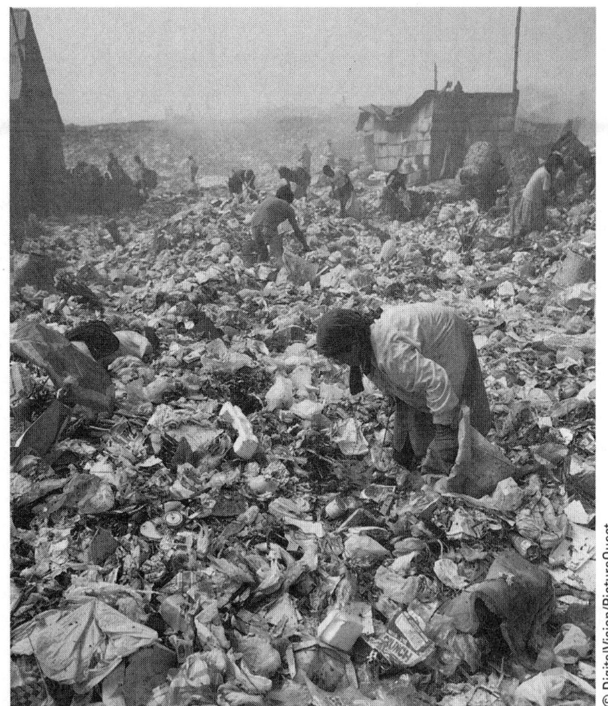

The problem of solid waste accumulation requires a multifaceted approach: recycle, reuse, refurbish.

Without the greenhouse effect, the earth's temperature would plunge to a frigid 3°F, and all living things would freeze to death.

However, burning fossil fuels increases the concentration of greenhouse gases in the atmosphere, adding to the greenhouse effect. Approximately 80 percent of the carbon dioxide emissions can be attributed to the burning of fossil fuels and is a major component of greenhouse gases.

Deforestation, the destruction of forests to make room for crops and grazing animals and to harvest timber, also has a significant impact on global warming. It reduces the number of trees available to absorb carbon dioxide. The carbon dioxide stored in trees is released into the atmosphere when the trees decay, are cut, or burned. Some scientists predict that, because this destruction adds to the greenhouse effect, temperatures will rise, polar ice caps will melt, and sea levels will rise, flooding coastal areas. These effects can occur worldwide, thus causing changes in climate that can affect agriculture.

Household temperature control, through the use of furnaces, air conditioners, and hot water heaters, accounts for 90 percent of the energy used in most American homes. Conserving energy in the home can prevent thousands of pounds of carbon dioxide from entering the atmosphere, thus reducing the impact of the greenhouse.

Solid Waste Accumulation

Solid waste is a byproduct of the technology that supports a rapidly increasing population. By the year 1999, Americans produced an estimated 230 million tons of garbage. Garbage disposal is a growing problem. Currently, nearly 67 percent of the solid waste in the United States ends up in landfills and dumps. An additional 16 percent of our trash is incinerated. Unfortunately, we recycle only 17 percent of our waste. Nearly 40 percent of our trash consists of paper, newspapers, magazines, books, packaging material, and junk mail. Food and yard clippings account for 25 percent of our waste. The remaining 35 percent consists of plastic, metal, glass, and other materials.[12] Figure 13.2 gives a breakdown of solid waste generation in the United States. Reduction and control of solid waste requires a concentrated, multifaceted approach to reduce the sources of waste and to recycle, reuse, and refurbish the products.

Hazardous Wastes

Hazardous wastes include the toxins that pollute our air and water and also the pesticides sprayed on crops, the chemicals transported on roads and rails, and those found in household

For Your Health

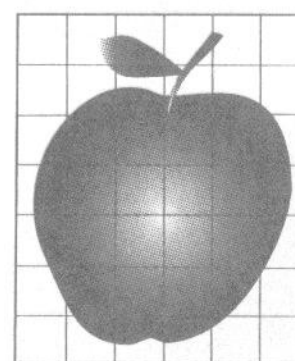

The Three R's: Reduce, Recycle, Reuse

- Buy only what you need and use it up.
- Buy durable products.
- Avoid packaging made of more than one material, because it is more difficult to recycle.
- Choose items that are packaged in recycled material.
- Select products that are recyclable in your community.
- Reuse what you buy.
- Line your trash can with paper.
- Make rags of old clothing to use instead of paper towels.
- Donate unwanted clothing and furniture rather than throw it away.
- Reuse gift boxes and wrapping paper.
- Recycle products such as aluminum cans, glass, plastics, and paper.
- Buy foods in bulk or economy-size containers and wrapped in the least amount of packaging.
- Purchase items sold in refillable or recyclable containers.
- Buy milk and juice in paper rather than plastic cartons.
- Request paper rather than plastic bags at the supermarket or carry groceries in a reusable bag.
- Avoid buying disposable items.
- Use fluorescent lights.
- Use both sides of scrap paper.
- Save glass jars and plastic containers for reuse.
- Use the recycle bins.
- Buy recycled paper products.
- Carry your lunch in a box or reusable bag.

To Save Energy:

- Turn off lights when not needed.
- Do not run water while brushing your teeth.
- Take brief showers rather than baths to save water.
- Repair drips and leaky pipes.
- Walk, ride bikes, and use public transportation to reduce air pollution.

products. Many hazardous wastes end up in the water supply and become water pollutants. Household hazardous waste such as cleansers, polishes, and pesticides can be toxic, corrosive, inflammable, caustic, volatile, or explosive. Toxins can enter the body through ingestion, inhalation, or absorption through the skin, causing damage to the nervous system, liver, kidneys, or reproductive system.

PCBs are found in garbage and industrial waste landfills and dumps. PCBs are absorbed by fish and birds and may cause cancer or liver damage. **PVC** (polyvinyl chloride), used by the plastics industry, is toxic to fish and can enter the food chain, thus affecting

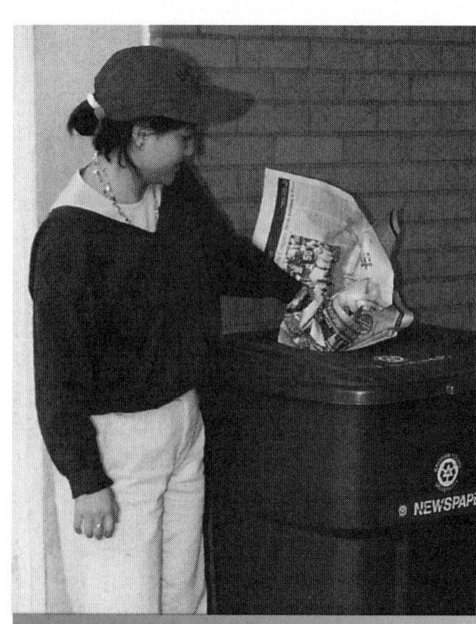

Only about 10% of the trash in the United States is recycled.

For Your Health

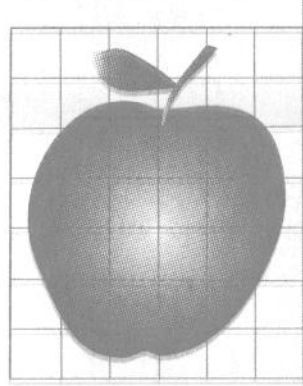

Anti-Pollution Measures

To conserve and preserve:

- Don't pour household chemicals or pesticides down the drain. Take them to a collection site.
- Use low-phosphate detergents.
- Leave lawn clippings on the lawn or compost yard trimmings.
- Never use your toilet as a trash can. The septic system is designed to handle liquid and solid human waste, not materials meant for the trash can.
- Install water-saving faucets and shower heads.
- When washing your car at home, use a bucket, not a running garden hose.
- Carpool or use public transportation if you can.
- Don't pour used oil or antifreeze down the drain or into drainage ditches. Take them to a service station.
- Get involved in neighborhood and community clean-up projects.
- Recycle!

humans. PVC can cause liver damage and cancer and can be transmitted to babies during breast feeding. CFCs from aerosol sprays, fire extinguishers, air-conditioning equipment, and refrigerators may damage the protective ozone layer. Children are especially sensitive to each of these toxic hazardous wastes. Much less solid waste will accumulate if we practiced the 3Rs: Reduce, Reuse, and Recycle.

Pesticides

Each year, weeds, insects, bacteria, fungi, viruses, birds, rodents, mammals, and other organisms considered pests consume or destroy an estimated 48 percent of the world's food production. In an effort to reduce this loss, 1,500 different substances are used in more than 33,000 commercial products.

In 1962, Rachel Carson published *Silent Spring,* which drew attention to the hazards of **pesticides**. Widespread use of chlorinated hydrocarbons—such as aldrin, dieldrin, and DDT—is dangerous, not only because they are toxic but also because these chemicals accumulate in human tissue, decompose slowly, and remain toxic for a long time. One of the best-studied pesticides is DDT, an insecticide composed of chlorinated hydrocarbons used in agriculture and lawns. Although its use is now banned in the United States, traces of DDT can still be found. DDT contaminated many terrestrial and aquatic ecosystems, where it passed through food chains from one organism to another. DDT consumed by fish and birds entered the tissues of human consumers. Environmentalists and other researchers publicized the hazards of DDT, convincing the EPA to ban its use in 1973. However, more than one-fourth of the fruit and vegetables sold in the United States is imported and may contain several different types of pesticide residues.

Carbonates, such as Sevin and Temik, are insecticides that inhibit an important enzyme in the central nervous system (acetylcholineaterase), making them nerve poisons. They are highly irritating to the eyes and may cause leukemia and lung cancer. They have been shown to cause birth defects and aplastic anemia in children.

Organophosphorous pesticides such as diazinon, parathion, and malathion are water-soluble and,

Some Non-Hazardous Alternatives to Frequently Used Household Products

- Air freshener: Set vinegar in an open dish.
- Drain cleaner: Pour boiling water down the drain, using a plunger or metal snake as needed.
- Furniture polish: Mix 1 teaspoon of lemon oil with 1 pint of mineral oil; or rub crushed raw nuts on wood surfaces.
- Household insecticides: Wash leaves of house plants with mild soapy water and rinse well.
- Moth control: Use cedar chips or place clothes in cedar chest.
- Oven cleaner: Mix equal parts of salt, baking soda, and water.
- Roach control: Use one chopped bay leaf mixed with cucumber skins.
- Silver cleaner: Soak silver in 1 quart of warm water mixed with 1 teaspoon salt and a piece of aluminum foil.
- Window cleaner: Mix 2 tablespoons vinegar in 1 quart of water, and use newspaper to wipe glass.

therefore, easily absorbed into the body. Humans exposed to low levels of organophosphorous pesticides may suffer from drowsiness, confusion, cramps, diarrhea, vomiting, headaches, and difficult breathing. Higher levels of exposure can cause convulsions, paralysis, tremors, coma, and even death.

Nontoxic alternatives to pesticides include pulling weeds instead of using herbicides and fertilizing with manure rather than chemical fertilizers. Leaves and shrub clippings can be composted rather than burned or bagged.

Endangered Species

More than 1.4 million species of plants and animals have been identified and named. Thousands of plant species are edible and more nutritious than many of the plant foods we eat today. Many plants have pharmaceutical value and could cure dreaded diseases that still threaten us.

The rain forests, located in a geographic zone that encircles the equator, are home to half of all species on earth. Deforestation caused by cattle ranching, logging, fuel wood collecting, mining, agriculture, burning, and construction of roads and dams destroys many of these species. Although some of the loss of species stems from the natural course of events, humans are the cause of most extinction. The challenge of striking a balance between protecting endangered species and solving economic concerns is a major environmental issue.

Personal Environmental Efforts

A quick and effective way to make more land available for growing food is to change our eating habits and to eat lower on the food chain. This means eating more vegetables, grains, and fruit and limiting our consumption of red meat. The typical American diet consists of almost 35 percent meat products. The United States has fewer than 5 percent of the world's population, but consumes more than 25 percent of its agricultural resources.

Other measures include avoiding processed foods and foods that contain additives; eating fewer foods that contain sugar; reducing the intake of foods high in fat; eating fresh produce when possible; and eating organically grown food when possible (see for example Learning Experiences in Chapter 3 on nutrition). If all of these strategies were implemented, harmful pollutants would be reduced, thereby improving personal and environmental health.

Summary

Ecology consists of living things interacting in their natural environment. Ecosystems consist of plants, animals, and other organisms interacting with the nonliving environment to form a self-sustaining unit. Through certain destructive acts, such as the various forms of pollution, people can degrade the environment and create health problems for themselves in doing so.

The Environmental Protection Agency is responsible for enforcing the Clean Air Act and recycling strategies. Air pollutants include carbon monoxide, sulfur oxides, nitrogen oxides, hydrocarbons, and ozone. Indoor air pollutants include lead (primarily from lead-based paints, which are now illegal), asbestos, and radon.

Pollutants also enter the water supply and can cause eutrophication in lakes and other inland water bodies. Other forms of pollution include thermal pollution and oil pollution. Noise pollution can have negative effects when people are exposed to high decibel levels over time, even from brief exposure. Deforestation produces a greenhouse effect and also threatens endangered species. The accumulation of solid wastes creates overflowing landfills. Hazardous waste contains toxins from pesticides and radioactivity.

Individuals can sustain resources by taking measures to reduce waste, conserve energy, recycle, and reuse products. They also can encourage people they know to do the same.

Web Sites

Acorn Naturalists: Science and Environmental Education
www.acorn.group.com

American Council on Science and Health
www.acsh.org/environment/index/html

Center for Environmental Education
www.cee-ane.org

Centers for Disease Control: National Center for Environmental Health
www.cdc.gov/nceh

Environmental Health Coalition
www.environmentalhealth.org/index1.html

Environmental Health Now: Medline Plus Health Information
www.nlm.nih.gov/medlineplus/environmentalhealth.html/oc/factsheets

Especially for Kids: Office of Response and Restoration, National Ocean Service, National Oceanic and Atmospheric Administration
www.response.restoration.noaa.gov/kids/kids.html

Green Brick Road—Environmental and Global Education Resources
www.abr.org

Health, Environment and Work
www.agius.com/hew/index.htm

John Heinz III Center for Science, Economics and the Environment
www.us-ecosystems.org

Let's Get Growing—Environment and Nature Educational Materials, K–12
www.letsgetgrowing.com

National Environmental Education & Training Foundation
www.neetf.org/Health/index.shtm

National Environmental Health Association
www.neha.org

National Institute of Environmental Health Sciences, U. S. Department of Health and Human Services, National Institutes of Health www.niehs.nih.gov/oc/factsheets/fskids.htm

National Kids Safety Council
www.nsc.org/ehc.html

Resource Center of Environmental and Occupational Health Sciences in Association with Rutgers University
www.eohsi.rutgers.edu/rc

U. S. Department of Agriculture: Natural Resources Conservation Service: Ecosystem Management Resources
www.nhq.nrcs.usda.gov

U. S. Environmental Protection Agency; Office of Children's Health Protection
www.epa.gov/children

Resources

Grades K–2

Cole, J. *The Magic School Bus Hops Home.* New York: Scholastic, 1995.

This imaginatively illustrated TV tie-in book is about animal habitats.

Cole, J. *The Magic School Bus on the Ocean Floor.* New York: Scholastic, 1992.

This colorfully illustrated book describes aquatic life.

Cole, J. *The Magic School Bus at the Waterworks.* New York: Scholastic, 1986.

This award-winning book (*Boston Globe*/Horn Book for Nonfiction) helps young children understand water.

MacDonald, S. *We Learn All About Protecting Our Environment.* Carthage, IL: Fearon Teacher Aids, 1993.

This teacher's resource book contains information and 40 activities that will help students practice readiness skills while learning about the environment.

Ryder, J. *Where Butterflies Grow.* New York: Lodestar Books, 1989.

Through this imaginative story, young students will observe the metamorphosis from caterpillar to butterfly.

Ryder, J. *The Snail's Spell.* New York: F. Warne, 1982.

This story helps children develop an appreciation for nature.

Dr. Seuss. *The Lorax.* New York: Random House, 1971.

This book, written in verse, describes one man's impact on the environment.

Sheekan, K., and M. Waidner. *Earth Child.* Tulsa: Council Oak Books, 1991.

320 pages of suggested games, stories, activities, experiments, and ideas about living lightly on Earth.

Grades 3–4

Dee, C. *Kid Heroes of the Environment.* Berkeley, CA: Earth Works Press, 1991.

This book contains explanations of simple things that students have done to help the environment.

Jeffers, S. *Brother Eagle, Sister Sky.* New York: Dial Books, 1991.

This award-winning book presents the words of wisdom in verse attributed to Chief Seattle. Beautifully illustrated, it will nurture an appreciation for the environment.

McHarry, J. *The Great Recycling Adventure.* Atlanta: Turner Publications, 1994.

Students gain an appreciation for "old things" in this imaginatively illustrated, lift-a-flap book on recycling.

Ortleb, E. P. *Air Quality and Pollution.* St. Louis: Milliken, 1990.

This teacher's guide provides visual aids, worksheets, and activity pages that will increase student awareness of air quality.

Roettger, Doris. *It's A Child's World: Pollution, Recycling, Trash, and Litter.* Carthage, IL: Fearon Teacher Aids, 1991.

This teacher's guide provides resource information that will help teachers design lessons on pollution, recycling, trash, and litter using nonfiction to promote literacy across the curriculum.

Seabury, D. *Earth Smart.* West Nyack, NY: Center for Applied Research, 1994.

Ready-to-use environmental science activities for the elementary classroom.

Simon, Seymour. *Earth Words.* New York: HarperCollins, 1995.

A beautifully illustrated dictionary of the environment.

Taplin, A. *Recycling in the Environment*. St. Louis: Milliken, 1991.

This teacher's guide is part of an environmental series designed to help teachers of third-, fourth-, or fifth-graders provide lessons that develop an awareness of basic ecological principles. Included in this book are color transparencies, reproducibles, and a teacher's guide.

Grades 5–6

Allen, J. *Earth Matters*. Torrance, CA: Frank Schaffer, 1994.

This teacher's guide contains strategies and activities for an interdisciplinary approach to teaching environmental issues.

Bonnet, R., and D. Keen. *Environmental Science: 49 Science Fair Projects*. Blue Ridge Summit, PA: McGraw-Hill, 1990.

This book introduces students to ecology through easy-to-understand procedures and experiments.

Children's Task Force on Agenda 21. *Rescue Mission Planet Earth*. New York: Kingfisher Books, 1994.

Butterfield, M. *1000 Facts About the Earth*. New York: Kingfisher Books, 1992.

Christie, T. *Global Alert!* Carthage, IL: Good Apple, 1988.

This activity book focuses on radon, hazardous waste, acid rain, water pollution, and other environmental issues; includes numerous word games and activities.

Croall, S., and W. Rankin. *Ecology for Beginners*. New York: Pantheon Books, 1982.

A humorous history of ecology.

Ortleb, E.P., and R. Candice. *Environment and Pollution*. St. Louis: Milliken Publishing, 1986.

This teacher's guide book contains background information, 12 color transparencies, and 20 reproducible pages to help students understand the relationships between living things and the environment.

Savan, B. *Earthwatch Earthcycles and Ecosystems*. Reading, MA: Addison-Wesley, 1991.

This book contains activities that will help students explore ways by which they can make the earth safer for all its inhabitants.

Environmental Health Resources

Cousteau Society, Inc.
930 W. 21st Street
Norfolk, VA 23517

Defenders of Wildlife
1244–19th Street, NW
Washington, DC 20036

Earth First!
PO Box 7
Canton, NY 13617

Friends of Animals
PO Box 1244
Norwalk, CT 06856

Greenpeace USA
1436 U Street, NW
Washington, DC 20009

Kids Against Pollution
PO Box 775, High Street
Closter, NJ 07624

National Arbor Day Foundation
211 North 12th Street
Lincoln, NE 68508

National Audubon Society
700 Broadway
New York, NY 10003

National Wildlife Federation
1400–16th Street, NW
Washington, DC 20036-2266

Sierra Club
730 Polk Street
San Francisco, CA 94104

U. S. Department of Agriculture
U. S. Forest Service
PO Box 96090
Washington, DC 20077

Notes

1. D. Chiras, *Environmental Science Action for a Sustainable Future*, 4th ed. (Redwood City, CA: Benjamin/Cummings, 1994).
2. S. Boyd, *Global Warming and Energy Choices*, A Community Action Guide (Washington, DC: Project Concern, 1991).
3. National Institute of Environmental Health Sciences, *Fact Sheet #2. How Do You Study Environmental Health?* Washington, DC: U. S. Department of Health and Human Services, National Institutes of Health, August, 1996).
4. National Institute of Environmental Health Sciences, *A Family Guide. 20 Easy Steps to Personal Environmental Health Now*. Washington, DC: U. S. Department of Health and Human Services. National Institutes of Health, 2000).
5. J. Palmer and P. Neal, *The Handbook of Environmental Education* (New York: Routledge, 1994).
6. Cited in S. Jeffers, *Brother Eagle, Sister Sky: A Message from Chief Eagle* (New York: Dial Books, 1991).
7. See note 1.
8. N. Meyers, *Gaia: An Atlas of Planet Management* (New York: Anchor Books, 1993).
9. See note 6.
10. S. Dashefsky, *Environmental Literacy* (New York: Random House, 1993).
11. See note 8.
12. G. Scott, "Reducing, Reusing, Recycling," *Current Health* (October 2, 1993), 24–26.

Learning Experiences

The following describes environmental health concepts and principles that can be incorporated into interdisciplinary lessons, and the resulting outcomes expected of children at different grade levels. If students understand the relationship between the quality of the environment and the quality of life for the individual and society, they will accept responsibility for protecting and improving the environment.

Grades K–2

Young children delight in the discovery of nature. They are likely to benefit from hands-on experiences that will increase their sensory awareness of the natural world. They should begin to recognize that environmental factors have a direct effect on the health of the individual and of society and grasp the importance of taking action to protect and improve the environment. The following competencies are offered to help develop lesson plans that will nurture an appreciation for an ecological balance. Students will demonstrate the ability to advocate for personal, family, and community health.

Students will be able to

1. Recognize those characteristics of the environment that contribute to health.
2. Identify ways to protect and preserve a healthy environment.
3. Identify several ways their surroundings affect their feelings.
4. Identify how the senses interact with the environment to produce positive or negative feelings.
5. Identify natural resources and describe their uses, including
   a. water—we use to drink, bathe, swim, feed plants
   b. air—we breathe
   c. refuse—garbage disposal
   d. animals—pets, food
   e. plants—decorations, food
6. Observe and describe simple plant and animal communities including these elements:
   a. solar energy
   b. air
   c. moisture
   d. soil
   e. plants
   f. scavengers (worms, insects, and so on)
   g. decomposers (bacteria and fungi)
7. Describe the various needs of plants and animals.
8. Define pollution including
   a. air pollutants
   b. water pollutants
   c. litter
   d. noise
9. Identify how our actions affect components of the environment:
   a. water
   b. air
   c. refuse, garbage disposal
10. Identify the personal, emotional, social, and physical elements of the environment that contribute to an individual's safety, well-being, and enjoyment of life.
11. Demonstrate ways of caring for the home, school, and community environment.
12. Describe wise uses of natural resources.

Grade 3–4

Students in grades 3 and 4 can learn their role and the role of the family, class, and school within the environment. They can learn to use resources and to assess how their personal actions contribute to development of a safer and healthier environment. In addition, they should learn how to communicate the need for a quality environment to others. Elementary-level students should identify how they may use resources to make decisions that improve the quality of their personal environment. They learn to accept limited responsibility for their personal impact on the environment.

Students will demonstrate the ability to advocate for personal, family, and community health.

Students will be able to

1. Recognize characteristics of the environment that contribute to health.
2. Identify ways to protect and preserve a healthy environment.
3. Discuss ways to help promote a healthy environment in the neighborhood.
4. Identify forms of pollution: air pollutants, water pollutants, noise, land pollutants.
5. Describe how pollution is harmful to the health of the individual and the community.
6. List the ways individuals contribute to pollution.
7. Identify ways of controlling pollution to protect our community.
8. Describes ways to conserve water, land, and wildlife.
9. Describe how the physical, social, and emotional elements of the environment affect feelings.
10. Distinguish between the personal actions that enhance the environment and those that harm the environment.
11. Describe how personal decision making effects the environment.
12. Initiate changes in the personal environment that contribute to development of a safer and healthier environment.
13. Demonstrate and communicate the need for personal involvement in improving the environment.
14. Observe and describe plant and animal communities.
15. Describe and discuss individuals' rights and responsibilities as they relate to the environment.
16. Describe the role of the family and home within the environment.
17. Describe the role of the class and school within the environment.

Grades 5–6

Students should demonstrate ways the individual and the community can contribute to the solution of environmental problems. They should identify how people interact with the environment and how those interactions produce positive or negative feelings in an individual. Further, they should identify resources that individuals may consult for accurate information concerning the environment. They should accept responsibility for making a positive impact on the environment.

Students will be able to

1. Demonstrate the ability to advocate for personal, family, and community health.
2. Understand the need for personal involvement in improving the environment.
3. Identify the personal, emotional, social, and physical elements of the environment that contribute to feelings of safety, well-being, and enjoyment.
4. Relate the concept of ecological balance to the survival of the individual and society.
5. Identify potential hazards to the environment: radiation, pesticides, natural disaster, contaminants.
6. Relate how destructive elements in the environment can threaten the quality of life.
7. Discuss the need for protecting and improving the environment.
8. Explain personal responsibility for promoting environments that contribute to feelings of safety, well-being, and enjoyment.
9. Identify how individuals, community groups, and governmental agencies can protect and improve the environment.
10. Explain how technological changes have altered the environment.
11. Explain the interrelationship between individuals and the environment.
12. Describe ecological factors that may favorably or unfavorably influence an individual's health.
13. Identify health problems that have ecological implications.
14. Describe how conservation helps maintain a healthful environment.

For suggestions on creating a rubric with which to evaluate student performance of Learning Experiences, see page 13.

Learning Experience 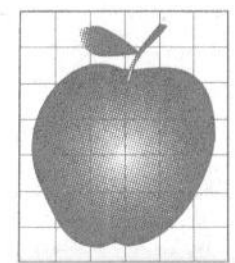 13-1

Sorting and Classifying Trash and Litter

Grade Level

K–2

Primary Disciplines

Math, Science, Technology

Learning Objectives

Following this activity, students will be able to

- Compare the similarities of their groupings.
- Chart their findings.

Time Required

40 minutes

Materials

Rubber gloves for each student

Description of Activity

Divide the class into cooperative working teams and take them on a trash-collecting expedition around the school or neighborhood. After returning to class, have the teams sort the litter and trash they've collected. A spokesperson for each team explains why the team members classified the items as they did. The teams compare the similarities of their groupings and then chart their findings. Here are some suggestions for classifications:

- Items that are part of nature
- Items that people make
- Items than can be recycled
- Broken items
- Items that can be fixed

Homework

Students collect and bring to class a medium-sized bag filled with paper, aluminum, cardboard, wood scraps, and other items around the home that have been discarded but can be reused in a new way.

Evaluation

The groups are assessed according to the chart below.

	4	3	2 1	
Teamwork	Worked well together. Stayed on task. Each member was involved.	Worked together. Stayed on task most of the time. Each member was involved.	Attempted to work together. Often off-task. Not all members were involved. Responsibility was unevenly shared.	Little or no teamwork. Did not respect each other's opinions. Disagreed. Relied exclusively on one person.
Active learning	Sought different solutions. Explored different approaches and strategies in an original or creative way.	Occasionally sought different solutions. Occasionally explored different approaches and strategies in an original or creative way.	Sought a single solution.	Relied on the first solution and used only one strategy to find it.
Communications	Asked questions. Discussed ideas. Listened, offered constructive criticism.	Asked questions. Discussed ideas. Listened. Attempted a summary of ideas.	Communicated through processes and strategies, but did not listen to constructive criticism.	Members worked individually. Did not communicate. Lacked respect for each other.

Learning Experience 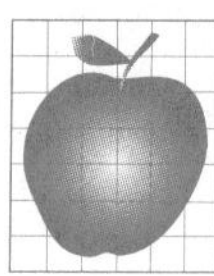 13-2

Recyling Relay

Grade Level

K–2

Primary Disciplines

Math, Science

Learning Objectives

Following this activity, students will be able to:

- Sort and separate objects.
- State the difference between recyclable and non-recyclable materials.

Time Required

20 minutes

Materials

Set of labeled recycling bins labeled "paper," "plastic," and "non-recyclable" for each team, recyclable items

Description of Activity

In teams of four, have students examine unsorted refuse (plastic bottles, papers and magazines, empty cartons, and so on). Place labeled recycling bins in front of each team. The teams place the refuse from their piles in the proper bins. The class examines the bins and discusses the rationale for placing each item in the specific bin.

Homework

Students will find out what is done with recyclable material in their home and bring in safe items for the activity.

Evaluation

When all teams have sorted their trash piles into the bins, the class will know the contents of each bin. In addition, the group will be assessed according to the chart below.

	4	3	2	1
Charting findings	Found one or more litter items from each of five categories.	Found one or more items from four of the five categories.	Found one or more litter items from three of the five categories.	Found one or more litter items from two of the five categories.
Classifying items	Was able to classify each item correctly.	Classified correctly four of the five items in four different categories.	Classified correctly three of the five items in three different categories.	Classified correctly two of the five items in two different categories.
Safety and health	Did not pick up dangerous items (broken glass, needles). Wore rubber gloves at all times.	Picked up two items or fewer that were considered somewhat dangerous or unhealthy. Not all members wore gloves at all times.	Picked up three items or fewer that were considered somewhat dangerous or unhealthy. Most members rarely wore gloves.	Picked up several items that clearly are unhealthy or dangerous (broken glass, needles). Did not wear gloves.

Learning Experience 13-3

Recycled Art

Grade Level

K–2

Primary Disciplines

Art, Social Science

Learning Objectives

Following this activity, students will be able to:

- Describe various ways to recycle.
- Demonstrate eye-hand coordination and fine-motor skills.

Time Required

30 minutes

Materials

Styrofoam, paper scraps, Popsicle sticks, string, glue

Description of Activity

Have students use Styrofoam, paper scraps, Popsicle sticks, aluminum foil, string, cardboard milk or juice cartons to create an artistic display.

Homework

Students bring in a cleaned cardboard milk or juice carton.

Evaluation

Students present and discuss their artwork and explain how it relates to recycling activities. Students are assessed according to the chart below.

	4	3	2	1
Use of material	Students used all material provided in a creative way.	Students used four of the items provided in a creative way.	Students used three of the items provided in a creative way.	Students used two of the items provided.
Describe ways to recycle	Students could name different ways to recycle each item.	Students named four different ways to recycle.	Students named three different ways to recycle.	Students named two different ways to recycle.
Presentation	Students clearly described their art objects. Students clearly explained how their art project related to recycling.	Students described their art objects. Students explained how their art project related to recycling.	Students described their art objects.	Students' description of their art object was unclear.

Learning Experience 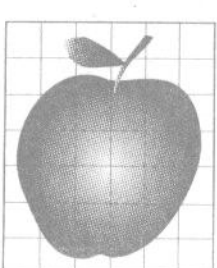 13-4

Milk Carton Birdhouse

Grade Level

K–2

Primary Discipline

Art

Learning Objectives

Following this activity, students will be able to:

- Describe a new way to recycle.
- Discuss an appreciation for nature.

Time Required

30 minutes

Materials

Clean half-gallon milk cartons (enough for every class member to receive one), string

Description of Activity

Introduction

Before class, cut a 1-inch hole in the side of each half-gallon milk carton approximately 2 inches from the bottom. Cut a strip from the side of another carton for a perch.

Activity

Discuss ways to recycle. Have students fold the strip and staple it to the milk carton below the opening. Have them use paper punches to punch two holes in the top of the carton and then thread string through the holes.

Homework

Students bring the birdhouses home. Parents help students tie their birdhouse to a tree near the home. Students observe and report on the activity surrounding the birdhouse.

Evaluation

Students are assessed using the chart below.

	4	3	2	1
Following Directions	Student correctly implements steps described in the activity.	Student follows directions but needs some help in one step.	Student follows directions but needs help in two steps.	Student needs help in all three steps.
Knowledge	Student gives three or more examples of ways to recycle.	Student gives two examples of ways to recycle.	Student gives one example of a way to recycle.	Student describes the project.

Learning Experience 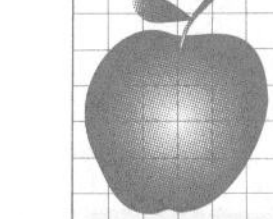 13-5

Miniature Landfill

Grade Level

3–4

Primary Discipline

Science

Learning Objectives

Following this activity, students will be able to

- Identify biodegradable litter.
- Demonstrate an understanding of landfills.

Time Required

Several 30-minute sessions (total duration is 6 months or longer)

Materials

Wooden match, apple core, plastic milk carton, short piece of cotton string, candy wrapper, foil gum wrapper, green leaf, glass marble, piece of newspaper, enough soil to fill milk carton, label

Description of Activity

1. Have students cut off the top of the plastic milk container.
2. Fill the milk carton with soil and bury the listed objects in it. Layer all objects in soil, so each object has its own space and is surrounded by soil.
3. Write the date and the list of buried objects on the label and attach it to the container.
4. Keep the milk container in a warm place for at least 6 months. Keep the soil moist throughout the experiment.
5. After 6 or more months, dump out the contents of the container. Note and record the appearance of each buried object.

Homework

None

Evaluation

Students are evaluated according to the chart below.

	4	3	2	1
Following directions	Student correctly implements all instructions.	Student needs assistance in implementing one of the steps.	Students need some assistance in implementing two of the steps.	Student needs assistance in implementing most of the steps.
Classification	Student correctly indicates which of the 8 items are biodegradable.	Student correctly indicates which of the 8 items are biodegradable.	Student correctly indicates 6 of the items presented.	Correctly identifies 4 of the items presented.
Knowledge	Student clearly describes a landfill; shows a clear understanding of the purpose of landfills; relates landfills to this project.	Student discusses landfills; shows some understanding of the purpose of landfills; describes the project.	Student discusses landfills and the project.	Student discusses the project.

Learning Experience 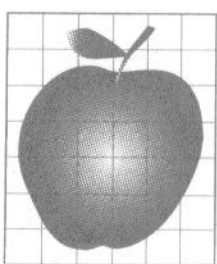 13-6

Creating Litmus Paper

Grade Level

3–4

Primary Disciplines

Math, Science

Learning Objectives

Following this activity, students will be able to

- Make litmus paper.
- Test for acidity.

Time Required

30 minutes

Materials

Chopping board, knife, half a red cabbage, bowl, sieve, measuring cup, saucer, scissors, blotting paper, two jars (one for water, one for vinegar), three small jars, labels, pencil, notebook

Description of Activity

Have students follow these steps:

1. Chop cabbage roughly and place in bowl.
2. Pour hot water over cabbage, just enough to cover cabbage.
3. Leave cabbage to soak until water turns purple.
4. Hold the sieve over the jar and slowly pour the cabbage water through it.
5. Cut out small strips of blotting paper. Dip both ends of blotting paper into cabbage water and lay dipped paper on a saucer for a few hours to dry.
6. Fill three small jars halfway to the top with water.
7. Label jar #1 "pure water." Label jar #2 "slightly acidic" and add a few drops of vinegar. Label the third jar "stronger acid" and fill to top with vinegar.
8. Place dried litmus paper into jar #1. (The color of the litmus paper remains blue.) Place new strips of litmus paper in jars #2 and #3. (The higher the acid content, the pinker the litmus paper.)

Homework

None

Evaluation

The chart below is used to assess the students.

	4	3	2	1
Following directions	Student correctly implements steps 1–8.	Student needs some help to implement some of the steps.	Student needs help to implement four or more steps.	Student needs help to implement most steps.
Knowledge	Student clearly describes the purpose of the project; fully describes the function of litmus paper; describes two or more testing situations using litmus paper.	Student describes purpose of the project; describes the function of litmus paper; gives one example of how litmus paper can be used for testing.	Student describes the project; shows an understanding of the function of litmus paper.	Student discusses the project.

Learning Experience 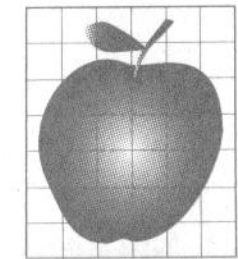 13-7

Air Pollution

Grade Level

3–4

Primary Disciplines

Math, Science

Learning Objectives

Following this activity, students will be able to explain air pollution.

Time Required

30 minutes

Materials

4" × 6" index card, scissors, transparent tape, thumbtack, magnifying lenses

Description of Activity

Have students implement the following procedure:

1. Fold a 4" × 6" index card in half so it is 4" × 3".
2. In the center of one-half of the folded card, cut a hole 2 × 2 cm.
3. Put a piece of transparent tape across the hole in the card so the sticky side faces inside.
4. Leave the card folded until you are ready to use it. Choose a place where you want to sample the air. Keep the card shut so it will not collect dirt in the meantime. Open the card and lay it near a tree, window frame, door frame, or other place. The tape should be sticky side up, showing through the hole.
5. Leave the card in place for 24 hours before you collect it. Do not leave it out in the rain. Look at the tape with a magnifying lens.
6. Observe and evaluate what you see.

Homework

None

Evaluation

Students are assessed according to the chart below.

	4	3	2	1
Following directions	Student correctly implements steps 1–6 with little or no assistance.	Student implements steps 1–6 with some assistance.	Student implements steps 1–6 with much assistance.	Student has difficulty implementing steps.
Knowledge	Student discusses air pollution; discusses the experiment.	Student describes air pollution; describes the experiment including observation.	Student shows some understanding of pollution; describes the experiment.	Student shows some understanding of air pollution or the experiment.

Learning Experience 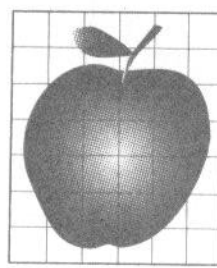 13-8

Feeding the Birds

Grade Level

5–6

Primary Discipline

Science

Learning Objectives

Following this activity, students will be able to

- Describe the relationship between animal populations and food supply.
- Report which bird will be attracted to a given type of food.

Time Required

45 minutes

Materials

Six aluminum pie plates with holes in them, three 2-liter plastic soda bottles with metal caps, scissors, three bolts and six corresponding nuts, mixed bag of wild bird seed, string, brass paper fasteners, box of crackers, bird identification book

Description of Activity

Have the students construct three identical bird feeders as follows:

1. Cut the bottom off a 2-liter plastic soda bottle. Cut 1"-long tabs in four equally spaced "sides" of the bottle. These tabs will be pushed through slots cut in an aluminum pie plate and fastened to it. The bird food will rest in the pie plate, and the holes in the plate will let rain drain through.
2. In the spaces between each tab, cut small V-shaped openings. When the bottle is filled with bird seed, the seed will come out the openings as the birds eat it.
3. Cut four slots in a pie plate that line up with the four tabs in the bottle. Push the tabs through the slots in the pie plate. Fold each tab up under the pie plate.
4. Punch a small hole with the end of the pair of scissors (or an awl) in each tab and through the pie plate. Place a brass paper fastener through each to hold them together. This attaches the base of the feeder to the bottle.
5. Punch a hole in a soda bottle cap, then punch a hole in the center of a second pie plate. This pie plate will go on top of the feeder and help shelter the food from rain. Place a bolt up through the inside of the cap and through the pie plate resting on top. Screw a nut into the bolt to hold the pie plate to the bottle cap. Tie a piece of string around the bolt. Screw another nut on top of the existing nut to secure the string tied between them. The other end of the string will be tied to a tree limb.
6. Separate the mixed bird seeds into piles, putting each kind in its own pile. Fill one feeder with one type of seed. Fill the second feeder with another type. Fill the third with crushed crackers. Tie the three feeders to a tree limb.
7. Observe and record the activity in the three bird feeders on a regular basis.

Homework

None

Evaluation

Students will be assessed according to the chart on page 467.

	4	3	2	1
Following directions	Student correctly implements all seven steps with little or no assistance.	Student implements all seven steps with some assistance.	Student implements all seven steps with much assistance.	Student is unable to implement the steps.
Knowledge	Student can describe the relationship between animal populations and food supply; is able to identify the bird types attracted to each food.	Student can describe the relationship between animal populations and food supply; can identify most of the bird types attracted to each food.	Student can provide simplistic connection between animal populations and food supply; can identify some of the bird types attracted to each food.	Student cannot describe the relationship between animal populations and food supply; can identify only one or two of the bird types attracted to each food.

Learning Experience 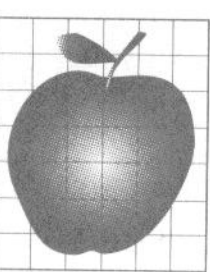 13-9

An Acrostic Poem

Grade Level

5–6

Primary Discipline

Language Arts

Learning Objectives

Following a nature field trip, students will write an acrostic poem based on their observations.

Time Required

20 minutes

Materials

Paper, pencils

Description of Activity

Have students write the name of an element of nature vertically on their papers. The word (pond, field, ocean, lake, forest) may appear in any location on the paper. Have students use the letters in that word to construct a poem expressing their feelings and ideas about the site of the field trip. The lines of the poem do not have to rhyme. Rather, the poem reflects students' feelings about the field trip site.

Examples:

Finding lots of
Interesting
w**E**eds
Look! A
bir**D** flies overhead

or

Flowers,
l**O**gs,
Robin
Eating
worm**S** and
na**T**ure all around.

Homework

None

Evaluation

The students will be able to

- Identify the elements of nature.
- Construct a poem.
- Describe their feelings and ideas about their field trip.

Source: J. Galle and P. Warren, *Ecology Discovery Activities Kit*. Copyright 1989, Prentice Hall. Reprinted with permission.

14

Safety, Injury Prevention, and First Aid

Carol Alberts and Suanne Maurer

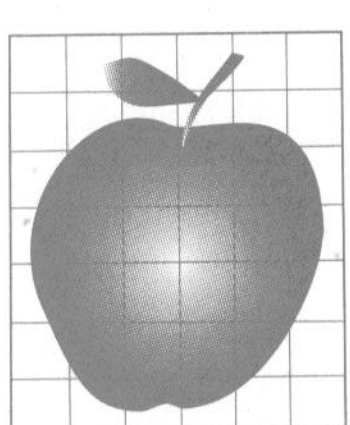

Chapter Outline

Safety Awareness

First Aid

Objectives

- Promote safety awareness in students and families
- Be able to activate the Emergency Medical Services (EMS) system
- Identify and practice first-aid procedures consistent with students' developmental level
- Demonstrate vehicular and pedestrian safety
- Show familiarity with the school emergency action plan
- Identify provisions of state Good Samaritan laws
- Demonstrate how to assess the victim and the accident scene
- Identify the symptoms of choking and know how to respond with the Heimlich maneuver
- Identify signs and symptoms of a heart attack
- Demonstrate the first aid procedure for shock
- Categorize the severity of internal and external signs of bleeding, including nosebleeds, and describe applicable first-aid procedures
- Describe the differences between first-, second-, and third-degree burns and first-aid treatments for each
- Describe what to do if a person has an asthma attack
- Define hyperglycemia and hypoglycemia and explain the differences between insulin shock and a diabetic coma

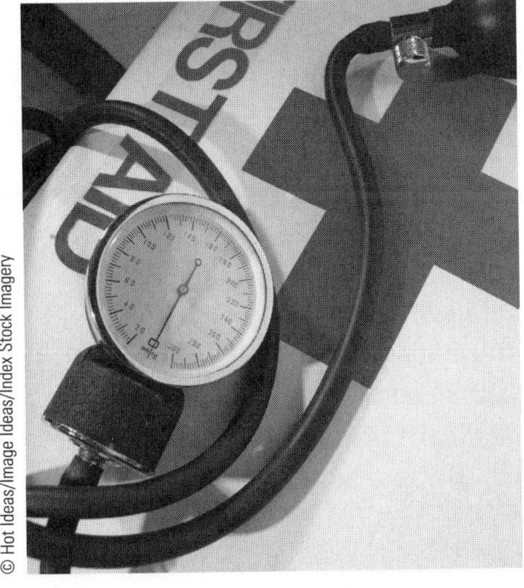

Kim's family bought her the best dirt bike she ever saw. It was red with silver stripes. She couldn't wait to go riding with her friends in the sand hills at the end of the street. When Samara came, Kim was all set to go, wearing her new matching helmet. Samara laughed and said, "Take off that silly helmet. You don't need it, and besides, all the kids will make fun of you." Kim's dad had told her that she could not ride the bike unless she wore a helmet. She tried to explain that to Samara, who laughed and said, "C'mon! All our parents want us to wear helmets, but we never do." Kim took off the helmet and hung it on the side of the bike. On the way to the dunes, the bike skidded out from under her and Kim hit the ground hard. She was dizzy and was bleeding from a wound on the side of her head. Samara ran to Kim and stood her up, trying to assist her down the street to the nearest house to get help.

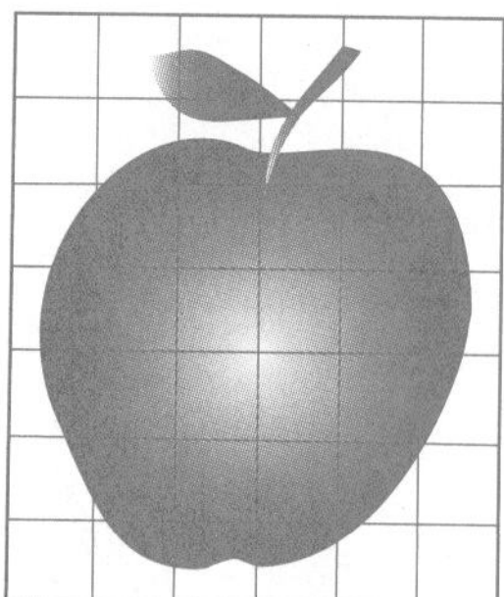

Because accidents happen when we least expect them, knowing what to do in the event of an emergency can lessen the extent of injury. With this knowledge, Samara would not have suggested that Kim get up immediately after her accident, and she might have showed Kim how to stop the bleeding by applying pressure while Samara went for help.

Most people at one time or another become involved in emergencies of varying severity and may not know what to do or how to help. Learning how to keep these emergencies from happening at all and how to access health emergency systems is important. This chapter provides the classroom teacher with a specific protocol for assessing a victim and summoning medical help. Teachers should use these measures for medical emergencies in the classroom and also teach them to students so that they are able to assist in medical emergencies when someone more qualified is not available.

All teachers and students should know how to activate the emergency medical services (EMS) system and how to assess a victim's status in a first-aid emergency. In addition, teachers who have had no first-aid or safety training should take a course prior to teaching any actual first-aid treatment procedures because improper treatment could harm an individual.

The American Red Cross, the National Safety Council, and the American Heart Association have certification courses that provide individuals with the knowledge and skills needed to respond effectively to medical emergencies. These include introductory, advanced, and teaching certification courses in safety education; first-aid training in cardiopulmonary resuscitation (CPR); and first aid for injuries and sudden illnesses. In some states, teachers can take these courses as part of a continuing education program; the courses may be required in other states.

Safety Awareness

Accidents account for a high percentage of injuries to children. Early educational experiences that promote safety are the best way to reduce the incidence of accidents and injuries. The following discussion identifies some of the situations and activities that have been found to be particularly applicable to children. Standards of safety-conscious behaviors in the areas of pedestrian, vehicular, fire, and home safety are in place in most locations. Specific safety concerns for recreational or environmental issues vary across the United States, though. Therefore, additional safety awareness lessons have to be designed to meet the needs of specific student populations.

Child Safety

The following statements represent an awareness of child safety that can reduce the chances of injury to your child. Check each statement that reflects your lifestyle.

- ☐ I buckle my child into an approved automobile safety seat even when making short trips.
- ☐ I teach my child safety by behaving safely in my everyday activities.
- ☐ I supervise my child whenever he or she is around water and maintain fences and gates that act as barriers to water.
- ☐ I have checked my home for potential fire hazards, and smoke detectors are installed and working.
- ☐ I have placed foods and small items that can choke my child out of his or her reach.
- ☐ I inspect my home, day-care center, school, babysitter's home, or wherever my child spends time for potential safety and health hazards.

If you checked only one or two statements, you should consider making changes in your lifestyle now.

Source: Adapted from American Red Cross, *First Aid: Responding to Emergencies*, 3d ed. (San Bruno, CA: Staywell, 2001), 464–465.

Approaches to Teaching Safety Awareness

In the early elementary school years, safety awareness education begins with identifying potentially dangerous situations in the school environment. Children need to understand the potential risk of physical harm in case of fire and when entering, exiting, or riding in cars and buses and crossing streets. After identifying these risks, students can practice appropriate behaviors and procedures for minimizing physical harm in these situations.

Walking children through fire-drill procedures and practicing bus and pedestrian safety are essential to children's forming an early conceptualization of personal safety. Among the measures that can be explored are crossing the street at the corner, looking both ways before crossing, riding bikes on the correct side of the road, and wearing bright colors (and reflective gear at night) to be more visible.

As soon as children are cognitively ready, they should be encouraged to discuss and participate in decision-making exercises regarding basic parameters of safe behavior and the reasons for basic rules in a safety-conscious lifestyle. Teachers should take advantage of teachable moments to reinforce positive student behaviors that demonstrate awareness and respect for safety-conscious behavior. For example, when children are running toward an area where cars are moving and remember to stop and look before entering that area, the behavior should be positively rewarded. Teachers on duty when school lets out should be alerted to these behaviors.

As children's knowledge of safety procedures becomes internalized, teachers should take advantage of opportunities for students to generalize the information and make decisions in other safety situations. Because we cannot teach children what to do in every potentially dangerous situation, the goal is to develop awareness of and sensitivity to risk of physical harm and the ability to make decisions that minimize that risk.

Vehicular and Pedestrian Safety

Once a child enters school, the ratio of adult-to-child supervision becomes more disparate. A teacher cannot hold every child's hand when crossing a street or walking to a bus stop. Therefore, children need to learn pedestrian and vehicular safety rules as soon as they begin school. One of the most significant adjustments they make in the school environment is to learn behaviors that will keep them physically safe.

One area of particular vulnerability is getting to and from school. K–2 students need to learn how to enter and exit vehicles, where to wait for cars and buses, and what to do when crossing a street. Lessons should include information on traffic lights and looking before crossing parking lots and driveways.

Home Safety

The following statements represent a safety-conscious lifestyle that can reduce your and others' chances of being injured. Check each statement that reflects your lifestyle.

- ☐ The stairways and halls in my home are well lit.
- ☐ I have nonslip tread or securely fastened rugs on my stairs.
- ☐ I keep all medications out of reach of children and in a locked cabinet.
- ☐ I keep any poisonous materials out of the reach of children, and in a locked cabinet.
- ☐ All rugs are firmly secured to the floor.
- ☐ I store any firearms, unloaded, in a locked place out of the reach of children and ammunition is stored separately.
- ☐ I keep the handles of pots and pans on the stove turned inward when I am using them.

If you checked only one or two statements, you should consider making changes in your lifestyle now.

Source: Adapted from American Red Cross, *First Aid: Responding to Emergencies*, 3d ed. (San Bruno, CA: Staywell, 2001), 464–465.

Recreational Safety

The following statements represent a safety-conscious lifestyle that can reduce your and others' chances being injured during recreational activity. Check each statement that reflects your lifestyle.

- ☐ I follow the rules laid down for any sport I take part in.
- ☐ I wear any recommended safety gear, such as a helmet or goggles, for any sport or activity.
- ☐ I wear a life jacket when I am in a boat.
- ☐ I enter the water feetfirst to check unknown water depths.
- ☐ I keep my recreational equipment in good condition.

If you checked only one or two statements, you should consider making changes in your lifestyle now.

Source: Adapted from American Red Cross, *First Aid: Responding to Emergencies*, 3d ed. (San Bruno, CA: Staywell, 2001).

Many cars and buses pick up students at the same time. Students need to know how to identify the correct bus or vehicle. Students who cannot read or identify numbers have to be given an alternative method of locating the correct bus. Students also need to recognize the importance of leaving the school only with the appropriate parent or individual assigned to pick them up. Children should be given a specific protocol for checking with a teacher or bus supervisor if they are offered a means of getting to or from school that departs from the usual plan.

The importance of wearing seat belts and putting them on properly is another aspect of safety education. According to statistics reported by the Centers for Disease Control and Prevention, 16.4 percent of high school students rarely or never wear seat belts.[1] Early education can help young people develop safety-conscious behavior and good decision-making skills. Appropriate behavior for riding on buses should be taught to children because school represents the first experiences on buses for most of them. Learning Experiences 14-4 and 14-6 identify information that children in grades K–2 need to know regarding pedestrian and vehicular safety. Once the children have learned appropriate safety behaviors in each of these areas, they should be given activities that require them to make decisions based on the safety rules for a variety of situations.

Home, School, and Recreational Safety

Safety-conscious behavior is needed in home, school, and recreational environments. Safety education in the home begins by creating a safe environment. Focusing on injury prevention by removing dangers from the home is a key element of safety education. This can include placing all medicines in areas where children cannot reach them, eliminating poisonous plants, labeling medicines and distinguishing them from candy, and covering electrical outlets. These safety measures, along with vigilant supervision, can reduce the incidence of preventable injuries.

Once students can identify which items are safe and which are not, they are ready to learn the reasons why poisonous substances are dangerous. The teacher might describe how some poisons affect the body. For example, some poisons make people sick to their stomach, some burn their throat as they swallow, others burn their skin if spilled, and so on. Students also should be made aware of why medicines and cleaners are kept in a safe place away from easy access and that they should respect parents' and teachers' rules for safety reasons. The safety reason for each rule should be explained.

Safety in the home includes lessons about picking up toys so no one trips over them or gets hurt. Children can learn about the dangers of using kitchen appliances and tools without parental supervision and the risks involved in playing with their older siblings' and others' things without first asking permission. The dangers of playing with or touching guns, knives, and other weapons should be emphasized. Children can be taught to stay away from areas that are locked or designated off limits by describing the dangers and offering alternatives.

As children get older and cognitively capable, they can expand their knowledge of safety awareness and learn first-aid concepts and procedures. For example, as students reach second grade, safety training can take them beyond their own personal safety behavior to include the attention to safety of others. Please review the boxes on safety.

A guest speaker might talk about bicycle and scooter safety, or a fire department representative might speak to the class about fire safety at home and at school. Reading and art projects that require students to recognize potentially dangerous situations reinforce what they have learned. Sending children home with a checklist or questions to ask their parents about safety also reinforces the development of safety-conscious behaviors in the home by making parents more aware of overlooked areas that are potentially dangerous. Adults may tend to take for granted some safe behaviors that children do not. Recommended areas for specific lessons on safety for grades K–2 are listed below:

Home	**School**
Fire hazards	Fire drill
Fire drills	Bus
Poisons	Playground
Guns	
Toys	

Recreational

Water activities
Bicycle/Scooter
Skating (inline/ice/roller)

Workplace/School Safety

The following statements represent a safety-conscious lifestyle that can reduce your and others' chances of being injured at your workplace/school. Check each statement that reflects your lifestyle.

- ☐ I know the fire evacuation procedures at my workplace/school.
- ☐ I know the location of first aid supplies and the nearest fire extinguisher at my workplace/school.
- ☐ I wear any recommended safety equipment and follow any recommended safety procedures.
- ☐ I know how to report an emergency at work/school.
- ☐ I know how to activate the emergency response team.

If you checked only one or two statements, you should consider making changes in your lifestyle now.

Source: Adapted from American Red Cross, *First Aid: Responding to Emergencies*, 3d ed. (San Bruno, CA: Staywell, 2001).

Strangers

As they grow, children rapidly expand their contacts with other children and adults. Prior to going to school, most children have found that adults and older children are trustworthy. They tend to transfer this trust and respect, naturally, without discretion, to other people in their expanding world, which usually includes teachers, participants in community life, and strangers.

Children need to be made aware of appropriate behavior with strangers, particularly in situations where they are alone. "Stranger" has to be defined. For example, if a child walks through a park from time to time and sees and talks with the same people, several times, should he or she consider them strangers? Should children converse with, or accept gifts from, or accept a ride with adults when a parent or guardian is not with them? Should children answer the door if a parent is not home?

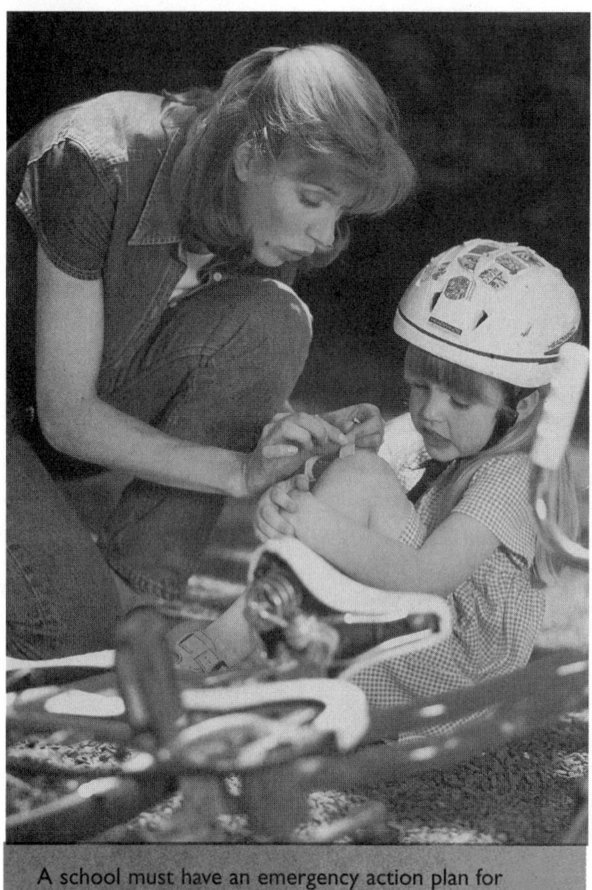

A school must have an emergency action plan for responding to injuries and accidents.

Teaching children appropriate behaviors in these and similar situations is a component of safety education. In addition to teaching children appropriate verbal responses to strangers, children need to be taught the boundaries for appropriate physical contact with other people. Because teachers, nurses, and other trusted family members often accompany children to the bathroom, they can be easily confused by what is appropriate and inappropriate contact from adults. These subject areas are sensitive. Possibly, some children in the class may already be victims of child abuse. Therefore, teachers should receive special training for working with students to help identify and prevent child abuse (see Chapter 11).

The information presented in this chapter represents only some safety issues that are of universal high risk for young children. Many other areas also could be covered. Because the classroom teacher cannot address every potentially dangerous activity, emphasis should be placed on students' being able to recognize potentially dangerous situations and being able to make sound decisions. Lessons also should include how to activate the EMS system (in the "First Aid" section, on the next page). Many cases have documented that a 5-year-old child calling 911 saved the life of a parent or sibling.

School Emergency Action Plan

Most schools have standard procedures for dealing with all forms of emergencies. Classroom teachers can contact the school nurse or other administrator to learn about the school's emergency action plan. Please review the box about Workplace Safety. Teachers also should know of any chronic medical conditions or health concerns of their students. For example, if a student has an allergy to bee stings, teachers should be aware of this and know what to do until the nurse or other medical professional arrives.

Included in this chapter is information about some common medical emergencies, their signs and symptoms, and first-aid treatment. This information may motivate some teachers to get additional first-aid training and prompt them to communicate with the school nurse about the school's emergency action plan. It can enable teachers to recognize an emergency in the earliest stage and thereby prevent more serious consequences. In addition, it provides information for teachers to pass on to their students so they can, in turn, apply it if a classmate has a medical emergency.

"Good Samaritan" Laws

Teachers are often concerned about their legal liability in the event students are injured or become ill while under their supervision, particularly if they administer first aid. Although laws vary from state to state, most states have Good Samaritan laws that protect an individual who makes a good-faith effort to help another person in an emergency. Those providing emergency treatment usually are not held liable for their first aid efforts, even when these are unsuccessful or do not represent the best care. These statutes do not always protect people with formal medical training, such as physicians or nurses, but they do apply to nonmedical professionals such as teachers. Teachers with concerns about liability should check their state laws to determine if their state has a Good Samaritan statute or if the school will protect them from potential lawsuits.

Personal Safety

In the Kitchen

1. Store knives with points away from the hand, or in special holders.
2. Keep curtains away from the cooking range.
3. Keep electrical appliances away from water.
4. Keep floors clean of grease and dirt.

Risk Factors

1. Accidents are the leading cause of death among those under 44 years old.
2. Accidents are the fourth most common cause of death in this country ranking behind heart disease, cancer, and stroke.

Awareness Counts

1. It is especially important that potential problem areas at home, on the road, and at work be identified so that you can create a relatively accident-free environment. Improving your accident-prone behavior is the only way to decrease your risk of accidents.
2. Your home or apartment should be regularly checked for safety hazards:
   a. Fix unfastened carpets.
   b. Repair faulty fixtures or outlets.
   c. Store poisons, firearms in safe place.
   d. Have safety guardrails on upper-level windows.
   e. Place smoke detectors in strategic areas.
   f. Have emergency numbers posted by the phone.
3. Know where fire extinguishers are located.
4. Is there a fire emergency plan in your home, office, or school?

Follow-Through

For information regarding safety procedures and requirements on the job, write to

The U.S. Department of Labor,
Washington DC 20212

or get in touch with the Department of Labor office in your region.
Or write to:

The National Institute for
Occupational Safety and Health,
Post Office Building
Cincinnati, Ohio 45202

For information regarding the safety of consumer products, write to

U.S. Consumer Product Safety
Commission Office of Washington,
DC 20207

For information regarding all kinds of accidents, write to

The National Safety Council,
444 N. Michigan Avenue
Chicago, Illinois 60611

First Aid

Teachers need basic first-aid information. How successfully they disseminate this information varies. For example, the section on the signs and symptoms of a heart attack contains information that students in grades 4–6 can readily comprehend, and its dissemination requires no practical first-aid training. On the other hand, performing abdominal thrusts (**Heimlich maneuver**) to help a choking victim or performing rescue breathing and CPR require specific hands-on training. Classroom teachers without formal training should not teach these techniques, but students still can learn that CPR is required to treat a heart-attack victim who has no signs of circulation. Guest speakers or mini-units taught by trained personnel from community agencies could be incorporated into the elementary school curriculum.

The "how to" information contained in each of the following first aid discussions could be presented to students by the classroom teacher, but the descriptive information is intended primarily for the teacher to increase his or her knowledge of basic medical emergencies. Teachers can decide whether to pass along this information to students to expand their knowledge and understanding of how to help others.

The most vital part of first aid training is learning to recognize an emergency situation and begin the procedure for summoning medical help as quickly as possible. Teachers who know the medical history of students can prevent medical emergencies. For example, if a teacher knows that a student is diabetic and that student's behavior changes in certain ways, the teacher is more likely to pay attention to that behavior. A call to the school nurse prior to the student's losing consciousness could mean immediate treatment and prevention of a more serious medical emergency. Often, the time elapsed between the onset of a medical emergency and the arrival of medical help is the critical factor in the victim's prognosis. The signs and symptoms of heart attacks or asthma, for example, is information that teachers and students can understand and apply without actually giving first aid treatment themselves.

Activating the EMS System

The emergency medical services (**EMS**) system is a community networking chain designed to help the sick and injured in emergency situations (see Figure 14.1). The first and most important link in the chain is the 911 call that activates the system. The 911 operator continues the chain by dispatching appropriate medical help to the scene. The medical personnel sent to the scene provide immediate emergency medical care, stabilize the victim when possible, and may transport the victim to the hospital. After the victim has been treated, the final step in the EMS chain is to provide rehabilitation for the victim.

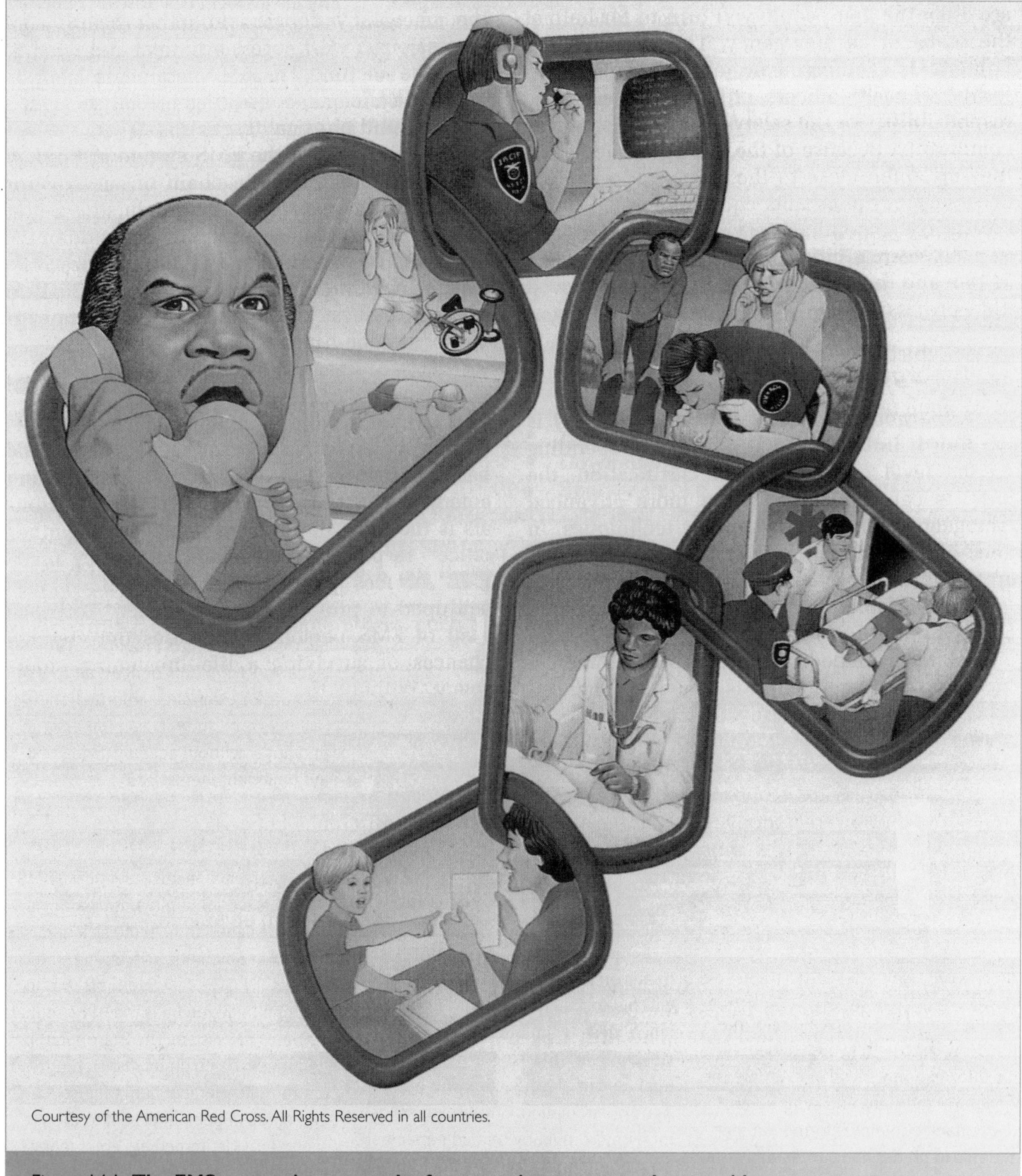

Figure 14.1 **The EMS system is a network of community resources that provide emergency care.**

For the EMS chain to be most effective, an individual, with or without first aid training, has to recognize that an emergency exists and make the 911 call. The speed with which the call is made may make the difference between life and death. In addition, the more information the caller can provide regarding the victim and the situation, the more likely the EMS team will be able to effectively treat and transport the victim. For example, if the 911 caller tells the dispatcher that the victim is trapped in a car, the dispatcher can be sure that the response team has appropriate equipment for extrication. Or, if the caller indicates that the victim has the signs and symptoms of a heart attack, a special response unit for cardiac emergencies would be dispatched.

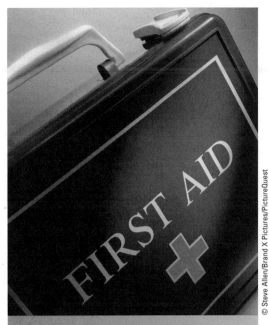

© Steve Allen/Brand X Pictures/PictureQuest

Knowledge of basic first aid measures is essential for school personnel.

The 911 caller should provide the dispatcher with the following information:

- the exact location of the emergency, including the town, street names, landmarks, the building, room, floor, and any other information that will expedite response time;
- the telephone number from which the call is being made and the caller's name;
- a description of what happened (for example, car accident, sudden illness);
- the number of people involved;
- the condition of the victim(s) (for example, unconscious, not breathing, has a pulse); and
- what first-aid treatment is being given.

The caller should confirm that the dispatcher has all the information before returning to the victim to give first aid.

The caller should allow the dispatcher to hang up first. This allows the dispatcher to give any additional directions and/or information to the first aider. Prior to making the call, the first aider needs to assess the scene and the victim. Assessment of the victim requires basic first aid knowledge, but the initial survey can be done quickly.

Assessing the Victim and the Accident Scene

Children should learn how to recognize that an emergency situation exists. Clues from the environment—such as unusual sounds, sights, smells, and behaviors—can help to identify an emergency. As soon as the first aider realizes that an emergency exists, he or she should begin to assess the scene. Using the clues from the environment, the first aider should try to identify the location, what happened, and how many victims are involved in the emergency. Teachers can use class exercises to help students learn to use environmental clues to identify key information about an emergency.

1. *Checking the Scene for Safety*

It should be emphasized that the first aider's safety is the most important priority. If the scene is unsafe, a first aider should remain clear of the situation. No attempt should be made to give first aid if there is a danger to the first aider's personal safety. For example, if there is a fire in a neighbor's home, no attempt should be made to go in the house.

2. *Assessing Victims*

When there is more than one victim at an accident scene, once the first aider determines that the scene is safe, the first aider must decide who to treat to first. The most severely injured person should be attended to first. Any victim who is conscious and breathing and is not in immediate danger (such as in a burning house) should not be moved.

The first step in assessing a victim is to determine whether he or she is conscious. Any victim who can speak or respond visually to the first aider is conscious. When consciousness is not immediately obvious, the first aider should approach the victim, tap him or her gently, and ask, "Are you okay?" If the victim does not respond, the first aider should look, listen, and feel to see if the victim is breathing. If the first aider suspects injuries, he or she should check consciousness and breathing without moving the victim, if possible.

Unconsciousness has different levels. For example, a **fainting** episode is usually considered to be a light stage of unconsciousness. A **coma**, on the other hand, is a deep stage of unconsciousness. The last of the five senses an unconscious person loses is usually hearing, and it is the first to return. Therefore, first aiders need to be careful what they say about the victim and his or her injuries, because, although the victim may not be able to respond, he or she may be able to hear what people are saying.

If the victim's position prevents the first aider from checking consciousness and breathing, the victim should be rolled onto his or her back: The first aider places one hand on the hip and one on the neck for stabilization. If the victim has a neck or a back injury, care should be taken to roll him or her as one unit (instead of moving shoulders then hips, for instance) to prevent spinal cord damage.

If the initial breathing check indicates the victim is not breathing, he or she must be rolled onto his or her back and the airway opened. This is done by placing two fingers on the bony part of the chin and the palm of the other hand on the forehead and tilting the head back while lifting the chin. Just opening the airway may restart breathing in a victim who has been injured. Once the airway has been opened, the first aider should kneel next to the victim and look for the rise and fall of the chest, place his or her cheek next to the victim's mouth to feel if air is being exhaled, and listen for any sound of air coming from the victim. This check should be made for 5 to 10 seconds.

If the victim is breathing and has a pulse, the pulse should be monitored. If the victim is not breathing and has a pulse, the first aider should begin rescue breathing immediately.

If the victim is not breathing, the first aider should check for signs of circulation. This may include checking for a pulse (an indicator of heartbeat). If someone has stopped breathing, his or her heart may continue to beat for a short time. Without sufficient oxygen to the brain and the heart muscle itself, however, the heart will stop beating.

The pulse is checked at the carotid artery in the neck for adults and children. The carotid artery is located by kneeling next to the victim's neck and placing the index finger and third finger on the Adam's apple and sliding the fingers approximately 1½ inches across the neck toward the spine and inline with the Adam's apple. For infants under 1 year of age, the pulse is taken at the brachial artery in the upper arm. The brachial artery is located halfway between the shoulder and elbow joints in the center of the upper arm on the inside part of the arm. The pulse should be taken with the index and third finger, as it is with an adult or older child. The pulse should be checked for a full 5 to 10 seconds. The pulse should not be taken with the thumb, because it has a pulse of its own and the first aider may confuse his or her own pulse with the victim's.

Once the victim's consciousness, breathing, and pulse have been checked, the final check is for severe bleeding. Severe bleeding is defined as arterial bleeding that pulses or spurts with each heartbeat (if the victim has a pulse). It does not mean profuse bleeding such as in a head wound. Severe bleeding is found in amputations or partial amputations when an artery is severed. Like absence of breathing and heartbeat, severe bleeding is life threatening. If a major artery has been severed, an individual can bleed to death in 2 minutes.

These four steps are commonly referred to as the ABCS: A = airway check, B = breathing check, C = circulation (pulse) check, S = severe bleeding check. In addition, these steps make up the primary survey.

A person can go without oxygen to the brain for up to 4 minutes without brain damage. Between 4 and 6 minutes, some brain damage is probable; between 6 and 10 minutes, brain damage is highly likely; and more than 10 minutes without oxygen almost certainly produces irreversible brain damage. Bleeding should be treated after breathing and heartbeat have been established unless it is rapid arterial bleeding from a major artery. In this case, treatment for bleeding should precede restoration of breathing and heartbeat. Given the short time available to treat breathing, pulse, and severe bleeding problems, the EMS system must be activated as soon as the first aider arrives at the scene.

Because emergency situations are almost always emotionally charged, those who respond have to stay as calm as possible. Confusion and indecision can produce panic. Practicing the decision-making process with a variety of different scenarios can reduce the chances that a first aider will panic and make incorrect decisions regarding actions to be taken.

Choking

Choking is a complete or partial blockage of the airway that prevents breathing. People who can speak or cough may be having difficulty breathing, but they are not choking. Coughing is the body's way of clearing the airway. People who are coughing should be left alone (not assisted or treated) until they can no longer cough or speak. In most instances, coughing clears the airway, or the victim stops coughing and eventually loses consciousness. A cough should not be confused with a high-pitched wheeze, which indicates that attempts to inhale are meeting with resistance and the victim probably is getting little, if any, air. Victims who are wheezing are choking and need immediate treatment.

The universal sign of choking is clutching the throat with one or both hands. This is the natural reaction of someone who is having difficulty breathing. Usually airways are obstructed by food or other small objects. In some cases, such as burns, poisoning, or allergic reactions, the throat swells up and closes the airway.

Choking can be life threatening if the airway is blocked and the victim cannot breathe. The first aider should ask the victim, "Are you choking? Can you speak?" If the victim does not respond or is coughing, action is needed and EMS should be activated. The Heimlich maneuver, often referred to as "abdominal thrusts," can be used on a victim to expel a foreign body from the airway.

Abdominal thrusts can be performed on individuals over 1 year of age who are standing or sitting down. To perform the procedure, stand behind the person who is choking and put your arms around his or her waist. Place the thumb side of one fist against the victim's abdomen, about 1 inch above the navel. Cover the fist with the other hand. With a quick inward and upward motion, press your hands against the choking person's abdomen. Be sure your hands are in the center of the abdomen.

No contact should be made with the sternum (breast bone) or the ribs. To be effective, the thrusts must be made on soft tissue. Repeat abdominal thrusts until something is expelled from the mouth or the victim becomes unconscious.

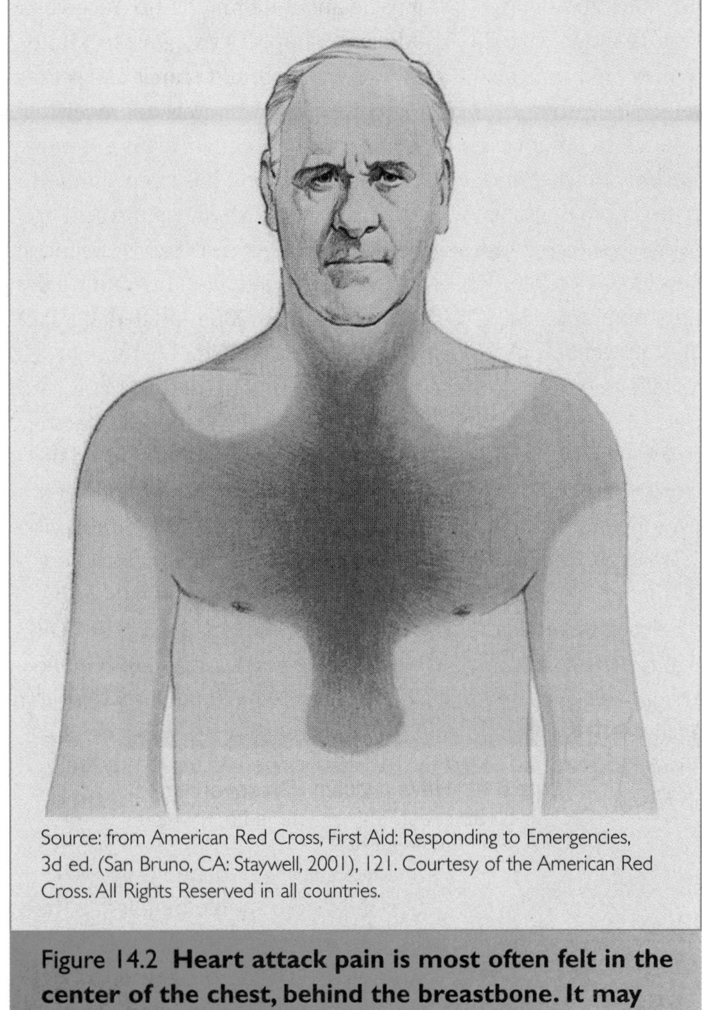

Source: from American Red Cross, First Aid: Responding to Emergencies, 3d ed. (San Bruno, CA: Staywell, 2001), 121. Courtesy of the American Red Cross. All Rights Reserved in all countries.

Figure 14.2 **Heart attack pain is most often felt in the center of the chest, behind the breastbone. It may spread to the shoulder, arm, or jaw.**

Signs and Symptoms of a Heart Attack

The heart needs a constant supply of oxygen to continue to beat steadily and effectively (see Chapter 2). If the oxygen that is supplied to the heart muscle is disrupted by a blockage in an artery or the heart muscle is damaged in some other way, a person experiences a heart attack. In some cases the heart may be beating during a heart attack, but it is not beating regularly or effectively.

When the heart muscle is malfunctioning, certain signals are present. During a heart attack, a person often has pain in the chest area, which can range from discomfort to an intense crushing sensation. Anyone who feels chest pain that is intense (even at rest) and lasts for more than 10 minutes should be checked by a doctor. The crushing feeling in the chest also might be described as a squeezing tightness or aching or a "heavy" type of pain. Frequently the pain spreads from the center of the chest to the shoulder, arm, neck, and jaw (see Figure 14.2). The pain is not usually relieved by changing positions or taking medication.[2] The victim may have difficulty breathing or exhibit shortness of breath and faster or noisy breathing. Sometimes the victim's skin appears pale or bluish, and he or she sweats profusely. In women, the first heart attack signals are often confused with feelings of indigestion.

If the heart stops beating, a heart attack can lead to cardiac arrest. The chances of surviving a heart attack are much better if it is treated prior to cardiac arrest. Most deaths from heart attacks occur within 2 hours of the onset of the first signals.[3] Sometimes the signs of a heart attack resemble indigestion or soreness and victims do not recognize that they are having a heart attack. Therefore, they do not seek medical assistance. In other cases, people deny the severity of what they are feeling and try to ignore the signals, hoping that the pain will subside. Just being aware of the signals of a heart attack and seeking prompt medical assistance is the best prevention of serious, often debilitating consequences or even death.

After a heart attack, the heart may continue to beat for a short time. Without oxygen, however, the already weakened heart will shortly stop beating altogether. Rescue breathing and/or cardiopulmonary resuscitation (CPR) should be started immediately and continue until medical help arrives.[4] (Rescue breathing and CPR certification courses are given by the American Red Cross and the American Heart Association.)

Shock

The circulatory system, which delivers oxygen to the body, is a complex, autonomically controlled system that responds to changes in the body and the mind (see Chapter 2). In stressful situations, the heart rate normally speeds up to increase the circulation of blood bringing oxygen to the vital body organs, such as the heart and the brain. The circulatory system also shunts blood away from the extremities such as the arms and legs, thereby providing more blood to the vital organs. The body can continue this state of increased circulatory output for a time. If, however, the body must sustain it for too long or if an injury affects the circulatory system itself, such as severe bleeding or a heart attack, the stress response (explained in Chapter 8) cannot meet the oxygen demands of the body without medical treatment. When the heart muscle and the brain do not receive an adequate supply of oxygen, the whole body is affected, and **shock** can set in.

If the heart or brain is not receiving enough oxygen, certain signs are present. Because blood has been shunted away from the extremities, the skin appears pale and cool. In more advanced shock, the lips and the area around the eyes may appear blue, indicating a lack of oxygen to the head.

Pain is an internal stressor, so it can accelerate the shock reaction. Placing the victim in a comfortable prone position (that is, lying on the back) that minimizes pain is important. If the victim is bleeding, it must be controlled. Normal body temperature should be maintained, which may require covering the person if the skin feels chilled. To increase circulation to the heart and head, the victim's legs should be elevated about 12 inches unless a head, neck, or back injury is present or the victim's legs or hips are broken. If the first aider is in doubt about the position, the victim should be left flat. The victim should not take in fluids, even if he or she is thirsty. Even though first aid treatment for shock can slow its progression, the EMS system should be activated as quickly as possible.

Minor Wounds and Bleeding

Any injury to the soft tissue of the body is considered to a **wound**. Wounds such as bumps and bruises are caused by breaks in blood vessels underneath the skin. People can bleed without a break in the skin. Bumps and bruises often swell because of the fluid that accumulates at the site of the injury. Bruises later may turn a black and blue color (a hematoma) because of the blood and fluid just below the skin surface.

Closed Wounds

For internal or closed wounds (without external bleeding) such as bumps and bruises, the affected body part should be elevated above the level of the heart and ice and a pressure bandage applied. If the individual complains of pain as the body part is being elevated, the first aider should place the body part back to its original position and apply ice and compression. A **pressure bandage**—an elastic bandage—can be wrapped snugly around the wound to help constrict the blood vessels and control internal bleeding and swelling. The first aider should wrap the injury starting from the part of the wound farthest away from the body and wrapping toward the body. Reducing the swelling of an injury will reduce the pain, increase the mobility of the affected area, and speed up the healing process.

Open Wounds

Open wounds, which break the skin, also need to be treated with elevation and ice. Depending on the severity of the break in the skin, however, controlling the bleeding may be the first priority. (Because someone else's blood and other body fluids may carry infectious organisms, the first aider should not touch the victim's blood without wearing latex gloves.) To control bleeding, direct pressure is applied to the wound, preferably with a sterile gauze pad or, if something sterile is not available, with a clean piece of cloth.

Once material has been placed over the wound, it should not be removed. If more layers are needed for absorption, more should be added to what is already there to avoid disturbance of any clotting that has started. Direct pressure should be maintained until the bleeding stops. To keep the pressure constant, a bandage can be wrapped over the wound. If direct pressure does not control the bleeding, the wound should be elevated above the level of the heart. This will reduce the blood pressure in the affected area, and gravity will slow down the bleeding, which helps the clotting process. If a fracture is suspected, the body part should not be elevated until the affected limb has been immobilized.

Open wounds should be kept clean to prevent infection. Minor wounds, such as scrapes and cuts, should be washed with soap and water and protected from further injury. More serious wounds, such as gashes, lacerations, and partial or complete amputations, should not be cleaned until the individual has been taken to the hospital. The first aid treatment for more severe wounds is to control bleeding, protect from further injury and contamination, treat for shock, and quickly have the victim transported to a hospital or emergency clinic.

Puncture Wounds

Puncture wounds, such as bites, stings, and nail wounds, are prone to infection. Because puncture wounds are deep and do not usually bleed, any infection or germs present at the puncture site are not carried out of the body by bleeding. Surface cleaning of puncture wounds may be insufficient to prevent infection. Therefore, careful cleaning with an antiseptic or hydrogen peroxide is important. A tetanus shot is often recommended. No attempt should be made to remove any object that is embedded in the body.

Nosebleeds

Nosebleeds are usually easily controlled and in most cases do not need medical assistance. Some individuals are more susceptible to nosebleeds than others for a variety of reasons, such as high blood pressure or thin mucoid tissue in the nasal passages. The first aid procedure for a nosebleed is to have the victim sit down to lower the blood pressure, lean forward, and apply pressure directly over the nostrils as if pinching the nostrils shut with his or her thumb and forefinger. A clean cloth or tissue can be used to absorb the blood. Leaning forward prevents blood from flowing down the back of the throat, which could cause the victim to choke. Pressure over the nostrils should be maintained for about 5 minutes. Releasing the pressure too soon to check to see if the bleeding has stopped will disrupt the clotting process and will increase the time needed to stop the bleeding. The victim should be reassured and reminded to breathe through his or her mouth. If the bleeding does not stop after 5 minutes, medical assistance should be sought.

Burns

Burns are classified by the depth of tissue destruction and the size of the body area affected. When a severe burn destroys the skin, it may be life threatening. Other factors that establish the severity of a burn are the specific body parts affected, the age of the burn victim, and any preexisting medical conditions.

The skin acts as a barrier against infection. When the skin is damaged, the body is vulnerable to infection. The most serious burns are those on the face, especially the mouth, nose, eyelids, hands, feet, and genitals. Respiratory tract burns are also serious. Victims under age 5 and over age 60 are more severely affected by burns than any other age group. All of these factors should be taken into consideration when trying to decide what first-aid action to take.

Following are the definitions of burn severity:

1. **First-degree burns** are characterized by redness, swelling, pain, and tenderness. They are superficial and affect only the outer layers of the skin. A sunburn is a common example.
2. **Second-degree burns** involve deeper layers of skin damage. The burn is characterized by blisters, swelling, and fluid loss from the capillaries in the inner layers of the skin. Second-degree burns are very painful.
3. **Third-degree burns** are characterized by a charred, white, or cherry red appearance. There are no blisters or fluids oozing from the affected area because the capillaries in the inner layers of the skin have been destroyed. The burn may have affected the underlying fat, muscle, and bone and destroyed these deep tissues. Pain may be absent because the nerve endings to the affected area have been destroyed. Any pain the victim feels is from surrounding areas that are less severely burned.

The first priority for all burns is to immediately remove the heat source and any clothing that may be continuing to burn the victim. Any clothing that is stuck to the burn site should not be removed, as this could cause further tissue destruction and introduce infection. Any jewelry should be removed as soon as possible because swelling likely will prevent removal later.

The first aid treatment for burns is to cool the affected area by flushing the area with copious amounts of cool water. Ice may be used for minor burns such as a finger burned from touching a hot stove. For more severe burns or burns that involve a larger surface area of the body, ice is not recommended. Once the area has been cooled, the burned area should be covered with a dry, clean, sterile dressing.

The greatest vulnerability of burn victims is the risk of infection. Thus, great care should be taken to keep the affected area from contamination. Ointments should not be used except for very minor burns. Because ointments may actually seal in heat, they inhibit the healing process. If blisters develop, they should not be broken. Blisters are a protective covering that help prevent infection.

In cases where the burn involves an open wound that is not severe enough to require medical treatment, the affected area should be washed with soap and water and covered with a dry, sterile dressing. When the burn area is completely cooled, an antibiotic ointment may be applied. The victim should be monitored for signs of infection.

A burn victim should be watched for shock. Except in cases of very minor burns, the victim should be instructed to lie down. The heart and respiration should be monitored, the burned area elevated above the level of the heart when possible, and normal body temperature maintained.

Seizures

Epilepsy is a brain disorder characterized by seizures that can range from a momentary blank stare to a total loss of consciousness and muscle spasms that can last for up to 5 minutes. Although an epileptic seizure may be a medical emergency, epileptics diagnosed without complications do not necessarily require medical assistance. For someone who is known to be an epileptic (usually the person is wearing a medic alert bracelet or necklace), medical assistance should be summoned only if (1) the seizure lasts more than 10 minutes, (2) an injury results from the onset of the seizure, (3) the individual is pregnant or has another medical condition that could be affected by the seizure, or (4) the seizure occurs in water. If a seizure occurs for an unknown reason or in conjunction with another condition—such as high fever, head injury, pregnancy, poisoning, low blood sugar, or heat stroke—the EMS system should be activated immediately.

As soon as the first aider realizes that a seizure is occurring, he or she should protect the victim from falling or getting hurt by assisting him or her to the ground. Hazards around the victim should be removed. This is particularly important to hazards around the victim's head. If the clothing around the neck is constricting, the collar should be loosened. No attempt should be made to restrain the tongue. The first aider should not attempt to put anything in the victim's mouth, give liquids, or attempt to perform rescue breathing. The victim should be reassured and monitored until the seizure subsides. After the seizure is over, the victim should be placed onto his or her side to prevent any fluids from going down the back of the throat. Usually a seizure victim can return to normal activity after a brief rest. If the cause of the seizure is unknown and lasts longer than 5 minutes or if the victim has multiple seizures, the EMS system should be activated or the victim should be encouraged to seek medical assistance.

Asthmatic Attacks

An asthmatic attack occurs when the bronchial tubes in the lungs go into spasms, making it very difficult for the person to breathe. Most asthmatics carry medication to relax the bronchial spasms. In severe asthma attacks, the victim's skin may turn blue from the lack of oxygen.

A first aider can help the victim by providing reassurance and helping to locate his or her medication, which is usually an inhaler or pills. Because bronchial spasms can be brought on by environmental allergens such as dust, feathers, smoke, or paint fumes, the first aider may want to move the victim to an irritant-free environment. The asthmatic will probably have an easier time breathing if he or she is in a sitting rather than a reclining position. The victim should be encouraged to drink water if possible.

Medical attention is necessary if an asthma attack is severe or prolonged, if the victim does not respond to medication, if the skin continues to be blue, or if the pulse rate exceeds 120 beats per minute. If a precipitating event, such as a bug bite, has produced an allergic reaction, medical attention is recommended. A severe allergic reaction can result in swelling of the respiratory tract, which, in extreme cases, can lead to respiratory arrest. For an asthmatic individual, this could be life threatening.

Diabetic Emergencies

Changes in diet and exercise can alter the amount of sugar in the blood of a diabetic, whether the sugar is too high (**hyperglycemia**) or too low (**hypoglycemia**). If untreated, it can result in a life-threatening medical emergency.

Two types of diabetic emergencies have similar signs and symptoms:

1. **Diabetic coma**. If a diabetic does not take his or her injections or eats more carbohydrates than usual, the blood sugar can become too high. The excess sugar in the blood gives the breath a fruity odor. The person becomes tired and drowsy (because the body cells do not have fuel for energy), is extremely thirsty, urinates frequently, and may vomit. The skin may appear flushed, and the individual may have difficulty breathing. These signs and symptoms come on gradually. If left untreated, diabetic coma can lead to unconsciousness and even death.
2. **Insulin shock**. Too much insulin or vigorous exercise can remove too much sugar from the blood. The signs and symptoms of insulin shock or low blood sugar include staggering and poor coordination, anger, bad temper, confusion, disorientation, sweating, pale color, and

Common Causes of Poisoning (by age group)

Under 6	6–19	Over 19
Analgesic medications	Analgesic medications	Analgesic medications
Cleaning substances	Bites and stings	Antidepressant drugs
Cosmetics and personal care products	Cleaning substances	Bites and stings
Cough and cold remedies	Cosmetics	Chemicals
Gastrointestinal medications	Cough and cold remedies	Cleaning substances
Plants	Food products/food poisoning	Food products/food poisoning
Topical medications	Plants	Fumes and vapors
Vitamins	Stimulants and street drugs	Insecticides
		Sedatives and hallucinogenic drugs

Source: Adapted from American Red Cross, *First Aid: Responding to Emergencies*, 3d ed. (San Bruno, CA: Staywell, 2001), 310. Courtesy of the American Red Cross. All Rights Reserved in all countries.

sudden hunger. In contrast to the slow onset of diabetic coma, insulin shock comes on quickly.

The signs and symptoms of diabetic coma and insulin shock are easily confused. Also, both conditions resemble many of the signs and symptoms of alcohol or drug intoxication. Both diabetic conditions are serious medical emergencies that require immediate medical attention.

Without insulin, an individual in a diabetic coma will die.

First aid treatment for people with low blood sugar or insulin shock is to feed them sugar. As long as the victim is conscious and can swallow without choking, any food or drink containing sugar, such as fruit juices, soft drink, or candy can be given. Within 10 to 15 minutes the condition should be improved. If there is no response, the victim should be given immediate medical treatment.

Poisoning

A **poison** is any substance that causes illness or injury when it enters the body. Poisons can enter the body in four ways: ingestion, inhalation, absorption, and injection. The most common type of poisoning in young children is ingestion, and it occurs primarily in the home. Common types of poisons that children ingest include household cleaners, gasoline, medicines, laundry products, alcohol, and perfumes; others are listed in the box on the next page.

The first aid treatment given for poisoning victims varies with the type of substance ingested. With food and medicine overdoses, the stomach must be emptied quickly to avoid absorption of the poison into the body's systems. With corrosive poisons (strong acids and alkalis) such as bleach, gasoline, lighter fluid, household ammonia, toilet bowl cleaners, and lye products, vomiting should not be induced. These substances cause burns in and around the mouth and esophagus. Inducing vomiting with these victims can result in more extensive burns of the mouth and throat. Corrosive poison victims often vomit spontaneously. In cases of severe damage, victims' throats may swell, possibly affecting respiration.

Most corrosive poisons have an antidote. The antidote is dependent on the specific type of acid or alkali ingested. Therefore, even individuals with first aid training are advised to contact the Poison Control Center for first aid instructions and information on antidotes. When calling the Poison Control Center for help, it is best to know the specific ingredients of the substance swallowed.

Summary

When children enter kindergarten, they find themselves in an environment with new safety issues including how and where to get into cars and buses, use crosswalks, and make decisions regarding strangers. They also learn school rules such as fire drills and regulations concerning weapons. Other safety issues include bike, skating, and water safety and identifying and avoiding poisons. The school usually has an emergency action plan with which the teacher and students alike should be familiar.

First aid information is taught according to the students' ability to learn and apply the information. Rudimentary information, such as when and how to dial 911, can begin at the lowest grade levels. Later, students can learn actual emergency procedures such as CPR and the Heimlich maneuver.

Before applying first aid, the first aider has to know how to assess the victim and the accident scene. This requires determining consciousness, breathing, signs of circulation, and any obvious bleeding. Knowledge of first aid procedures can prevent more serious consequences and even save lives. Among the more common emergency situations are choking, heart attack signs, shock, various forms of bleeding, burns, seizures, asthma attacks, and diabetic emergencies. The first step in dealing with safety and emergency issues is to acquire the fundamental knowledge. This can progress to hands-on practice as the curriculum and school system deem appropriate.

Resources

American Red Cross. *Community First Aid and Safety.* St. Louis: Mosby Lifeline, 1993.

Bever, D. L. *Safety: A Personal Focus,* 3d ed. St. Louis: Mosby Year Book, 1992.

Faber, D. S., and C. A. Sears. *The Life You Save: A Safety and First Aid Text.* Winston-Salem, NC: Hunter Textbooks, 1990.

Merrick School District. *Comprehensive Health and Safety Curriculum, Grade 5.* Merrick, NY: 1990.

National Safety Council. *Accident Facts,* 4th ed. Boston: Jones and Bartlett, 1994.

National Safety Council. *First Aid and C.P.R.* Boston: Jones and Bartlett, 1991.

New York Board of Fire Underwriters. *Fire Prevention and Safety: A Teacher's Handbook.* New York: Board of Education and Fire Department, 1993.

New York State Education Department. *Safety Education Syllabus: Grades K–12.* Albany, NY: Bureau of Curriculum Development, 1986.

Notes

1. Centers for Disease Control and Prevention, *Youth Risk Behavior Surveillance, United States* (1999). www.cdc.gov/mmwr/pdf/ss/ss4807.pdf
2. ARC, First AID. American Red Cross, First Aid: Responding to Emergencies, 3d ed. (San Bruno, CA: Staywell, 2001), 121.
3. American Red Cross. *Community C.P.R.* (St. Louis: Mosby Lifeline, 1993).
4. See note 2.

Learning Experiences

Safety-conscious actions cannot prevent all accidents or sudden illnesses; but they can reduce their incidence and severity. Children should learn first aid care for the sick and injured to minimize the consequences of delayed medical treatment. Deciding what action to take in an emergency situation requires knowledge, logical thinking, and decision-making skills. First aid training can be the means to developing cognitive skills. Everyone can learn to activate the EMS system and learn an emergency action plan. Some knowledge of basic first aid enables children to help in an emergency when medical help is not readily available. Individuals who learn basic first aid have the tools to save lives.

Teaching children about safety, first aid, and prevention of injuries should be one of the central themes of the early elementary school curriculum. Some safety lessons have to be taught directly, such as walking through a fire drill. Other lessons can be taught across the curriculum. These learning experiences might include reading stories that include safety issues, writing stories, or creating an art project to reinforce basic safety principles.

Grades K–2

The main goal for grades K–2 is to develop an awareness of appropriate safety-conscious behaviors in the home, school, and recreational environments. The students should be encouraged to discuss and participate in decision-making exercises that allow them to understand safe behaviors and the reasons for the basic rules they need to follow. These rules will serve as their guide for developing a safety-conscious lifestyle. They need to understand the potential risk of physical harm in case of fire; when entering, exiting, and riding in cars and buses; when waiting for cars and buses; and when crossing a street. After lessons in safety, first aid, and injury prevention, these students should be able to

1. Relate safety procedures to important wellness concepts.
2. Indicate knowledge of safety practices during fire drills; crossing streets; and entering, exiting, and riding in buses and cars.
3. Draw the universal symbol for poisons and identify poisonous and nonpoisonous materials.
4. Demonstrate appropriate responses to strangers.

5. Describe safety hazards when playing with toys, recreational equipment, and other children.
6. Summon help by calling 911 and giving the operator the correct name, address, age, phone number, and safety problem.
7. Treat minor injuries.
8. Choose behaviors that prevent accidents and promote wellness.

Grades 3–4

The major goal for students in grades 3–4 is to expand the notion of safety to new activities they are capable of participating in and increasing their understanding of why safety rules are important. They are now cognitively ready to learn basic first aid concepts and procedures. Students who have had safety training in K–2 should expand their knowledge of safety beyond their own personal safety to include the care of others. Once they know the rules, they should be taught why the rules are important and should be given opportunities to apply safety principles in situations that have not been discussed specifically. After these experiences, students should be able to:

1. Apply knowledge of safety procedures by participating in decision-making activities involving fire, bus, car, and pedestrian safety.
2. Describe safety procedures for activities such as bicycling, swimming, and running.
3. Describe fire safety procedures at home.
4. Report a fire while at home.
5. Call for help when home alone.
6. Describe how weather can affect personal safety.
7. Activate the EMS system.

Grades 5–6

Students at this level are becoming skilled in first aid practices. These students can readily comprehend the signs and symptoms of a heart attack, for example. They should be able to help others by calling health personnel, activating the EMS system, or providing first aid or CPR. The most important goal is to behave in ways that will prevent injury to themselves and others. After lessons in safety, first aid, and injury prevention, these students should be able to:

1. Apply first aid procedures for a child and an adult with an obstructed airway.
2. Report when a victim is conscious or unconscious, is breathing, and has a pulse.
3. Describe the signs and symptoms of a heart attack.
4. Perform first aid procedures for a burn, a seizure, asthma attack, minor wound, nosebleed, shock, diabetic episodes, and poisoning.

For suggestions on creating a rubric with which to evaluate student performance of Learning Experiences, see page 13.

Learning Experience 14-1

Learning About the Telephone

Grade Level

K–2

Primary Disciplines

Math, Art

Learning Objectives

Following this activity, students will be able to

- Point to the different parts of the telephone and the numbers that appear on the phone.
- Dial their own telephone number.
- Dial 911 and respond to questions.

Time Required

20 minutes

Materials

Crayons, picture of a phone to color, phone

Description of Activity

Introduction

Students become familiar with the different parts of the phone by demonstration.

Activity

- Identify the different parts of the phone. On their pictures, the students color the phone, using a different color for each identified part.
- Have the students practice writing and then dialing their phone number. You can role-play an emergency telephone call with them. Have students give their name, address, telephone number, and information about the emergency.

Homework

Students will ask their parents to post emergency numbers next to the phone. Have students complete the following Emergency Telephone Numbers form with assistance from parents.

Evaluation

Students will be able to

- Demonstrate their ability to call 911.
- Describe situations when 911 should be called, including bleeding, unconsciousness, heart attack, fire, and so on.

EMERGENCY TELEPHONE NUMBERS

Police ______________________________

Fire ______________________________

Ambulance ______________________________

Poison Control Center ______________________________

Have your students work with their parents to assemble a first aid kit. Include the following items.

___ Bandages, several sizes

___ Sterile pad, 2 x 2 inches

___ Rolled gauze

___ Antiseptic

___ Adhesive tape (for use on skin)

___ Alcohol

___ Tongue depressor

___ Triangular bandage

Optional items:

___ Flashlight

___ Batteries

___ Candles

___ Matches

___ Bottled water

___ Battery-operated radio

Learning Experience 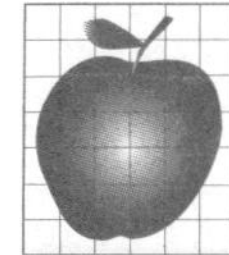 14-2

Bulletin Board for Safe Places

Grade Level

K–2

Primary Disciplines

Art, Language Arts

Learning Objectives

Following this activity, students will be able to

- List safe places to go when in danger.
- Tell where their own areas of safety are.
- List safe places on their route to and from school.

Time Required

25 minutes

Materials

Old magazines, scissors, construction paper, tape, thumbtacks

Description of Activity

Have the class make a bulletin board consisting of cutout pictures of places to be if in danger. These pictures could include a police station, fire station, school, friend's house, and so on. Discuss with students their reasons for selecting pictures of safe places and explain the danger.

Homework

Students identify safe places they can go to when in danger and report to class.

Evaluation

Students will be able to

- Recognize in writing the safe places they have identified.
- Spell the new words correctly.
- Explain why some places are safer than others.
- Describe dangerous situations.

Learning Experience 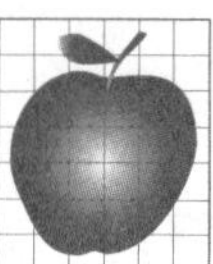 14-3

Safety Walk

Grade Level

K–2

Primary Disciplines

Geography, Spelling

Learning Objectives

Following this activity, students will be able to

- Identify streets observed on a walk.
- Tell the meaning of street signs.
- Perform safe behaviors while walking.

Time Required

10 minutes

Materials

None

Description of Activity

Introduction

Invite a local police officer or crossing guard to accompany the class on a safety walk.

Activity

During the walk, have students identify street signs. The police officer or crossing guard also demonstrates the proper way to cross the street.

Homework

None

Evaluation

Students will be able to

- Recognize and explain common street signs (stop signs, traffic lights, crosswalks, and so on).
- Walk safely, including looking both ways when crossing a street.

Learning Experience 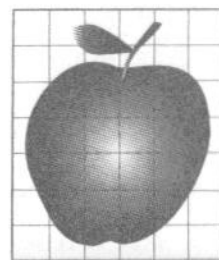 14-4

Understanding Street Signs

Grade Level

K–2

Primary Disciplines

Art, Math

Learning Objectives

Following this activity, students will be able to

- Describe the information on specific street signs.
- Identify shapes of triangle, octagon, rectangle, diamond, round, and crosswalk.

Time Required

30 minutes

Materials

Large paper grocery bags, scissors, construction paper, markers, paste

Description of Activity

Have the class make and explain costumes of the six basic traffic signs listed in the second learning objective, as follows:

1. Cut head and arm holes in large paper bags.
2. Paste on traffic signs.
3. Have each child act as a designated sign and explain its function.

Homework

Students draw the shapes of street signs they saw on the way home. They bring the list to school the following day for discussion.

Evaluation

Students will be able to

- Recognize and explain the common street signs.
- Identify and name the shapes of common street signs.
- Correctly replicate the shapes and symbols of common street signs.

Learning Experience 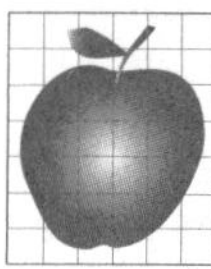 14-5

Safe Biking/Rollerblading

Grade Level

K–2

Primary Discipline

Social Studies

Learning Objectives

Following this activity, students will be able to demonstrate safe biking and rollerblading techniques.

Time Required

30 minutes

Materials

None; outdoor activity

Description of Activity

On the playground, have students discuss and demonstrate the following safety considerations when riding a bike and rollerblading:

- Watching for cars.
- Not going between parked cars.
- Crossing at designated areas.
- Wearing safety equipment.
- Role-play and walk children through these activities.

Homework

None

Evaluation

Students will be able to

- Describe and demonstrate safe street behaviors when participating in outdoor activities.
- Identify equipment that will keep them safe when biking or rollerblading.

Learning Experience 14-6

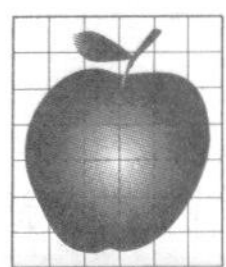

Automobile Safety

Grade Level

K–2

Primary Discipline

Language Arts

Learning Objectives

Following this activity, students will be able to

- Distinguish safe from unsafe behaviors in a car and bus.
- Describe the safest way to get in and out of a car and bus.

Time Required

30 minutes

Materials

Police officer, car (if car is not available, use chairs)

Description of Activity

Introduction

Invite a police officer to discuss automobile safety with students.

Activity

The officer takes the students into the school parking lot and demonstrates the safest way to get in and out of a car and a bus.

If a car is not available, use chairs on the sidewalks near the curb and practice entering and exiting. Have students role-play ways to enter, exit, and behave in an automobile.

Following the activities, direct a class discussion about use of a seat belt, not standing in buses, safe behavior on the bus or in a car, and so on.

Homework

None

Evaluation

Students will be able to

- Describe and demonstrate safe behaviors in parking lots, cars, and buses.
- Explain why the use of seat belts is important.
- Demonstrate ability to use seat belts properly.

Learning Experience 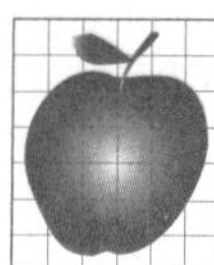 14-7

Who Are My Friends?

Grade Level

K–2

Primary Disciplines

Art, Spelling

Learning Objectives

Following this activity, students will be able to

- Identify people who help (police, firefighters, and so on).
- Describe the differences between friends and strangers.
- Report the colors of police officer and firefighters' hats, trucks, and cars.

Time Required

45 minutes

Materials

Colored construction paper (red, blue, black, white), police officer, firefighter

Description of Activity

To encourage students to think of police officers, firefighters, bus drivers, and school personnel as friends, invite these community servants to demonstrate their equipment at the school. Alternative: Schedule a field trip to a police or fire station to allow children to become familiar with these professionals.

Have each student make a "hat" corresponding to the actual colors used by local police and fire departments.

Homework

None

Evaluation

Students will be able to

- Identify people in the community that represent safety.
- Distinguish between friends and strangers.
- Learn new spelling words.
- Identify uniforms or other symbols (hats, badges, and so on) of helpers in the community.

Learning Experience 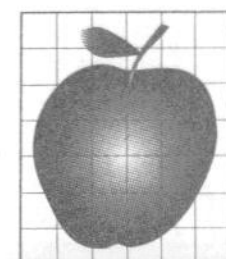 14-8

All About Me

Grade Level

K–2

Primary Disciplines

Language Arts, Creative Arts

Learning Objectives

Following this activity, students will be able to

- State their name, address, and telephone number.
- Give that information in an emergency.

Time Required

30 minutes

Materials

Glue, crayons, scissors, construction paper

Description of Activity

At the beginning of the school year, make address tags for each student. Have students color them or glue them on colored paper. Name tags could have the following information:

I am ________________________.

I live at ______________________.

My phone number is ____________.

Have each student recite the information on his or her tag after completing it. Also, have students fill out an identification card they can place near their phone at home.

Take attendance by calling students' first name and asking the students to answer with their last name.

Homework

Students draw a picture of the outside of their home, with the street number on the house and a street sign with the name of the street. At the bottom they state their city or town.

Evaluation

Students will be able to

- Write their name, address, and telephone number.
- Recite their name, address, and telephone number when asked by a helping official.
- Draw a picture of their immediate home area (house, street, and so on).

Learning Experience 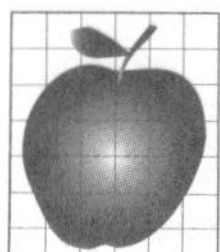 14-9

Safety on the Road: Using Reflectors

Grade Level

3–4

Primary Discipline

Science

Learning Objectives

Following this activity, students will be able to

- Report the meaning of the term "reflection."
- Explain the importance of wearing light colors to give others better vision at night.
- List objects that can reflect light.

Time Required

30 minutes

Materials

Flashlight, piece of 2" × 2" reflection tape for each student, glue, piece of 4" × 4" material for each student

Description of Activity

Lead a discussion on reflection, as follows:

1. Shine the flashlight on the places that reflect light at different intensities (toward the front windows, in a dark corner, on a piece of reflective material).
2. Have the students make reflective patches they can pin onto their clothing by putting a piece of reflective tape onto a piece of cloth.

Homework

Students take their reflective tape home and place it on their bicycles.

Evaluation

Students will be able to

- Describe how light reflection works.
- Identify commonly available reflective materials.
- Explain the importance of wearing outfits that reflect light when out in the dark.
- Describe the importance of using recreational equipment with reflective materials.

Learning Experience 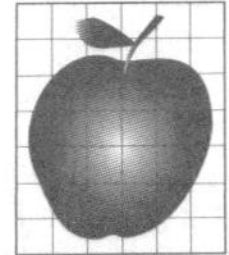 14-10

Meet the Fire Department

Grade Level

3–4

Primary Discipline

Social Studies

Learning Objectives

Following this activity, students will be able to

- Describe fire safety precautions.
- Develop a list of fire safety rules for home.

Time Required

20 minutes

Materials

Fire Department representative, home safety check

Description of Activity

Invite a local fire department representative to speak about home fire safety. Have students generate a list of fire safety rules for the home and post them on the bulletin board.

Homework

Students take home the safety checklist that was developed in class and review it with their parent(s). The parent(s) will initial the form and the student will bring the form back to school.

Evaluation

Students will be able to

- Identify fire safety personnel.
- Describe fire safety guidelines for the home and school, including dangers of using matches, playing near stove, and so on.
- Identify fire escape routes from home and school buildings.
- Explain the importance of smoke detectors in the home and how to maintain them.

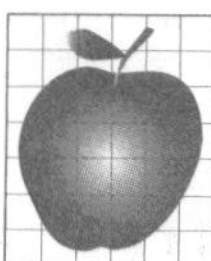

Learning Experience 14-11

Class Fire Drill

Grade Level

3–4

Primary Discipline

Geography (maps)

Learning Objectives

Following this activity, students will be able to

- Describe safe and proper protocol during a fire drill.
- Outline the school's escape plan.
- Explain the importance of a "fire buddy."

Time Required

30 minutes

Materials

Map of the school, highlighter, escape routes from classroom, cafeteria, gym, and so on

Description of Activity

Have students highlight escape routes on the map. They can practice by walking through each of the possible routes. Assign student pairs to be responsible for each other during fire drills or a real evacuation. The escape route map can be posted on the bulletin board.

Homework

None

Evaluation

Students will be able to

- Describe fire safety guidelines for the school.
- Identify fire escape routes from the school.
- Describe the importance of having a "fire buddy" in school.
- Produce a simple map showing escape routes.

Learning Experience 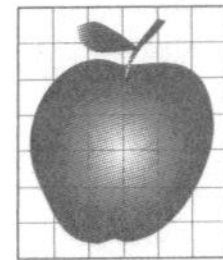 14-12

Family Fire Drill

Grade Level

3–4

Primary Discipline

Geography (maps)

Learning Objectives

Following this activity, students will be able to

- Describe the safest escape route from their home.
- Report on their family practice escape plan.

Time Required

45 minutes

Materials

Construction paper, crayons, markers, handout

Description of Activity

Have students make a map of their home and then designate the safest escape route for family members. The teacher can use the handout as a template for the students.

Homework

Students discuss escape route with their parents.

Evaluation

Students will be able to

- Describe fire safety guidelines for the home.
- Identify fire escape routes from the home.
- Describe the importance of having a "fire buddy" at home.
- Identify escape routes at home.
- Produce a simple map.

Fire Safety at Home

Directions: With the help of your teacher, locate the primary and secondary exit routes from the bedrooms of this house in case of fire.

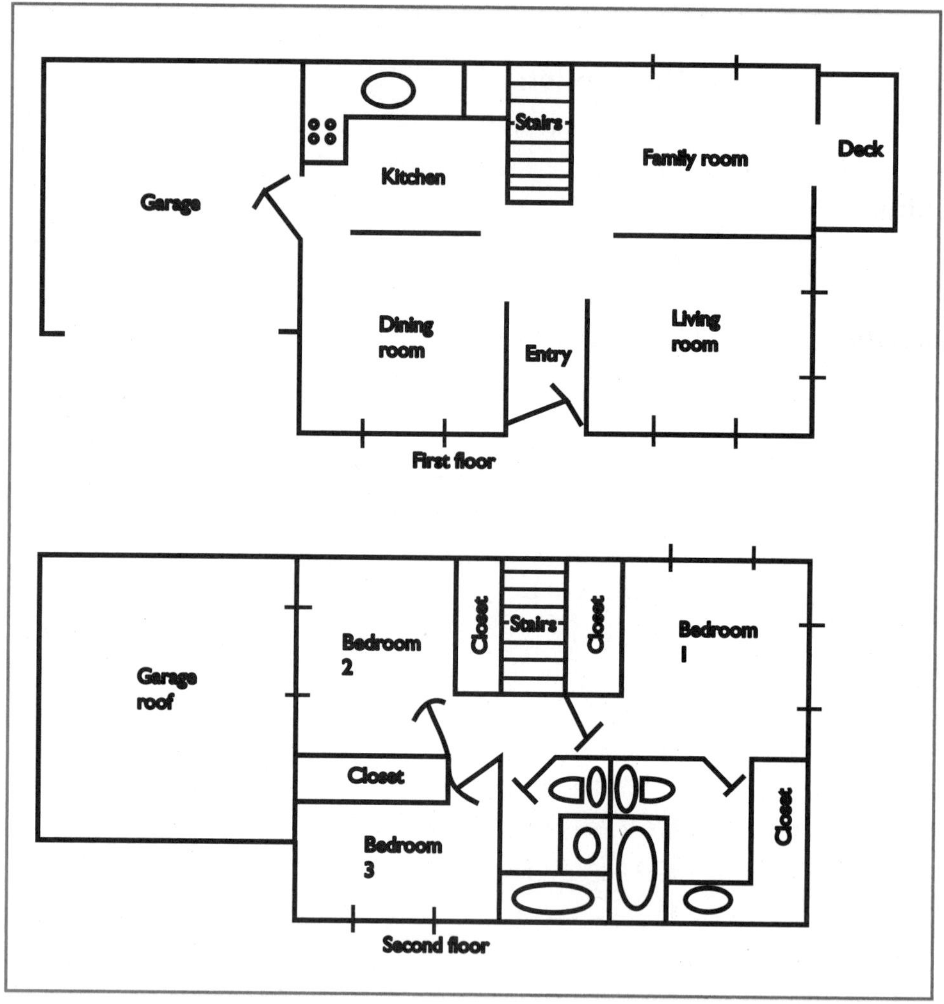

Learning Experience 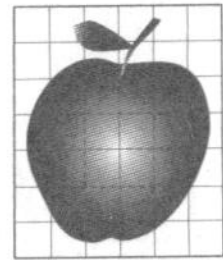 14-13

Fire Safety

Grade Level

3–4

Primary Discipline

Science

Learning Objectives

Following this activity, students will be able to

- Describe proper safety procedures if someone's clothing catches on fire.
- Explain why a person should stay low to the ground during an escape from fire.

Time Required

Varies according to extent of instruction and practice

Materials

Step 1: a piece of material, a jar, a match; Steps 2–4: gymnasium or large room with mats, rugs, two cones with ropes across them

Description of Activity

1. Ignite a piece of material and cover it with a nonflammable object. Discuss with the students how the fire was put out because of lack of air.
2. In a large room, have students practice "stop, drop, and roll" techniques on command. Discuss how this activity can put out a fire on a person's clothing.
3. Discuss with students how smoke fills a room and how it affects people's ability to breathe.
4. Have students practice "stay low and go" by crawling under the rope (which represents the imaginary smoke level). The rope should be about two feet off the ground.

Homework

Students bring in pictures from newspapers about fires and people escaping from them. The rope should be about 2 feet off the ground

Evaluation

Students will be able to

- Describe emergency actions when clothing is on fire.
- Demonstrate the "stop, drop, and roll" and the "stay low and go" techniques.
- Explain how fire is extinguished by lack of air.

Learning Experience 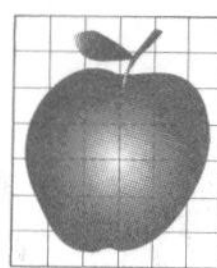 14-14

Little Red Riding Hood

Grade Level

K–2

Primary Discipline

Language Arts

Learning Objectives

Following this activity, students will be able to

- List people whom children should classify as strangers.
- Report why strangers might be bad people.
- Avoid talking with or accompanying strangers without an adult they know.

Time Required

25 minutes

Materials

Little Red Riding Hood book

Description of Activity

After reading the story of Little Red Riding Hood, have the class discuss strangers and how children should act around strangers. Ask the children to share stories about meeting strangers while they were with their parents or other familiar adults. The children share the rules they have received from their parents about strangers. Explain that not all strangers are bad people.

Homework

Students discuss this topic with their parents.

Evaluation

Students will be able to

- Demonstrate reading comprehension skills by identifying, from a story, characteristics of a stranger.
- Distinguish between good and bad strangers.

Learning Experience 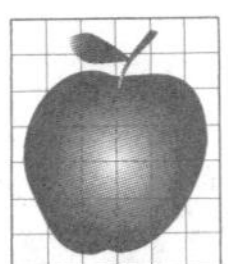 14-15

The Safest Way Home

Grade Level

3–4

Primary Disciplines

Geography, Art

Learning Objectives

Following this activity, students will be able to

- Describe a safe route to their home from school.
- List the potential areas of danger they may face on the way home (street crossings, open lots, wooded areas, and so on).

Time Required

30 minutes

Materials

Chalkboard, chalk, construction paper, pencils, crayons

Description of Activity

Select a favorite spot several blocks from the school with which the students are familiar (for example, a park or convenience store). Draw a simple map on the chalkboard, with the students' help, identifying the route that could be taken to get from the school to that location including safe crossings, unsafe areas, and so on. The class discusses the safest route and what makes it safe.

Homework

Students draw a simple map of the route they take home and identify the safe areas and the unsafe areas.

Evaluation

Students will be able to

- Label and read simple maps.
- Describe safe routes from home to school.
- Identify potential areas of danger in their commonly traveled routes.

Learning Experience 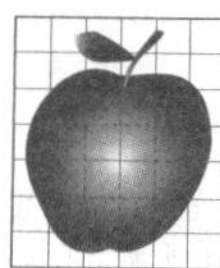 14-16

School Fire Safety Features

Grade Level

3–4

Primary Discipline

Social Studies

Learning Objectives

Following this activity, students will be able to

- List equipment in the school building that is designed to protect them from injury from fire.
- Describe the route they would take out of the building in case of fire, from different locations.

Time Required

45 minutes

Materials

Paper, pencils

Description of Activity

Take the students on a tour of the school building to familiarize them with the equipment and construction features designed to protect them from fire injuries (for example, nonflammable stairwells, panic bars on exits, emergency lighting, public address system, exit signs, fire alarms, smoke detectors, safe rooms). Have students describe how they would exit the building from the lunch room, gymnasium, bathrooms, and so on. Have the class discuss how the building is designed to protect students with disabilities. Have the students walk through these various exits and identify safety features along the way.

Homework

Students develop a list of safety equipment and construction features in their own homes.

Evaluation

Students will be able to

- Identify fire safety equipment, including fire doors, exit signs, public address systems, panic bars, and so on, and explain how they are used.
- Describe common exit routes from various locations in the school and home.

Learning Experience 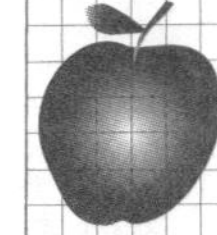 14-17

Seat Belt Safety

Grade Level

3–4

Primary Disciplines

Science, Language Arts

Learning Objectives

Following this activity, students will be able to

- Explain the importance of wearing a seat belt.
- Wear a seat belt whenever they are riding in a car.
- Remind others when they do not wear their seat belts.

Time Required

30 minutes

Materials

Strollers with safety belts, dolls, masking tape

Description of Activity

Put the doll inside a play stroller and demonstrate the following:

1. Collision with a wall with no safety belt.
2. Head-on collision with another vehicle with no safety belt.
3. Turning the stroller sharply, causing the doll to fall from the carriage.
4. The class discusses what can be done to prevent these accidents. The activities are repeated using a fastened belt or tape securely around the doll.

Homework

None

Evaluation

Students will be able to

- Demonstrate and explain the importance of safety belts in collisions.
- Identify places where safety belts are necessary (high chairs, swings, strollers, and so on).

Learning Experience 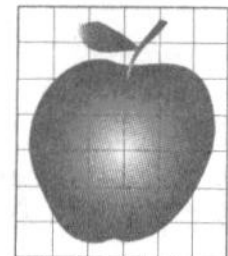 14-18

Smoke Detector Safety

Grade Level

3–4

Primary Discipline

Science

Learning Objectives

Following this activity, students will be able to

- List the different kinds of detectors.
- Locate detectors in school and home.

Time Required

60 minutes

Materials

Local smoke detector salesperson, different smoke detectors

Description of Activity

Invite a local salesperson to demonstrate different types of smoke detectors. This person illustrates the proper places to put smoke detectors and stresses the importance of maintenance (check battery each month, change battery every 6 months, and so on). Have students take a walk around the school and identify locations of smoke detectors in the building.

Homework

Students write a description of where smoke detectors are located in their apartments and houses.

Evaluation

Students will be able to

- Explain how smoke detectors work and why they are important.
- Describe where smoke detectors should be placed in the home and in the school.
- Describe the maintenance of smoke detectors.

Learning Experience 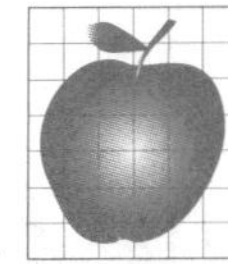 14-19

In Case of a Heart Attack

Grade Level

5–6

Primary Disciplines

Science, Language Arts

Learning Objectives

Following this activity, students will be able to

- List the early signals of heart attack.
- Contact the EMS.

Time Required

30 minutes

Materials

Telephone

Description of Activity

After a science lesson about the heart and how it works, lead a discussion of what happens when the heart cannot beat properly. Include the signs and symptoms of a heart attack (persistent chest pain; crushing feeling in the chest; pain radiating from the jaw, neck and shoulder; perspiring; difficulty breathing). The students role-play a heart attack and a call to 911 to report the need for further medical assistance.

Homework

As a follow-up activity, if desired, students interview an EMS doctor, nurse, or fire department person and write a report on the signs and symptoms of a heart attack.

Evaluation

Students will be able to

- Explain how the human heart works.
- Describe signs and symptoms of a heart attack.
- Explain when to call 911.
- State the appropriate information to give 911 operator.

Learning Experience 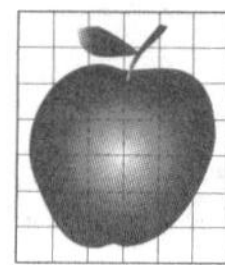 14-20

Minor Wounds and Bleeding

Grade Level

5–6

Primary Discipline

Science

Learning Objectives

Following this activity, students will be able to

- Apply direct pressure and elevation.
- Describe the location of pressure points.
- Describe how to control bleeding.
- Name potential barriers between a rescuer and a victim's body fluids.
- Identify good places to keep latex gloves for emergencies.

Time Required

30 minutes

Materials

Latex gloves for each student; 4" or 2" gauze pads.

Description of Activity

After teaching about the blood supply and circulation, demonstrate how to elevate and apply direct pressure to a bleeding wound. Also demonstrates how to apply pressure to other pressure points (at brachial artery in mid-arm and femoral artery in groin). The sequence is as follows:

1. Put on latex gloves, apply direct pressure, elevate, and then apply pressure to the pressure point.
2. Allow students time to practice finding pressure points and applying direct pressure.
3. Role-play several mock injuries in which the victim is bleeding and the students are responding as rescuers.
4. Discuss the importance of latex gloves and important places to store them (in car, garage, kitchen, athletic bag, and so on).

Homework

None

Evaluation

Students will be able to

- Describe procedures for controlling bleeding.
- Explain the importance of using latex gloves when responding to bleeding.
- Identify the basic components of the circulatory system.
- Identify pressure points and demonstrate how to use them to control bleeding.

15

The Consumer of Health Products and Community Health Services

Estelle Weinstein

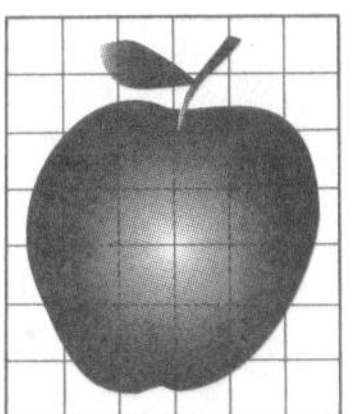

Chapter Outline

Consumer Health Education
Drug Information
Vitamin Use
Food Labels
Consumer Advocacy
Quackery
The Practitioner–Patient Relationship
Components of Community Health
The Community Health Care System
Government Health Care Agencies
Health Care Providers
Payment Systems
Managed Care/Health Maintenance Organizations (HMOs)

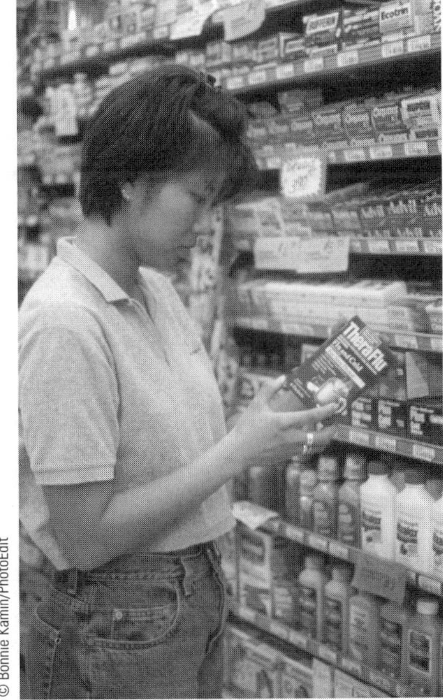

© Bonnie Kamin/PhotoEdit

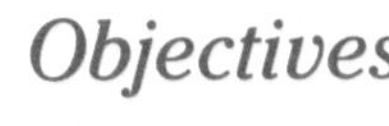

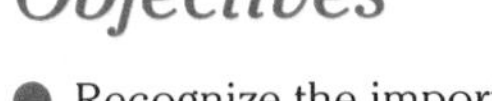

Objectives

- Recognize the importance of making wise consumer decisions
- Recognize reliable sources of health information
- Understand product labels and how to relate them to personal health
- Evaluate the effectiveness of vitamin supplementation
- Identify health care agencies and their roles in maintaining the nation's health
- Identify the various medical and allied health practitioners
- Be able to make decisions about traditional and complimentary medical practices
- Identify the various mental health practitioners
- Recognize and evaluate the various health care payment systems

Every morning when Brendan and Alex eat their breakfast, their mother gives them a chewable vitamin. It looks like candy and tastes good, but they are never permitted to have more than one a day. They really don't know what vitamins do, but they do know that vitamins have something to do with keeping them healthy. Sometimes, when one of them is sick, their pediatrician gives their mother a piece of paper with a prescription on it that a person in the supermarket takes and gives them medicine. They know they have to take the medicine only when it is given to them. They are not sure why it works, but they do start to feel better.

Whenever they go grocery shopping with their dad, they notice that he reads the labels on the cans and boxes, especially when he is buying something they don't usually buy. Often they ask for cereals they have seen advertised on TV and their dad tells them these are unhealthy because they have too much sugar. The children can't figure out why the TV program tells them the exact opposite. This is all confusing!

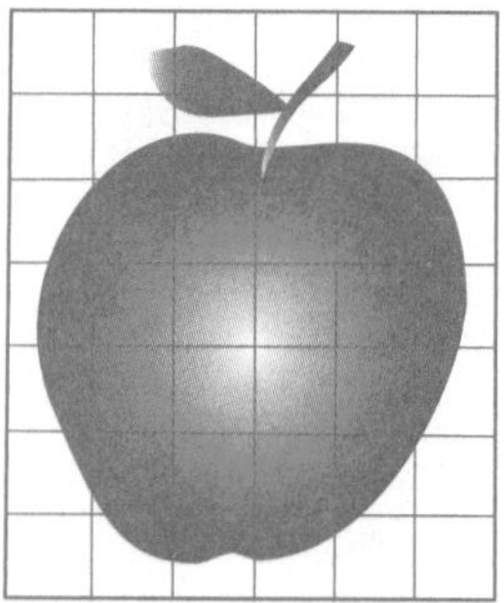

What do Brendan and Alex need to know about taking vitamins and other medications, as they become old enough to make decisions about their own health? What information on food labels is important for them to understand? How do they distinguish reliable and useful information from that which they receive from the media and other sources?

How do children learn about the difference between vitamins and drugs? How do they know which products are "good" and which are "bad" for them? Where do they learn how to determine if information they hear is true or untrue, real or myth? What and who should they believe? They need to become informed consumers.

Now, as in no other time in history, consumerism has become more important. Today, through sophisticated advertising and the media, people are bombarded with often-conflicting information about a vast array of products and services. The sexy and convincing marketing strategies (often targeted at young children) make products appealing and frequently avoid, if not outright misrepresent, their capabilities and confound people's ability to make informed decisions that ultimately affect their health.

As families disperse internationally for long periods and travel extensively with children for leisure or business, they become a part of the larger global community. As a result, the part the community plays in maintaining an individual's or family's health and the part the individual or family plays in the health of the community become important for individuals or families to understand and take responsibility for.

Children need to know where health services are, what their purposes are, which services are of high quality and which are not, and which services are lacking. Knowing about individual providers of health services, health service

For Your Health

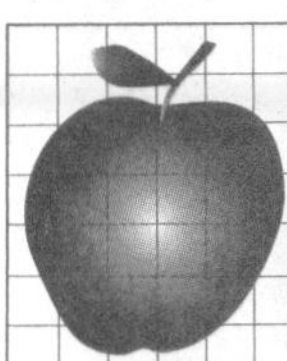

Hints for Taking Medications

A spoonful of sugar helps the medicine go down.

To take tablets or capsules: Stand or sit up straight. Sip some water to moisten your mouth and throat first, then swallow the tablet with a mouthful of water. Follow up with another glass of water. If the tablet feels "stuck," eat a piece of bread or a banana, then drink more water. Capsules float, so tilt your head slightly forward for easier swallowing.

To use nose drops: Tilt your head back. Breathing through your mouth, put the drops in your nostrils. Gently breathe in through your nose. Keep your head tilted back a few minutes.

To use eye drops or ointment: Tilt your head back. Pull down your lower eyelid and look toward the ceiling. Put the drops or ointment in the "pouch" formed by your lower lid, then close your eye gently. Wipe away any excess with a tissue.

To use ear drops: Tilt your head so the ear points up; grasp your earlobe and pull it down and back to straighten the ear canal. Put in the drops. Keep your head tilted a few minutes, then place a loose cotton plug at the opening of your ear to keep the drops from running out.

Note: Wash your hands thoroughly before and after using any nose, eye, or ear drops, and never let the dropper touch your body.

delivery systems, how to access them, and how to pay for them are valuable consumer tools for children to master before adulthood. This knowledge and how to use it makes the difference between quality care and poor care. Sometimes it makes the difference between life and death.

People, as advocates for their own health who watch out for themselves and their loved ones, will be better prepared to negotiate the new and sometimes complicated health delivery systems, especially managed care. They will be effective in advocating for themselves and their local and global community's health. This chapter will provide teachers with a framework for teaching about consumerism, including appropriate student goals, objectives, and activities and to educate classroom teachers to become knowledgeable consumers. With the necessary information, teachers can increase their students' abilities to implement effective consumer behaviors. Teachers will need the following information when incorporating these topics into their curriculum.

Consumer Health Education

Too often, consumers believe that some federal agency or other official source is responsible for monitoring health-related products. Given this naïve belief system about consumer protection agencies and government-sponsored programs, uneducated consumers may believe that unsafe products are not available in the over-the-counter market or think that a licensed practitioner is automatically looking out for the patients' best interests.

Thinking that they are protected, consumers misuse health care products and have unrealistic expectations about health services. Yet, the true source of power over goods and services lies with consumers themselves, who not only pay for them but also have the capability of choosing them from a variety of possible alternatives. Recognizing the limitations of government to monitor all services, educated consumers do their own investigations. Thus, the challenge of consumer health education is to help people become savvy about which products and services actually match their health-related needs and learn how effective the products or services will be when compared to others.

How does one become an educated consumer? It requires knowing where and how to access accurate and dependable information and apply it to one's own personal situation; becoming familiar with the variety of items available, their uses, effectiveness, and prices; recognizing the influences of others on their own consumer decisions; and knowing their rights as consumers and how to access consumer protection agencies. Educated consumers advocate for their own health and the health care of their community.

The political and socio-medical climate in the medical and health care communities is changing. Nontraditional treatments, especially holistic approaches based on valid scientific evidence, are becoming acceptable interventions. Because new products and services often originate outside of conventional medical traditions, consumers understandably have difficulty figuring out which are useful and which are quackery.

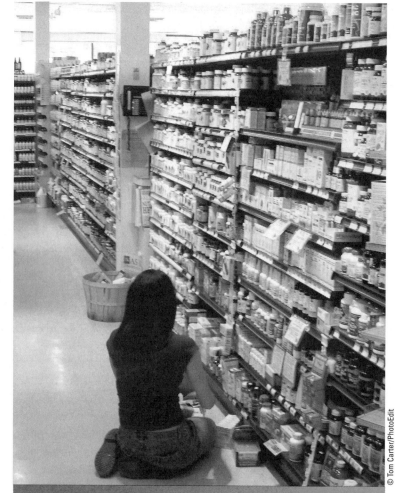

© Tom Carter/PhotoEdit

Over-the-counter drugs fill many shelves in supermarkets and pharmacies.

Drug Information

Although the federal system of making a drug available to the general public is tedious, drawn out, and sometimes controversial, it does ensure a substantial amount of accurate information. Only recently has this drug information become readable and understandable to the public. Nevertheless, the information provided on drug containers is still complicated. An easier source of information for the consumer is the physician or pharmacist.

Drugs are either prescription (must be prescribed by a medical provider) or purchased over-the-counter (OTC). When a physician recommends a drug, whether it's prescription or OTC, the consumer must ask several questions about how that drug relates to his or her personal situation. For example: "What is this prescription for? How often and for how long should I take it? Will it interact with any of the other drugs I'm taking? Are there any warnings I should know about, or any side effects? If I experience any of these, what should I do? Do I need to know anything else about this drug? Is there a generic version that is equally effective and less expensive?" Educated consumers should be prepared with pencil and paper so they can write down the answers. If the physician does not have the time to answer the questions, the consumer should seek another physician. Moreover, doctors do not always discuss the synergistic effect of prescribed drugs with foods or other drugs their patient may be taking. These combinations sometimes result in life-threatening reactions and even death. Wary consumers know to ask for additional information to match their unique needs and circumstances. Another effective means of achieving that information is through the pharmacist. With the computerizing of pharmacies, printouts contain a great deal of information about medications, their potential side effects, and their interactions.

Government-Accepted Definitions

- **Light (Lite).** May refer to calories, fat, or sodium. Contains 1/3 fewer calories, or no more than 1/2 the fat of the higher-calorie, higher-fat version; or no more than 1/2 the sodium of the higher-sodium version.
- **Calorie-free.** Fewer than 5 calories per serving.
- **Fat-free.** Contains less than 0.5 grams of fat per serving.
- **Low fat.** Contains less than 3 grams of fat per serving.
- **Reduced or less fat.** At least 25% less fat per serving than the higher-fat version.
- **Lean.** Fewer than 10 grams of fat, 4 grams of saturated fat, and 95 milligrams of cholesterol per serving.
- **Extra lean.** Fewer than 5 grams of fat, 2 grams of saturated fat, and 95 milligrams of cholesterol per serving.
- **Cholesterol-free.** Contains fewer than 2 milligrams of cholesterol and 2 grams (or less) of saturated fat per serving.
- **Low cholesterol.** Contains 20 milligrams of cholesterol (or less) and 2 grams of saturated fat (or less) per serving.
- **Reduced cholesterol.** At least 25% less cholesterol than the higher-cholesterol version; contains 2 grams (or less) of saturated fat per serving.
- **Sodium-free.** Fewer than 5 milligrams of sodium per serving and no sodium chloride (NaCl) in ingredients.
- **Very low sodium.** Contains 35 milligrams of sodium (or less) per serving.
- **Low sodium.** Contains 140 milligrams (or less) per serving.
- **Sugar-free.** Fewer than 0.5 grams of sugar per serving.
- **High-fiber.** Contains 5 grams of fiber (or more) per serving.
- **Good source of fiber.** Contains 2.5 to 4.9 grams of fiber.

Hence, consumers are advised to use the same pharmacist whenever possible so that their drug history can be assessed each time a new prescription or OTC medicine is suggested. Furthermore, families should maintain a drug history for their children until they are old enough to maintain one for themselves. When families move around frequently and change doctors and pharmacies just as frequently, maintaining a lifetime drug history helps ensure against allergic reactions, synergistic effects, and drug ineffectiveness.

Vitamin Use

Vitamin supplementation is a growing industry that is undergoing much scrutiny. This is particularly confusing for the consumer. Vitamins are not considered drugs but, rather, food supplements. Therefore, they have not fallen under the same governmental control and restrictions as other drugs. Taking vitamins as treatments for specific conditions or to alleviate health problems is still not scientifically supported or accepted by conventional medicine or the Food and Drug Administration. Yet, with minimal labeling restrictions, they are sold with controversial promises.

Alternative and conventional medical professionals are presently studying the claims of vitamins as effective treatments for all sorts of medical problems. The results are not yet confirmed. Some vitamins are relatively benign, and their use is less problematic than others that are thought to have serious side effects especially if taken in higher-than-recommended doses.

Children are introduced to vitamins in infancy. They are usually covered with a candy or other sweet casing. Often, children do not associate vitamins with drugs. Thus, part of their education is to learn about vitamins and other drugs, their interactions and their risks.

Food Labels

Foods can have a serious impact on health. Some foods are touted to cure all sorts of ailments—increase sexual appetites and sexual capabilities and do all sorts of other magical things. In some cases, foods contain ingredients that can cause serious allergic reactions. Although labels on foods have been available for several decades, consumers' recent interest in dietary fat, sugar, and salt intake, as they relate to their health, has motivated many changes.

In the past, a person would need a degree in chemistry or nutrition to understand food labels. The new federal labeling requirements are considerably less confusing. By reading the food labels on commercial products, consumers can relate the information to their own health status. For example, people who have been asked to control their cholesterol by limiting their fat intake to less than 30 percent of daily calories need to know the relationship of fat calories to total calories in the product, the amounts of saturated and unsaturated fats, and how these relate to the amount of fat in their total daily diet. People with diabetes or hypertension need to know how many grams of sugar or salt are in a food product and how that translates to total sugar or salt intake for their specific dietary needs (see also Chapter 3).

Food manufacturers have used all sorts of advertising tricks, designed solely for the purpose of increasing sales, to sway (and sometimes totally mislead) the public. Words such as "free" and "lite," although meant to describe certain qualities of food, have sometimes been incorporated into the name of the product, further confusing the public. Sometimes compelling language, such as "guarantee" or coupons with "your money back" are used. A guarantee that a medication or health product will work in all instances is not possible.

In addition, foods on menus in restaurants that might otherwise seem like healthy choices are often prepared by chefs who have little understanding of nutrition. The foods can contain ingredients that make them health risks, such as high salt or fat. Being an educated consumer is a difficult task for anyone who frequently eats out or doesn't have the time to study food labels.

Children—if taught about food labels, how to read them, what they mean, and what to look for—are less likely to fall prey to sophisticated advertising and more likely to become consumer advocates.

Consumer Advocacy

The frequent absence of consumer representation on professional decision-making bodies that determine costs and ensure quality of medical products and services is a problem. More often than not, the quality and cost of health care are managed through a system of professional peer review. In the case of medical treatment, physicians and other health care practitioners establish whether services or products are medically necessary or appropriate for a given treatment. The power given to professionals in this system, coupled with government involvement in health care delivery, has created a need for consumer advocacy groups to give consumers a voice. Raising students' awareness of effective and trustworthy consumer groups is a component of consumer health education. Teaching students to seek opinions from consumer-driven magazines like *Consumer Reports* is also helpful.

Young people tend to get their information about products and services from one another. Children are particularly vulnerable because they have been mesmerized by television advertising during the many hours they watch TV. What they buy and how they are persuaded by media appeals comes from testimonials presented by their heroes or authority figures. Advertisers use various tactics—including their knowledge of people's desire to be like others, claims of "scientific proof," snob appeal, fear, promises of sexuality and attractiveness, low price, and cultural factors—to market their products.

Even though purposely advertising false information about a product or service is illegal, advertising experts are skilled at manipulating words and pictures that appeal to the public. When the press reports the results of a scientific study, the message is often exaggerated or misleading. Reporters are not scientists: Their job is to write stories that sell newspapers and TV features. For example, almost every day an article can be found about a new "breakthrough" that will cure one kind of cancer or another. Yet, the medical community would argue that, though we are making many advances, we still have a long way to go.

One day the local press carried an advertisement about the cholesterol-lowering effects of walnuts. The very next morning all of the walnuts in the local supermarkets were sold out. There was no search for the accuracy of this information by readers to the paper. Some took the time to seek advice from their physician before they purchased and consumed the walnuts. Educated consumers would have sought answers to some of the following questions: Who said this? How many walnuts would I have to eat? How much would eating walnuts lower my cholesterol? What other outcomes of eating walnuts could be expected? What implications does eating walnuts have on my health profile? These questions are rarely answered in the lay press.

Information about health products and services can be obtained from several reliable sources. In addition to federal, state, and local consumer protection agencies (U. S. Public Health Service, Consumer Product Safety Commission, Federal Trade Commission) and state and local health departments of consumer affairs, local voluntary agencies (for example, the American Public Health Association and the American Lung Association) and licensed or certified medical practitioners (physicians, nurses, dieticians, and so on) can provide people with accurate information. Information released by an official health arm of the federal or state government is generally accurate and useful as a guideline. Consumer-protection groups are not only good resources for consumer information; they also produce useful written pamphlets and brochures about consumer protection strategies.

Some health newsletters are affiliated with medical education institutions (for example, *Mental Health Letter, Women's Health Watch,* Harvard's *Health Newsletter,* and the Mayo Clinic *Health Letter*). They publish accurate information about health studies and health topics in easy-to-read language. Also, hospitals and voluntary agencies offer national and local hotlines, providing both verbal and written information. These often are specific to a health problem. For example, the American Cancer Society provides accurate, current information about products, treatments, and services associated with cancer. The American Heart Association does the same for heart disease. Many of the hotlines can be found in the telephone directory of toll-free 800 numbers. These agencies often provide online services.

Developing awareness and strategies that question what one reads, what one hears, and what one takes at face value is a challenging task for children. Asking questions and thinking critically about what they see and hear are basic processes students must learn to become educated and informed. If these critical analytic skills are in place before adolescence, the power of peer pressure and blind trust of the written or spoken word can be diminished. Then, when a friend says, "Don't worry—it's perfectly safe," students will know how to respond.

Quackery

Quackery occurs when health care is administered by unlicensed or unethical providers; when promises of cures are made about products that are actually useless; and when ineffective procedures or diagnostic or therapeutic processes, products, remedies, or devices are used before they are scientifically validated. Often quacks prey on the seriously ill or the elderly because they are particularly vulnerable. This vulnerability emerges when they have received unsuccessful treatment from the conventional medical system and are therefore ready to accept any magical cure.

The strategies that quacks use include advertising through mass-produced literature and well designed home mailings. Rarely does their promotion appear in professional medical or health care journals. Quacks sometimes refer to studies that do not apply scientific methods and are designed to confuse the unsophisticated public. The advertisements, like the quacks themselves, fool consumers by photographing models in medical settings dressed in medical-type uniforms. Sometimes they display bogus credentials that appear in frames similar to recognized degrees or training certificates commonly displayed in doctors' offices.

One must be wary of promises about simplistic, magical cures and painless treatments for otherwise complicated or painful problems—especially if these alternative products and services completely reject conventional medicine.

Among the most common forms of quackery are drugs, cosmetics, nutritional substitutes, exercise or electronic devices, because consumers seek quick solutions to complicated problems. Some of these have a place in effective treatment, when they are scientifically validated or administered by capable and trained practitioners. For example, the preoccupation with quick weight loss and an instantaneous lowering of cholesterol is a source of much quackery that markets dietary supplements and cholesterol-lowering drugs in supermarkets and health food stores. Although some of these products are benign and may someday prove to have scientific validity, many can harm the body and can be quite costly.

To counteract quackery, people who suspect it should report it to agencies such as the Better Business Bureau, Office of Consumer Affairs, or a medical professional group such as the American Medical Association. Young students can be taught to question what they are told about health care, how to ask questions, and who is reliable.

The Practitioner–Patient Relationship

In addition to personal variables—including family attitudes, personal experiences, and cultural or religious factors—one's choice of physician or health care provider frequently depends upon one's address and income. A factor that contributes greatly to effective medical care is the practitioner–patient relationship. Selecting a trustworthy practitioner or medical group requires knowing their availability and accessibility and feeling comfortable with the doctors, nurses, and other staff.

If the family doctor is not one who is handed down from one generation to another, a good place to start is by identifying a doctor that meets the patient's needs through recommendations from friends, the local medical society, physicians or nurses, and the like. An interview with a prospective physician is helpful to identify communication styles, office ambiance, and professional credentials (education, licensure/certification, fellowships, length of time in practice, and so on). At such an interview, prospective patients can find out about availability for appointments and emergencies, how telephone questions are answered, hospital affiliations, and payment schedules.

During regular office visits, good communication between patient and practitioner becomes important. Being prepared with written questions before an office visit is effective. Also, because of the anxiety and sometimes embarrassment associated with a medical examination, people may not effectively communicate their symptoms. It is best to write them down beforehand.

Sometimes gender differences influence how people will behave. For example, some men learn that complaining is a weakness. Thus, they may not communicate symptoms as readily as women. Male doctors may expect more complaints from women and therefore not take them as seriously as they would from male patients. Also, cultural factors sometimes interfere with the practitioner–patient relationship. Certain diagnostic procedures and treatments are not acceptable in some religious and ethnic groups. Thus, cultural traditions may interfere with treatment recommendations.

When a diagnosis is made, the doctor and the patient should select treatment approaches together. Physicians should be supportive of second opinions and willing to make information and records readily available to patients who request them. When a treatment or recommendation is acceptable, patients should take notes or receive written material that confirms what they have agreed to. Sometimes the practitioner is busy and cannot take the time at that moment to fully explain or give directions. If this happens, arrangements should be made for an appropriate time when all questions can be answered. If the physician or his or her representative (sometimes the nurse or health counselor) is not willing to take the time, the consumer should consider a change in physician.

Thus, educated consumers are also educated patients who take responsibility for their own health and care. As educated consumers, students can begin to contribute to the community's health by making healthy decisions, choosing healthy behaviors, and advocating for comprehensive services accessible to all.

Joshua and **Tammy** grew up in the Midwest on a small farm not far from a small town. Everyone in the neighborhood knew one another. They knew when a neighbor was ill, and they knew what the illness was. One local doctor took care of everyone's family, delivered babies, set broken bones, wrote prescriptions, and sometimes gave medicines to those with colds and flu. Not too far away, in a nearby town, was a small hospital and an ambulatory surgery center. People went there only if Dr. Gregg said it was necessary.

Sometimes, if a person was really sick, he or she would be helicoptered to a hospital in the big city. When Joshua and Tammy were in elementary school, their family moved to the big city. Here, they had a choice of more doctors, several hospitals, and more voluntary agencies than their parents could think about. The health problems in the city also were different from those in their small town. But choosing a physician and getting an appointment when they needed one was a big problem, as was having enough money to pay the medical bills. Joshua and Tammy often heard their parents talk about their "HMO," but they didn't know what that meant. They knew their new doctor was a pediatrician and did not treat adults in their family like Dr. Gregg did. Their parents had a different doctor. The new pediatrician seemed okay, but they didn't know her very well, so they did not want to ask her personal questions or even tell her when they were afraid. They couldn't imagine picking up the telephone and calling the office any time they needed to, as they had back home. They learned about 911 and other emergency procedures. Things certainly did change for them.

What are some of the strategies Joshua and Tammy's family can use to select a health provider? Who are some of the various providers they might choose from? What do they need to know in order to create a healthy patient–practitioner relationship? What other community health services are available to children and their families? How will they pay for health care?

Components of Community Health

At one time, an area or region was considered to be a **community** by political or geographic boundaries alone. A community's health status and health problems were confined to the people who lived within those boundaries. More recently, the notion of community has expanded dramatically to include a designated area in which the people who live or work have similar needs and interests or belong to a similar culture or ethnic group.[1] Moreover, it is a place with some evidence of a common life, some common behavioral norms, and an organized approach to health resources.[2] A community also is designated as such "by the boundaries within which a problem can be defined, dealt with and solved."[3]

As the world becomes more and more accessible and people move readily from one place to another, sometimes a great distance, community health takes on a more global nature. What happens in one community—whether it involves an outbreak of a dangerous communicable disease such as HIV/AIDS, West Nile virus, or mad cow disease, or an environmental catastrophe such as Chernobyl—may result in a health problem that has implications for the whole world.

A community's health is looked at collectively rather than individually. Components of the health services of a community are the range of services available to its people, the promotion of public health and prevention efforts, and the planning and delivery of health services based on its special needs. These may differ from one community to another. For example, some communities have environmental pollution problems because they are situated in industrial areas. Other communities, at a low socioeconomic level, have nutritional and substance abuse problems and problems of inaccessibility to medical care. Still other communities have a disproportionate number of infirm elderly people with special health needs. The community's range of services necessary to meet its own unique needs is a measure of the quality of the community's health.

Medical care and health care are often confused with one another. They are different. Medical care or "sick care" is a direct service (treatment) administered to people who are ill or think they are ill. The medical delivery system, however, is moving toward health care, which is the promotion of health and prevention of health problems by controlling social and environmental contributors to disease. The focus of medical care is on illness, repair, and prevention of further illness from the same cause, whereas the focus of health care is on wellness and the maintenance of good health. A measure of a community's health is the availability of both health care and medical care services to all constituents.

The philosophy that all citizens have a right to some measure of medical care and health care is widely accepted. Nevertheless, accessibility to services is too often related to people's ability to pay or their ability to negotiate the complexities of the health system. A familiar saying is "You can't buy good health." Although that may have been true in the past, it is no longer the case. People with financial means often have access to better health care products, medical services, and knowledge about how to maintain their health. People of low economic status often have little or no access. For example, early maternal and child health care, which results in better outcomes of childbirth and childhood illnesses, is much more readily available to people who can pay for the services than to those who cannot. The ability to live longer and to have a better quality of life while living with a chronic disease is more likely for people with financial means. As medical costs increase dramatically (which they have done over the past few decades), fewer and fewer people have the ability to pay for services. Moreover, people who can afford health care are not dispersed evenly across communities. Therefore, the nature of community health problems is uneven within the same community and from one community to another. Because these problems have implications for the health of school-aged children, they must be considered when planning educational health lessons in the schools.

The Community Health Care System

A vast substructure of health services that provide for and promote a community's health exists, to some extent, within each small community. Many of these health services interact with the larger city, state, and federal systems. A community's ability to serve the health needs of its constituents is measured against national standards for similar communities and includes information about the health status of the population and the availability of health services in that community. Local, national, and federal agencies maintain this information. Hence, interested consumers can determine the health of their community by looking at its services and health statistics as compared with other similar communities.

Community health services, agencies, and organizations make up the subsystems of the **health care delivery system**. The delivery system employs health care providers who play many different roles in their respective subsystems. A **health care provider** is a professional (doctor, dentist, and so on) who delivers health care services directly to the consumer. A health care delivery system may provide direct services, such as medical or nursing care, or indirect services, such as education or advocacy. These services are supported by tax dollars (through government agencies) or through non-tax dollars (donations, out-of-pocket payment for care, insurance companies, and so on).

Elementary schoolchildren are consumers of health services in their community. They are also future advocates for health in the political and social system. This chapter emphasizes the services in the local community health care system, preparing them for these roles.

The following is a brief synopsis of the structure of the federal, state, and local agency system.

Government Health Care Agencies

Official health care agencies are found at the federal, state, and local levels. The role of each is discussed briefly.

Federal Agencies

How much responsibility the federal government has in the health care of its citizens shifts with changes in administration. Through a system of agencies, the federal government makes several kinds of contributions; some are regulatory, others support research and/or direct services.

Official or public health agencies are organizations that are legislatively sanctioned and supported by government revenue. Federal health care functions include developing national standards for health care, identifying international health problems that affect the United States, disseminating information, and providing tax revenue to support statewide and local health care initiatives. Although not necessarily affecting local citizens directly, federal control of payment systems (the way health care is paid for) in the delivery of health care, grants for services, research, and health education initiatives have enormous implications for how the local community health care system operates and prioritizes its programs. Figure 15.1 shows the agencies of the federal system under the Department of Health and Human Services, with a further breakdown of the Public Health Service.

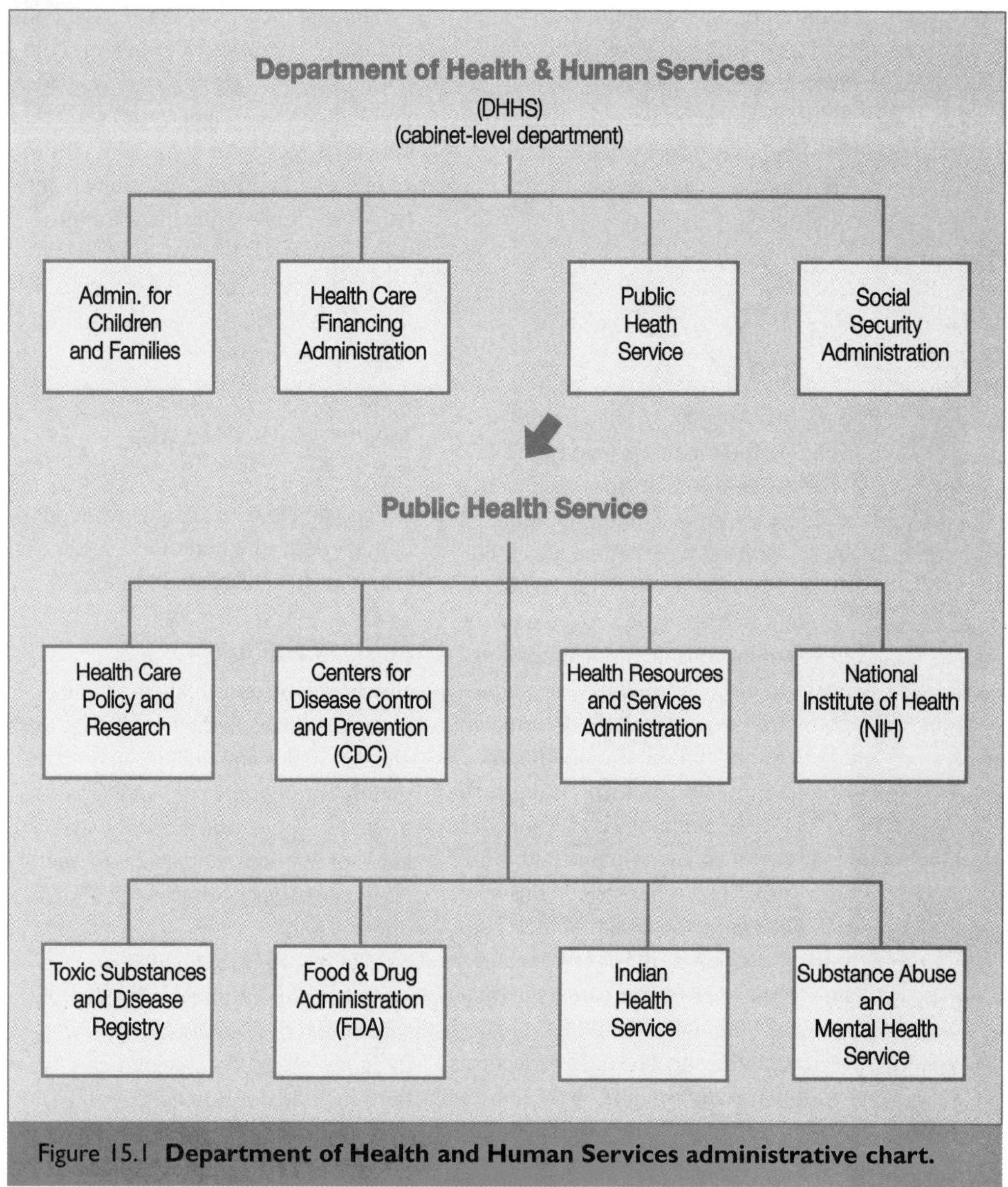

Figure 15.1 **Department of Health and Human Services administrative chart.**

State and Local Health Departments

Official state and local health departments provide a variety of health services within a political jurisdiction. They promote the health of people within the state, particularly the under-served. They monitor and maintain a healthy environment, control diseases and disabilities, and attempt to ensure accessibility and adequacy of health-care services and resources.

State health departments are responsible for ensuring implementation of rules and regulations established by that state's legislature. Through state health departments, the local health departments, as branches of the state, carry out direct services to the local communities within their jurisdiction. In so doing, the local health departments have the greatest impact on the health problems of the community. Thus, these are the agencies with which students should become familiar.

The local health department is an important resource for schools. Its network of medical centers provides direct medical, dental, nursing, and mental health services to the public. It is concerned with maintenance and improvement of the community's health through screening, immunization, laboratory diagnosis and treatment services, alcohol and other drug abuse programs, control of chronic and communicable diseases, dissemination of public health information, and education provided in both inpatient and outpatient clinics. Local health departments monitor community health through constant vigilance and statistical analyses.

Because of fiscal constraints and an outgrowth of voluntary health care

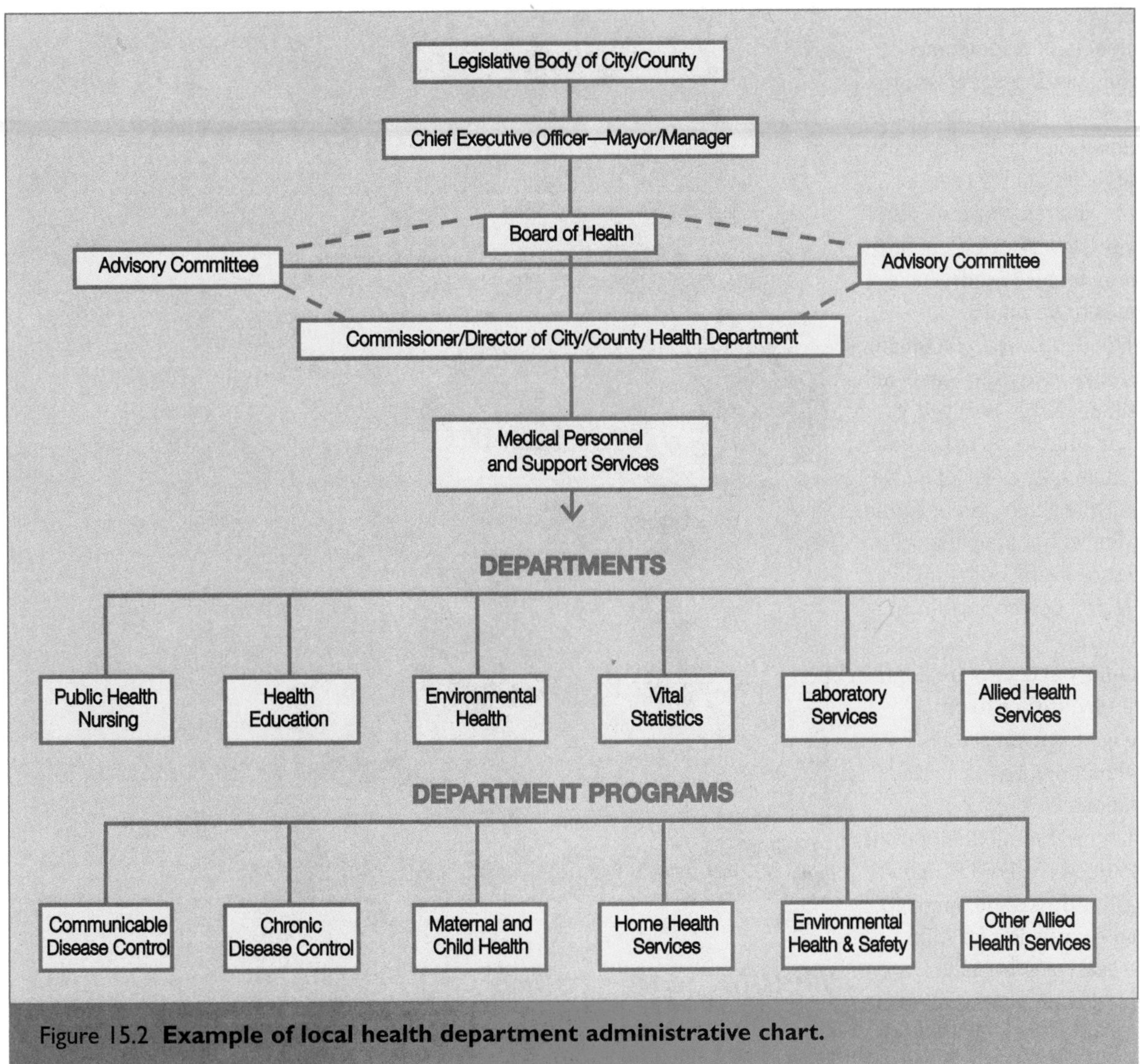

Figure 15.2 **Example of local health department administrative chart.**

agencies in the community that also provide health care services, local health departments have taken leadership roles in collaborative efforts, diminishing overlap and overcoming gaps in services. Recently they have developed associations with school districts to seek funding and establish health care centers on school premises. These associations present innovative and resourceful ways to provide services for under-served children and reluctant, hard-to-reach populations. Elementary school teachers will find the health education division of their local health department to be a useful resource for speakers and educational materials (see Figure 15.2).

The Private Sector

In addition to the official government health network, a substantial number of health care agencies and individual providers deliver direct medical and other health care services to their communities through the private sector. Many voluntary agencies, organizations, and foundations make important contributions. Each has individual goals and objectives. Because these **voluntary organizations** are independent of each other, their services may overlap. Voluntary agencies may be organized to deal with a specific illness or disease (such as the American Diabetes Association and the American Cancer Society); a body organ or system (for example, the American Lung Association and the American Heart Association); a health care issue (for example, Planned Parenthood and Alcoholics Anonymous); or general health concerns (such as the American Red Cross and United Way). They are either independent agencies or local branches of state, national, or international units of an umbrella organization.

Typically, these agencies are governed by boards of directors, are staffed by paid employees, have a large network of volunteers, and sometimes employ consultants. The agencies provide one or several of the following services: medical, mental health, dental, or nursing services; financial support for individuals with health problems; research (direct or supported); political advocacy for their cause; and educational programs or training for the community. Frequently, when an organization has a single focus and that health problem is eliminated or resolved, it tends to find another focus rather than disband. When an agency is not located in a community, it usually can be found in a surrounding community that extends services to several communities. The service region covered is known as a "catchment area."

Some voluntary agencies are established and run by **philanthropic groups** or religious organizations. Philanthropic foundations are supported through donations, corporations, or family foundations through their private financial resources. The Ford Foundation, Robert Wood Johnson Foundation, and American Foundation for AIDS Research are examples. Religious organizations (one of the oldest forms of voluntary agencies) provide health care services either directly to patients through funded and staffed hospitals or to individuals and communities through donations. Philanthropic and religious organizations, like others in the voluntary sector, commit large sums of money to research, new and creative health-care projects. and initiatives for special populations.

The organizations described are an integral part of health care delivery and can be excellent resources for referrals and educational materials. Because of the multitude of programs they implement or support, they provide opportunities for school-aged children to visit and learn about volunteerism and about how to get their health needs met. This can be the beginning of children's involvement in their community's health.

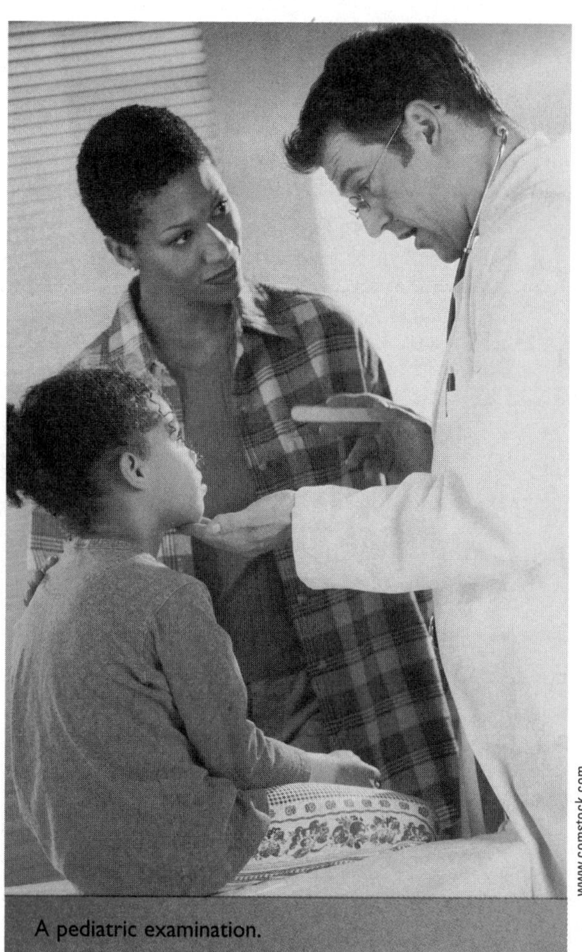
www.comstock.com

A pediatric examination.

Health Care Providers

Medical care and other health care services are housed in hospitals, clinics, health care centers, individual health care offices, and other settings. These may be public or private and may provide one or many health care services. Patients can be treated within the setting, where they stay overnight (inpatient care) or as an outpatient (ambulatory care, where the patient comes for treatment and then leaves).

Within these settings, depending on the type of services offered, are many different types of medical practitioners and other health care providers. Traditional medical practitioners are those trained in what is known as **allopathic medicine**, sometimes called conventional or orthodox medicine. The following is a brief description of the more common classifications of health care providers.

Medical Practitioners

Medical practitioners have received a prescribed course of training that qualifies them to practice medicine. The main types are outlined briefly below; others are listed in the box on page 521.

Physicians are people who are trained and licensed in allopathic medicine and have earned the right to have an MD after their name as a symbol of their academic degree. Physicians differ in their practices by virtue of any specialized training and the populations they commonly serve. Some have chosen additional training in **alternative medicine** and combine the two practices.

General practitioners and **family practitioners** are physicians who have

Selected Medical Specialties

Practitioner:	Specializes in:
Allergist	allergies
Anesthesiologist	sedating patients for surgery
Cardiologist	heart and blood vessel diseases
Dermatologist	skin disorders and diseases
Endocrinologist	gland disorders
Gastro-enterologist	diseases and disorders of the stomach and intestinal tract
Gerontologist	diseases and disorders of elderly people
Gynecologist	female reproductive health
Hematologist	diseases and disorders of the blood and blood-forming tissues
Internist	diagnosis and treatment of diseases of the internal organs by nonsurgical means
Neurologist	diseases of the nervous system
Obstetrician	prenatal care and childbirth
Oncologist	cancer
Ophthalmologist	conditions of the eye
Orthopedic surgeon	bone and joint disorders; bone fractures and injuries
Otolaryngologist	ear, nose, and throat diseases
Pathologist	study of the nature and cause of disease
Pediatrician	diseases of children
Physiatrist	physical disabilities
Psychiatrist	mental and emotional disorders
Radiologist	diagnosis and treatment using radiation
Surgeon	manual and operative procedures to correct defects
Urologist	diseases of the urinary tract and male reproductive tract

had training in general medicine and are interested in overall prevention, diagnosis, and treatment regardless of the patient's age or other classification. Recently, in the environment of managed care, these practitioners have become known as primary-care doctors, the gatekeepers of individual and family health. They refer their patients to specialists and other health care providers for consultation when necessary.

Medical specialists are physicians whose training has gone beyond general medicine to include specialized training in a certain medical area. Examples of medical specialists are obstetricians, gynecologists, pediatricians, geriatric doctors, surgeons, cardiologists, gastroenterologists, neurologists, psychiatrists, ophthalmologists, and so on. Sometimes these specialists have additional training in a sub-area of their specialty, such as cardiovascular surgeons, hematologists, pulmonologists, and immunologists. In most cases these medical specialists see only patients referred to them by general practitioners or other doctors after the patient has been diagnosed with a problem associated with that specialty. The box above lists examples.

Dental specialists are practitioners who have had additional training in a specialized area within dentistry, such as orthodontics (tooth alignment), endodontics (care of gums), or oral surgery (special tooth extractions, apicoectomies, root canals, and the like).

Allied Health Care Providers

Chief among allied health care providers are nursing professionals and physicians' assistants:

Nurses are medical professionals who administer treatment prescribed by medical doctors and offer other services, including health instruction and health counseling. The registered nurse (RN) designation is awarded to those who successfully complete a course of study at the diploma, associate, bachelor, or master's level of nursing and pass a licensing examination. Nursing assistants provide ancillary nursing services under the supervision of a licensed nurse. These assistants include LPNs, nurses' aides, and home health care aides. They are regulated through government programs and educated through a variety of courses.

Nurse practitioners are medical professionals with a degree in nursing and a master's degree or other advanced training in specialties, such as childbirth, pediatrics, and others. In some states, nurse practitioners are permitted to perform as independent providers.

Physician assistants are medical personnel with training similar to that of nurse practitioners who can also perform diagnostic procedures, some types of suturing, and some direct care, generally under the supervision of a physician. This specialty, and that of nurse practitioners, often supplement health care in areas that have a scarcity of medical personnel. In some states they are also licensed to perform as independent providers.

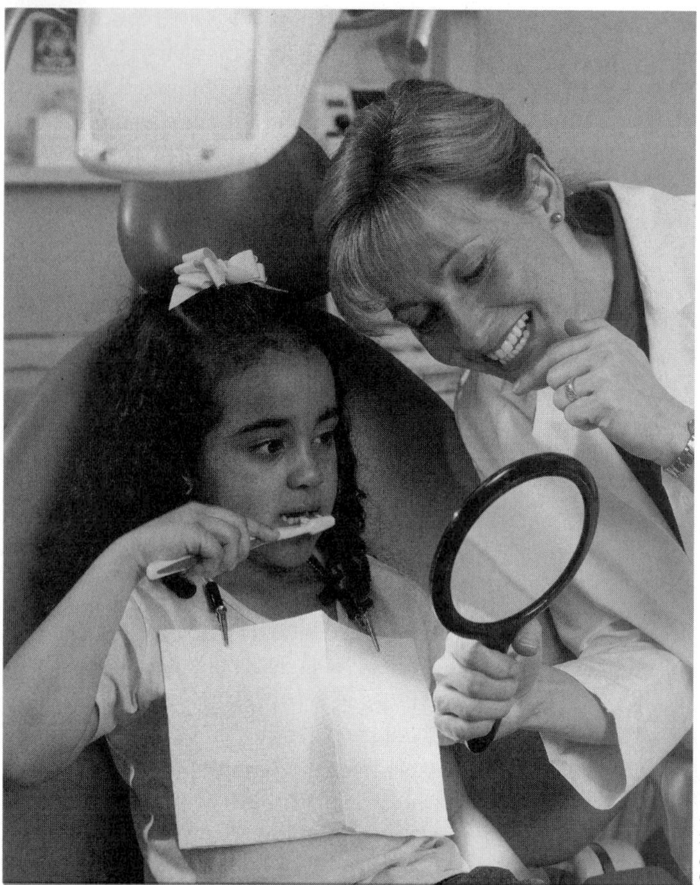
© Corbis Images

Dental specialists help children learn fundamental techniques for dental hygiene.

Other allied health professionals are trained to perform specific medical services that complement direct care. Though too numerous to describe here, they include physical therapists, radiologists, respiratory therapists, lab technicians, and so on.

A network of allied dental providers participates in dental health care. These include dental hygienists (who clean teeth) and dental lab technicians (who make false teeth and other dental appliances). Like medical specialists, these specialists usually receive referrals from the primary provider—in this case, the family dentist.

Alternative/Complementary Medicine

Some practitioners, who may or may not be trained in allopathic medicine, treat medical problems with methods commonly called alternative medicine or complementary medicine. Alternative medical providers may be MDs or osteopaths, homeopaths, Chinese medicine specialists, chiropractors, and naturopaths, and so on. They may provide several different types of treatments in conjunction with, or exclusive of, conventional medicine, including acupuncture, herbals, reflexology, and nutritional supplementation. This segment of practitioners is growing rapidly and insurance companies are just beginning to consider payment for their treatment. The most popular allopaths are described below.

Osteopaths (DO) are practitioners that use the same methods of treatment as conventional physicians, including dispensing of drugs and surgery, but integrate them with personal hygiene, manipulation of the musculo-skeletal system, and nutritional counseling. These professionals practice in settings similar to that of conventional physicians. Taking a more holistic approach to medicine, they emphasize creating a sense of harmony within the person and between the person and his or her environment.

Chiropractors are licensed providers whose practices are limited to mechanical disorders of the back and musculo-skeletal system. Because they believe that health is achieved by maintaining a specific relationship between the nervous system and the spine, their treatment focuses on realigning the vertebrae. Like osteopaths, they practice a more holistic form of medicine, which often emphasizes nutrition, stress reduction, and similar health concerns. Unlike MDs and ODs, they are not allowed by law to perform surgery or provide prescriptive drugs.

Mental Health Care Practitioners

Mental health care is provided to individuals, families, and groups in many different settings (inpatient hospitals, outpatient clinics, community health care centers, homes, halfway houses, and so on) by a variety of professionals who are identified by the training they receive, the theoretical framework in which they work, and sometimes by membership in a professional association or by the state license they hold. Although licensure ensures some qualifications, states do not license all qualified mental health practitioners equally, because of political and economic issues unrelated to the quality of training. For example, in some states, couple and family therapists are graduates of professional programs and are approved by the American Association of Marriage and Family Therapists (AAMFT), but are not permitted to sit for licensing examination.

Psychiatrists are medically trained mental health care practitioners (that is, they hold an MD degree) with special medical training, who also have knowledge of counseling theories and of the relationship between the biophysiological functioning of the body and mental and emotional conditions in a cause-and-effect relationship. At this time this is the only category of mental health care practitioners authorized to prescribe medication as a treatment approach. Therefore, these professionals often work in conjunction with other mental health care providers. Because their orientation is based on a medical model, they are inclined to treat most mental disorders with drugs.

Psychologists are licensed practitioners with a Ph.D. in Clinical Psychology who diagnose and treat people with personality problems and other mental health disorders using psychological testing and talk therapies. Though they may specialize in a specific counseling modality, they usually are trained to understand several theories associated with mental health, including behavioral, cognitive, psychoanalytical, rational-emotive, and more. They also may specialize in the treatment of one segment of the population, such as children, adolescents, substance abusing and battered people.

Marriage and family therapists (MFTs) have completed either a master's or a Ph.D. in this or a closely related specialty and are trained in diverse theories and practices associated with **systems theory**. When possible, they work with couples, families, or groups of people who have influence on or are influenced by a problem, rather than with individuals. If a state does not license MFTs, their qualifications can be established by clinical membership in the AAMFT.

Social workers are professionals with training in social problems, such as substance abuse, eating disorders, chronic illness, family planning, bereavement, and so on. Social workers are trained at the bachelor's (BSW), master's (MSW), or doctoral (DSW) level, incorporating extensive clinical supervision that dictates their eligibility for licensure. If they are certified, they are designated certified social workers (CSWs). They practice in inpatient settings, outpatient clinics, schools, and individual or group practices.

Counselors encompass an extensive array of professional and paraprofessional counselors with academic degrees and training in specific counseling areas. These include pastoral counseling, school guidance counseling, community counseling, alcohol and substance abuse counseling, abortion counseling, and peer counseling, among others.

The wide acceptance of many different diagnostic and treatment options in the health care delivery system has created this broad spectrum of medical and health care providers and services. Knowledge of these definitions will help students use the system effectively, as well as broaden their own career options.

Payment Systems

Medical and related health care services are paid for in several different ways, including government-sponsored payment systems, private insurance, and direct or out-of-pocket payments.

Government Payment Systems

The federal government, most often in conjunction with a state, provides several different health payment programs for consumers. The two major programs are Medicare and Medicaid. Beyond these are hospitals and clinics that provide direct health care services to people in the military and their families, special populations such as American Indians, and people with certain illnesses that are part of funded research or experimental treatment programs.

Medicare is a federal health insurance program that provides coverage for hospital (Part A) and medical (Part B) services for people over the age of 65 and some other special populations (for example, kidney dialysis patients).

Medicaid is a federally funded program providing payment for services for economically disadvantaged citizens including people who are eligible for welfare, dependent children, and people who receive supplemental income because they are blind, aged, or disabled. Neither of these programs is all-inclusive, but they both represent the notion that all U.S. citizens deserve at least minimal medical care.

Private Insurance

People used to go to the doctor or hospital and pay directly for their services (commonly known as out-of-pocket payments). As medical and health care systems became more complicated and expensive, people could no longer afford to pay for services this way. Thus, they often did not use medical services until they were very ill.

Then, private insurance became available, where individuals or groups (mostly businesses) pay a premium to an insurance company with whom they have a contract. These annual contracts (insurance policies) with private insurance companies for individuals and groups designate how much money will be paid out-of-pocket (through deductibles and co-insurance), what are considered reasonable charges, and which health care services are and are not included.

Insurance companies also offer a host of policies that cover services not included in the usual policies. These include coverage for extended care in a nursing home (long-term care), psychiatric inpatient, home care, outpatient mental health, disability, and catastrophic illness.

Managed Care/Health Maintenance Organizations (HMOs)

As a result of the continuing rise in medical and health-related costs, prepayment plans for reimbursement have been designed by insurance companies and the federal government. In the past this meant that a person or family would contract (on an individual or group basis) with an insurance company to pay a premium for all medical care over the term of the policy (usually 1 year) with no (or very low) out-of-pocket deductibles or co-payments. The person or family knew exactly what their annual medical costs would be, regardless of how often they needed care. For that privilege, they must use the facilities (hospitals, offices, labs) and doctors who are part of the plan. These insurance plans are known as health maintenance organizations (HMOs). Because they limited the selection of a doctor or facility to those in the plan, many people did not want to participate.

To capture the rest of the market, insurance companies, private medical groups, and hospitals have modified the HMO to include alternatives such as independent practitioner associations (IPAs), private practice organizations (PPOs), and point of service. Today people can choose from a number of prepaid programs. One plan uses doctors employed by and facilities owned by the plan only. In another plan, people select a primary care doctor who is reimbursed by the insurer but has the privilege of sending patients to specialists in or outside of the plan when and if it is deemed necessary. If the doctors used are within the plan, the patient pays no additional charges, but if patients want to select services or doctors outside the plan, they pay additional deductible and co-insurance fees out-of-pocket. Selecting a payment system that is right for any one individual or family has become a complicated and personal matter.

Summary

The modern world poses many challenges for consumers, particularly with regard to their health. Widespread quackery is testament to the pitfalls to which consumers often succumb. The temptation for quick fixes must be replaced by carefully reasoned and informed decisions regarding health products and services. In the area of vitamin supplements, in particular, consumers are essentially on their own because, at this time, government agencies do not monitor these products, which are not defined as medicines. Food labeling offers some help, although the information on labels is still somewhat technical, confusing, and hard to understand for the average person.

Consumers need to network to obtain the best medical services and products. Resources are available through government agencies, consumer protection organizations, professional journals, hotlines, and Internet services. The doctor–patient relationship is important enough to warrant extra effort. Consumers can help the relationship by writing down questions and symptoms and requiring doctors to address their questions and concerns.

The health of a community encompasses the range of medical and health services available to people within the community, the promotion of public health and prevention efforts, and the planning and delivery of health services. These programs and services are under the umbrella of an interrelated network of federal, state, and local agencies and organizations. At the federal level, the Department of Health and Human Services authorizes the U. S. Public Health Service to oversee state departments of health, which are responsible for monitoring and maintaining a healthy environment, controlling disease agents, and promoting accessibility and adequacy of health care, particularly for under-served people. Local health departments have the greatest impact on a community, because they carry out the direct services.

In addition to governmental efforts are health services provided through the private agencies, the best known of which are the American Cancer Society, American Heart Association, United Way, and American Red Cross. Voluntary associations, such as the Ford Foundation and Robert Wood Johnson Foundation, provide health care services either directly or indirectly through their donations.

Traditionally, health care practitioners were divided into conventional (or allopathic) practitioners and alternative (or complementary) medical practitioners. The former include physicians, dental specialists, and nursing professionals. Alternative medicine specialists include osteopaths, chiropractors, homeopaths, Chinese medicine specialists, and naturopathists, among others. This division between conventional and alternative medical practice is blurring (albeit slowly), and traditional medical schools are offering education in complementary practices.

Mental health care is provided through a network of psychiatrists, psychologists, marriage and family therapists and social workers, among other counseling professionals. Understanding the boundaries their training, licensure and accreditation establishes helps consumers to make informed choices about their mental health care.

Payment for health care is made through the federal systems of Medicare and Medicaid, or through a host of private insurance plans including prepaid managed care programs and HMOs.

Web Sites

Alternative Care
www.altcare.com/welcome.html

Alternative Medicine Home Page
www.pitt.edu/~cbw/altm.html

American Dental Association
www.ada.org/index.html

American Heart Association
www.amhrt.org/

American Lung Association
www.amlung.org/

American Psychological Association: PsychNet
www.apa.org

Better Business Bureau
www.bbb.org/index.html

Centers for Disease Control and Prevention
www.cdc.gov/

Dental Consumer Advisor Home Page
www.pe.net/~iddpc`/

Environmental Protection Agency
www.epa.gov

Federal Trade Commission
www.ftc.gov/index.html

Food & Drug Administration
www.fda.gov

Harvard Health Publications
www.harvardhealthpubs.org
www.harvardhealthpubs.org/Harvard_Search

Health Care Information Resources
www-hsl.mcmaster.ca/tomflem/top.html

Health Policy Page
epn.org/idea/health.html

Holistic Health
www.hir.com/

MedAccess
www.medaccess.com

Medscape
www.medscape.com/

National Cancer Institute
www.nci.nih.gov/

National Clearinghouse for Alcohol and Drug Information
www.health.org

National Health Information Center: Office Of Health Promotion/Disease Prevention
nhic.nt.health.org

National Institute of Allergy and Infectious Disease
www.niaid.nih.gov/

National Institutes of Health
www.nih.gov

National Institute on Drug Abuse
www.nida.hih.gov

Surgeon General's Report
www.surgeongeneral.gov/

The Chiropractic Home Page
www.mbnet.mb.ca/~jwiens/chiro.html

The Heart: An Online Exploration
www.fi.edu/biosci/heart.html

Notes

1. D. Miller and J. H. Price, *Dimensions of Community Health*, 5th ed. (New York: McGraw Hill, 1998).
2. L. Green and C. Ottoson, *Community and Population Health with Power Web: Health & Human Performance*, 8th ed. (New York: McGraw Hill, 1999).
3. National Commission on Community Health Services, *Health Is a Community Affair* (Cambridge, MA: Harvard University Press, 1967), 20.

Learning Experiences

Students as consumers, particularly at the elementary-school level, are governed by their family patterns and the media. Each family is embraced by a local and regional community. Like a family, each school or district represents a component of that community with special health concerns, unique political and social designs, attitudes, values, and behavioral characteristics. The global and local ethno-cultural patterns of consumerism influence the use of community health services, creating rich and powerful curriculum material for teaching. The following Learning Experiences represent concepts and principles in interdisciplinary lessons with expected outcomes for students at the different grade levels. The developmental stages of students in each class should also be considered when planning curricula. Armed with this information, the teacher can use these lessons and activities as guidelines and a starting point for teaching consumerism and understanding of community health care information.

The following are the concepts and outcomes one would hope to develop in students as they mature.

Grades K–2

Very young children are rarely consulted when they are given medications or asked to submit to health examinations. They are simply expected to take them as given. This subtle passive behavior, which is encouraged in the young, often sets the course for lifelong compliance without a questioning process and leaves decisions regarding health to others. The marketing media are acutely aware of this early childhood conditioning, and advertisers are known to focus on children in their media pitch for sales. Hence, consumer education at this level of education prepares children to become active participants in the use of goods and services.

Moreover, students in the earliest grades do best when they are moving around. Therefore, they are likely to learn about their community from assignments and class field trips that encourage out-of-classroom explorations. Their exploration of the community should be limited because their notion of community does not go much beyond their extended family, immediate surroundings, and neighborhood school. With this in mind, lessons can be planned to develop the following competencies. They will be able to

1. Identify health products commonly used in their homes and how they are used.
2. Ask questions about products and services as they relate to their own health (for instance, "Why are certain foods good for me and others not? When do I need to go to the doctor [dentist]? What does the label say? How much does that cost? What are vitamins?").
3. Ask questions of their health care providers and of their parents about their own health care ("How often do I have to take that medicine? How much of a fever do I have? How will I know when I'm ready to go back to school? How come we have different doctors?").
4. Recognize the various health care providers the family commonly uses and what they do.
5. Identify some of the more common health care services their family or friends use in the community (for example, emergency services, hospitals, clinics).
6. Locate the health care providers in their school and know when and how to contact them.

7. Identify how other children in their class, especially those from different ethno-cultural backgrounds, use different providers and services.
8. Identify local pharmacists and the role they play in health care.
9. Reach emergency medical services and their own medical provider.

Grades 3–4

In these grades, children can build on the concepts of K–2 and be more familiar with their own use of products and services. At this grade level, the boundaries of the students' community are expanding, as are their communication skills. They are increasingly independent about things they want, people they want to listen to, and so on. As they become more familiar with the school setting (in much the same way that a newcomer develops comfort in a new community), they feel safer and freer to create relationships outside of their immediate classroom during the school day. Some of the other teachers and support personnel in the school then become resources.

By the end of these grades, students will be able to

1. Distinguish products that are safe and beneficial from those that are harmful.
2. Identify several sources to provide them with accurate information.
3. Evaluate the usefulness and accuracy of information about products and services.
4. Recognize product labels and advertising and understand what they mean to an individual's health.
5. Ask questions about their health and give accurate simple information about symptoms.
6. Identify health care professionals and health care agencies (specialists, alternative medicine providers, and the like) and the roles they play in health and medical care.
7. Recognize community health problems.
8. Effectively use the school health network (nurses, social workers, school psychologists).

Grades 5–6

As students reach the conclusion of their elementary school years, they increase their access to products. They have greater opportunities to visit local stores and supermarkets with friends and when running errands. They also have some money, from allowances or babysitting, with which to buy products. They become more aware of, and have greater access to, the contents of their own medicine cabinet. This is a time when students can develop a feeling of control over their own health through critical questioning and participation in decision making. Building on earlier years, these children continue to expand their community boundaries and their participation in and interactions with their community. Their ability to have a say in how they are treated and in what they are asked to take or use should become more and more refined as they mature. The ability to access school health care services will spill over to include the local community's services. The way their community fits into the larger society, neighboring communities, and state and federal government agencies will become part of their sphere of understanding.

After these grades, students will be able to

1. Critically evaluate advertisements of health care products and services.
2. Identify quackery and how to avoid it.
3. Ask questions of medical and health care practitioners about their recommendations.
4. Describe their rights as consumers of health products and services.
5. Assess the reliability of health information.
6. Recognize labels on food products and understand what they mean.
7. Make decisions about which products and services to use.
8. Recognize symptoms and accurately describe them to a practitioner.
9. Identify different cultural values, attitudes, and behaviors that influence the purchase of products and services.
10. Identify medical specialties and other health care providers.
11. Identify health agencies and their services and responsibilities at the federal and state levels.
12. Identify hotlines and other information sources and how to use them.
13. Describe methods of paying for health care.
14. Identify various careers in health.

The Learning Experiences presented next utilize teaching strategies frequently used in the elementary school in all disciplines including creative artwork, drama, experimentation, interviewing, discussions, class trips, and the like. Elementary schoolchildren, free from the constraints of maturity and political correctness, like to role-play, hear stories, daydream, and fantasize. They particularly like to relate stories about themselves and their families. Some of these stories handed down from grandparents and parents are about products, places, and cultural habits. They are usually hospitable to friendly visitors (especially from local voluntary agencies) and to visiting places of interest, such as a hospital or clinic.

They learn from touching and seeing. Hence, school visits to stores that sell products may also be effective. When they draw or cut and paste, they appreciate having their work displayed. This affords an excellent opportunity to demonstrate the information a class gains in consumer and community health to the entire school community.

For suggestions on creating a rubric with which to evaluate student performance of Learning Experiences, see page 13.

Learning Experience 15-1

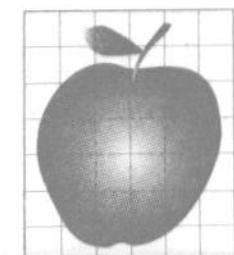

Getting to Know Drugs and Medicines

Grade Level

1–6

Primary Disciplines

Reading, Spelling

Learning Objectives

Following this activity, students will be able to

- Identify medicines used frequently in their family.
- Recognize the difference between OTC and prescription drugs.
- Ask questions about a drug prescribed to them.
- Explain the information on drug labels.

Time Required

45 minutes

Materials

Over-the-counter drug containers, a medical prescription, prescription drug containers, pencils/pens and writing paper, magazines

Description of Activity

Previous homework required (see below).

Grades 1–2

Each student will show two empty medicine containers to the class, one an OTC drug and the other a prescriptive drug that a family member has used.

Students state the name of the drug and describe what the drug is used for. They also describe how the drug was to be used (how many per day, for how many days, and so on). They describe the "directions for use" given on the container.

You might discuss how an OTC drug label describes use for the general public and how directions for a prescription drug are determined by the health-care practitioner prescribing it.

Grades 3–4

In addition to the above, the students will describe the symptoms warranting use of the drug. For the OTC drug, they will read the label carefully and, from it, describe what the manufacturer suggests for its use, in what doses, for what age levels, when it is contraindicated, and what side effects might signal a problem.

You might want to discuss things such as allergic reactions, synergistic effects, and the difficulty of understanding the chemistry of drugs from the labels.

Grades 5–6

The students will compare a list of drugs found in their home medicine cabinet: How many are outdated? How many are prescription and how many OTC? You might want to discuss keeping drugs after their expiration date, using drugs by one person prescribed for another person with similar symptoms and the like.

Each student will present an OTC drug he or she has used, an advertisement that describes it, and the cost of the drug as described in the ad or stores in which it is sold. Students will describe to the class the intended use as described on the container, and how that compares with the advertising pitch. (You might want to explore with students advertising strategies and subtleties that contribute to drug misuse.)

Homework

Grades 1–2

Students each bring in two empty drug containers, one OTC and one prescription drug. They identify the drug on a piece of paper, with the help of parent/guardian. The parent tells the student what it is used for.

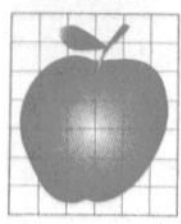

Learning Experience 15-1 continued

Grades 3–4

Students bring in the same containers as indicated for grades 1–2, are able to read the label and understand it, and identify proper use of the drug.

Grades 5–6

Students prepare a chart with three columns, as shown on page 531. Go through your medicine cabinet to identify each drug. In the first column identify the drug by name. In the second column identify the date the drug expired (and should have been discarded). In column 3 identify each drug by whether it is an OTC or prescribed by a medical practitioner.

They select one OTC drug and find a newspaper or magazine advertisement for that drug.

Evaluation

A rubric can be developed to measure students' ability to

- Describe symptoms of illness in a clear manner.
- Identify common drugs their family uses and what they are generally used for.
- Identify how often the most common drugs are to be taken.
- Explain the difference between OTC and prescription drugs.
- Read and understand the directions on the drug container.
- Explain how to read an advertisement about drugs and distinguish between advertising pressure and facts.

Drugs in My Medicine Cabinet	Expiration Date	OTC or Prescription?
____________________	__________	__________
____________________	__________	__________
____________________	__________	__________
____________________	__________	__________
____________________	__________	__________
____________________	__________	__________
____________________	__________	__________
____________________	__________	__________
____________________	__________	__________
____________________	__________	__________
____________________	__________	__________
____________________	__________	__________
____________________	__________	__________
____________________	__________	__________
____________________	__________	__________
____________________	__________	__________
____________________	__________	__________
____________________	__________	__________

Total in medicine cabinet __________

Total OTC __________

Total expired __________

Total prescription __________

Learning Experience 15-2

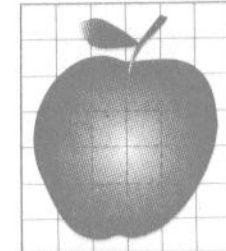

My Doctor and Me

Grade Level

K–6

Primary Disciplines

Language Arts, Science

Learning Objectives

Following this activity, students will be able to

- List symptoms and prepare questions for a visit with their medical practitioner.
- Decide what conditions are necessary for them to see or call a medical practitioner.
- Be able to get in touch with their doctor or health care facility.
- Identify which diagnostic tests and equipment doctors commonly use.

Time Required

30 minutes.

Materials

Lab coat, stethoscope, syringe/needle, medical history form, telephone, scale, height chart, thermometer, and any other available equipment common to a medical office

Description of Activity

First, write on the chalkboard a list of questions students would ask a doctor if they were going for a regular preventive health check-up, and a list of questions they would be expected to be asked. Then, have students participate in several role-play scenarios as described below, to learn about the practitioner–patient relationship. (The fish-bowl role-play is a particularly good technique because it allows all of the students to participate, and it allows you to constantly change the story-line or roles. The students sit in a circle, and the role-play starts with the players in the center. They are given the story line and begin the role-play. If a student in the circle wishes to take the part of a character, he/she raises his/her hand, and when you permit, the student taps the player on the shoulder and they exchange places. The role-play continues with the new player in the original player's seat. You may stop the role-play at any time and change the scene or the participants to get at the various issues.)

Possible Scenarios

1. A child is sick or hurt at home, and someone in the family has contacted the medical office (or the emergency room or clinic). (The students may actually identify the telephone number to be dialed.)
2. The students pretend that they have just arrived at the clinic for a regular office visit (roles include medical practitioner, child, parent[s], nurse).
3. The doctor describes the various pieces of equipment (stethoscope, thermometer, x-ray machine, etc.), and the various tests that may be taken (blood, urine, blood pressure, and so on).
4. Family members interview a doctor to see if they want him/her to be their family doctor. The doctor explains what his/her procedures are.
5. The patient and the practitioner talk after the patient has been diagnosed with the flu. The doctor prescribes several medications.
6. The patient is at the pharmacy with a prescription from the doctor.

Homework

Students in grades 3–6 could bring in a list of diagnostic tests they or family members have had. What is the test for? What does the test entail? What kind of practitioner takes the test or does the diagnostic procedure?

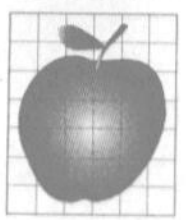

Learning Experience 15-2 continued

Evaluation

A rubric can be developed to measure students' ability to

- Formulate questions they would ask a medical professional on a routine office or clinic visit.
- Identify the questions they think they would be asked (including symptom descriptions).
- Provide clear and accurate information and responses to the questions they are asked.
- Identify the situations or symptoms that would make it necessary to call a doctor.
- Identify commonly used equipment they would find in their doctor's office, and the uses of that equipment.
- Identify their practitioners and where and how to get in touch with emergency services, their doctor, and the like.

Learning Experience 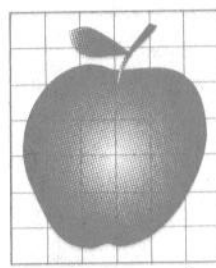 15-3

How Sick Am I?

Grade Level

3–6

Primary Disciplines

Language Arts, Science

Learning Objectives

Following this activity, students will be able to

- Describe symptoms of illnesses.
- Recognize when symptoms require medical attention.
- Identify someone they can tell when they feel ill.

Time Required

30 minutes

Materials

Chalkboard, paper, crayons, magazines for cut-outs (Pictures/symptoms in each situation should become more complicated as grade level increases.)

Description of Activity

- Students are instructed to bring in pictures of different places one could go if they had symptoms of an illness. Include: doctor, nurse, hospital, clinic, pharmacy, eye doctor, etc.
- Write a list similar to the following on the chalkboard (less complicated for lower grades, more complicated for higher grades): runny eyes; red and itchy mosquito bite; runny nose; headache, body temperature above 100°F; wheezing; stomachache; blurred vision; a rash all over; feeling tired; green or pussy discharge; swollen glands; giant hives; feeling numb; earache; swelling and red after a fall; bleeding; severe pains in chest; any severe pain; sore throat; constant vomiting; unconsciousness; coughing, choking; disorientation/stupor; swollen bee sting.
- Give each student four pieces of paper on which they draw or paste their responses.
- Read one symptom at a time from the list, and ask the students to select one of the pictures on their desk that best describes where they would go if they had the symptom.
- Encourage discussion about why particular choices are made. Instruct students to keep a record of how they answered their question.

Homework

This is a good activity for the students to take home to do with their parent/guardian. Encourage discussion with parents and ask for feedback the following day. The students keep a record of their own answers and their parents' answers and compare the two. As part of their homework, have students answer the following questions:

- I learned ______________________.
- I was surprised to find out ______________________.
- My parents/guardian and I differed about ______________________.

Evaluation

A rubric can be developed to measure students' ability to

- Identify symptoms of illness and appropriate ways to respond to them. (One might look for responses that include stay home, go to school, call the doctor, call emergency, or go to the hospital.)
- Identify people in the family, school, and community to whom they can go when they are feeling ill.
- Identify their health providers and important health services in the community. (With young children one might look for [pictures of] a house, a school, a doctor's office, a hospital.)

Learning Experience 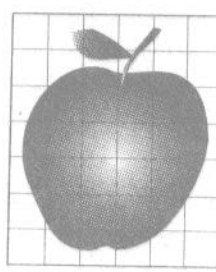 15-4

Truth in Advertising/ Truth in Labeling

Grade Level

5–6

Primary Disciplines

Math, Reading Comprehension, Science

Learning Objectives

Following this activity, students are able to

- Read and understand labels.
- Describe advertisers' marketing strategies.
- Make critical decisions about the products and services they use and the relationship of the product to their health.

Time Required

30 minutes

Materials

Magazines, scissors, masking tape, videos of commercials (optional)

Description of Activity

See Homework for description of preparation for classroom activity.

Introduction

Students each have an opportunity to sell their product. After they have explained about it convincingly (see Homework assignment), they answer questions asked by their classmates.

Activity

During the presentation, have the class take notes about what interested them, what they liked or didn't like, and so on. Then have the students discuss whether they will buy the product (or use the service), what appealed to them (or turned them off), and why. After all of the students have had a turn (this may be done in small groups if the class is large), have the class review several of the advertisements to determine what professional advertising appeals were used. Some of those that should be discussed are the appearance of the models (do they look like doctors or friends?), what senses were being appealed to (smell, sight, and so on), what values were being appealed to (having fun, keeping young, and so on), what story was being told, what language made the ad believable (for example, scientific or familiar?), and so on.

Finally, ask the students to determine what the product/service is supposed to be used for, who should use it, under what circumstances, and so forth. They might also discuss how often the commercial appears when they watch TV. (It is effective to have them report on this the very next day.)

Homework

In preparation for the activity, have each student select a product or service related to health that they will sell to the rest of the class. In addition to bringing a sample (where appropriate), they will collect advertisements and pictures of their product/service, develop slogans, and make appeals that will convince the class of the worth, usefulness, or effectiveness of it. They do not have to tell everything, and they can slant the information, but they must be truthful, not fraudulent. Class members will be permitted to ask questions, which presenters also have to answer truthfully.

Evaluation

Develop a rubric to measure students' ability to

- Identify and explain the important information on a drug label.
- Describe marketing strategies commonly used in health-related advertisements and present examples of each.
- Recognize the myths, misinformation, and accurate information presented in advertisements.

Learning Experience 15-5

How Much Does It Cost?

Grade Level

4–6

Primary Disciplines

Math, Science

Learning Objectives

Following this activity, students are able to

- Apply the information about weights and measurements.
- Explain the cost of goods as they relate to amount purchased.
- Describe dosage in medications.
- Report on the cost of medications and other health products and prescriptions.

Time Required

45 minutes

Materials

Samples of products in different sizes, product labels, prescription and OTC directions, sales slips

Description of Activity

Review common measurements that appear on medications and other health products (percentages, micrograms, grams, fluid ounces, teaspoon dose, tablespoon dose, and so on).

Given a prescription or over-the-counter suggested dosage, ask the class to determine how many, or how much, will be taken in one dose, daily, over the life of the prescription. Using the cost identified by the bill or sales marker on the item, ask students to determine how much a single dose costs, how much a daily dose costs, how much will be spent on the product yearly (if it is required for ongoing use), how beneficial is it to buy the product in larger/smaller (or generic) containers. Insurance reimbursements can be discussed. You could invite a local pharmacist to speak to the class, telling him/her beforehand the objectives of the lesson. The pharmacist may bring several samples.

Homework

Students bring to class two or three products related to health. If they bring a medicine bottle, they should bring only the empty container or bottle.

Evaluation

Develop a rubric to measure students' ability to

- Understand and explain weights and measurements that relate to dose amounts.
- Calculate the cost of an item by size of container and equate the cost to each dose.
- Explain what a generic drug is and how it may differ from a name-brand drug.
- Identify the costs of some of the more typical drugs and health-related items they and their family use and calculate the average use over a week and month.

Learning Experience 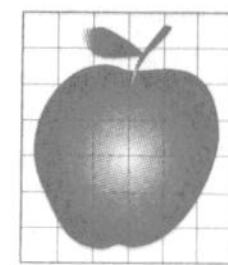 15-6

The Teddy Bear Clinic at a Community Hospital

Grade Level

K–2

Primary Disciplines

Science, Social Studies

Learning Objectives

Following this activity, students will be able to

- Locate their local hospital and contact the emergency department.
- Recognize medical procedures (and thereby become less fearful of any medical attention they may receive).
- Identify various medical equipment and how it is used to help people.
- Describe elementary self-care strategies.
- List medical services and medical practitioners.

Time Required

On-site 1½ hours plus transportation time to local hospital

Materials

- A teddy bear or other stuffed animal, materials for drawing, pasting, coloring; class trip arrangements
- All other materials supplied by the local hospital:

  Respiratory equipment: table, display bear with oxygen, drawing of lungs, "no-smoking" oaths, oxygen tank equipment and masks

  Suturing: table with injured bear, syringe with small needle, Novacain bottle, straight 2–0 sutures, sterile suture set-up, band-aids, antibiotics

  X-ray: view box to illuminate x-rays, stretcher for the large teddy bear with arm in cast, demonstration x-rays, portable x-ray machine

  Casting: table towels, container for water, large "airship" balloons, casting materials, stocking and wrapping materials, gloves
- Teddy Bear Clinic Diplomas

Description of Activity

Introduction

The following describes a complete program, designed by a local hospital in partnership with a school district, wherein children are walked through a Teddy Bear Clinic set up in a hospital's conference room: Children bring their own toys or teddy bears, which are then x-rayed, receive sutures, and have casts placed on injuries.

You can bring this program to your local hospital educators for replication.

The hospital educators and the classroom teachers who arrange this program design classroom sessions to take place 1 week before the students will make their visit to the hospital. The class discusses what they will see at the hospital. If the students cannot furnish their own teddy bears, they share those that are available. They rotate taking care of their teddy bear, changing its diapers and caring for its other needs, for 1 week in class prior to the visit.

Approximately 90 students and their teddy bears can be accommodated at one time in a main conference room or emergency clinic on the day of the program, set up as shown in Exhibit A.

When the children are seated, a wheelchair with a large panda bear circles the room at the same time a siren is sounded (which gets their immediate attention). The students are then shown the emergency room sign on the wall. They are told that the demonstrations are what they might experience if they were hurt and brought to the emergency room for care.

A team of approximately six health professionals (nurses, doctors, technicians) then examine the students' dolls, teddy bears, Ninja Turtles, Care Bears, or

Source: Robin Grass, RN, M.A., Director of Community Medicine, South Nassau Communities Hospital, Oceanside, New York, 1996. Reprinted with permission.

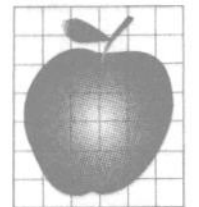

Learning Experience 15-6 continued

whatever stuffed animals they have brought. The professionals are selected to represent varied ethnicities and cultures whenever possible. Attempts are also made to select female physicians and male nurses to dispel stereotypical notions about health professionals.

The students are instructed to pretend they are parents of the bears and tell the professionals the animals' name and medical condition. The students are encouraged to come up with conditions such as sore throat, high fever, and broken bones. During the examination, stethoscopes and tongue blades are used on the animals, with the students' assistance.

When the examinations have been completed, approximately 22 students are assigned to one of the four areas of the room, where they sit on the floor in front of the following demonstrations:

- *Oxygen therapy:* They observe a teddy bear receiving oxygen therapy for choking or for an asthma attack. They learn about oxygen. They feel the cool mist from the mask, and they take an oath never to begin smoking.
- *Suturing:* After approximately 5–7 minutes, they move into the next area, where a teddy bear receives stitches after "cutting" its leg. The students observe the needle with Novacain and discuss their previous cuts, falls, and sutures. After 5–7 minutes, the students proceed to the next station.
- *X-ray:* A portable x-ray machine is used to demonstrate x-rays on a large Yankee (or your own sports team) team bear with a colored cast on its arm. The x-ray procedure is demonstrated, and a number of x-rays are illuminated at the view board. An x-ray of the head is shown, and the children identify the eyes, nose, and mouth. (This is a good time to instruct students to wear safety helmets when bicycle riding.) One x-ray with a needle in a foot is shown, and the students are educated about wearing shoes at the beach and other outdoor places. Another x-ray of a bullet in a thigh is shown, and the students are told of the dangers of playing with guns and knives. The last x-ray shows a coin located in the stomach, and the children are cautioned about placing toys and other foreign objects in their mouths.
- *Casting:* The students move to the next station, which features a bear with a cast. They are shown the different stages of casting (demonstrated on a long, inflated balloon). They watch the initial padding being applied and feel the heat generated by the new casts.

When the four stations have been completed, the students return to their original seats. The teachers and staff serve refreshments. The teachers then distribute the Teddy Bear Clinic diplomas (an example is shown in Exhibit B), Future Doctor hats, and a questionnaire for the students to take home to their parents (who are requested to mail them to the hospital) (shown in Exhibit C). When they return to their classroom, the students develop a "thank you" collage, which can be displayed in the hospital lobby.

Homework

None

Sources

Children's booklets from Positive Promotions, Teacher's Collection:

- Teddy Goes To The Emergency Room (educational coloring and activities book)
- A Visit to the Emergency Room (educational coloring and activities book)
- About Same-Day Surgery

Evaluation

The hospital will usually do an evaluation of the programs they offer.

Exhibit A

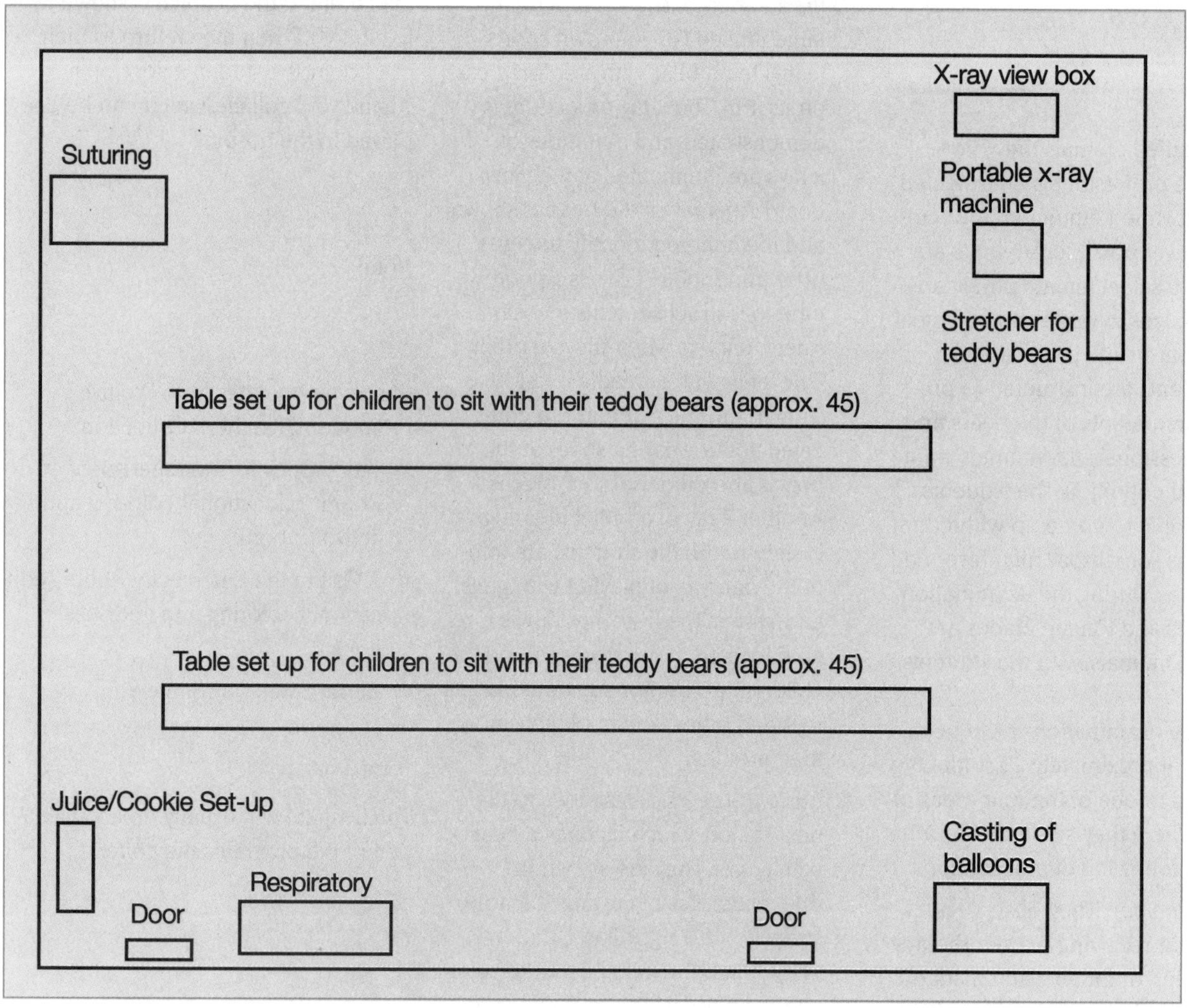

X-ray view box

Suturing

Portable x-ray machine

Stretcher for teddy bears

Table set up for children to sit with their teddy bears (approx. 45)

Table set up for children to sit with their teddy bears (approx. 45)

Juice/Cookie Set-up

Casting of balloons

Respiratory

Door

Door

Exhibit B

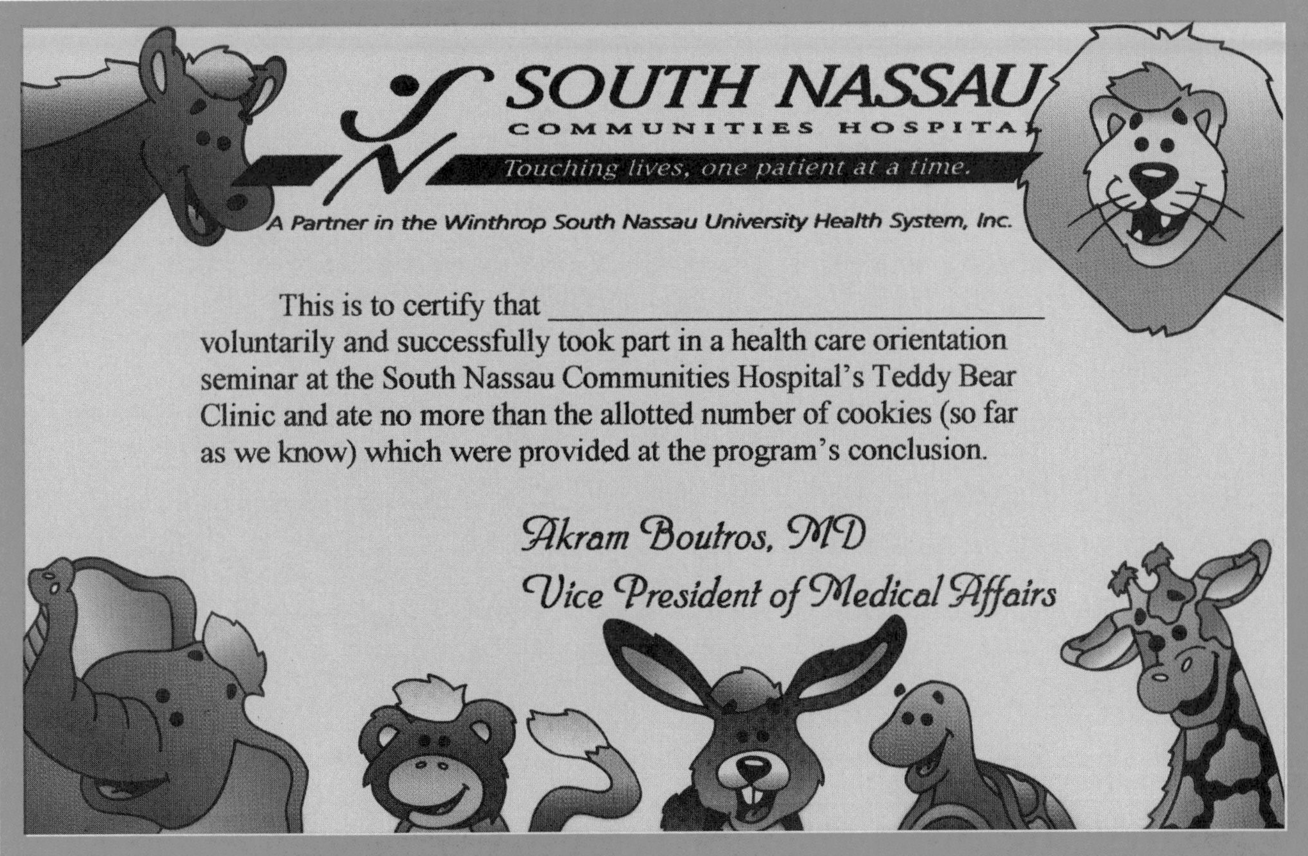
SOUTH NASSAU
COMMUNITIES HOSPITAL
Touching lives, one patient at a time.
A Partner in the Winthrop South Nassau University Health System, Inc.

This is to certify that ______________________________
voluntarily and successfully took part in a health care orientation seminar at the South Nassau Communities Hospital's Teddy Bear Clinic and ate no more than the allotted number of cookies (so far as we know) which were provided at the program's conclusion.

Akram Boutros, MD
Vice President of Medical Affairs

Exhibit C

Dear Parent,

Your child recently attended a Teddy Bear Clinic at the Community Hospital. We hope he/she has already shared his/her experiences with you.

This program is part of the hospital's commitment to community health education and is designed specifically for grades K–2 to give them a better understanding of how common emergencies are diagnosed and treated in a hospital environment.

We encourage you to discuss the program with your child. We would appreciate it if you would take a few moments to complete the following survey and return it to your child's teacher. This response will assist us in improving future Teddy Bear Clinics.

What was your child's reaction to the program? ______________________________

Did the clinic help to alleviate some of his/her fears associated with a hospital? ________

Is your child less anxious about injuries and treatment? _________________________

____

What part(s) of the clinic was your child most impressed with?

☐ Respiratory treatment ☐ Suturing ☐ X-ray ☐ Casting

Other comments/suggestions: ____________________________________

____

Name ____

Address ____

Phone ____

Please check the areas that interest you, and we will send you additional information:

☐ Support groups/lectures ☐ Volunteering ☐ Fund raising ☐ Special events

Thank you.

Sincerely,

Date: ______________________

A parent permission slip

Keep running and walking.
Keep playing and jumping.
Keep biking and hiking.
Have races and play ball.

Ride surf boards and
boogie boards.

You're great.
You're fantastic.
You're soooo awesome!

Keep that strong and healthy heart

FOREVER.

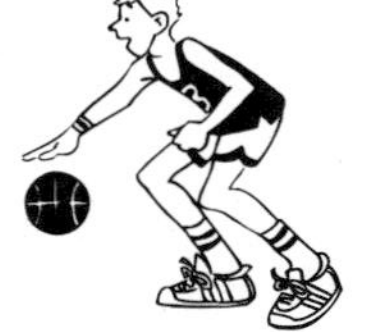

Dolores Clancy, RN CCRN

Source: Center for Cardiac Rehabilitation, 440 Merrick Road, Oceanside, NY 11572. Reprinted with permission.

Fold Here

For Kids Only:

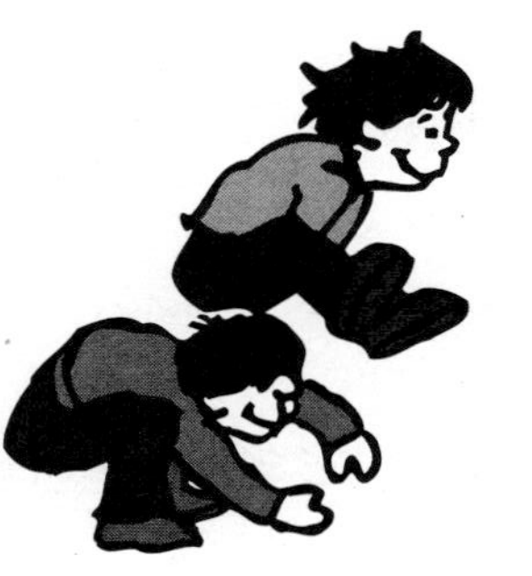

A Message From
A Heart Nurse

Kids are great.
Kids are fantastic.
Kids are soooooo awesome!

Kids run and play.
Kids can bike all day.
Kids ride surf boards
and boogie boards
and skate boards.

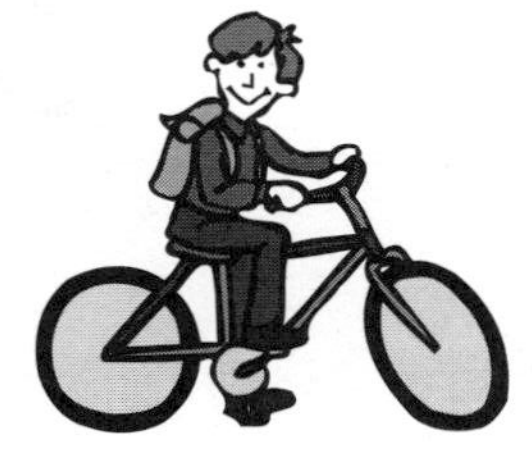

Kids exercise in gym class.
Kids climb and jump and dive and swim.
Kids play ball and have races.
Kids dance and jump rope.
Kids ice skate and roller blade.

Kids have strong and healthy hearts.

But something happens to
some kids when they turn into
teenagers and grown-ups.

Some of them don't run or walk
anymore. They always want to
ride in a car.

Some sit and play video games
all day.

Some of them start to smoke.
They think it's cool — big mistake.

Some of them drink beer and
booze and try drugs.

Some of them eat too much
fast food and too much
junk food.

SOOOO, KIDS . . .

Keep doing the
things you are doing
even when you turn
into a teenager and
grown-up.

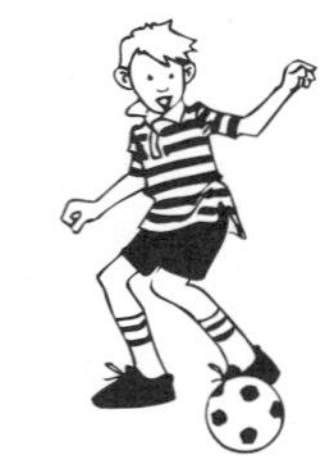

Learning Experience 15-7

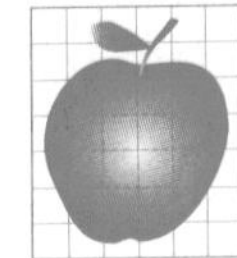

Locating Medical Resources

Grade Level

1–6 (The neighborhood map can be more detailed as the students mature).

Primary Disciplines

Social Studies, History

The study of world maps and the locations of continents, countries, cities, and other features can begin with a simple map of the student's immediate area. The concepts of east/west/north/south can develop at the same time as students learn about locations associated with health.

Learning Objectives

Following this activity, students will be able to

- Identify the location of medical and health care facilities in their neighborhood.
- Develop a directional map.
- Understand maps as guides.
- Identify the medical resources that their family uses and their location.

Time Required

One classroom session; one morning or afternoon local trip

Materials

Magazines, coloring books, crayons, scissors, paste, posterboard or large coloring paper

Description of Activity

This activity can be done in groups or individually. The following is a guideline for how this activity can be adapted to the various grade levels, along with samples.

Grades 1–2

Ask students if they and their family have ever used a map. They can relate times when they used maps. Together with the children, draw a simple map that identifies some of the facilities in the school that relate to their health and how they get there from their classroom (Exhibit A provides an example). This could include the nurse's office, the lunchroom, the social worker, school psychologist or school guidance counselor's office, bathrooms, and so on. With a copy of the map in hand, the students will walk through the building together and locate the different facilities from the map. At the nurse's office, the students will be invited in for an on-site visit, where they will be introduced to the nursing staff and the facility.

Grades 3–4

Have students cut out pictures from magazines of different kinds of medical and health care facilities they are familiar with (doctor's office, clinic, dentist's office, hospital, pharmacy). Provide each student with a simple street map, similar to the one in Exhibit B, identifying three or four main streets in their neighborhood that house some of these services. Have students prepare a collage by pasting pictures of the various services onto the map in their appropriate places and, using crayons, identify them by name. They will then take a walk through those streets in the neighborhood, using their map as a guide. One of the facilities could be identified for an on-site visit (for example, the pharmacy, a pediatrician's office).

Grades 5–6

Take students on a morning trip (preferably walking) from the school to the nearest hospital, where they will go on a tour of the hospital. These tours can usually be planned by the hospital's community relations or community education department. When the students return from their visit, have them prepare a map in collage form in groups, identifying the various streets that led them to the hospital and other health care facilities they encountered along the way. Exhibit C provides an example.

Homework

Students can each develop a simple map that guides them to the hospital from their home. With the help of their family, they may be able to identify

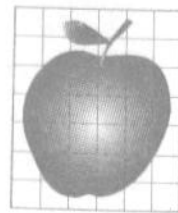

Learning Experience 15-7 continued

other facilities the family uses (dentist's office, pharmacy, doctor's offices, and so on). Students can also be invited to study an actual neighborhood map and identify health services that are on the map and add others that are not.

Evaluation

Upper Level: Develop a rubric for each map whereby the students receive a grade for their map, as follows:

- A = 4 points if they have the path correctly outlined for their grade level.
- B = 3 points if they have spelled words correctly.
- C = 2 points if they can identify all of the expected sites.
- D = 1 point if the sites are properly marked/project is creative.
- F = 0 points if none are correct or map is not submitted.

Exhibit A

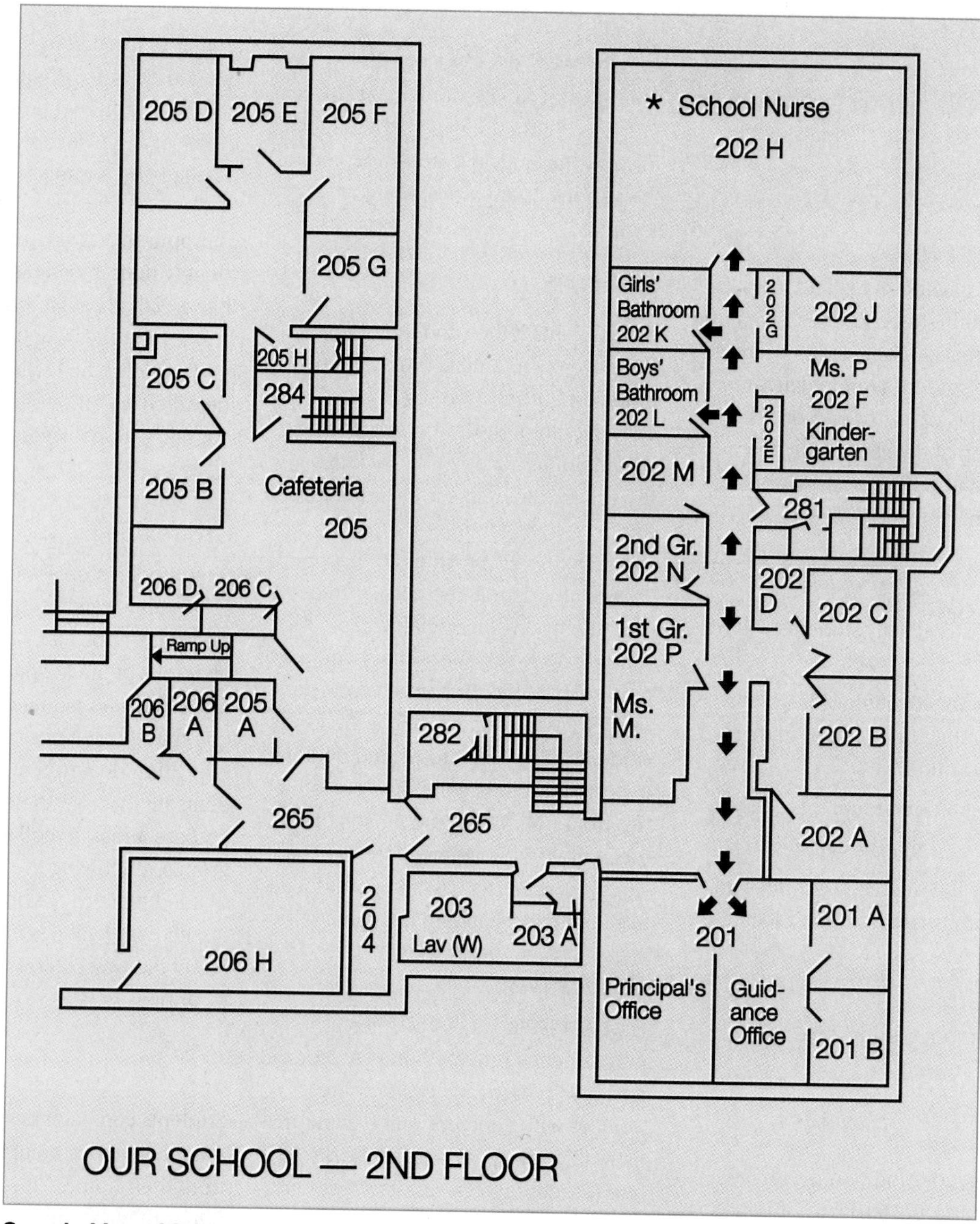

OUR SCHOOL — 2ND FLOOR

Sample Map of School

Exhibit B

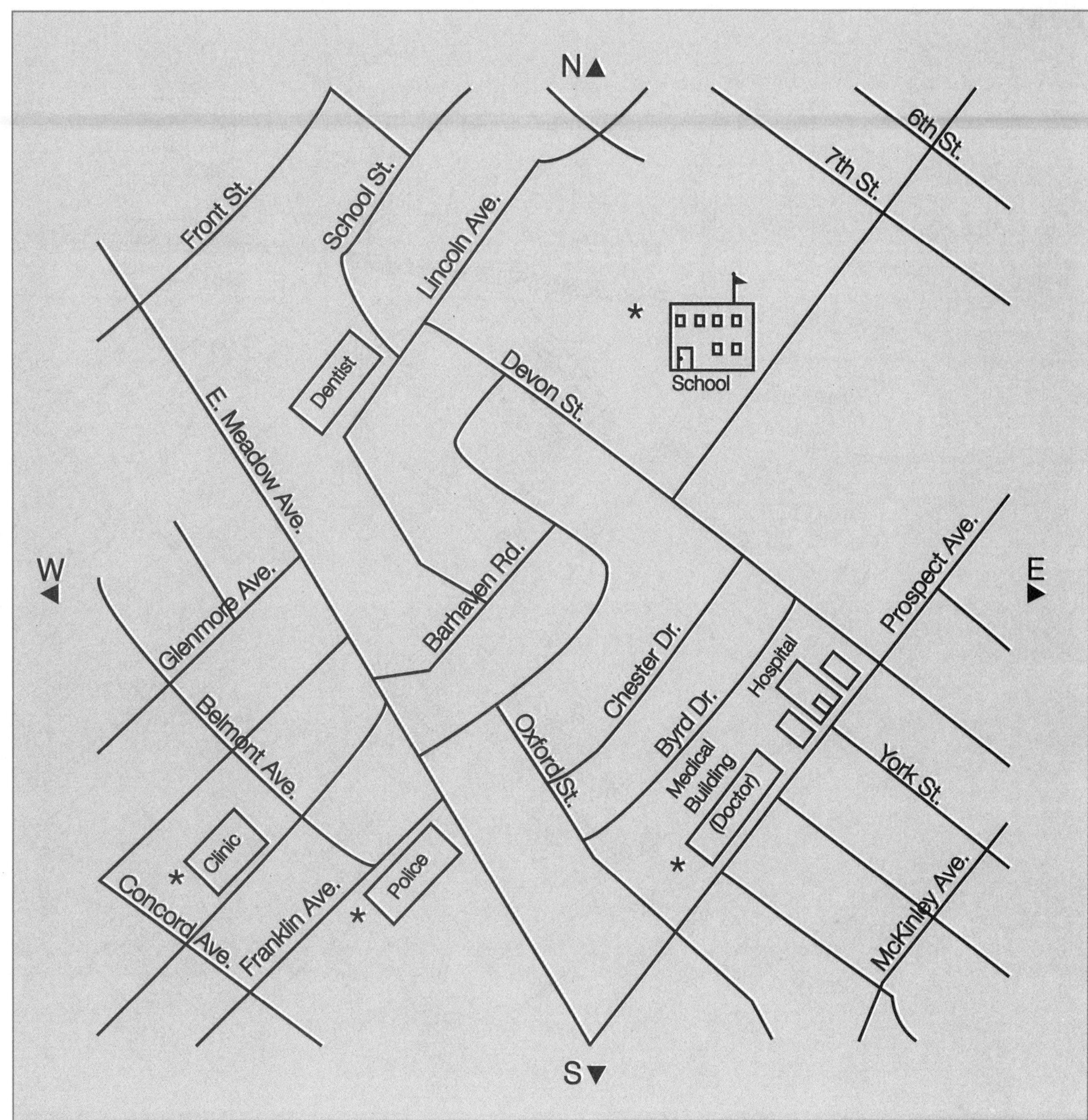

Sample Street Map

Exhibit C

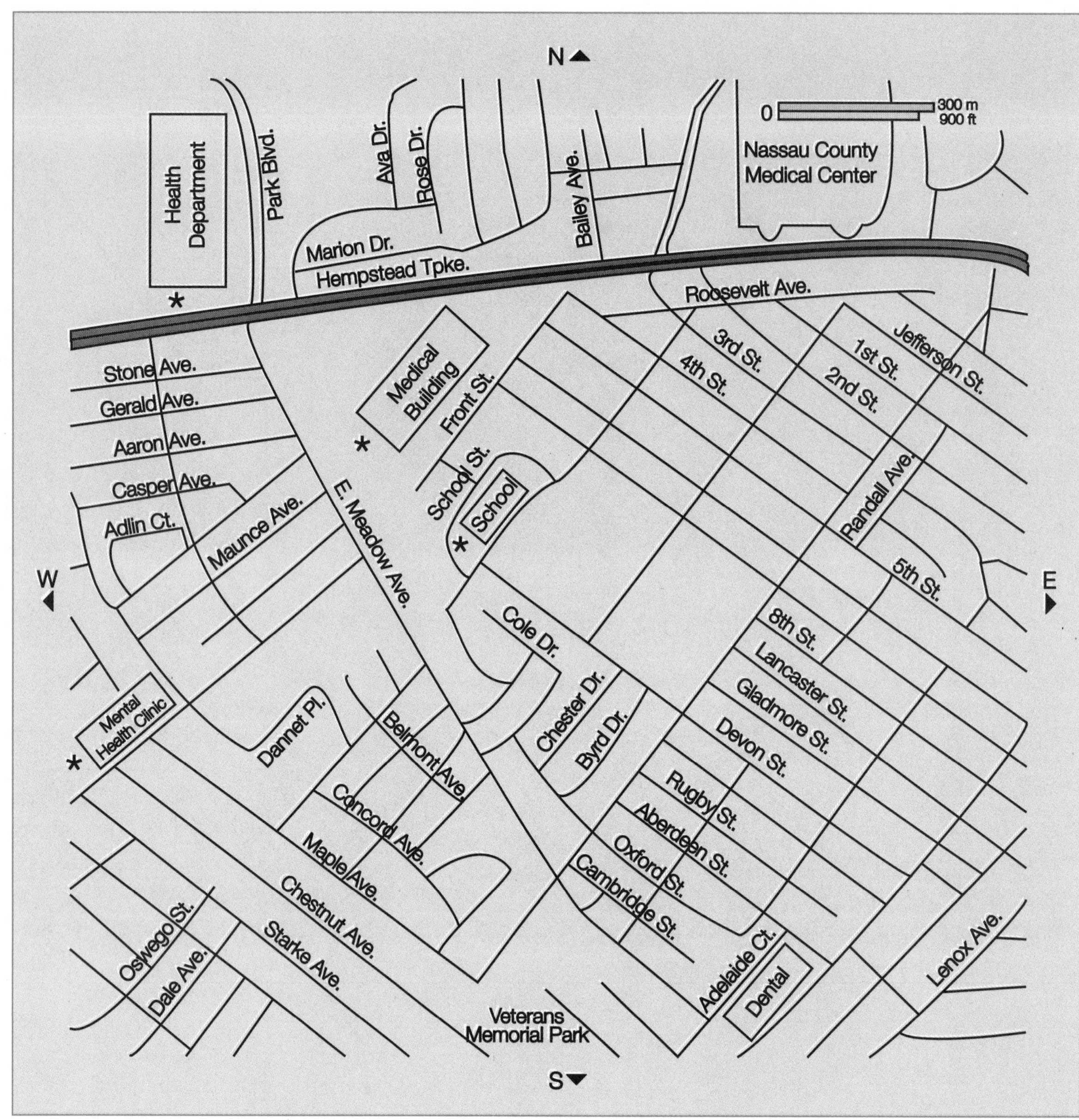

Sample Map for Grades 5–6

Learning Experience 15-8

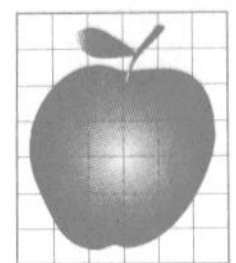

Guess Who I Am

Grade Level

4–6

Primary Disciplines

English, Language Arts

Learning Objectives

Following this game, students will be able to

- Identify the services associated with specific health care provider specialists.
- Understand questions asked by their physician.
- Perform elementary research on health care providers.

Time Required

1 hour

Materials

Color-coded card sets (described below)

Description of Activity

This is a questioning game to be played after a classroom discussion of health care providers.

Introduction

Prepare three sets of 10 different color flashcards each—10 blue, 10 yellow, and so on. One side of each card will contain only the color; the other side will identify a health care provider. The 10 cards in each set will have the same 10 providers (for example, pediatrician, obstetrician, surgeon, chiropractor, nurse, pharmacist, family practitioner, psychiatrist, orthopedist, psychologist).

Two Days Before

Divide the class into groups of 10 by color-coded flashcards. Each group of 10 students with the same color flashcards will be divided into two teams (A team and B team) with five students in each.

When the groups of A teams and B teams are set up, give students each a flashcard and instruct them not to show their card to anyone. Assign the homework as described on page 550 and tell them that they will participate in a game two days hence. If they give their information away beforehand, they will lose game points for their team.

Activity

Each color-coded group will participate in a Guess Who I Am game. At the conclusion of the game, the scores for all the A teams will be added together, as will the scores for all B teams. The combined A and B teams with the highest combined score win the game.

The day of the game, instruct students to get into their color-coded teams of 5 A's and 5 B's in a group and sit opposite one another. One person will be scorekeeper.

Tell the students that when their turn comes, the opposite team will ask them three questions about their practitioner (for example, "Do you take care of young children?" "Can you prescribe medication?"). Then the questioning team will collaborate and make one guess at identifying the practitioner the opposite team member is representing. After the student has answered the three questions and has acknowledged if the guess is correct or not, the student "practitioner" must present three important facts about the practitioner.

Each correct guess scores 5 points for the questioning team. Each correct piece of information given by the practitioner scores 1 point for that team. Each incorrect piece of information or lack of information scores 1 point for the opposite team.

Beginning with the first Team A student on the left, in each color-coded group, one A member will have a turn, then one B member will have a turn, until all of the students have had a chance to participate.

After each student has had a chance, the scores for all the A teams

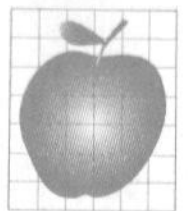

Learning Experience 15-8 continued

are added and the scores for all the B teams are added to determine the group winner (As or Bs).

Homework

In preparation for this session, each student will be given a color-coded card with the name of a health care provider identified on it. Students should be given 2 days to do the assignment, and they should be instructed to keep the identity of their health care provider a secret for the upcoming game.

They are to write a one-page summary (that will be collected and graded) about their provider, including the services provided, where this practitioner may be located, the type of patient or client they serve, and any other descriptive information they can find. Their paper could include information such as the following:

I take care of people with ______________________________.

I usually see people who are/have ______________________________ (age, illness, and so on).

Sometimes I see my patients in my office, and other times I see them in

______________________________.

My services are paid for by insurance. I can prescribe medications when necessary. Sometimes I send people for ____________________ tests. I am a (medical doctor, dentist, allergist, podiatrist). I have a license to practice in ______________

____________________________.

Evaluation

The game itself is an evaluation tool by including the scoring of information about the provider. The homework assignment is a means of evaluating students' ability to research and do written work.

Learning Experience 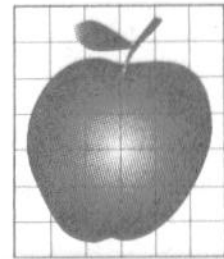 15-9

Who Am I and What Do I Do?

Grade Level

K–3

Primary Disciplines

Language Arts: Spelling, Art

Learning Objectives

Following this activity, students will be able to

- Identify reliable health care providers and facilities.
- Increase their vocabulary and be able to recognize the spelling of health care providers and facilities.
- Identify some of the activities of health care providers.
- Recognize newspapers and magazines as resources.
- Produce a piece of artwork with cut-and-paste medium.

Time Required

About 30 minutes

Materials

Sets of cards (described below), paste, paper, magazines

Description of Activity

Grades K–1

Make a set of cards with a picture of the health care provider or facility and the correct spelling of the title or name written across the bottom of the card. Distribute the cards to the students. Each student with a card (one at a time) will come up to the front of the room, hold up the card while the rest of the students (with your help) pronounce the name of the provider or facility aloud together. The students will then write the name of the provider or facility in their notebook, and the student with the card will write it on the board and hang the card below it.

Grades 2–3

Prepare two sets of cards: one with the name of a provider or a facility on each card (enough for half of the class), and the other with an identifying picture of the provider or facility for each card (enough for the rest of the class). Distribute all of the cards. Then one student at a time will come forward, and the student with the identifying picture card to match it will also come forward. The class will then speak the title aloud and discuss that provider. The students can talk about the services; whether their family or they have ever been to that provider/facility; what questions they would ask if they were to use that provider or facility; and so on.

Homework

Grades K–1

This assignment should be sent home in writing so the students can get help from their parents. If appropriate, the homework should be planned for the weekend. Each student will be asked to pick one provider or facility from the ones identified during the lesson. At home, they will cut out letters that spell the name of the provider/facility and pictures that represent something about that provider or facility and paste them on a piece of colored paper (making a collage). The collages can be hung around the room.

Grades 2–3

The students will make a list of the various health care facilities/providers they or their families use. They are to prepare a brief picture-and-word scrapbook containing words and pictures that are associated with the provider or facility.

Evaluation

Grading of the homework; spelling bee, or quiz.

Learning Experience 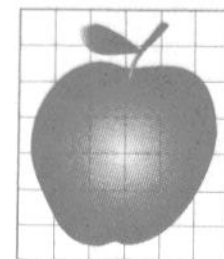 15-10

The Untold Story

Grade Level

K–6

Primary Disciplines

Language Arts, Social Studies

Learning Objectives

Following this activity, students will be able to

- Identify other cultures and lifestyles as they relate to people's health.
- Make decisions about health-related issues.
- Write more creatively.

Time Required

This can be fill-in time or part of other sessions or a story time of 45 minutes.

Description of Activity

Prepare or select several stories that relate to health services or products. Two usable stories follow (the example here is intended for grades 4–6, but the stories and language can be adapted to lower grade levels).

Grades K–2

1. Instruct the students to read (or read to them, depending upon their abilities) the story and answer the questions that follow (in writing or verbally).
2. Have the students write questions that might be asked at the end of the story. Call on one student at a time to read their question and have the other students answer them. Add your answer where necessary.

Billy came to school last week, and he looked very tired. He was sneezing and coughing all day long. The teacher kept saying, "Billy, please cover your nose when you sneeze." The teacher sent Billy to the school nurse. Billy didn't come to school the next day. We heard he went to the local hospital. The teacher helped us to make get-well cards for Billy, and we sent them in one package. Billy had a communicable disease. The principal gave us notes about Billy to take home to our parents. Our parents were invited to come to school and listen to a health department public nurse explain what happened to Billy. After that, some of us had to take shots.

Questions for Discussion

- Where is the hospital that Billy went to?
- What is a communicable disease?
- What kind of medical doctor takes care of children Billy's age?
- What is a health department?
- What does a public health nurse do?
- What do people get shots for?
- When Billy comes home, he will need to take medicine. Where will his family buy their medicine?

Questions students might ask:

- What is wrong with Billy?
- Can I catch it?
- Why did Billy go to the hospital?
- What happens in the hospital?
- Does Billy have to take medicine?

Grades 3–6

Read the following story to the students. Then lead a discussion about the questions asked below.

The Chi family just moved in down the street. Five people make up the family: two boys (Sam, 6 years old, and John, 3 months old), their mom, their grandma, and their aunt.

Mrs. Chi works as a nurse practitioner who specializes in midwifery, and Aunt Lucie is a chiropractor. Grandma Chi came from Asia many years ago and brought Mom Chi and Aunt Lucie with her when they were children. Many of the people in the neighborhood will use Aunt Lucie's services, because she will have an office in the house and it is convenient.

I overheard my mom talking with Mrs. Chi about doctors and other health services our family uses. My mom was telling her what a wonderful pediatrician we have. Dr. Roberts has been a friend of the

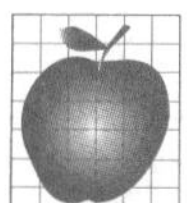

Learning Experience 15-10 continued

family for many years. Mom also told her about an excellent pharmacist in the neighborhood. Mrs. Chi asked my mom if she knows any doctor who practices alternative medicine. My mom was confused about what alternative medicine is. Mrs. Chi said she was interested in someone who had experience with nutrition, herbal medicine, and acupuncture. My mom said we use only "regular" doctors. Mrs. Chi said that alternative medicine doctors can be "regular" doctors, too. They talked for quite a while. I wondered what alternative medicine is myself.

Questions for Discussion:

- What does a nurse practitioner who specializes in midwifery do?
- What does a pediatrician do?
- What does a chiropractor do?
- What did Mrs. Chi mean by "alternative medicine?"
- Do you have to be of Asian descent to use alternative or complementary medicine?
- What is acupuncture?
- How do I know if the treatment I am getting is good treatment?
- What did the Mom mean when she said, "We use "regular" doctors?"

Have the students develop a list of questions that might be asked of practitioners:

- Where were you trained? Are you licensed to practice in this state?
- Will my medical insurance cover your bills?
- Do you practice allopathic and alternative medicine?
- How would I know if acupuncture (or herbal, nutritional treatment) is right for me?
- What kind of treatment can I expect to have if I use your chiropractic services?

Homework

After the storytelling is over, the students can do research about different kinds of medical practices. They might prepare a one-page report about a type of medical practitioner (pediatrician, obstetrician, nurse practitioner, chiropractor, acupuncturist, and so on).

Evaluation

- Homework is graded for spelling, grammar, accuracy of information, and so on.
- Students' answers to discussion questions are graded as they are called upon. Some of the discussion questions can be used as a brief in-class test.
- Students can be grouped for discussion and the group with the best answer could receive extra credit.

Learning Experience 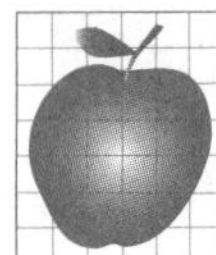 15-11

What Are the Rules?

Grade Level

K–2

Primary Discipline

Health

Learning Objectives

Following this activity, students will be able to

- Explain school rules about medication use.
- Explain home rules about medication use.

Time Required

One lesson (30 minutes)

Materials

Large sheets of paper, markers

Description of Activity

Read the following brief story:

> Bakari has just come from visiting the doctor. She has not been feeling well and the doctor gave her medicine to take every four hours. Her mommy gives her one when she gets up in the morning at 6 AM. Bakari is in the first grade and must take her medicine at 10 AM and 2 PM while at school. What should her mommy/daddy/parent/guardian do and how can she take her medicine at school?

- Ask: What does Bakari's mommy/daddy/parent/guardian need to do?
- Ask: What does Bakari's teacher need to do?
- Ask: Who should give the medicine to Bakari?
- Ask: What do you think Bakari's mommy/daddy/parent/guardian will tell her about taking her medicine at home?

Answers to the questions should be continued until all students are clear that first her mother/daddy/parent/guardian must tell the school and make sure the person who will be responsible (probably the nurse) knows what the schedule is.

The teacher must know that this is going on. No one else in the class needs to know about Bakari's medicine. At home, Bakari should take medicine only from her mommy/daddy/parent/guardian.

Evaluation

Students are able to:

- Explain what the rules are for taking medicine in school.
- Explain what the rules are for taking medicine at home.

The students will work on decorating the rules that have been generated by this activity.

Learning Experience 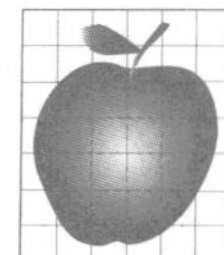 15-12

What's the Difference?

Grade Level

K–2

Primary Discipline

Health

Learning Objectives

Following this activity, students will be able to

- Describe the difference among foods, poisons, and medicines.
- Demonstrate how to avoid unknown and potentially harmful jars, bottles, and substances

Time Required

One lesson (30 minutes)

Materials

Activity sheets with pictures of different foods, household cleaners, pills, and medicine bottles (both over-the-counter medications and prescription drugs), crayons

Description of Activity

- Ask: Who can tell me what a food is?
- Ask: Who can tell me what a poison is?
- Ask: Who can tell me what a medicine is?

Continue this activity until all students can identify examples of each item.

Hand out the activity sheet. Ask the students to color each food item on the sheet green; each poison on the sheet red; and each medicine on the sheet yellow.

- Ask: Why were you asked to use those colors?
- Have students share their work.
- Correct any incorrectly colored items.

On the back of the sheet, ask the students to draw where they think each type of item should be stored.

Evaluation

Students are able to:

- Identify foods, poisons, or medicine.
- Describe how each item should be handled.
- Describe where each item should be stored.

NAME: ____

Color any food green; color any medicine yellow; color any poison red.

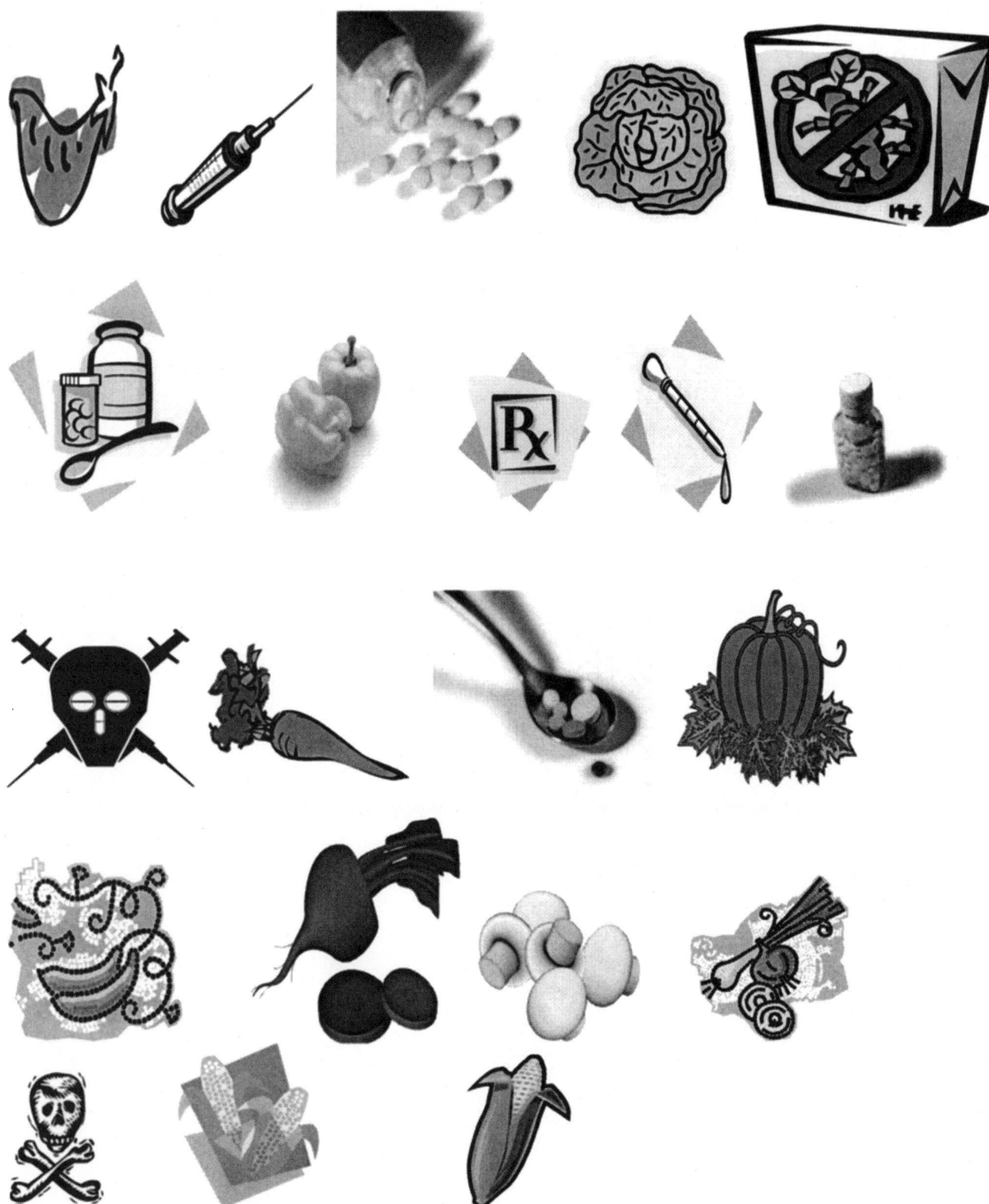

Appendix A

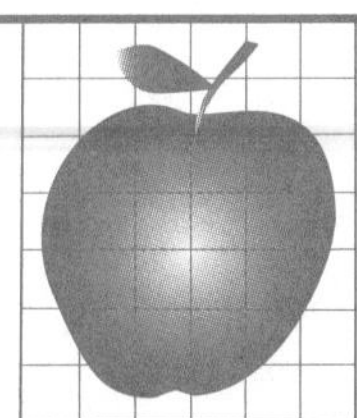

Report on the 1990 Joint Committee on Health Education Terminology

November 1, 1990

One of the essential underpinnings of any profession is a body of well-defined terms used to enable members to communicate easily and with the clarity necessary for understanding among themselves and with others. The field of health education has changed dramatically in the past two decades. The definitions in this report provide a common interpretation of terms frequently used by health educators in a variety of settings. Therefore, the terms presented here are defined for use by the professional health educator as well as by other individuals and groups.

The Committee recognized that other health professionals (e.g., physicians, nurses, etc.) are concerned with and involved in health education as a part of their professional role and that they may have a different orientation. Consequently, they may use different terminology from that contained in this report. It is hoped, however, that the terms defined will be of help to these groups to clarify terminology used by health education professionals.

Words referring to health service and related personnel (e.g., patient educator, health counselor) or words which are in general use and understood by a variety of professionals (e.g., mass communication, objectives, self-help, self-care, evaluation) are not included. The Committee chose to define community and school health education and associated terminology, because degrees are offered in these areas. Other areas (e.g., patient and worksite health education) were omitted because they tend to be areas of emphasis rather than degrees.

There may be other interpretations of the words defined; however, those presented in this report are as many health educators view them today. The terms included reflect trends, concepts, and practices. They help to explain what the profession is, who its practitioners are, and how they function. Additional uses might include the following:

- Articulating the health education professional preparation program to other units on college and university campuses
- Assisting governmental agencies in planning effective health education policies and programs
- Assisting editorial boards in determining appropriate health education word usage
- Guiding accrediting and credentialing agencies
- Explaining the field of practice to other professionals
- Establishing a basis for consistency of language usage in the professional literature and in research endeavors and grantsmanship

Historically, the Public Health Education Section of the American Public

This report was received and acknowledged in November 1990 by the Board of Directors of the Association for the Advancement of Health Education.

Joint Committee on Health Education Terminology 1990 Committee Members

Evelyn E. Ames, Ph.D., CHES
Western Washington University
(American Public Health Association, SchoolHealth Education and Services Section)

Harriet H. Barr, M.P.H., CHES,
Committee Co-Chair
University of North Carolina at Chapel Hill, School of Public Health (American Public Health Association, Public Health Education and Health Promotion Section)

Bradley J. Bradford, M. D.
Pediatrician
(American Academy of Pediatrics)

Chet E. Bradley, M.S., CHES
Wisconsin Department of Public Instruction (Society of State Directors of Health, Physical Education, and Recreation)

Peter A. Cortese, Dr. P.H., CHES,
Committee Co-Chair
California State University, Long Beach
(Association for the Advancement of Health Education)

Karen A. Gordon, M.P.H.
Princeton University
(American College Health Association, Health Education Section)

Marian V. Hamburg, Ed.D., CHES
Professor Emeritus, New York University
(Society for Public Health Education)

Cheryl C. Lackey, M.P.H., CHES
Texas Department of Health
(Association of State and Territorial Directors of Public Health Education)

Paul Mico, M.P.H., CHES
(Attended the August meeting as alternate delegate for Dr. Hamburg) Third Party Associates, Inc. (Society for Public Health Education)

John Seffrin, Ph.D., CHES
Indiana University
(American School Health Association)

Health Association (APHA) developed a statement of terminology about 1927 (1). The first committee report on terminology was published by the American Physical Education Association in 1934 (2). The American Association for Health, Physical Education, and Recreation (AAHPER) presented a report on health and physical education terminology in 1950–51 (3). Another AAHPER joint committee was appointed in 1962 to foster and improve understanding on the part of school and public health educators (4). After nine years, AAHPER again took the lead which resulted in a 1973 joint committee terminology report (5). In 1990, the Association for the Advancement of Health Education (AAHE), an Association of the American Alliance for Health, Physical Education, Recreation and Dance, continued this leadership by convening a joint committee of delegates of the Coalition of National Health Education Organizations (CNHEO)* and a representative from the American Academy of Pediatrics to update the earlier terms and to add relevant new definitions.

The Association for the Advancement of Health Education provided staff support as well as funding for the Terminology Committee meeting. Additional financial support for dissemination of the report was contributed by the majority of organizations represented. The meeting was convened at the AAHE/AAHPERD headquarters in Reston, VA, August 2–5, 1990.

Process of Formulating the Definitions

The charge to the Committee was to review the 1973 Report of the Joint Committee on Health Education Terminology, to determine which terms are still relevant, to delete those considered outdated, to revise as deemed appropriate, and to add new terms currently used in the health education field. Individual members came with reference documents to be used in the process. AAHE library materials also were available. The committee was co-chaired by the coordinator of the Coalition and the AAHE delegate to the Coalition.

A draft document was completed during the meeting and subsequently circulated to a select number of outside reviewers for comment. The final document was presented as a Committee Report to the AAHE Board of Directors.

After acceptance by the AAHE Board of Directors, the Report was published in the Journal of Health Education and copies were provided to organizations whose delegates served on the Joint Committee. Each organization was encouraged to disseminate the final report to a wide audience.

Criteria

The 1973 report was reviewed carefully. Some terms from this report were excluded, some repeated verbatim, some revised, and new terms were added based upon the criteria listed below.

Essentialness is basic to the field of health education and necessary for communication.

Authoritativeness is recognized or accepted by the profession as official language.

Significance is so important in communication within and among groups that its use requires common interpretation.

Encompassment is sufficiently broad and inclusive to eliminate unnecessary additional definitions but is restrictive enough to have clear meaning.

Usage occurs frequently enough to affect and effect communications.

Adaptability can be used effectively by various health professions and other individuals and groups.

Clarity definition is necessary to maintain consistency of use among disciplines.

A. Contextual Definitions

Health education takes place within the broad context of health. Certain health terms are defined to clarify how health education functions. These are:

Health

There are many definitions written for the word "Health." Three examples are provided.

> "A state of complete physical, mental, and social well-being, and not merely the absence of disease and infirmity." (6)

> "A quality of life involving dynamic interaction and independence among the individual's physical well-being, his (*sic*) mental and emotional reactions, and the social complex in which he (*sic*) exists." (7)

* The Coalition was established in 1973 to provide a vehicle for collaboration of all major national health education organizations. Its primary mission is to mobilize the resources of the Health Education profession in order to expand and improve health education, regardless of the setting. Each member organization appointed one delegate and one alternate. The following organizations are members: American Public Health Association, School Health Education and Services Section and the Public Health Education and Health Promotion Section; American College Health Association; American School Health Association; Association for the Advancement of Health Education, American Alliance for Health, Physical Education, Recreation and Dance; Association of State and Territorial Directors of Public Health Education; Society for Public Health Education, Inc.; and the Society of State Directors of Health, Physical Education and Recreation. The Coalition facilitates national level communication, collaboration and coordination among the member organizations; provides a forum for the identification and discussion of health education issues; formulates recommendations and takes appropriate action on issues affecting member interests; serves as a communication and advisory resource for agencies, organizations and persons in the public and private sectors on health education issues; and serves as a focus for the exploration and resolution of issues pertinent to professional health educators.

"An integrated method of functioning which is oriented toward maximizing the potential of which the individual is capable. It requires that the individual maintain a continuum of balance and purposeful direction with the environment where he (*sic*) is functioning." (8)

Health Promotion and Disease Prevention

Health promotion and disease prevention is the aggregate of all purposeful activities designed to improve personal and public health through a combination of strategies, including the competent implementation of behavioral change strategies, health education, health protection measures, risk factor detection, health enhancement and health maintenance.

Healthy Lifestyle

A healthy lifestyle is a set of health-enhancing behaviors, shaped by internally consistent values, attitudes, beliefs and external social and cultural forces.

Official Health Agency

An official health agency is a publicly supported governmental organization mandated by law and/or regulation for the protection and improvement of the health of the public.

Voluntary Health Organization

A voluntary health organization is a nonprofit association supported by contributions dedicated to conducting research and providing education and/or services related to particular health problems or concerns. (Note: Private voluntary organization—PVO—is the term used outside the U.S.A. to denote a voluntary health organization; in some countries and in connection with the United Nations, the term nongovernmental organization—NGO—is used.)

Private Health Agency

A private health agency is a profit or nonprofit organization devoted to providing primary, secondary, and/or tertiary health services which may include health education.

B. Primary Health Education Definitions

Certain health education terms are generic and are defined here, as follows:

Health Education Field

The health education field is that multidisciplinary practice, which is concerned with designing, implementing, and evaluating educational programs that enable individuals, families, groups, organizations, and communities to play active roles in achieving, protecting, and sustaining health.

Health Education Process

The health education process is that continuum of learning which enables people, as individuals and as members of social structures, to voluntarily make decisions, modify behaviors, and change social structure in ways which are health enhancing.

Health Education Program

A health education program is a planned combination of activities developed with the involvement of specific populations and based on a needs assessment, sound principles of education, and periodic evaluation using a clear set of goals and objectives.

Health Educator

A health educator is a practitioner who is professionally prepared in the field of health education, who demonstrates competence in both theory and practice, and who accepts responsibility to advance the aims of the health education profession.

Examples of settings for health educators and the application of health education include, but are not limited to, the following:

- Schools
- Communities
- Post-Secondary Educational Institutions
- Medical Care Institutions
- Voluntary Health Organizations
- Worksites (Business and Industry)
- Rehabilitation Centers
- Professional Associations
- Governmental Agencies
- Public Health Agencies
- Environmental Agencies
- Mental Health Agencies

Certified Health Education Specialist (CHES)

A Certified Health Education Specialist (CHES) is an individual who is credentialed as a result of demonstrating competency based on criteria established by the National Commission for Health Education Credentialing, Inc. (NCHEC).

Health Education Coordinator

A health education coordinator is a professional educator who is responsible for the management and coordination of all health education policies, activities, and resources within a particular setting or circumstance.

Health Education Administrator

A health education administrator is a professional health educator who has the authority and responsibility for the management and coordination of all health education policies, activities, and resources within a particular setting or circumstance.

Health Information

Health information is the content of communications based on data derived from systematic and scientific methods as they relate to health issues, policies, programs, services, and other aspects of individual and public health, which can be used for informing various populations and in planning health education activities.

Health Literacy

Health literacy is the capacity of an individual to obtain, interpret, and understand basic health information and services and the competence to use such information and services in ways which are health enhancing.

Health Advising**

Health advising is a process of informing and assisting individuals or groups in making decisions and solving problems related to health.

C. Definitions Related to Community Settings

The terms that relate more specifically to community or public health education are defined here, as follows:

Community Health Education

Community health education is the application of a variety of methods that result in the education and mobilization of community members in actions for resolving health issues and problems which affect the community. These methods include, but are not limited to, group process, mass media, communication, community organization, organization development, strategic planning, skills training, legislation, policy making, and advocacy.

Community Health Educator

A community health educator is a practitioner who is professionally prepared in the field of community/public health education who demonstrates competence in the planning, implementation, and evaluation of a broad range of health promoting or health enhancing programs for community groups.

D. Definitions Related to Educational Settings

The terms that relate more specifically to school health education are defined here, as follows:

Comprehensive School Health Program

A comprehensive school health program is an organized set of policies, procedures, and activities designed to protect and promote the health and well-being of students and staff which has traditionally included health services, healthful school environment, and health education. It should also include, but not be limited to, guidance, counseling, physical education, food service, social work, psychological services, and employee health promotion.

School Health Education

School health education is one component of the comprehensive school health program which includes the development, delivery, and evaluation of a planned instructional program and other activities for students pre-school through grade 12, for parents and for school staff, and is designed to positively influence the health knowledge, attitudes, and skills of individuals.

School Health Services

School health services are that part of the school health program provided by physicians, nurses, dentists, health educators, other allied health personnel, social workers, teachers, and others to appraise, protect and promote the health of students and school personnel. These services are designed to insure access to and the appropriate use of primary health care services, prevent and control communicable disease, provide emergency care for injury or sudden illness, promote and provide optimum sanitary conditions in a safe school facility and environment, and provide concurrent learning opportunities which are conducive to the maintenance and promotion of individual and community health.

School Health Educator

A school health educator is a practitioner who is professionally prepared in the field of school health education, meets state teaching requirements, and demonstrates competence in the development, delivery, and evaluation of curricula for students and adults in the school setting that enhance health knowledge, attitudes, and problem-solving skills.

Comprehensive School Health Instruction

Comprehensive school health instruction refers to the development, delivery

** The Committee believes that Health Counseling is a term that should be defined by the health counseling profession.

and evaluation of a planned curriculum, pre-school through 12, with goals, objectives, content sequence, and specific classroom lessons which includes, but is not limited to the following major content areas:

- Community Health
- Consumer Health
- Environmental Health
- Family Life
- Mental and Emotional Health
- Injury Prevention and Safety
- Nutrition
- Personal Health
- Prevention and Control of Disease
- Substance Use and Abuse

Post-Secondary Health Education Program

A post-secondary health education program is a planned set of health education policies, procedures, activities, and services that are directed to students, faculty and/or staff of colleges, universities, and other higher education institutions. This includes, but is not limited to:

- General Health Courses for Students
- Employee and Student Health Promotion Activities
- Health Services
- Professional Preparation of Health Educators and Other Professionals
- Self-Help Groups
- Student Life

ERRATA

References for the Report on the 1990 Joint Committee on Health Education Terminology

1. Mabel Rugen. (1972). *A fifty year history of the public health section of the American Public Health Association, 1922–1972.* American Public Health Association, Inc. Washington, DC, p. 9.
2. Jesse Feiring Williams (Chair). (1934, Dec. 10). Report of the Health Education Section of the American Physical Education Association. Definitions of terms in health education, *Journal of Health and Physical Education*, 5(16–17), 50–51.
3. Bernice Moss (Chair). (1950). Joint Committee on Health Education Terminology. *Journal of Health and Physical Education*, 21(41).
4. Robert Yoho (Chair). (1962, Nov). Joint Committee on Health Education Terminology. Health education terminology, *Journal of Health, Physical Education, Recreation*, 33(27–28).
5. Edward B. Johns (Chair). (1973, Nov/Dec). Joint Committee on Health Education Terminology. Report of the Joint Committee on Health Education Terminology, *Health Education*, 4(6), p. 25.
6. World Health Organization. (1946). *Constitution of the World Health Organization*. Geneva, World Health Organization.
7. *Health education: A conceptual approach to curriculum design, school health education study*. 1967. Washington, DC: 3M Education Press, p. 10.
8. Halbert Dunn. (1967). *High level wellness.* Virginia: R. W. Beatty, 4–5.

Appendix B

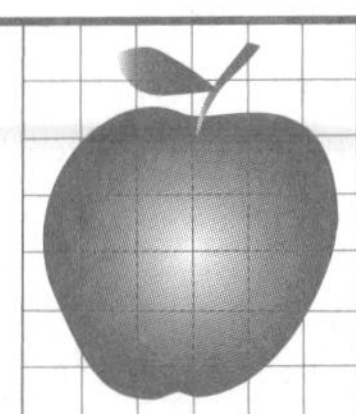

Healthy People 2000—National Health Priority Areas and Objectives Which Target Health Education of the School-Age Population

The numbers preceding each statement refer to the national health priority areas (e.g., priority area 1 refers to Physical Activity and Fitness, 2 refers to Nutrition). Each priority area has its own set of objectives; several objectives are to be accomplished in more than one priority area. Therefore, some objectives have several priority numbers listed. Those asterisked are specific objectives measured by the Youth Risk Behavior Surveillance System (Division for Adolescent and School Health, 1993).

National Health Priority Area 1: Physical Activity and Fitness

1.2, 2.3, 5.10, 17.12

Reduce overweight to a prevalence of no more than 20 percent among people ages 20 and older and no more than 15 percent among adolescents ages 12 through 19.

***1.3, 15.11, 17.13**

Increase to at least 30 percent the proportion of people aged 6 and older who engage regularly, preferably daily, in light to moderate physical activity for at least thirty minutes per day.

***1.4**

Increase to at least 20 percent the proportion of people aged 18 and older and to at least 75 percent the population of children and adolescents aged 6 through 17 who engage in vigorous physical activity that promotes the development and maintenance of cardiorespiratory fitness three or more days per week for twenty or more minutes per occasion.

***1.6**

Increase to at least 40 percent the proportion of overweight people aged 6 and older who regularly perform physical activities that enhance and maintain muscular strength, muscular endurance, and flexibility.

1.7, 2.7

Increase to at least 50 percent the proportion of overweight people aged 12 and older who have adopted sound dietary practices combined with regular physical activity to attain an appropriate body weight.

National Health Priority Area 2: Nutrition

2.19

Increase to at least 75 percent the proportion of the nation's schools that provide nutrition education from preschool through 12th grade, preferably as part of quality school health education.

National Health Priority Area 3: Tobacco

***3.5**

Reduce the initiation of cigarette smoking by children and youth so that no more than 15 percent have become regular cigarette smokers by age 20.

***3.9**

Reduce smokeless tobacco use by males aged 12 through 24 to a prevalence of no more than 4 percent.

3.10

Establish tobacco-free environments and include tobacco use prevention in the curricula of all elementary, middle, and secondary schools, preferably as part of quality school health education.

3.14

Increase to 50 percent the number of states with plans to reduce tobacco use, especially among youth.

National Health Priority Area 4: Alcohol and Other Drugs

*4.5

Increase by at least one year the average age of first use of cigarettes, alcohol, and marijuana by adolescents aged 12 through 17.

*4.6

Reduce the proportion of young people who have used alcohol, marijuana, and cocaine in the past month.

*4.7

Reduce the proportion of high school seniors and college students engaging in recent occasions of heavy drinking of alcoholic beverages to no more than 28 percent of high school seniors and 32 percent of college students.

4.9

Increase the proportion of high school seniors who perceive social disapproval associated with the heavy use of alcohol, occasional use of marijuana, and experimentation of cocaine.

4.10

Increase the proportion of high school seniors who associate risk of physical or psychological harm with the heavy use of alcohol, regular use of marijuana, and experimentation with cocaine.

*4.11

Reduce to no more than 3 percent the proportion of male high school seniors who use anabolic steroids.

4.13

Provide to children in all school districts and private schools primary and secondary school educational programs on alcohol and other drugs, preferably as part of quality school health education.

National Health Priority Area 5: Family Planning

*5.4, 18.3, 19.9

Reduce the proportion of adolescents who have engaged in sexual intercourse to no more than 15 percent by age 15 and no more than 40 percent by age 17.

*5.5

Increase to at least 40 percent the proportion of ever sexually active adolescents aged 17 and younger who have abstained from sexual activity for the previous 3 months.

*5.6

Increase to at least 90 percent the proportion of sexually active, unmarried people ages 19 and younger who use contraception, especially combined method contraception, that both effectively prevents pregnancy and provides barrier protection against disease.

*5.8

Increase to at least 85 percent the proportion of people aged 10 through 18 who have discussed human sexuality including values surrounding sexuality, with their parents and/or have received information through another parentally endorsed source, such as youth, school, or religious programs.

National Health Priority Area 7: Violent and Abusive Behavior

*7.8, 6.2

Reduce by 15 percent the incidence of injurious suicide attempts among adolescents aged 14 through 17.

*7.9

Reduce by 20 percent the incidence of physical fighting among adolescents aged 14 through 17.

*7.10

Reduce by 20 percent the incidence of weapon carrying by adolescents aged 14 through 17.

7.16

Increase to at least 50 percent the proportion of elementary and secondary schools that teach nonviolent conflict resolution skills, preferably as part of quality school health education.

National Health Priority Area 8: Educational and Community-Based Programs

8.4

Increase to at least 75 percent the proportion of the nation's elementary and secondary schools that provide planned and sequential kindergarten through 12th grade quality school health education.

8.9

Increase to at least 75 percent the proportion of people aged 10 and older who have discussed issues related to nutrition, physical activity, sexual behavior, tobacco, alcohol, other drugs, or safety with family members on at least one occasion during the preceding month.

National Health Priority Area 9: Unintentional Injuries

*9.12

Increase use of occupant protection systems, such as safety belts, inflatable safety restraints, and child safety seats, to at least 85 percent of motor vehicle occupants.

*9.13

Increase use of helmets to at least 80 percent of motorcyclists and at least 50 percent of bicyclists.

9.18

Provide academic instruction on injury prevention and control, preferably as part of quality school health education, in at least 50 percent of public school systems.

National Health Priority Area 18: HIV Infection and National Health Priority Area 19: Sexually Transmitted Diseases

*18.4, 9.10

Increase to at least 50 percent the proportion of sexually active, unmarried people who used a condom at last sexual intercourse.

*18.4a, 19.10a

Increase to at least 60 percent the proportion of sexually active young women aged 15 through 19 (by their partners) who used a condom at last sexual intercourse.

*18.4b, 19.10b

Increase to at least 75 percent the proportion of sexually active young men aged 15 through 19 who used a condom at last sexual intercourse.

19.12

Include instruction in sexually transmitted disease transmission prevention in the curricula of all middle and secondary schools, preferably as part of quality school health instruction.

Appendix C

Health Resources for Teachers

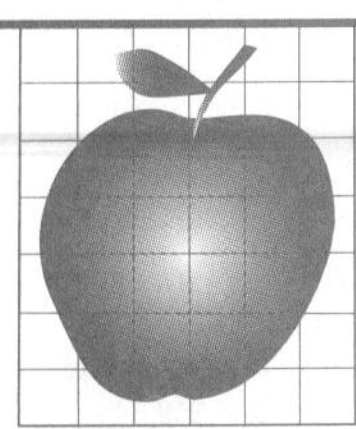

At-Risk Resources, The Bureau for At-Risk Youth, 135 Dupont Street, PO Box 760, Plainview, NY 11803-0760, 800-999-6884: teen sexuality, peer mediation, elementary guidance, drug prevention, parenting, staff development, pre-teen guidance, books, pamphlets, posters, computer software.

Be Smart About Germs (1994), by S. Kleinsinger, Educational Activity Books, published by Positive Promotions, Brooklyn, NY, 800-635-2666: a coloring and activity book.

The Buying Guide for Fresh Fruits, Vegetables, Herbs & Nuts. Educational Department, Blue Goose, Inc., PO Box 46, Fullerton, CA 92632: pictures of foods.

Child Abuse Prevention Services, PO Box 176, Roslyn, NY, 11576: information and education about child abuse.

Childhelp USA, 6463 Independence Avenue, Woodland Hills, CA 91367, 800-422-4453: outreach for child abuse.

Clearinghouse on Child Abuse and Neglect Information, PO Box 1182, Washington, DC 20013, 703-385-7565: information and brochures.

Creative Food Experiences for Children (1974), by M.T. Goodwin & G. Pollen, available from CSPI, 1755 S Street, NW, Washington, DC: activities for children.

Early Childhood Nutrition Program (1979), by J. Randall & C. Olson, available from the Cornell University Distribution Center, 7 Research Park, Ithaca, NY 14850: developing nutrition education for children.

ETR Associates, PO Box 1830, Santa Cruz, CA 95061-1830, 800-321-4407: a wide variety of health materials, comprehensive health catalogs for teachers and health professionals, school health K–12, books, pamphlets, videos.

Family Life Educator, published by ETR Associates, PO Box 1830, Santa Cruz, CA 95061-1830, 408-438-4081: articles, news and reviews, teaching tools, abstracts.

Films for the Humanities and Sciences, PO Box 2053, Princeton, NJ 08543-2053, 600-257-5126: psychology and mental health, addiction, human sexuality, death and dying, AIDS films, videos, and videodiscs.

Inside-Out National Instructional TV: 30 videotape programs for relaxation, dealing with day-to-day problems of children.

Intermedia, 1300 Dexter Avenue North, Seattle, WA 98109, 800-553-8336: substance abuse, teen suicide, teen parents, sexuality, violence prevention, videos.

Journeyworks Publishing, Health Promotion, PO Box 8466, Santa Cruz, CA 95061-8466, 800-775-1998: fitness, women's health, abstinence, rape, pregnancy prevention, STDs/HIV, caregiving, mental wellness, smoking cessation, pamphlets.

Kiddie Quieting Reflex, A Choice for Children (1980), by E. and C. Stroebel and M. Holland, published by Lippincott Co., Whetersfield, CT: illustrated book for children.

Kidsrights, 10100 Park Cedar Drive, Charlotte, NC 28210, 800-892-KIDS: counseling, games, booklets on self-esteem, play therapy, life skills, violence prevention, videos on substance abuse, parenting.

Meaningful Movement for Children (1985), by H.A. Hoffman, J. Young, and S.E. Klesius, published by Kendall/Hunt, Dubuque, IA: physical activities for children.

Meeks/Heit Publishing Company, Blacklick, OH: textbooks with activities for K–12 in several health areas.

A Moving Experience: Dance for Lovers of Children and the Child Within (1987), Zephyr Press, Tucson, AZ: physical activities.

National Center for Missing and Exploited Children, 2101 Wilson Boulevard, Suite 550, Arlington, VA 22201-3052: information about finding missing children.

National Center for Drug Abuse, Violence, and Recovery, a division of NIMCO, PO Box 9, 102 Highway 81 North, Calhoun, KY 42327-0009, 800-962-6662: videos, software, displays, booklets, games, posters, CD-ROM.

National Child Abuse Coalition, 733–15th Street, NW, Suite 938, Washington, DC 20005, 202-347-3666: information and brochures on child abuse and neglect.

Noteworthy Creations, PO Box 335, Delphi, IN 46923, 800-305-4167: nutrition education resources for young children —songbooks, tapes, training video.

Nutrition Comes Alive (1985), by S. Nelson and M.C. Maples, available form Cornell Cooperative Extension, NY (see local county listings): activities and workbook.

Physical Education for Elementary School Children, 9th edition, (1995), by G. Kirschner and G. J. Gishburne, published by WCB Brown & Benchmark, Madison, WI: yearly programs, units, and daily lesson plans for elementary school children.

STDs!: Sexuality Transmitted Disease Guide (1995), Educational Activity Books, published by Positive Promotions, Brooklyn, NY, 800-635-2666: educational activities for children.

Sunburst Communications, Dept SG57, 33 Washington Avenue, Pleasantville, NY 10570, 800-431-1934: health and guidance videos on conflict resolution, respect, drug education, sex and AIDS, and careers, for grades K–12.

Tiger Juice (1981), by Stuart Bedford, Scott Publishing, Chico, CA: a book about stress for kids of all ages.

Tricon Publishing, 2150 Enterprise Drive, Mt. Pleasant, MI 48851, 517-772-2811: human growth and development curriculum series about kids' health: books, models, charts.

Understanding AIDS (1992), by G. Umland, Educational Activity Books, published by Positive Promotions, Brooklyn, NY, 800-635-2666: a coloring and activity book.

Appendix D

Key Documents

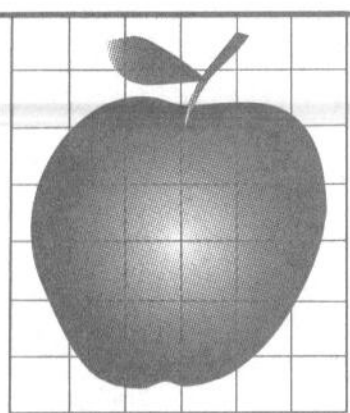

American Association of School Administrators. (1991). *Healthy Kids for the Year* 2000: An Action Plan for Schools. Arlington, VA: American Association of School Administrators

Association for the Advancement of Health Education. (1992). Healthy Networks: Models for Success. Reston, VA: Association for the Advancement of Health Education

Association for the Advancement of Health Education. (1991). Strengthening Health Education for the 1990's. Reston, VA: Association for the Advancement of Health Education

American Cancer Society. (1992). National Action Plan for Comprehensive School Health Education. Atlanta: American Cancer Society

American Medical Association. (1990). AMA Profiles of Adolescent Health. Chicago: American Medical Association

Association for Supervision and Curriculum Development. (1994). ASCD Yearbook. Association for Supervision and Curriculum Development. Alexandria, VA: ASCD

Boyer, E.L. (1983). High School: A Report on Secondary Education in America. New York: Carnegie Foundation for the Advancement of Teaching

Center for the Study of Social Policy. (1993). Kids Count Data Book: State Profiles of Child Well-Being. Greenwood, CT: Annie E. Casey Foundation

Council of Chief State School Officers. (1991). Beyond the Health Room. Washington, DC: Council of Chief State School Officers

Council of Chief State School Officers. (1993). Survey Report Council of Chief State School Officers. Washington, DC: Council of Chief State School Officers

Department of Health, Education and Welfare. (1971). The Report of the President's Committee on Health Education. Washington, DC: DHEW

The Gallup Organization. (1994). Values and Opinions of Comprehensive School Health Education in U. S. Public Schools: Adolescents, Parents, and School District Administrators. Atlanta: American Cancer Society

Guttmacher, Alan. (1991). Today's Adolescents: Tomorrow's Parents: A Portrait of the Americas. New York: Alan Guttmacher Institute

Joint Committee on Health Education Terminology. (1991). Report of the 1990 Joint Committee on Health Education Terminology. Reston, VA: Association for the Advancement of Health Education

Lavin, A.T., Shapiro, G.R., and Weill, K.S. (1992). "Creating an Agenda for School-based Health Promotion: A Review of 25 Selected Reports." *Journal of School Health* 62 (60)

Metropolitan Life. (1988). Health: You've Got to Be Taught: An Evaluation of Comprehensive Health Education in American Public Schools. New York: Metropolitan Life Foundation

National Commission on the Role of the School and the Community in Improving Adolescent Health. (1990). Code Blue: Uniting for Healthier Youth. Alexandria, VA: National Association of State Boards of Education

National Educational Commission on Time and Learning. (1994). Prisoner of Time. Washington, DC: U. S. Government Printing Office

National Professional School Health Education Organization. (1984). Comprehensive School Health Education. Journal of School Health 54(8), 312–315

National School Boards Association. (1991). School Health: Helping Children Learn. Alexandria, VA: National School Board Association

Northwest Regional Education Lab. (1993). We Can't Teach that Here— Or Can We? Portland, OR: Northwest Regional Education Lab

Office of the Surgeon General. (1992). Parents Speak Out for America's Children. Washington, DC: U. S. Government Printing Office

Pine, P. (1995). Promoting Health Education in Schools —Problems and Solutions. Arlington, VA: American Association of School Administrators

Seffrin, J.R. (1994). America's Interest in Comprehensive School Health Education. Paper presented to the Second Annual School Health Leadership Conference, Atlanta, GA

Task Force on Education of Young Adolescents. (1989). Turning Points: Preparing American Youth for the 21st Century. Washington, DC: Carnegie Council on Adolescent Development

U.S. Public Health Service. (1990). Healthy People 2000: National Health Promoting and Disease Prevention Objectives. Washington, DC: U. S. Government Printing Office

U.S. Department of Health and Human Services. (1987). Setting Nationwide Objectives in Disease Prevention and Health Promotion: The U. S. Experience. Washington, DC: U. S. Government Printing Office

Glossary

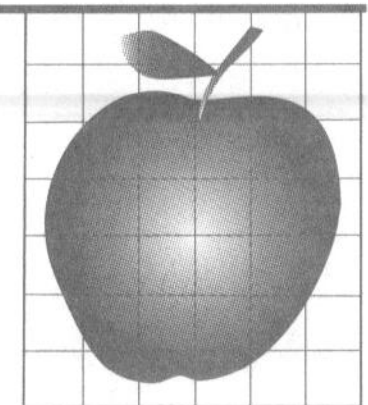

Acquired immunity Form of immunity that results from memory T cells' "remembering" antigens that previously invaded the body and activating a defense response

Addiction Reliance on something (often used with reference to drugs) to maintain homeostasis

Adrenal glands Glands that secrete hormones involved in various body functions and developmental characteristics

Agoraphobia Anxiety about or avoidance of places or situations from which escape may be difficult or embarrassing

Air pollutants Contaminants in atmosphere in quantities and of a duration that render them potentially hazardous to living things

Alcoholism Addiction to alcohol

Alimentary canal Hollow, muscular tube that is the defining component of the digestive system, beginning with the mouth and ending with the anus

Allergy Overreaction of body's immune system to a substance in the environment

Allopathic medicine Conventional or orthodox medicine

Alternative medicine Medical treatments provided in conjunction with, or exclusive of, conventional medicine, including acupuncture, herbals, reflexology, and nutritional supplementation, among others. Also called complementary medicine

Alveoli Tiny air sacs in lung

Amenorrhea Two or fewer menstrual periods a year

Amino acids Nitrogen-containing building blocks of body tissue; components of proteins

Amniocentesis Fetal test in which fluid is removed from the uterus through a long, thin needle inserted into abdominal wall and uterus into amniotic sac

Amylase Enzyme in saliva that begins breaking down starch into sugar

Anabolic steroids *See* Steroids

Anaphylactic shock Allergic reaction characterized by difficulty breathing, producing an extreme drop in blood pressure

Angina Pain in region of heart resulting from blockage of nutrients to heart tissues

Anorexia nervosa Eating disorder involving extreme weight loss, putting the individual at high health risk

Antibodies Agents capable of destroying specific organisms invading the body

Anticipatory grief Grieving before death occurs when it is known to be imminent

Antigen Any substance that triggers the immune response

Anus End of intestinal tract, from which bodily wastes are excreted

Aorta Main artery from the heart, leading to network of arteries in the body

Arteries Vessels that carry blood away from the heart

Arterioles Smallest of arteries

Arteriosclerosis Narrowed arteries caused by build-up of plaque inside artery walls

Asthma Periodic episodes of breathing difficulty, wheezing, and shortness of breath resulting from swelling of membranes or mucous build-up in and around bronchial tubes

Atrium *See* Auricle

Attitudes Constellation of related beliefs

Auditory canal Part of ear that directs sound into middle and inner ear

Auricle Compartment in upper heart

Authenticity Feeling of being autonomous and separate

Autogenic training Relaxation technique using elements of meditation, progressive muscle relaxation, and self-hypnosis

Autoimmune Any of the diseases in which the immune system fails to discriminate between foreign and normal body substances and attacks itself

Autonomic nervous system Peripheral nerves that control involuntary responses

Axon Appendage to neuron that receives information from cell body and relays it to a neuron

B cells Form of white blood cell originating in the bone marrow

Behavioral objectives Objectives that determine the selection of content, activities, and evaluation procedures for units of study

Beliefs A person's acceptance of something as true or real

Benign Noncancerous

Bereavement Intense grief associated with death or loss of a significant person

Bile Digestive enzyme, manufactured in liver and stored in gallbladder, that aids in breakdown of fat and pancreatic juices

Binge eating Eating disorder characterized by eating a lot of food in a short time

Biofeedback Technique used to gain voluntary control over certain physiological responses

Biological impedance analysis Method using variances in electrical current to assess body composition

Biosphere Global ecosystem

Birth defect Any inherited disease condition that begins during embryonic development and is present at birth

Bisexual Sexual orientation in which the person is attracted to individuals of either gender

Blood Fluid component of circulatory system

Blood pressure Force of circulating blood against wall of blood vessels

Body composition Proportion of fat weight to lean weight in body

Body mass index (BMI) Measure of body surface area used to assess body composition

Body system Group of organs working together to perform a specific bodily function

Bronchioles Tubes leading from bronchi into alveoli in lungs

Bronchus (pl., *bronchi*) Tube leading to each lung from windpipe

Bulimia nervosa Eating disorder characterized by binge eating followed by purging

Bully Busters A plan of actions for controlling bullying

Bullying Tormenting, being cruel or mean to people perceived as weaker or more vulnerable

Cancer Any of the diseases caused by rapid, uncontrolled growth and reproduction of abnormal cells

Capillaries Tiny blood vessels that connect arteries and veins

Carbamates Nerve poisons that have been shown to cause birth defects

Carbohydrates Nutrient that is the body's primary source of energy

Carcinogens Biological irritants that potentially cause cancer

Carcinomas Cancerous tumors that develop in secretory organs

Cardiovascular Pertaining to heart and blood vessels

Carriers Individuals who have a gene mutation and are capable of passing it to offspring even though carriers are not symptomatic themselves

Cell metabolism Process whereby respiratory system and heart supply body cells with oxygen and dispose of carbon dioxide

Central nervous system (CNS) Brain, spinal cord, and peripheral nerves

Cerebellum Portion of brain involved with movements and equilibrium

Cerebral cortex Portion of human brain with uniquely human mental and emotional capacities

Cerebrum Largest part of brain, divided into two hemispheres

Cervix Opening to uterus

CFCs Chlorofluorocarbons from aerosol sprays, fire extinguishers, air-conditioning equipment, and refrigerators, thought to damage the ozone layer

Chance locus of control Belief that luck or fate determines one's health status

Child neglect Condition characterized by failure to provide for a child's physical, educational, or emotional needs

Chiropractor A health professional who manipulates the body to adjust the spine

Choking Complete or partial blockage of the airway, preventing breathing

Cholesterol Yellow, waxy substance produced by the liver and found in animal products used by the body for metabolism and production of certain hormones

Chromosome Set of genes that carry hereditary information

Chronic Diseases that continue over time and tend to gradually become worse

Chyme Pasty substance that results from partial digestion of food in stomach

Cilia Small, hairlike projections lining membranes of bronchioles in lungs

Clitoris Pea-sized part of female genitalia that is highly sensitive to sexual stimulation

Cocaine White crystalline powder used illegally for its stimulant effects

Cochlea Part of ear that picks up vibrations from ossicles and sends the information to the brain

Cognitive functioning Human intellectual abilities including short- and long-term memory, attention, focus, judgment, and problem solving

Colon Large intestine

Coma Deep stage of unconsciousness

Communicable Diseases that are transmitted by germs or pathogenic organisms from an infected person or animal to an uninfected person, directly or indirectly; also called contagious or infectious

Community Group of people with similar needs and interests or belonging to a similar culture or ethnic group, with some evidence of a common life, behavioral norms, and an organized approach

Complementary medicine *See* Alternative medicine

Congenital Present at birth, as in congenital heart defect

Contagious *See* Communicable

Cornea Part of eye where light enters

Coronary heart disease Condition involving damage to blood vessels or heart

Cowper's glands Two pea-size male organs that produce a pre-ejaculation fluid

Cystic fibrosis Genetic disease of respiratory system and sweat and mucous glands

Decibel Measurement system for loudness of sound, or noise

Decision making Mechanism by which people take responsibility for their behavior

Deforestation Destruction of forested areas for enterprises such as crops, grazing animals, and timber

Degenerative Diseases that progressively result in more deterioration

Delusions Misinterpretations of either real or imagined events; can be induced by mind-altering drugs

Dendrites Branches of neurons that convey impulses to cell bodies

Denial Defense mechanism that places the unpleasant thought or experience out of mind

Depressants Drugs that slow down the central nervous system, enabling relaxation and sleep

Deprivational stress Form of stress caused by lack of stimulation

Dermis Layer of skin, just beneath epidermis, that contains sweat glands, oil glands, hair follicles, muscle fibers, blood vessels, and sensory nerve endings

Development Maturation process whereby body systems increase in complexity and ability to perform more complicated functions

Diabetes mellitus Disease in which the body cannot metabolize carbohydrates because pancreas cannot produce insulin at all (Type I, sometimes called "juvenile") or produces insufficient amounts (Type II, or adult-onset)

Diabetic coma Unconsciousness resulting from abnormally high level of blood sugar

Diaphragm Muscle at bottom of chest cavity

Diastolic pressure Blood pressure at relaxation; the lower of two blood pressure measurements

Disaccharides Complex sugars

Disease *See* Illness

Distress Negative stress

DNA Chemical make-up of genes that has been called "genetic blueprint"

Dose-response time Time from administration of a drug to first response

Down syndrome Chromosomal defect with characteristic physical features, cardiovascular problems, and some degree of mental retardation

Drug Any chemical that has no food value and, when taken into the body, causes changes in the structure or function of the body

Drug abuse Chronic, deliberate, and excessive use of any drug, prescription, or over-the-counter medicine, legal or illegal, that results in impairment of the user's physical, mental, emotional, or social functioning

Drug dependence Physical or psychological need to use a drug despite adverse consequences

Drug misuse Inappropriate or improper use of a drug that results in impairment of physical, mental, social, or emotional well-being

Duodenum First section of small intestine

Eardrum Part of ear that vibrates when sound reaches it

Ecology Study of living things in their natural environment

Ecosystem Natural association of populations of plants and animals that persists over time

Educational objectives Objectives that determine the selection of content, activities, and evaluation procedures for units of study

Ejaculation Release of semen in spurts through the urethra in the penis

Electro-encephalograph Electrical measurement of certain body functions

Emotional abuse Psychological maltreatment; any act that results in impairing a child's psychological growth and development

EMS Acronym for emergency medical services

Endocrine glands Glands that transport hormones within the body

Endocrine system A body system that produces hormones

Endometrium The internal lining of the uterus

Enuresis Bed-wetting

Epidermis Outer layer of skin

Epididymis Storage structure on testicles where sperm cells mature

Epilepsy Brain disorder characterized by seizures

Equilibrium Balance

Erogenous zones Areas of the body that bring sexual pleasure when touched or stimulated

Esophagus Tube that carries food from mouth to stomach

Essential hypertension High blood pressure that has no known cause

Essential nutrients Nutrients that must be obtained from foods, as the body cannot manufacture them

Estrogen Female sex hormone

Etiology Cause(s) of a condition or disease in a population

Eustress Positive, or "good" stress

Eutrophication Accelerated growth of algae, which thrive on inorganic pollutants, in nonflowing bodies of water

Exocrine glands Glands that release substances into the digestive tract or to the outside of the body rather than into the bloodstream

Extensors Muscles that straighten the joints

External locus of control A point of control that comes from the environment

Fainting State of light unconsciousness

Fallopian tubes Tubular passages leading from uterus to each of two ovaries

Family life education Teaching/learning about all aspects of the family

Family practitioner A primary care physician who treats the entire family

Farsightedness Eye condition in which a person cannot see close objects clearly

Fertilization Union of sperm and an ovum

Fetal sonography *See* Ultrasound

Fiber (dietary) A form of carbohydrate including cellulose, hemicellulose, and pectin

Fight or flight Physical response to situations perceived as dangerous or a threat that enables humans to face the situation or flee

First-degree burn Least severe category of burn, superficial; characterized by redness, swelling, pain, and tenderness

Flexors Muscles that bend the joints in the arms and legs

Food chain Arrangement of organisms of an ecological community in which each uses the next (usually lower) member as a food source

Food labels Federally mandated listing of certain nutrients, calories, and other information on commercially packaged products

Friendship Relationship between people involving mutual trust, support, respect, and intimacy that may or may not be sexual

Fructose A simple sugar found in fruit

Galactose A simple sugar

Gallbladder Digestive organ that stores bile and releases it into small intestine as needed

Gametes Sperm or eggs

Gay Homosexual; sexual orientation toward members of the same gender

Gender Biological condition of being male or female, identified by an X (female) or a Y (male) chromosome

Gender identity Sexual identity; a person's conviction about being male or female

Gender roles Culturally established norms that determine how people should present themselves according to whether they are biologically male or female

Gender role stereotypes Behaviors, characteristics, and nuances ascribed to men and women regardless of whether they actually possess them

General adaptation syndrome (GAS) Sequence of bodily changes in response to stress: general alarm reaction, resistance, exhaustion

General practitioner A physician who does not specialize in one body system

Genitals Body organs responsible for reproduction

Global warming *See* Greenhouse effect

Glucose A simple carbohydrate, also known as "blood sugar"

Greenhouse effect A natural process that occurs when certain gases in the atmosphere allow much of the sun's visible radiation to pass through to the earth but trap infrared heat reflected from the sun-warmed earth and redirect much of it back to the Earth's surface

Grief Emotional suffering caused by loss

Growth Division and enlargement of body cells, which occurs most rapidly during the earliest stages of life

Guided fantasy Method of relaxation in which the person visualizes a peaceful scene or happening

Habituation Psychological dependency on a drug

Hallucinations False perceptions of reality; can be induced by psychedelic drugs

Hashish Dried resin of marijuana plant

Hatha yoga Form of yoga combining breathing, stretching, and balance

HDLs High-density lipoproteins; the "bad" form of cholesterol in the blood

Health State of being that renders a person physically able to withstand the onset of disease and readily heal itself; a mental state that copes well with stress, has a high self-esteem, and has a sense of control over one's life; a social well-being that supports healthy and positive relationships and sense of community; and a sense of spirituality that gives meaning to life

Health behavior Any activity undertaken for the purpose of preventing or detecting disease

Health care Promotion of health and prevention of health problems by controlling social and environmental contributors to disease

Health care delivery systems Community health services, agencies, and organizations

Health care providers Professionals who deliver health care services directly to consumers

Health risk factors Characteristics or patterns of behavior associated with the potential for developing an illness

Heart attack Death of heart muscle

Heimlich maneuver Abdominal thrusts used to expel a foreign body from a person's airway

Helper T-cells *See* T cells

Hemoglobin Protein that gives blood its red color

Heroin Semisynthetic drug made from morphine

Heterosexual Sexual orientation in which the individual prefers members of the opposite gender

Homeostasis Harmonious balance among the various body systems

Homosexual Gay or lesbian sexual orientation

Hormones Chemical messengers of endocrine system

Human growth hormones Chemicals found naturally in the body or produced synthetically that induce build-up of proteins in body tissue

Hymen Small membrane covering opening to vagina

Hyperglycemia Level of sugar in the blood that is too high, which could result in a life-threatening diabetic episode

Hypersomnia Sleeping too much; can be a sign of depression

Hypertension High blood pressure

Hypoglycemia Level of sugar in the blood that is lower than normal and could result in a diabetic emergency

Hypothalamus Part of brain that is the control center for the endocrine system

Illness Sickness or lack of well-being

Immune system Blood and lymphatic systems working together as a defense against invading pathogens

Infectious *See* Communicable

Inhalants Volatile chemicals such as nitrous oxide or nondrugs such as paint thinners or model airplane glue that affect the brain similar to central nervous system depressants

Insomnia Difficulty falling and staying asleep

Instructional objectives Learner outcomes of a lesson

Insulin A hormone produced by the pancreas that aids in the digestion of sugar

Insulin shock Too much insulin in the blood, resulting from low blood sugar; a diabetic episode

Integumentary system Body system consisting of skin, hair, and nails

Internal locus of control Belief system in which people believe in their own ability to affect their health

Intramuscular Form of drug administration directly into muscle tissue

Intravenous Form of drug administration directly into bloodstream

Involuntary muscles Muscles that are not consciously controlled; smooth muscles

Iris Colored part of eye that surrounds pupil and regulates its diameter

Ketosis Potentially dangerous medical condition that results from acid-base imbalance in body

Kidneys Organs of urinary system that filter wastes from the blood in forming urine

Killer T cells *See* T cells

Lactose Milk sugar

LDLs Low-density lipoproteins; the "bad" form of cholesterol in the blood

Lens Part of eye that refracts light and focuses it on retina

Lesbian Homosexual orientation in which females prefer other females

Leukemias Cancerous tumors of bone marrow and blood-forming cells

Lifestyle Choices, actions, habits, and communication patterns that are within our control and that increase or decrease our risk for illness

Lipids Blood fats, consisting of triglycerides, free fatty acids, phospholipids, and sterols

Liver Digestive organ that produces bile, removes some waste from the body, and produces and stores glucose

Locus of control Continuum representing how much control a person feels he/she has over what happens in life

Lymph Clear, watery fluid that circulates throughout the body and drains debris from the bloodstream

Lymphocytes Type of white blood cell found in lymph nodes

Lymphomas Cancerous tumors of lymph glands or nodes

Macrominerals The seven minerals the body needs daily

Macrophages Specialized white blood cells that fight invading pathogens

Malignant Cancerous

Maltose A complex sugar

Marijuana Drug derived from the plant *Cannabis sativa*

Marriage Legally sanctioned, permanent arrangement between a man and a woman

Masturbation Touching one's own genitals deliberately in an attempt to derive sexual pleasure

Meditation Relaxation process that increases awareness of the inner self and produces an altered state of consciousness

Medulla Part of brain located just above spinal cord that controls breathing, heart rate, blood pressure, and swallowing

Melanin Dark brown substance in epidermis that helps determine a person's skin color

Melanoma Most virulent of skin cancers

Memory T cells *See* T cells

Menarche First onset of menstruation during puberty

Menstrual cycle Monthly process in which egg and uterus prepare for fertilization and pregnancy

Menstruation Discharge of unfertilized egg in a mixture of blood and other fluids, as part of menstrual cycle

Mental illness Problems or disorders related to psychological processes or organic functions of brain

Metabolism Process of converting nutrients into body tissue and body functions

Metastasis Process of cancer cells spreading from an encapsulated tumor to other body sites

Methadone Synthetic opiate used in place of heroin as a treatment

Microminerals *See* Trace minerals

Midbrain Part of brain that regulates sleep and controls eye movement and pupil size

Minerals Inorganic nutrients essential to human health

Morphine Drug extracted from the opium poppy

Motor fitness Fitness standard comprising speed, agility, coordination, balance, power, and reaction time

Mourning *See* Grief

Mutations Changes in chemical make-up of genes

Myocardium Wall of heart

Narcotics Powerful painkillers that also induce sleep

Near-death experiences Accounts by people who were thought to have died and then were revived.

Nearsightedness Eye condition in which the person cannot see distant objects clearly

Neglect The failure to provide for the physical and emotional needs of a child by caregivers

Neurons Cells that are basic units of nervous system

Neurotransmitters Chemicals that send messages across a synapse from axon of a nerve cell to another nerve cell

Nocturnal emission Ejaculation during sleep, primarily among boys in puberty; more commonly known as "wet dream"

Noncommunicable diseases Diseases that are not contagious

Nonessential nutrients Nutrients that the body can synthesize itself and, therefore, do not have to be taken in food

Nuclear family A married man and woman and their children

Nutrient density A measure of the body's ability to proportionately use the various foods

Nutrition Acquisition and utilization of food, food products, and supplements for the purpose of achieving and maintaining optimal health, growth, and development

Obesity Body weight 20% or more above recommended weight

Objectives Measures or expectations about what students will be able to do upon completing an educational experience, unit of study, grade, developmental level, or individual lesson

Olfactory nerves Nerves involved with sense of smell

Open wound Injury that involves break in skin

Opiates Powerful painkillers that also induce sleep

Optic nerve Nerve that carries information from retina of eye to brain

Orgasm Climax; end result of sexual intercourse accompanied by ejaculation in males and series of vaginal contractions in females

Ossicles Three bones in ear (called hammer, anvil, and stirrup) that magnify vibrations from eardrum

Osteopath A medical practitioner who treats abnormalities of the body with therapeutic manipulation

Osteoporosis A disease characterized by loss of minerals in the bone

Ovaries Female organs that secrete hormones that promote development of reproductive organs and secondary sex characteristics

Over-the-counter (OTC) drugs Medications that a consumer can purchase commercially

Ovulation Release of female egg as part of menstrual cycle

Ovum (pl., *ova*) Female reproductive cell

Pancreas Digestive organ that secretes insulin and other digestive juices

Panic attack Sudden onset of intense apprehension, fearfulness, or terror, often associated with feelings of impending doom

Parasympathetic nerve impulses Sensations that reverse effects of sympathetic nerve impulses after the excitement or stress has passed, bringing body functions back to normal

Parenteral injection Administration of a drug intramuscularly, intravenously, or subcutaneously

Pathogens Bacteria, viruses, and other agents of disease

PCBs Polychlorinated biphenyls; carcinogenic compounds found in garbage and industrial waste landfills and dumps

Penis Male organ that expels sperm and urine

Peripheral nerves 31 pairs of spinal nerves and 12 pairs of cranial nerves

Peristalsis Involuntary, rhythmic contractions of stomach muscles that begin the process of digesting protein

Personality Sum of a person's feelings, beliefs, perceptions, attitudes, communication style, and behaviors

Pesticides Chemicals used to destroy insects that harm plants used for human consumption

Phagocytes Specialized white blood cells that fight invading pathogens

Phenylketonuria (PKU) Genetic disease identified by absence of an essential amino acid, resulting in severe mental retardation

Philanthropic groups Organizations supported through donations, corporations, or family foundations through private financial resources

Physical abuse Nonaccidental injury or threat of injury

Physician A medical doctor

Physician assistant A trained practitioner with limited medical practice working under the direction of a physician

Pineal gland Gland, located in brain, involved in body's internal clock and sleep

Pituitary gland Gland that releases hormones that regulate hormonal output of other endocrine glands

Plasma Liquid component in which blood cells are suspended

Platelets Component of blood that maintains walls of blood vessels

Poison Any substance that causes illness or injury when it enters the body

Pollution Harmful substances deposited in air, water, or land that cause dirty, unhealthy, or hazardous products

Polysaccharides Classification of carbohydrates consisting of starch, glycogen, and most fibers

Pons Bundle of nerve fibers linking spinal cord to brain

Post-traumatic stress disorder Emotional disorder characterized by frequent reexperiencing of an extremely traumatic event

Powerful-other locus of control Belief that one's health is controlled by someone other than the self

Premonition Foretelling an event that happens in the future

Prescription drugs Medications that only a licensed professional practitioner can order

Pressure bandage Elastic bandage wrapped around wound to constrict blood vessels and thereby control internal bleeding and swelling

Primary prevention Actions that preclude a health problem from developing

Progressive muscle relaxation Method of relaxation concentrating on relaxing specific muscle groups in an ordered sequence

Prostate gland Male organ that produces seminal fluid

Protein Nutrient consisting of amino acids the body needs to build and maintain tissue and other essential body functions

Psychedelics Drugs that can produce hallucinations and delusions

Psychiatrist A practitioner that treats psychological problems

Psychoactive Describes effects of a substance on the brain; mind-altering

Psychological dependency Habituation

Psychologist A licensed practitioner who treats mental and emotional problems

Puberty A time of rapid sex-related changes that marks the beginning of adolescence

Pulse Heartbeat externally felt at the radial artery or carotid artery

Pupil Dark opening in center of eye that permits light to enter

PVC Polyvinyl chloride, a compound found in furnaces, air conditioners, and hot water heaters that can cause liver damage and cancer

Quackery Unethical means to sell products or services

Recommended Dietary Allowances (RDA) An eating guideline set by Food and Drug Administration as a standard for energy and nutrient intake

Receptors Nerve endings

Rectum End of large intestine where wastes are excreted

Red blood cells Blood cells that contain a protein called hemoglobin

Respiration Breathing

Retina Inner layer of eye that contains color receptors

Reverse tolerance Psychological dependency in which the user requires less of a substance to achieve the desired results

Rheumatic heart Serious condition resulting from acute bacterial infections of throat or rheumatic fever

Risk Any behavior that people perceive as being associated with some danger or thrill

Risk factor *See* Health risk factors

Saliva Digestive juice that begins breaking down starches into sugars and moistens dry food

Sarcomas Cancerous tumors of connective body tissue

Satiety Feeling of fullness after eating

Saturated fat Nutrient found in all animal products and dairy products; increases level of blood cholesterol

Scrotum Muscular pouch containing the two testicles

Secondary prevention Early identification and treatment of a health problem to prevent it from worsening or reverse it

Secondary sex characteristics Visible bodily traits (beyond chromosomes) that differentiate males from females, such as facial hair in males

Second-degree burn Category of burn involving deep layers of skin damage; characterized by blisters, swelling, and fluid loss from capillaries in inner layers of skin

Sedatives Classification of drugs that slow down the central nervous system, enabling relaxation and sleep

Sedentary lifestyle A way of living characterized by lack of activity

Seizure Momentary to total loss of consciousness and muscle spasms; associated with epilepsy

Self-concept Uniquely human factor of self-awareness

Self-esteem Feeling of regard for oneself; confidence; self-worth

Self-worth The value or regard held about one's self

Semicircular canal Part of ear involved in maintaining a sense of balance

Seminal vesicles Male glands that produce a fluid suitable for sperm mobility

Separation anxiety disorder Inappropriate and excessive anxiousness when separated from a person to whom the person is emotionally attached

Septum Wall of muscle separating right and left chambers of heart

Sexual abuse Any contact or interaction between a child and an adult in which the child is used for the sexual gratification or stimulation of the adult

Sexual harassment Uninvited and unwelcomed sexual requests for sexual favors

Sexuality Aspect of one's total sense of self that relates to attitudes, values, feelings, and beliefs about gender, body image, expressions of intimacy, love, affection, fears, fantasies, and decisions about sexual behaviors

Sexuality education Formulation of sexual learning within an educational program that explores the biological, emotional, social, spiritual, and intellectual variables that make up the total person

Sexual orientation An individual's gender-specific interests for participating in sexual activity

Shock Lack of oxygen to heart and brain resulting from trauma or stress

Sickle-cell anemia Genetic blood disease characterized by blood cells with a sickle shape that impede blood flow and cause other debilitating symptoms

Skinfold thickness Method of assessing body composition using calipers to pinch the skin at certain body sites

Social worker A mental health practitioner who treats people with mental or emotional problems

Sociopath Person who lacks a sense of right and wrong and acts in antisocial ways

Somatic nervous system Peripheral nerves that control voluntary actions

Sperm Male reproductive cell

Spirituality Ethical and moral component of wellness that gives meaning to life by linking a person to a higher being

Starch Storage form of glucose in plants

Steroids Chemicals present in the body naturally or produced synthetically that induce the build-up of proteins in body tissue

Stimulants Drugs that speed up central nervous system reactions, increasing alertness and excitability

Stress Specific set of changes in the body caused by a wide variety of stimuli

Stressor Any of the stimuli that produce the bodily changes characteristic of stress

Stroke Blockage of blood vessel in brain from a blood clot

Subcutaneous Administration of a drug directly beneath the skin

Sucrose A complex sugar more commonly known as table sugar

Suppressor T cells *See* T cells

Survivor guilt Feeling of fault for having survived a circumstance in which someone else has died

Sustainable ethic Principle encouraging people to follow biological principles of conservation, recycling, use of renewable resources, restoration, population control, and adaptability

Sympathetic nerve impulses Sensations that adjust body functions when the person is under physical or emotional stress or excitement

Synapse A small space between neurons

Synergistic effect Response that is compounded, or greater than the sum of its parts; often refers to taking two or more drugs simultaneously

Systems theory In psychotherapy, the premise that treatment must occur in the context of the entire family, rather than individually

Systolic pressure Blood pressure during contraction, expressed as the higher of two blood pressure readings

Tai chi Eastern form of movement and balance exercises

Taste buds Nerve receptors on the tongue

T cells Form of white blood cells originating in the thymus gland; classified as helper T cells, killer T cells, memory T cells, and suppressor T cells

Tertiary prevention Actions to contain or minimize irreversible damage or contain and slow progression of disease

Testes Two male organs that secrete hormones and promote growth of reproductive organs and secondary sex characteristics

Testicles Two oval-shaped organs that produce sperm

Testosterone Male sex hormone

THC Tetra-hydro-cannabinol, the psychoactive ingredient in *Cannabis sativa* (marijuana)

Thermal pollution Degradation resulting from water warmed by power plants that use water as a coolant, which reduces oxygen in water and thereby kills animals and plants

Third-degree burn Most severe category of burn; characterized by charred, white, or cherry red appearance of skin

Threshold dose Lowest dose of a chemical at which the drug will work

Thymus Gland that promotes development of antibodies in children

Thyroid gland Gland that secretes hormones that regulate body's metabolic rate and affect growth

Trace minerals Minerals the body needs in very small amounts

Trachea Windpipe

Transcendental meditation (TM) Relaxation process based on repeating a mantra while in a comfortable sitting position, to reduce distracting thoughts and facilitate peaceful concentration

Type A Personality classification described as hard-driving, competitive, aggressive, easily angered, unable to relax, and, thus, prone to stress-related diseases

Type B Personality classification described as laid-back, easy-going, relaxed, and rarely angered

Ultrasound Technology using high-frequency sound waves to produce a visual image of developing fetus

Underwater weighing A means of assessing body composition by submersion in water; also called hydrostatic weighing

Unfinished business Things a person wishes he or she had said or done before a person's death

Universal values Values accepted by essentially all cultures

Unsaturated fat Form of dietary fat that is considered less detrimental than saturated fat

Ureters Tube from each kidney that transports urine from kidneys to bladder

Urethra Tube that transports urine and, in males, sperm to outside body

Uterus Pear-shaped muscular organ inside of which an embryo/fetus develops

Vagina Muscular canal leading from outside of body to cervix

Values Things or ideas that individuals hold in high regard; judgments people make about themselves and others

Vas deferens Tubular structures that carry sperm from epididymis to ejaculatory duct

Vegetarians People who do not consume animal products

Veins Vessels that carry circulating blood back to the heart

Ventricle Lower compartment in the heart

Villi Fingerlike projections from intestinal wall living that propel food along in the digestive process

Vitamins Carbon-containing nutrients the body must obtain to maintain health

Voluntary muscles Muscles that the individual can control; skeletal muscles

Voluntary organizations Collection of independent agencies, organizations, and foundations that contribute to a cause without obligation or compensation

Vulva Folds of tissue that cover the vagina

Wellness Optimal health, enabling a person to have a purposeful and enjoyable experience of living

White blood cells Blood cells whose primary function is to defend the body against harmful substances

Wound Injury to soft tissue of body

Yoga Form of meditation

Zygote Fertilized egg

Photo credits

ii: © Fitness & Wellness, Inc.
1: © 2002 Britt Erlanson/The Images Bank/Getty Images
5: © Corbis Images
10: www.comstock.com
25: © SuperStock
65: © Corbis Images
68: © Fitness & Wellness, Inc.
80: © Fitness & Wellness, Inc.
117: © Ariel Skelley/Corbis Stock Market
125: Michael Newman/PhotoEdit
151: © Aaron Haupt/Photo Researchers
159: www.comstock.com
197: © David Young-Wolff/PhotoEdit
207: © Fitness & Wellness, Inc.
210: © 2002 Augustus Butera/Stone/Getty Images
225: © Tom and DeeAnn McCarthy/Corbis Stock Market
228: John Crawley
237: Hillary and Greg Portnoy
269: © 2002 Mitch Kezar/Stone/Getty Images
278: © 2002 Erlanson Production/The Image Bank/Getty Images
281: © 2002 EyeWire/Getty Images
303: © 2002 PhotoDisc/Getty Images
305: © 2002 PhotoDisc/Getty Images
329: © David Young-Wolff/PhotoEdit
331: Mary Kate Denny/PhotoEdit
375: © Philip Condit II/Stone/Getty Images
378: © Bob Daemmrich/Stone/Getty Images
397: © SuperStock
401: © Fitness & Wellness, Inc.
441: © John Luke/Image Ideas/Index Stock Imagery
451: © DigitalVision/PictureQuest
452: © John Crawley
469: © Hot Ideas/Image Ideas/Index Stock Imagery
474: www.comstock.com
477: © Steve Allen/Brand X Pictures/PictureQuest
509: © Bonnie Kamin/PhotoEdit
512: © Tom Carter/PhotoEdit
520: www.comstock.com
522: © Corbis Images

Index

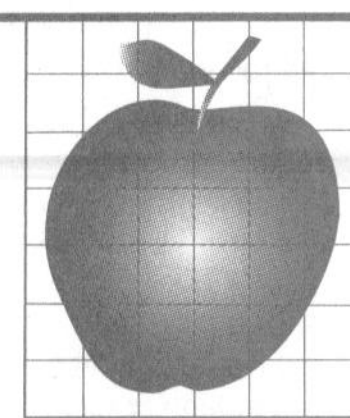

LE = Learning Experience